CLINICIAN'S GUIDE TO

# ASSISTIVE
# TECHNOLOGY

# CLINICIAN'S GUIDE TO

..................................................................

# ASSISTIVE TECHNOLOGY

Edited by

**Don A. Olson,** PhD
Associate Professor
Department Physical Medicine and Rehabilitation
Northwestern University Medical Schools
Director, Dixon Education and Training
Rehabilitation Institute of Chicago
Chicago, Illinois

**Frank DeRuyter,** PhD
Director and Associate Professor
Speech Pathology and Audiology
Duke University Medical Center
Durham, North Carolina

*with 6 part editors*
*with 35 contributors*
*with 128 illustrations*

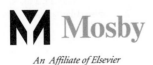 Mosby

*An Affiliate of Elsevier*

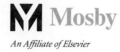

*Publishing Director:* John A. Schrefer
*Associate Editor:* Kellie F. White
*Developmental Editor:* Christie M. Hart
*Project Manager:* Linda McKinley
*Senior Production Editor:* Julie Eddy
*Designer:* Julia Ramirez
*Cover design:* Julia Ramirez

Mosby, Inc.
*An Affiliate of Elsevier*
11830 Westline Industrial Drive
St. Louis, Missouri 64146

Printed in the United States of America

**Library of Congress Cataloging-in-Publication Data**

Clinician's guide to assistive technology / edited by Frank DeRuyter, Don A. Olson.
   p. ; cm.
  Includes bibliographical references and index.
  ISBN 0-8151-4601-9
  1. Self-help devices for the disabled I. DeRuyter, Frank. II. Olson, Don A.
  [DNLM: 1. Self-Help Devices. 2. Disabled Persons–rehabilitation. WB 320 C64184 2001]
  RM950 .C554 2001
  617′.03–dc21

                                         2001045231

04 05  CC/RRD  9 8 7 6 5 4 3 2

# PART EDITORS

......................................................................................................

**Peggy Barker, MS**
Applied Assistive Technology Research
Santa Cruz, California

**Dudley S. Childress, PhD**
Director, NU Rehab Engineering & Prosthetics
Chicago, Illinois

**Michael L. Jones, PhD**
Director, Crawford Research Center
Shepherd Center
Atlanta, Georgia

**Carol Sargent, BSEE, OTR/L**
Instructor
Ohio Assistive Technology Distance Learning Project, ORCLISH
Toledo, Ohio

**Lawrence H. Trachtman**
Durham, North Carolina

**Jack Uellendahl, CPO**
Prosthetics Specialist
Hanger Prosthetics and Orthotics
Scottsdale, Arizona

# CONTRIBUTORS

**Jürgen Babirad, MSA, ATP, CDRS**
Rehabilitation Technology Associates, Inc.
Valatie, New York

**Peggy Barker, MS, ATP**
Applied Assistive Technology
Santa Cruz, California

**Diane Bristow, JD, MS, CCC-SLP**
Speech-Language Pathologist/Assistive Technology Specialist
Associate Attorney
Howarth & Smith
Los Angeles, California

**Diane Nelson Bryen, PhD**
Executive Director
Institute on Disabilities
Pennsylvania's University Center of Excellence in Developmental Disabilities
Temple University
Philadelphia, Pennsylvania

**Kevin Caves, ATP**
Director, RERC on Communication Enhancement
Duke University Medical Center
Durham, North Carolina

**Dudley S. Childress, PhD**
Director, NU Rehab Engineering & Prosthetics
Chicago, Illinois

**Frank DeRuyter, PhD**
Director and Associate Professor
Speech Pathology and Audiology
Duke University Medical Center
Durham, North Carolina

**Thomas DiBello, CO**
Private Clinical Practice/President Owner
Dynamic Orthotics & Prosthetics
Houston, Texas

**Molly Doyle, MS, CCC**
Rancho Los Amigos National Rehabilitation Center
Program Director
Las Floristas Center for Applied Rehabilitation Technology (CART)
Downey, California

**Julie Edwards, CO**
Scheck & Siress
Arlington Heights, Illinois

**Mark L. Edwards, CP**
Director of Prosthetics
Northwestern University Prosthetic, Orthotic Center
Chicago, Illinois

**Laura Fenwick, CO**
Glenview, Illinois

**Amy S. Goldman, MS, CCC**
Associate Director
Institute on Disabilities,
Pennsylvania's Initiative on Assistive Technology (PIAT)
Temple University
Philadelphia, Pennsylvania

**Susan Goltsman, FASLA**
Principal
Moore Iacofano Goltsman, Inc
Berkeley, California

**Kathleen Gradel, EdD**
Director, Baker Victory
Services Early Childhood
Primary Program
Buffalo, New York
Training/Marketing Director,
Assist Tech, Inc.
Stow, New York

**Cheryl Griebel, PT**
Children's Hospital of Denver
Assistive Technology Program
Denver, Colorado

**Craig Heckathorne, MSEE**
Research Engineer
Rehabilitation Engineering Research Program & Prosthetics Research Lab
Northwestern University Medical School
Chicago, Illinois

**Judy Henderson, MA, CCC-SP**
Lucile Salter Packard Children's Hospital
Stanford University Medical Center
Rehabilitation Technology Center
Palo Alto, California

**Alice E. Holmes, PhD**
Associate Professor of Audiology
Communicative Disorders
University of Florida
Gainesville, Florida

**Christine Jasch, OTR/L**
Rehabilitation Institute of Chicago
Alan J. Brown Center for Augmentative Communication
Electronic Aids to Daily Living and Computer Access
Chicago, Illinois

**Michael L. Jones, PhD**
Vice President, Research and Technology
Director, Crawford Research Institute
Shepherd Center
Atlanta, Georgia

**David Kreutz, PT**
Shepherd Center
Atlanta, Georgia

**Michelle L. Lange, OTR, ABDA, ATP**
Clinical Director
Assistive Technology Partners
The Children's Hospital
Denver, Colorado

**Richard G. Long, PhD**
Assistant Professor
Department of Blind Rehabilitation
Western Michigan University
Kalamazoo, Michigan

**Jean Minkel, MA, PT**
Minkel Consulting
New Windsor, New York

**Steve Mendelsohn**
New York, New York

**James Mueller**
J.L. Mueller, Inc.
Chantilly, Virginia

**Jessica Presperin Pedersen, MBA, OTR/L, ATP**
Governors State University
University Park, Illinois

**Linda Petty, OT(C)**
Clinical Specialist
Adaptive Technology Resource Centre
University of Toronto
Toronto, Ontario
Canada

**Gail L. Pickering, MA**
Speech Language Pathologist/Assistive Technology Specialist
Studio City, California

**Jon Sanford, M. Arch**
Research Architect
Rehab R&D Center
Atlanta VAMC
Decatur, Georgia

**Carol Sargent, BSEE, OTR/L**
Instructor
Ohio Assistive Technology Distance Learning Project, ORCLISH
Toledo, Ohio

**Marcia Scherer, PhD, MPH, CRC**
Director, Institute for Matching Person and Technology
Webster, New York
Senior Research Associate, International Center for Hearing and Speech Research
Associate Professor, Physical Medicine and Rehabilitation
University of Rochester Medical Center
Rochester, New York

**Susan Johnson Taylor, OTR/L**
Seating and Mobility Specialist
Rehabilitation Institute of Chicago
Seating & Positioning Clinic
Chicago, Illinois

**Lawrence H. Trachtman**
Durham, North Carolina

**Jutta Treviranus**
Director
Adaptive Technology Resource Centre
University of Toronto
Toronto, Ontario
Canada

**Jack Uellendahl, CPO**
Prosthetics Specialist
Hanger Prosthetics and Orthotics
Scottsdale, Arizona

**Richard F. *ff.* Weir, PhD**
Research Scientist
VA Chicago Health Care System, Lakeside Division
Research Assistant Professor
Department of Physical Medicine & Rehabilitation
Northwestern University Medical School
Chicago, Illinois

# FOREWORD

......................................................................................................................

*Justin Dart*

A ll persons with disabilities are encouraged to see the increased interest and new texts that have been appearing recently about assistive technology. For far too many years, we have heard repeatedly about the benefits of assistive technology. However, few of us have had the opportunities that can be afforded by its appropriate use.

Cost and availability of these devices seem to be the major factors impeding use. However, another major barrier to the successful transfer of technology to persons with disabilities has been the avoidance of active consumer involvement by clinicians. We appreciate and fully recognize the outstanding work of our professional colleagues in the field of rehabilitation. We value the knowledge that they have given us to train and take care of our own bodies. We have learned about the limitations of our bodies, how to compensate for what no longer functions, and new ways to achieve independence for work, recreation, and an improved quality of life.

However, frustration and failures still abound when we seek services, whether for acute medicine, rehabilitation, or maintaining good health. It is discouraging when services are available but the needed or relevant services are not rendered. Although we appreciate the advances that have been made, we continue to be critical of professional vie of our condition by our physicians, therapists, and clinicians. Although it appears simplistic, if you go to a surgeon, you can be assured that you will have surgery. If you go to a psychologist, you can be assured that you will get psychologic treatment. And if you go to a physical therapist, you can be assured you will get muscle conditioning. These services may or may not be what are needed. Likewise, far too often if we are referred to a technician specializing in seating and positioning, we will get a maximum evaluation focused specifically on that area. Again, it may or may not be the genuine need that the person with the disability desires to have met.

For instance, a friend of mine spent 2 weeks in a well-known rehabilitation hospital as an in-patient being evaluated for seating and positioning to correct or improve the seating for a scoliosis that she had lived with for more than 70 years. By the time her hospital stay was over, the professional staff had made significant changes in her wheelchair for positioning, but her main request—the need for a voice-activated computer to facilitate her research work more effectively—was not addressed. This woman had to endure a stay of an additional 3 days to obtain what she had come in to achieve initially. Unfortunately, this story can be repeated substituting different people and different problems.

It is true that cost and availability of equipment are impeding our successful use of technology in many cases. But fundamentally, it is the lack of consumer involvement and understanding of the consumer's *true needs* and the neglect to investigate all possible options that is the crux of the problem.

This new manual, designed to provide information for the clinician and the consumer who need to work together in a practical working relationship, will result in maximizing the use of technical aids. Basic principles and a philosophy for working with persons with disabilities are set forth in this manual. It also has a special feature: its material will be updated yearly. That way, the many changes that occur in assistive technology will be presented sooner, and people with disabilities and the professionals who work with them can benefit sooner. The specific suggestions given, when coordinated with those of the involved consumer, will result in achieving a mutually satisfactory goal. For all these reasons, this manual with its yearly updates is truly welcomed.

Finally, we have made great strides in the past few years by passing legislation, expanding programs, creating awareness of persons with disabilities in the community, and fostering acceptance of technology use in the home and workplace and in recreation. This new manual is yet another step in assisting persons with disabilities to return to the everyday world more capable and confident that they can function at a high level, be productive, and enjoy their active lives.

# INTRODUCTION

*Don A. Olson, PhD*
*Frank DeRuyter, PhD*

More than 49 million Americans demonstrate an ongoing disabling condition. Of these, over 13 million people, or about 5.3% of the U.S. population, use assistive technology. Clearly, many more people would welcome the improved quality of life that assistive technology (AT) can bring. Assistive technology allows the users to cope better with their disabilities and gives them the chance to compete in the arenas of their choice. Although some of the available devices are highly sophisticated and expensive, others are low tech and inexpensive and yet have amazing potential for the person with a disability.

This guide proposes a clinical and client/customer services approach that promotes a collaborative relationship between the person with a disability, the caregiver, and the rehabilitation professional. As technology progresses and new options are made available daily, the basics about assistive technology are not always clear to the rehabilitation professional, caregiver, or the person who could benefit from the assistive technology. This manual clarifies the relationship between the involved parties. Also, this guide is designed to help raise the level of awareness and knowledge of assistive technology in our field.

In recent years, several programs and activities have had a major affect on the growth of assistive technology. The progress in the field of assistive technology has been greatly enhanced through the research and development activities conducted at the outstanding Rehabilitation Engineering Research Centers funded by the National Institute on Disability and Rehabilitation Research. Although thousands of individuals have already experienced improvements in their quality of life, millions more need these services and devices. Still, the affect of the Rehabilitation Engineering Research Centers has resulted in the growth throughout the rehabilitation community of a focus on technology.

Secondly, the State Tech Act program and the more recent Assistive Technology Act have been another huge step forward in providing knowledge about available resources and the latest technology to the general public. These programs have provided accessibility, information, and services and have eliminated barriers that affect large numbers of persons with disabilities who are users or potential users of assistive technology. In addition, the Independent Living/Civil Rights Movement for people with disabilities has helped increase awareness and improve access to assistive technology.

Perhaps the most important impetus for change has come from the Americans with Disabilities Act (ADA). The ADA prohibits employers from discriminating against disabled persons and requires businesses to provide "reasonable accommodations." This legislation has significantly changed the lives of disabled persons as many reasonable accommodations have been managed through the implementation and use of assistive technology. Employers, businesses, and schools are responding to the demands of the law, and the needed changes are occurring and resulting in more employment for persons with disabilities and an improved quality of life socially.

Knowledge, practice, and the priority for assistive technology have not always kept up with the major movements in this area. All disciplines of rehabilitation therapists must be cognizant of the ongoing innovations. Unfortunately, most therapists do not receive in-depth assistive technology training in their curricula. As a result, many are overwhelmed with the prospect of having to develop a program of assistive support to aid in the independence of their clients. Although printed resources exist, many focus on the highly technical as opposed to the practical aspects, which this guide attempts to do. Specific training of the technical components is not the only aspect of assistive technology. Clearly the best way to start is to work closely with the people who have a disability when they first come for assistive technology services. Then, the process of understanding what the client goals are and what the clients would like to accomplish are important for successful outcomes as are understanding function and ability as they relate to different assistive technologies, understanding all of the possible considerations and options for various assistive technologies, and the way to validate successful outcomes.

All of these are important components that go beyond just understanding the technical aspects of technology. This guide attempts to provide that framework. Frequently, caregivers and/or support personnel will be the ones working most closely with the assistive technology user and will require knowledge. This guide also attempts to make information useful to those individuals. In other instances, the professional will find working more closely with nursing staff or referring physicians necessary. Because the nurses' or physicians' goals of for those with disabilities may not include assistive technology, they must be included so that they truly understand the importance of independence to their patients. This guide also attempts to meet those needs.

As new settings evolve in the assistive technology service delivery arena, an increasing need exists for greater awareness about assistive technology. Formerly, an assessment for assistive technology occurred either in a self-contained setting or as part of a rehabilitation unit. Today, they may occur in any of several settings, such as nursing homes, schools, home health situations, long-term care centers, vocational placement centers, or community clinics. In addition, through the use of telemedicine and telerehabilitation, assistive technology services are beginning to be provided to remote and rural locations through alternative service delivery means.

The National Institute on Disability and Rehabilitation Research has been instrumental in developing a new paradigm for all consumers and professionals as we attempt to work toward mutual goals. Their new paradigm moves us from the medical model to a societal model, which provides for full and equal participation in our communities for the persons who are considered able and persons with disability. The key to the model is ensuring that people with disabilities are a part of planning, developing, and implementing their respective needs. Nowhere is this more important than in planning, prescribing, and implementing a technology service or technology program for an individual with a disability.

To ensure ongoing use of the technology and more importantly ensuring that the correct technology is prescribed, active participation, practice, arrangement, and implementation with the individual needing the technology is mandatory. This begins with an in-depth discussion of what individuals perceive as their needs, what they want to do, and what they expect the technology to do.

This guide is planned to assist the professional in working with their clients and providing them with the total array of options that are available to solve their specific problems. Only when a person with a disability is actively involved in the planning of this program can an assistive technology program be successful. And only then will it meet the new paradigm of consumer empowerment currently prescribed by independent living and national agencies developing programs for persons with disabilities. We have started to meet the enormous needs for assistive technology that exist in our country. Bringing this great potential for added independence and improved quality of life to many more people is a worthy goal. It is up to each of us as we work with our clients/customers to explore the array of options in assistive technology and to help secure those that are the most appropriate.

# CONTENTS

# PART 1

......................................................................................................

## Assistive Technology Principles

......................................................................................................

*Lawrence H. Trachtman*

The assistive technology profession is at a crossroads. It has matured from the toddler and adolescent years of the 1970s and 1980s to young adulthood. In the formative period, it was a novelty and treated with excitement. As with young children, expectations were minimal yet accomplishments were reveled. Accountability, such as the time or money spent on solving individual problems, was almost nonexistent. Keeping pace with the many advances in assistive technology was difficult. Even though many of the solutions were still unique to the individual user, some sensed that assistive technology was on the verge of public acceptance. Two parallel events motivated this progress: the evolution of the technology, sustained largely by the surge in computer processing, and improved service delivery, or ways to effectively provide the technology to the end user. The profession also grew rapidly. Many people from a variety of educational backgrounds entered the field bringing with them an array of skills and experiences.

With young adulthood, however, came responsibility. Having to pinpoint exactly when changes began to occur is difficult. Perhaps it was when the Tech Act was passed in the late 1980s. However, progress and excitement began to wane. Two new forces became part of the evolution: increased consumer demand for technology that was becoming prevalent throughout society and payers' growing concerns about limited resources and demonstrable outcomes. These two forces often were at odds. Assistive technology professionals managed to avoid accountability for a long time. However, as consumer demand grew, spurred largely by the early success of the state Tech Act projects for increasing public awareness, resources diminished and payers began asking tougher questions. This trend was not limited exclusively to assistive technology—all of health care was scrutinized.

Today, the dialogue continues and many tough questions are still being asked. I am reminded of the parable of three blind men who come across an elephant. One finds the trunk and describes the animal as round and strong; the second feels the body and indicates it is large and heavy; and the third feels the tail and says the animal is slim and flexible. Of course, each man's observation is correct based only on his limited perception of the obstacle.

The provision of assistive technology today is not unlike this story. Replace the three men with an end user, a service provider, and a payer, with each asking to describe the benefits and outcomes of assistive technology. For the end user, unique goals and expectations exist that are shaped by individual abilities, predisposition to technology, the environment, financial resources, and family and community supports. The provider also contributes a unique set of knowledge and skills, whose outcomes are influenced by resources, expectations, time, and money. Finally, the payer's concerns must be addressed. Similar to the user, the payer also has goals and expectations. However, the payer's constraints can include predetermined mandates and demands for services that exceed limited resources.

Because of the history of the profession, now more than ever clinicians must be capable of not only just working with the user of products and services but also must be keenly aware of outside social and political forces, the need to measure and document outcomes, and to keep pace with professional and technologic changes. In addition, assistive technology users are more educated than they were just a few years ago. Similar to consumers of all products, assistive technology users should expect value and real benefits for their dollars.

The crossroads mentioned earlier are real. The profession can no longer conduct business as in the past and must rethink all current strategies, including multidisciplinary teams, technology demonstration centers, and mobile service vehicles. The core educational programs should even be reevaluated. The types of students graduating from today's programs are facing different work settings and expectations because a business rather than a clinical climate often prevails. Credentialing is now a pervasive topic. As health care changes, the clinicians' roles in providing assistive technologies also change. Currently, some assistive technology programs are being forced to discontinue.

In reading the chapters in this section, the following questions should be remembered:

- What is assistive technology? Do definitions need to be updated?
- Who benefits from assistive technology?
- When is assistive technology appropriate? When is it not appropriate? How can the clinician best match the technology to the end user's needs?
- How can the clinician ensure meaningful user input in the assessment and delivery process?
- How does the clinician know if assistive technology use is successful? What are the measures of success?
- What is the future of assistive technology and the assistive technology profession? How can the clinician adapt to the enveloping changes?

Each chapter in this part covers the questions and issues raised earlier in greater depth. In Chapter 1, Matching Consumers with Appropriate Assistive Technologies, Marcia Scherer explores the factors that influence the individual's and family's successful adoption of assistive technology. She presents the Matching Person and Technology model and illustrates through a case study how the end user can be involved in technology selection. In Chapter 2, Contexts: Assistive Technology at Home, School, and Work and in the Community, Diane Nelson Bryen and Amy Goldman present assistive technology applications within the contexts of everyday life, a common shortcoming when technology is provided solely in clinical contexts. Their tables, selection and implementation principles, and case studies are useful teaching tools. Michael Jones discusses human factors and environmental access in Chapter 3. Jean Minkel challenges the clinician's current thinking of service delivery in Chapter 4, Assistive Technology Service Delivery. After presenting critical considerations in service provision, she proceeds to suggest a change from the expert model to the interactive and consumer-directed models. Her discussion of points of entry suggests that funding sources rather than service location or disability type is delineating assistive technology services. In Chapter 5, Outcomes, Frank DeRuyter has studied outcomes measurement in assistive technology extensively. His chapter summarizes much of the current thinking on this timely subject. Finally, Steve Mendelson and Kathleen Gradel provide an excellent summary of current legislation affecting assistive technology provision and funding in Chapter 6, Funding and Public Policy. They highlight advocacy options and action strategies for making the most of existing resources.

The views presented by these distinguished authors represent the condition of assistive technology today, but change is unrelenting. The clinician should continue to be informed of all that is occurring in society and develop a unique approach to the successful application of assistive technology.

# CHAPTER 1

# Matching Consumers with Appropriate Assistive Technologies

*Marcia J. Scherer*

Various factors influence predispositions of individuals and family members to use assistive technology. The goal of assistive technology is to provide the most appropriate technology for a particular person, with minimal disruption to a user's accustomed and preferred ways of doing things, ultimately resulting in an enhanced quality of life.[1]

## Technophile versus Technophobe

Approximately 20% of persons with disabilities who work or attend school require help with daily self-care activities such as bathing, dressing, and eating.[2] Technologies are being developed to replace the need for assistance from other persons in the areas of self-care, mobility, communication, recreation, reading, and writing. These technologies have helped many individuals with severe disabilities and chronic health conditions live independently in their communities. However, people with disabilities who are consumers of assistive technology devices and services have differing views about the extent to which technology improves the quality of their lives. Users also differ in the degree to which they employ assistive technology.[3,4] Many individuals with disabilities reject technologies outright, whereas others try various devices only to abandon them later. Although unused and abandoned technologies represent wasted resources, people who are not performing at their functional best also abandon them.

Users of assistive technology devices and services include persons with disabilities (primary consumers) and their family members and care providers (secondary consumers). Primary and secondary consumers need to know the ways to use technology and feel comfortable with it.

In general, the potential users of technology appear as two broad groups: technophiles and technophobes. Research shows that technophobes outnumber technophiles by more than 2 : 1.[5] The technophile embraces technology, whereas a technophobe avoids it. Encouraging technophobes to use new technical products is just as challenging as preventing technophiles from using each new product.

Age and gender determine the makeup of the groups.[5,6] A technophobic person is typically 50 years old or older and avoids and even fears such technologies as VCRs and computers. In Western society (even more so in the rest of the world), many women have traditionally received little exposure to technology and tend to be uninformed about new advances.[7] They may be uninterested in complex and sophisticated high-tech products. Non–technically oriented men may also feel threatened by technologic devices because of embarrassment about their lack of skills and focus in interests traditionally held by men.

Statistics show that persons aged 60 and older have the fewest high-tech products in the home. This age group also is projected to grow dramatically within the next several decades. Older individuals have a high avoidance rate of assistive technologies, even though they might benefit significantly from their use.

Despite some people's reluctance and their avoidance of technology, the encouragement for home care as opposed to hospital stays or nursing facilities, as well as the desire people have to live in their own home and as independently as possible, mean that more technology is being used at home.

Although a sizable portion of the population may be considered technophobic, many people are encountering some of the most fear-inducing technologies of all—those used to support and maintain life (home health care technologies and durable medical equipment) and those designed to compensate for functional losses resulting from physical disabilities or limitations (assistive technologies).

## Assistive Technologies

Since 1988, all new federal legislation affecting persons with disabilities has mentioned assistive technology as an important service delivery component. The landmark legislation for assistive technology provision was the Technology-Related Assistance for Individuals with Disabilities Act of 1988 (PL 100-407), which was reauthorized most recently in 1998 as the Assistive Technology Act. This legislation defined an *assistive technology* device as "any item, piece of equipment, or product system, whether acquired commercially off the shelf, modified, or customized, that is used to increase, maintain, or improve functional capabilities of individuals with disabilities." This definition has remained basically the same in all subsequent legislation that affects people with disabilities.

Assistive technologies compensate for sensory and functional losses by enabling a person to do the following:

- Move with wheelchairs, lifts, braces, and quad canes
- Talk with manual communication boards and computerized communication systems
- Read with magnifiers and computers that have synthesized voice output for persons with vision loss
- Hear with hearing aids, personal FM systems, and vibrotactile pagers
- Manage self-care tasks with built-up eating utensils and environmental control systems

The available features and options in computerized and electromechanical devices have increased dramatically in recent years. In this chapter, they are referred to as *high-tech*, or *complex*, devices. Devices that have simple mechanical operations are referred to as *low-tech* devices, as are those without mechanical, electrical, or computerized components. By definition, all these devices are assistive technologies, and a simple device has as much value as a high-tech one for users who find that the device has enhanced their functioning, independence, and quality of life.

Individuals with the most severe disabilities require the most customized and computerized technologies—high-tech devices—for their enhanced independent functioning. In fact, if these technologies were not available, many people would not be able to live in their communities or homes.

## Matching Technologies to User's Needs

When technology use is more optional, some individuals and families may resist using any type of device. Others purchase anything they believe might help reduce the effects of a disability. This has been found to be particularly true for parents of children with disabilities. When technology is about to be used in the home by a family, involving everyone who is affected by it at the outset is important (Table 1-1). The characteristics of the physical and attitudinal environments in which it operates, the preferences and needs of the person who use and are affected by it, and the characteristics of the technology must be remembered.

Although the sample questions shown in Table 1-1 are directed to the person with a disability, concerns and needs of family members are similar. Providers also need to ad-

## TABLE 1-1

*Sample Questions and Technology Domains*

| TECHNOLOGY DOMAIN | MILIEU | TECHNOLOGY |
|---|---|---|
| *Mobility* | Where does the person want to go? | Is the assistive technology affordable for this person? |
| | What barriers exist to getting there? | Is the assistive technology safe, reliable, and comfortable? |
| | What forms of assistance are available? | Will the assistive technology eclipse the person using it? |
| | What in the environment needs to be changed? | Is the assistive technology aesthetically pleasing? |
| | What in the environment can be changed? | Is the assistive technology easy to use, repair, and maintain? |
| *Speech* | Is the person being asked to use an assistive technology? By whom? | What nontechnical options are available? |
| | With whom does the person most communicate now? | Is the assistive technology portable for this person? |
| | Who does the person want to communicate with more? | Can the assistive technology be set up and used independently? |
| | Will all the person's primary environments support use of the assistive technology? | Is the assistive technology fast enough? |
| | Will the assistive technology put demands on others? | Is the assistive technology easy to learn to operate? |
| | | Does the assistive technology require other devices? |
| *Hearing* | In what settings does the person spend a great deal of time? | Does the assistive technology do what the person expected? |
| | What communication situations are challenging? | Can the person easily use the assistive technology? |
| | Have frequently used public places been properly equipped? | Is the assistive technology comfortable? |
| | Is the workplace accommodating? | Does the person feel embarrassed to use this assistive technology? |
| | Are family members understanding? | Is maintenance complicated? |

*Modified from Scherer MJ: Living in the state of stuck: how technology impacts the lives of people with disabilities, ed 2, Cambridge, Mass, 1996, Brookline Books and Scherer MJ: Matching person and technology (MPT): model and assessment instruments, Rochester, NY, 1994, Scherer.*

dress the influence of assistive technology on family life, and vice versa. Family reactions need to be assessed when a person acquires a disability. Reactions are different if the person with a disability is a child, spouse, or parent. Family members may exhibit denial, guilt, or overattention to need satisfaction and may become hostile to professionals. The burden of emotion and care may lead to isolation of family members from extended family and friends. Concurrently, family members may feel that care providers have violated their privacy. In addition, after acute rehabilitation the individual and family members are often responsible to continue rehabilitation without emotional support and plans for respite.

Today's emphasis on self-determination, making choices, and independent living make the disabled person and family more in charge but gives them additional responsibilities. If a family was dysfunctional and chaotic before the onset of disability, family problems and struggles will probably exacerbate. A poor rehabilitation outcome is more likely if limited coping resources and inadequate follow through on rehabilitation plans occur.

Once home, users often find that the devices that worked so well in the rehabilitation facility do not function well in the home setting. The powered wheelchair may be tearing up the carpet or the speech device never can be found in the same room when needed. These situations lead to stress and frustration. For children and adolescents, nonuse of devices often occurs because such devices segregate them from their peers. Mature individuals may also stop using technologies that they view as stigmatizing.

## Mobility Technologies

Mobility-related devices represent the single largest category of assistive technologies. The most frequently encountered mobility products in the home are walkers, canes, manual and powered wheelchairs, leg braces, and crutches. Ramps, wheelchair accessories, and modified vehicles often complement personal mobility devices.

The use of a mobility device may result in decreased access around the house or reduced ability to enter and leave the home easily. Transportation often has to be rearranged, steps and stairs have to be eliminated, and carpeting has to be removed. Having potential users test devices in the home and involving all family members in product selection are important guidelines. The result is a minimal amount of undesirable modifications to the family's activities and to the home, in which everyone feels like a participant. Family members, however, may still feel stress from those physical or architectural changes that must be made to the home. When these changes to the familiar home environment are combined with changes in daily routines, an overwhelming sense of disruption may occur. The rehabilitation professional may encounter resistance to change, resentment toward the individual with a disability, or anxiety, insecurity, or depression resulting from the loss of familiar routines and surroundings.

## Speech Communication Technologies

Assistive technology devices used for speech may be either manual or electronic (computerized). Manual communication systems, or letter boards, can fit on a lap and be highly individualized. Boards for nonverbal children or illiterate adults may have pictures or icons on them. A manual communication board user communicates by pointing to a symbol (a letter, word, number, or picture) with a finger or pointer. Electronic speech devices are often computerized. The user's selection of a word or phrase can be displayed and may also be spoken. Words can be connected into sentences through a voice synthesizer before they are printed or spoken.

The most frequently heard complaint about manual and computerized speech devices is their slowness and the patience required by all conversation participants. Vocabulary constraints and the quality of the synthesized speech limit computerized systems. The devices also require significant training for the user and communication partners. Nonuse of computerized speech devices is often associated with family reluctance to use them and the existence of easier alternatives. For example, families may try to understand and adapt to a family member's speech before adopting a communication device. In addition, many people with disabilities have an aversion to replacing a natural function, however limited, with a device.

## Hearing Technologies

Technologies for persons with hearing loss can be categorized into the following four groups:

1. Hearing aids worn behind or in the ear to amplify sound
2. Devices that enhance communication when in a group or large-area situation (e.g., video-text display, infrared, FM and audio induction loop systems)
3. Technologies that allow communication over distances (e.g., TTY devices, television decoders, fax machines, paging devices, the Internet)
4. Alerting technologies (e.g., vibrating alarm clocks, flashing lights to indicate the ringing of a doorbell, telephone, or fire alarms)

A person may choose to use a combination of these technologies. Although many hearing-impaired individuals do use several of the technologies described, others with similar hearing losses may not use any devices.

According to studies conducted by Scherer and Frisina,[9,10] factors associated with the nonuse of hearing aids include the nature and extent of the hearing loss, discomfort with ear molds, the expense and visibility of the aids, and disappointment that perfect hearing was not restored. Additionally, hearing aid users often comment on difficulties in discriminating a speaker's voice from background noise. As the distance between the listener and speaker increases, discrimination decreases. This is exacerbated in an environment with considerable background noise.

Communication is fundamental to interpersonal relationships. Hearing loss may lead a person to avoid conversation and eventually become socially withdrawn and isolated. For a formerly gregarious person, loneliness, depression, and anger at having to change a lifestyle may occur. A person with hearing loss may also be unintentionally left out of discussions about family relationships because intimate conversations are usually conducted in soft, low voices or whispers.

Family, friends, and colleagues need to be attentive to including a person with hearing loss in conversations. Most available amplification technologies do not result in restored hearing, only varying degrees of improved communication capabilities. Thus the individual and significant others must make several emotional and social adjustments to hearing loss and learn techniques for handling a variety of communication situations.

## Implications for Practice

The rehabilitation professional is a crucial resource for identifying potential mismatches of people and technology. The incidence of nonuse or inappropriate use of assistive technologies can be reduced and the disappointment and frustration that often accompany less than ideal use can be minimized with successful matches. Assistive devices are meant to be helpful and enhance functioning, and the rehabilitation professional needs to foster this.

Over the years, assistive technology devices have become lighter, more attractive, and more flexible. Differences among individual users can now be accommodated that make the process of matching a person with the most appropriate technology quite complex. This is especially true because improved functioning does not ensure successful device use. The provision of a device is not an end. Rather, a piece of equipment is only a means to help individuals achieve high quality of life and personal goals while functioning in different environments. Individuals have psychologic and psychosocial needs that assistive devices also must accommodate. Assistive technology use should not require or result in compromising of personal goals and preferences.

### The Need for a Model When Matching a Person and a Technology

Successful assistive technology use requires adapting the device to the person's capabilities and temperament and also adapting the person, family, teachers, and co-workers to the realities and situations of the technology use. One method that has been found useful in organizing the myriad of influences on a person's predisposition to or readiness for the use of a high-tech yet optional technology is the Matching Person and Technology model[7] that advocates addressing the following:

1. Exact characteristics of the environment and psychosocial settings in which the assistive technology is used
2. Pertinent features of the individual's personality and temperament
3. Salient characteristics of the assistive technology

The Matching Person and Technology model consists of assessment instruments to document user goals and preferences, views of the benefits to be gained from a technology, and changes in self-perceived functioning and outcome achievement over time. These instruments assess the quality of the match between a person and a specific type of technology (assistive, educational, workplace, or health care). A general survey of technology use is also available to identify technologies that the person presently uses comfortably. Each instrument is a paper-and-pencil questionnaire on a single two-sided sheet, which can also be used as an interview guide, and requires about 15 minutes to complete. The questions originate from the actual experiences of technology users and nonusers, so they have content validity. Evidence exists that they are reliable and valid measures. Consumer and professional versions of each assessment are designed to be used as a set to ensure the following:

1. Consumer input drives the matching person and technology process.
2. Rehabilitation professionals are helped in their consideration of a variety of relevant influences on technology use.
3. Different perspectives of the professional and technology user become evident so that they can be addressed.

## Milieu

As mentioned, an assistive technology may create stress from changes made to the home or workplace, together with anxiety, insecurity, and depression at the loss or modification of familiar routines. Resistance to architectural changes and resentment from others may occur at work, home, and school and be directed toward the individual with a disability. Devices being tested in the settings where they are used and involving everyone who is affected are important factors.

Social interactions and cultural expectations shape self-concept, self-efficacy, motivation, personal aspirations, and other influences on the individual's predisposition to technology use. The attitudes and expectations of others can have a profound influence on the kinds of support given for assistive technology use. For example, a common reason for abandonment is that the individual was forced to use the device before being discharged from rehabilitation. The technology immediately became a focal point for resentment. Other factors such as environmental accommodations, available resources (e.g., private insurance for specialized treatment, availability of personal assistance), and special opportunities (e.g., placement in a rehabilitation center with the newest equipment, proper training for use) are also important milieu characteristics.

## People

People are dynamic and have changing needs and goals. Assistive devices must sometimes be considered relatively long-term solutions to functional limitations because of the expense and one-time funding requirements. Meeting the individual's current needs while attempting to project future ones can be a challenge.

Many people with disabilities have an aversion to replacing a natural function, however limited, with a technologic device. They may believe that technology use leads to a loss of remaining functional abilities and increasing dependence. Additionally, those without knowledge of or exposure to technologic devices may exhibit anxiety when faced with the possibility of using them. Anxiety increases the difficulty people have learning the skills needed to operate the devices.

Device use is more acceptable when low-tech and high-tech options are available and the person can exercise choice. Devices that require a great deal of cognitive ability from the user are frequently abandoned in favor of easier alternatives. Other obstacles to optimal technology use include giving a person a device that requires developing unusual or new skills, changing accustomed performance patterns, eclipsing of the person by technology because of undue attention directed to it, and having device use result in loss of privacy. If the user is already feeling conspicuous, they are compounded when the user feels stigmatized by assistive technologies.

## Technology

Assistive technologies have a high acceptance rate when they are lightweight and portable, easy to use and set up, and cost-effective to obtain and maintain. They are also well received when they are the same as or similar to devices used by the general population (more universally designed) and perform effectively and reliably.

Also important are a device's flexibility and the degree to which it can accommodate the addition of other devices. The increased practice of integrating multiple devices controlled by a single input device often results in a more streamlined appearance, but can also create cognitive overload.

Devices are unlikely to be used if they are not available when needed, are viewed as not worth all the effort, do not have enough practical applications, and create discomfort or inconvenience. Adequate training in operating and maintaining the technology is important, as is the availability of a backup system.

Assistive technology use is interactive. Altering one system affects other devices being used. For example, optimal use of one assistive technology can lead to improved functioning, self-esteem, and self-efficacy, and wider social contacts and enthusiasm for trying another technology. A person may also be new to one device but more experienced with another technology. The introduction of a new technology can make the use of an existing one more complicated or cumbersome. The following case study illustrates many of these points.

## CASE STUDY

## M.F.

This case discussion is one of many in the book *Living in the State of Stuck: How Technology Impacts the Lives of People with Disabilities*, which has been summarized to illustrate the changing role of assistive technologies in a single life span.[4]

I first met M.F. in early 1986 when she was 42 years old and being trained to use a computerized communication system. She was classified as having severe (athetoid) cerebral palsy and was preparing for her first full-time paid position at an independent living center. M.F. had a bachelor's degree in English. She was eager to learn the new computerized communication system because it would double as a word processor and enable her to communicate with others more efficiently than she could with her manual communication board.

M.F. had no recognizable unaided speech. Additionally, she required a powered wheelchair for mobility. Because she was the only child in an affluent family, her socialization, education, and rehabilitation were of the highest quality available to her and her family at the time.

Several years before I met her, M.F. was working in a sheltered workshop, where she met T.C., a woman with Down syndrome. M.F.'s parents were getting older and could not give her the care she required. Their capabilities so complemented one another that by working together they discovered that living independently in an apartment was possible. Recently widowed, M.F.'s mother, who worried about the care of her daughter during her lifetime, was considerably relieved. This arrangement enabled M.F. to live outside her family home for the first time in her life.

M.F.'s job with the independent living center lasted just 1 year because she said, "I didn't learn my responsibilities fast enough—I grew up in a world that didn't teach me how to handle responsibilities." After that, she began doing volunteer work helping special education students in a public school. In 1991, T.C. informed me that M.F. had been in and out of hospitals and rehabilitation facilities for most of that year. M.F. had neck surgery that left her paralyzed from the neck down. M.F. later wrote the following:

> It started off with loss of function in my left arm and hand, the two most important appendages of my body as I used them for pointing, directing my motorized wheelchair,

holding T.C. while she transferred me, and many more things that I took for granted. It ended about eight months later with the loss of function of my legs.

Because of M.F.'s changed condition, she and T.C. moved from their Chicago area apartment to M.F.'s hometown "to be close to family and friends." M.F.'s mother, who had been living in the same apartment complex until her back problems caused her to repeatedly fall, also moved with them. The caretaking role between M.F. and her mother had shifted. Concern over the welfare of M.F.'s mother and M.F. increased the burden for T.C. M.F. said the following:

> T.C. is doing extremely well considering all she has been through with me, especially the move, which she was not too happy about. She had spent almost every night with me in the hospitals and had spent every night at Memorial with me, so she just wanted things to be normal again. I, on the other hand, became extremely depressed because the only activity I could engage in was to think of all of what I used to do. There are times now, though, when I think she has accepted my new disability better than I have—or did until the past few months. Before I got my new wheelchair she would say, "Things will get better when your wheelchair comes" and "We will just have to struggle through it like I said before your surgery."

M.F. now requires new assistive technologies because her condition has changed so much. M.F. and T.C. needed to get used to these changes, which added more stress to what they were already feeling. M.F. explains as follows:

> After my neurologist ordered an MRI, it turns out I have what is called a swan-neck de-formity. When I put my head forward my spine closes and the fluid stops flowing. When I put it up the fluid starts again. I came home with a cervical collar and a corset, more for support than for correcting the problem as the doctors assured me I couldn't get any worse.
>
> Everyone was holding their breath when my motorized, reclining wheelchair arrived as I could still sit up when the seat and back were made and the chair was ordered. To every-one's relief, the doctor said I didn't need either the cervical collar or my corset when I used the wheelchair. I was especially glad, as I didn't like to look that disabled, or you could say, I wasn't accustomed to having that many people stare at me. Even though I've had a disability all my life, little did I know that the new chair would really cause people to stare—but more out of amazement than pity. The chair itself is the optimum in high-tech. It is controlled by using a joystick that I hold in my mouth. This enables me to be in the recliner mode, the drive mode, and the Light Talker mode, meaning I can use my communication device in this mode. I change modes by pushing a button at the side of my head. People have said it looks like a rocket, especially when I'm tilted all the way back.
>
> Luckily, there was a one-time grant given through the state, and people from UCP suggested I apply. The grant and Medicaid paid for the wheelchair. It paid less than one fourth of the cost of the Light Talker. Fortunately, I bought the van before all this happened or there would have been the additional expense of purchasing one and hav-ing it customized. Without it, I would be stuck at home as it is impossible to get my chair in a car. Mother helped pay for the Light Talker, which gives me a means of com-munication. UCP has a program to teach people how to use an IBM computer and then finds employment for them. I am going to enter it because I would like to have a part-time job writing or doing something along those lines. Anyway, it will do me good to learn more about IBMs and to know that I may be able to become productive again.

M.F.'s experience illustrates several challenges encountered when helping people with physical disabilities maintain their quality of life as they age:

- Added stress on already-burdened care providers occurs. Family members and other care providers who devote a major portion of their day to the care of their loved one with a disability may feel overwhelmed by the increased need for medical and technologic interventions. When they see the individual continue to deteriorate or become depressed in spite of such assistance, family members may experience their own sense of helplessness and despair.

- New device and equipment needs manifest. Aging persons with disabilities undergo changes in their physical capabilities and general health that require modifications in devices and heightened attention to their special needs.
- A dynamic interactive relationship among assistive device use, quality of life, functional capabilities, and temperament exists, which can change over time. Therefore this constellation of factors needs to be continually addressed, first from a person-centered perspective and second from the standpoint of functional limitations and capabilities.

## User Involvement in Technology Selection

The most recent laws regarding persons with disabilities recognize the importance of user involvement in rehabilitation services, including assistive technology. This emphasis advocates choice, self-determination, and independent living. The person with the disability and the family have more responsibilities than ever before.

As noted in Galvin and Scherer,[2] one key to achieving better person and technology matches is adopting a collaborative approach to technology selection, training, and support. Users and professionals cooperate in the matching process. With the user and professional working toward similar goals, each has particular strengths to contribute to the relationship. Technology users know their interests, likes and dislikes, priorities, and practical aspects of their living situations. Professionals know about different assistive devices and have access to a variety of resources and experience in evaluating technologies and people's functioning.

When a technology user and a professional form a partnership, each partner is responsible for completing certain tasks, gathering information, and making certain decisions. Professionals can stimulate discussion of the person's current capabilities and functioning and feelings related to technology use. Such consideration can include lifestyle, motivation, adjustment to disability, attitude toward technology, and values. Together, users and professionals can explore how these issues relate to technology acceptance. The Matching Person and Technology model is one means to support such a collaborative approach. Regardless of the way the model is used to assess the potential quality of the person and technology match, professionals must ensure that the following occurs:

- User needs drive the matching process, not technology availability.
- Professionals have the support they need to become knowledgeable about a variety of technologies and relevant resources.
- Different perspectives of the professional and user become evident so that they can be addressed.
- A range of low-tech and high-tech interventions is considered.
- Trial periods with the interventions in situations of actual use are arranged.
- Desirable interventions are selected with the necessary support systems established to ensure their success.
- Specific criteria and time frames by which to judge the intervention's usefulness to the person are identified.

Individuals with disabilities who are fully involved in their technology selection generally are more enthusiastic and independent technology users and are probably more satisfied with the overall rehabilitation services.

## Assessing the Achievement of a Good Person and Technology Match

How can the practitioner feel assured that the outcomes of the technology matching process result in user satisfaction and enhanced quality of life? The most obvious answer is to wait approximately 3 months and then follow up with the user and ask. For example, having users complete a prematching and postmatching assessment provides one measure of self-reported gains in many areas of functioning and overall quality of life.[1] Follow up requires time from both parties, either in person, over the phone, or through the mail. Additionally, the person may have moved or become so active and busy, thus avoiding follow-up contact. Yet efforts to obtain follow-up data are rewarded by new insights, improved ways of matching the person and technology, and satisfaction in knowing the practitioner did the best possible job.

If the practitioner asks only one question of the user, it should be "How has this technology made a difference in your life?" This open-ended question allows the person to provide positive and negative outcomes of technology use. The emphasis is also placed on whether the person's life has been enhanced by the technology—not on how well the person's life has incorporated and adapted to technology use.

## Summary

Not all people with disabilities are attracted to assistive technology. Many have endured years of dissatisfaction before getting the technology that best meets their needs and preferences. Rehabilitation professionals can provide a valuable service by identifying potential mismatches of person and technology so that modifications can be made to the technology and the environments where it functions. Although users need to make their own decisions and choices regarding device use, rehabilitation professionals need to be actively involved in the matching process or their professional obligations are not fulfilled. A collaborative approach to assistive technology selection offers the greatest likelihood of meeting the user's needs and most efficiently managing limited resources.

## References

1. Scherer MJ: Outcomes of assistive technology use on quality of life, *Disabil Rehabil* 18 (9): 439-448, 1996.
2. Galvin JC, Scherer MJ, editors: *Evaluating, selecting and using appropriate assistive technology,* Gaithersburg, Md, 1996, Aspen.
3. Phillips B, Zhao H: Predictors of assistive technology abandonment, *Assistive Technol* 5 (1):36-45, 1993.
4. Scherer MJ: *Living in the state of stuck: how technology impacts the lives of people with disabilities,* ed 2, Cambridge, Mass, 1996, Brookline Books.
5. Mitchell S: Technophiles and technophobes, *Am Demographics* 16 (2):36-42, 1994.
6. Enders A: *Questionable devices,* pp 271-276, presented at the second annual meeting of the rehabilitation engineering society of North America, Bethesda, Md, 1978, Rehabilitation Engineering Society of North America (RESNA).
7. Scherer MJ: What we know about women's technology use, avoidance, and abandonment. In Willmuth ME, Holcomb L, editors: *Women with disabilities: found voices,* New York, 1993, Haworth Press; *Women Ther* 14 (3/4):117-132, 1993.
8. Scherer MJ: *Matching person and technology (MPT): model and assessment instruments,* Rochester, NY, 1994, Scherer.

9. Scherer MJ, Frisina DR: Applying the matching people with technologies model to individuals with hearing loss: what people say they want—and need—from assistive technologies. In Scherer MJ, editor: *Technology & disability: deafness and hearing impairments,* vol 3, pp 62-68, Rochester, NY, 1994.
10. Scherer MJ, Frisina DR: Characteristics associated with marginal hearing loss and subjective well-being among a sample of older adults, *J Rehab Res Dev* 35 (4):420-426, 1998.

# CHAPTER 2

# Contexts: Assistive Technology at Home, School, Work, and in the Community

*Diane Nelson Bryen*
*Amy S. Goldman*

Technology is a lot like freedom—once it's uncorked, there's no putting it back. Its fruits are there for everyone's enjoyment and benefit. It is often said that assistive technology is liberating (for the individual with a disability), and that is certainly the case. However, it is time to be clear that assistive technology is liberating not just for the individual with a disability but indeed for America as a whole.[1]

In this chapter, we describe the way assistive technology can be used in the everyday contexts of home, school, work, and community to increase the independence, productivity and contribution, inclusion and participation, and quality of life of children and adults with disabilities. In addition, every context is described, technology applications and functional goals are listed, examples of technology are provided, and context considerations are illustrated. Principles for the selection and implementation of assistive technology are discussed, with a focus on the collaborative relationship between the intended user and provider. Finally, real-life examples of assistive technology solutions in varying circumstances are presented in short case studies.

## Technology in Everyday Life

As technology has come to play an increasingly important role in the lives of all persons in the United States, in the conduct of business, in the functioning of government, in the fostering of communication, in the conduct of commerce, and in the provision of education, its impact upon the lives of the more than 50,000,000 individuals with disabilities in the United States has been comparable to its impact upon the remainder of the citizens of the United States.[2]

Adults spend approximately one third of each day sleeping, another third working, and the rest divided between attending to basic needs and engaging in leisure. Technology is an important tool for work. Most people use some form of transportation technology such as cars, buses, or trains to travel to and from work. At work, many rely on the telephone, voice mail, fax, and computers so that work is easier and they are more productive or so that tasks can be performed quicker and more efficiently. At home, many use timesaving methods such as the microwave or the food processor to prepare dinner, answering machines for telephone messages, and an electric toothbrush. After dinner, some might rent a videotape, listen to a book on tape while performing household chores, talk to friends on the telephone, browse the Internet on a computer, exercise on a stationary bike or a treadmill, or go to the movies.

Technology surrounds everyone. It affects all aspects and contexts of everyday lives, from work, the ability to accomplish the chores that keep lives running smoothly, to the way people establish and maintain relationships and enjoy leisure. Technology makes lives easier and more efficient through access, environmental control, communication, mobilization, learning, self-care, and enjoying recreation and leisure.

Technology also has had a dramatic effect on children. It affects their communication and learning in school, their activity at home, and their play at home and in the community. Children use computers for early learning and literacy, whereas older students search the Web to gather information for reports and term papers. From early electronic games such as Nintendo using the television as a screen to complex computer or CD-ROM challenges requiring higher logic and reasoning skills, new technologies have captured the imaginations and free time of children. Similar to adults, children are connected through e-mail to their peers around the world. Although some adults are telecommuting to work, students with significant health disabilities or in rural areas are telecommuting to their classrooms. In some schools, unique learning opportunities that could not be offered otherwise such as Japanese language instruction are presented through distance learning. As with adults, technology is redefining what children do and the way they perform.

## Assistive Technology in Everyday Life

Assistive technology also is redefining everyday possibilities for children and adults who have a wide range of disabilities. In the home, classroom, workplace, and community, assistive technology is providing creative solutions that enable individuals with disabilities to be more independent, self-confident, productive, and included. These technology solutions, along with personal assistance services and environmental access, improve peoples' ability to learn, compete, work, volunteer, share in the goods and services of their communities, and interact with family and friends.[3]

Assistive technology was referred to in the congressional findings supporting reauthorization of the Technology-Related Assistance for Individuals with Disabilities Act Amendments of 1994 (referred to as the *Tech Act*) as follows[4]:

> For some individuals with disabilities, assistive technology is a necessity that enables them to engage in or perform many tasks. The provision of assistive technology devices and assistive technology services enables some individuals with disabilities to (1) have greater control over their own lives, (2) participate in and contribute more fully to activities in their home, school, and work environments, and in their communities, (3) interact to a greater extent with nondisabled individuals, and (4) otherwise benefit from opportunities that are taken for granted by individuals who do not have disabilities.

Assistive technology has clearly made a difference in the lives of many children and adults with disabilities. In 1993 The National Council on Disabilities conducted a 19-month study to better determine the cost and benefits of assistive technology devices and services. Some of the study's findings include the following[5]:

- Almost three quarters of school-age children were able to remain in a regular classroom, and 45% were able to reduce using school-related services.
- A total of 62% of working-age adults were able to lower dependence on family members, 58% were able to decrease reliance on paid assistance, and 37% were able to increase earnings.
- A total of 80% of the elderly individuals studied were able to curtail dependence on others, half were able to lessen dependence on paid assistance, and half were able to avoid entering a nursing home.
- Almost one third of assistive technology users indicated that their family saved an average of $1,110 per month with assistive technology. Simultaneously, one quarter of the users indicated that they experienced additional equipment-related expenses that averaged approximately $287 per month.
- A total of 92% of the 42 users of assistive technology who had paid jobs reported that the assistive technology enabled them to work faster or better. A total of 83% indicated that they earned more money, 81% noted working more hours, and 67% said that the equipment had allowed them to obtain employment. A total of 15% indicated that the equipment made keeping their jobs possible.

- Assistive technology users, when asked to estimate the effect of equipment on their quality of life on a scale from 1 to 10, disclosed that without the equipment their quality of life was about 3. As a result of the equipment, the number jumped to approximately 8.4.

The results of this study certainly underscore the opinion of Williams[1] in 1991, which was that assistive technology is liberating not only for the individual with a disability but also for all of America.

## Guiding Principles of Assistive Technology

A few guiding principles should be remembered when viewing everyday contexts. Assistive technology is a tool—just one important tool—to allow an individual with a disability to overcome or bypass a functional limitation that may result from a particular disability. Focus should be on the *functional goal* that the individual wants to accomplish, which may be increased independence with self-care at home, enhanced communication to increase classroom participation, more access to or interpretation of visual information at work, or greater mobility for better access to goods and services in the community.

Regardless of the context, relationships are important. Therefore whether assistive technologies are used in school (learning), at work (being productive), at home (increasing independent self-care), or in the community (accessing goods and services), they should promote *positive relationships* with family members, peers, co-workers, neighbors, and others.

For many assistive technologies, especially the more high-tech, sophisticated devices, provision of the assistive device is not sufficient. Necessary *services and support* also must be provided if the technology solution is to meet the expectations for which it was designed. With these additions such as an ecologically based and consumer-responsive evaluation, context-relevant training, or timely repairs, underuse or device abandonment is less likely.

Access to assistive technologies should complement the *removal of structural and programmatic barriers* on the job and in public accommodations as outlined in the Americans with Disabilities Act (ADA). Removal of architectural barriers (e.g., providing curb cuts and ramps) and reducing programmatic barriers (e.g., supplying assistive listening devices in a theater or providing written materials in large print or other accessible formats in a doctor's office) are mandated under the ADA so that people with disabilities have equal access to employment, schooling, and goods and services in the community. The ADA literally and figuratively "opens the doors" to schools, the workplace, the doctor's office, and public and private services. However, without needed assistive technology, people with disabilities may still not be able to "go through the doors" or participate and contribute once they have entered.

Finally, *consumer choice and preference* are critical to the successful selection of a particular assistive technology solution for a child or adult. Abandonment of the assistive device decreases when the choice and preferences of the users are considered.[6]

## Assistive Technology at Home

Young children, school-age children, adults, and older adults spend anywhere from one third to most of their time at home. They cook, eat, engage in self-care, participate in leisure and play, and enjoy many of the most intimate and enduring relationships within the home. Therefore people can use assistive technology at home to increase function, enhance independence and environmental control, promote communication, increase access to visual and auditory information for participation, increase self-esteem, improve mobility, and enhance play, leisure, and family interaction.

The following categories of assistive technology used in the home are based in part on work by Blackstone[7] and Wright and Goldman[8] (Table 2-1).

TABLE 2-1

*Assistive Technology at Home*

| APPLICATION/GOALS | EXAMPLES OF TECHNOLOGY | HOME CONSIDERATIONS |
|---|---|---|
| *Positioning*<br>Increased function, health, and safety through stable and comfortable positioning | Customized wheelchairs and inserts, standing aids, straps, trays, materials placed within reach, adjustment of table/desk, sidelying frames, beanbag chairs | Positioning aids increases function and participation, while reducing secondary disabilities such as hip displacement and scoleosis. May require multiple systems for each activity. |
| *Access*<br>Enhancement of speed, accuracy, endurance, independence, and effective functioning | Input devices (e.g., switch, expanded keyboard, mouse, trackball, touch window, speech recognition), head pointers, keyguards, key latches, keyboard emulators, reachers/grabbers | Access devices are key to independence/participation. Optimization of control requires delineation of input device (e.g., joy stick, single switch), selection technique, and rate enhancement. Integration of systems (e.g., mobility, communication, computer) needed. |
| *Environmental Control*<br>Effective control of the home environment (e.g., TV, household appliances) | Switch connections for battery operated items, control units for appliances/utilities, remote control units, robotics | Environmental controls used to turn computers, wheelchairs, and devices on/off. Use remote control to eliminate wires and optimize independent use of technology. |
| *Communication*<br>To be an active family member, to have more choice and control, and to live more independently | Electronic communication devices with or without speech, language boards, regular/adapted computers with regular/specialized software, CAD programs, Internet, Fax, speaker phone | Communication is necessary for effective family life. Communication devices promote face-to-face communication with family members and neighbors, support telephone use and in many cases support written communication. |
| *Assistive Listening Aids*<br>Access to auditory information needed for effective communication, independence, recreation, and leisure, including face-to-face and telephone conversations, listening to TV and radio | Hearing aids, personal FM systems, sound field FM systems, telephone amplifiers, captioning, TTD/TTY | Hearing is a core means for oral communication with family and neighbors. Hearing aids should be checked daily by user or family member. |

| Category | Description | Examples | |
|---|---|---|---|
| **Visual Aids** | Enhancement or interpretation of visual/print information for independence and recreation, including reading mail, participating in leisure activities (e.g., books on tape), or engaging in social interaction through the Internet | Screen readers, reading machines, screen enlarger, Brailler, large print books, high contrast materials, scanners with speech synthesizer, CCTV, audio tapes | Access to printed material is often needed for independent living and to participate fully in leisure activities at home. Social interaction through the Internet can be supported through enlarged text or with a screen reader. |
| **Mobility** | Movement within the home environment for maximal independence and social interaction | Manual walkers, crutches or wheelchairs, manual or powered mobility aids (e.g., wheelchairs, scooters), desk chairs on wheels | Mobility aids are important for independence, participation, socialization, communication, and control. Home may require modifications for wheelchair accessibility. |
| **Vehicle Modifications** | Ensure safe and often independent transportation from home to community | Tie downs for wheelchairs, wheelchair lifts, hand controls, visual signals, other driving aids | Without accessible transportation through vehicle modifications, participation with family and friends and inclusion in community life are greatly limited. |
| **Self-Care** | Increased independence and participation in activities such as cooking, dining, laundry, housecleaning, dressing, personal care, grooming, bathing | Electronic feeders and page turners, adapted utensils, adapted toilet seats, robotics, Velcro closures for clothing, built up handle on utensils and tools, reachers and grabbers | Self-care at home is critical for routine health, safety, and hygiene. Most can be accomplished by removal of architectural/structural barriers at home. |
| **Home Modifications** | Enable entrance, movement, and participation within the home | Widened doorways, ramps, stair glides, lowered shelves and light switches, grab bars in bathrooms, intercom systems, automatic door locks, lowering countertops, smoke detectors that flash | Home modifications are fundamental, whether a child with a disability is in the home, an adult is living alone or with a spouse, or an older person with physical or sensory limitations is at home. |

## Assistive Technology to Enhance Activities of Daily Living and Self-Care

Assistive technology to enhance activities of daily living and self-care consists of devices and adaptations to improve participation or increase independence in activities such as cooking and dining, laundry, housecleaning, dressing, personal care and grooming, and bathing. These devices may range from simple Velcro closures for clothing, built-up handles on utensils and tools, and reachers and grabbers to more technologically complex devices such as electronic feeding machines.

## Assistive Listening Devices and Access to Auditory Information

Assistive listening devices are used to amplify auditory signals, especially speech, and include hearing aids or personal listening devices. They also may include phone amplifiers. In addition, for people who are deaf, television captioning and text telephones transform speech to text, thus permitting the "listener" to have access to auditory information. These devices enable an individual with hearing loss to participate in conversations, talk on the telephone, or listen to the radio or television—each promoting access to information, recreation, and participation in family and social life at home.

## Vision Aids

Vision aids are devices that assist persons with limited vision by increasing contrast, enlarging images, or substituting tactile or auditory cues for visual information. Examples include Braillers, magnifiers, large-print books, tape-recorded materials, screen readers, scanners with voice synthesizers, and closed-circuit televisions. In many cases, some of these same vision aids assist a person with limited literacy skills in gaining access to printed information. In all circumstances the goal is to enhance or interpret visual information so that people can live at home more independently (e.g., reading their own mail and other written information), participate more fully in leisure activities at home (e.g., using Braille Scrabble, books on tape, or large-print books), or engage in social interaction through the Internet with a screen reader.

## Augmentative Communication Devices

Similar to assistive listening devices, augmentative communication devices permit a child or adult with significant communication disabilities to be active family members, to have more choice and control, and to live more independently. These devices, which supplement or replace natural speech, range from fabricated language boards with letters, words, or pictures to voice amplifiers and computers with speech synthesizers and specialized software. Communication devices promote face-to-face communication with family members and neighbors, allow the child or adult to use the telephone and other telecommunication systems such as the Internet, and in many cases support written communication.

## Environmental Controls

Environmental controls include electronic or computerized systems with switch controls (including voice recognition) that enable individuals without mobility or sufficient manual ability to control household appliances and devices such as the television or lights. Environmental controls include generic remote controls for the TV or stereo, switch connections for battery-operated items, control units for appliances, remote control units (e.g., infrared light beam, radio frequency), and robotics. They allow a child or adult to control the environment without help from family members or personal assistants whether for performing household chores, playing with toys, or enjoying leisure.

## Home Modifications

Home modifications include adaptations to the home to permit access or independent mobility and self-care, ensure safety, and increase independence and participation. Examples include widening entranceways and doorways, installing stair glides, ramps, grab bars in the bathroom, intercom systems, and automatic door locks, lowering countertops and cabinets, changing floor coverings, and providing adaptations to fixtures. They also include appliances that substitute one type of signal for another such as doorbells that activate a flashing light or smoke detectors that vibrate. Home modifications are fundamental if individuals with disabilities, whether a child with a disability, an adult living alone or with a roommate, or an older individual with physical or sensory limitations, are to live at home.

## Recreation, Leisure, and Play Modifications

Recreation, leisure, and play modifications can include specialized equipment or adaptations to accommodate a variety of leisure and recreational pursuits at home or in the community, access to materials and activities allowing peer interaction, hobby development and enjoyment, and good use of free time. Some examples include backyard playground adaptations to slides and swings, computer games, board-game modifications, built-up handles on gardening equipment, special mountings for fishing rods, knitting machines, page turners, hand-powered bikes or adapted tricycles, and drawing software for the computer. However, the modification also may be as simple as providing books on tape.

## Mobility Aids

Mobility aids may be manual or power operated and can support, replace, or augment walking. This category includes walkers, crutches, or canes, four-wheeled manual chairs with or without custom adaptations, or three-wheeled or four-wheeled battery-powered scooters or chairs. Each type of mobility aid permits independent movement that increases a person's personal mobility, ability to explore, and social interaction.

## Seating and Positioning Aids

Seating and positioning aids include modifications or adaptations to wheelchairs or other positioning systems that are used to support the trunk and head in an upright posture. Seating and positioning aids may be required for the safe, comfortable, and functional performance of activities of daily living, including eating and grooming. Certain positioning systems such as side-lying frames and floor sitters permit a user to more comfortably and functionally participate in play and recreational activities. They also reduce pressure on weight-bearing surfaces to prevent skin breakdown. Finally, seating and positioning aids are essential to making controls or other equipment accessible for increased independence. Examples include side-lying frames, crawling assists, floor sitters, chair inserts, customized wheelchairs that tilt in space, standing aids, beanbag chairs, sandbags, and simple floor mats. Each particular aid increases function and participation through stable and comfortable positioning. Proper seating and positioning also may reduce secondary disabilities such as hip displacement and scoliosis or health problems such as pressure sores.

## Access Devices

Access devices are used to interface a user to an augmentative communication device, a computer, a wheelchair, or battery-operated toys and appliances to enhance speed, accuracy, endurance, and independence when hand use is limited. Access technologies include input devices (e.g., switch, expanded keyboard, mouse, trackball touch window, joystick, speech recognition), head pointers, keyguards, and keyboard emulators. When access systems are integrated appropriately, maximum independence and effective functioning are ensured when an individual uses several types of assistive technologies (e.g., powered mobility, augmentative communication, computers, environmental controls).

## Vehicle Modifications

Vehicle modifications can occur in personal transportation such as cars and vans to ensure adequate, safe, and often independent transportation from home to work, school, into the community, and to visit family or friends. Devices or adaptations that may be required for driver control, passenger safety, or mobility device transport include tie-downs for wheelchairs, wheelchair lifts, visual signalers, hand controls, and driving aids. Without accessible transportation through vehicle modifications, participation with family and friends and inclusion in community life are severely limited.

Learning about the individual, the individual's current and preferred lifestyle at home, and the range of assistive technology solutions to accommodate functional limitations increases personal choice and control, independence and safety, and inclusion and participation at home. Relationships formed and sustained at home become more reciprocal because some of the time previously spent on personal care activities can be reduced.

## *Assistive Technology at School*

Infants, toddlers, and school-aged children may spend 3 to 8 hours each day or more in child-care settings, preschool, or school. These are environments where children learn, develop social skills through forming peer and other relationships, eat, and play. In addition to learning academic skills such as reading, writing, mathematics, and the sciences, children learn many lifelong skills about independence, productivity, contribution, and participation. Assistive technology can support each of these aspects of development for young children. For some children with disabilities, assistive technology devices and services also are a necessity, not a luxury, to access school life and learning. Assistive technology may be a needed service to promote development as part of an individualized family service plan (IFSP) within the context of early intervention, a related service or supplemental aid to ensure a free and appropriate public education (FAPE) under the Individuals with Disabilities Education Act (IDEA), or an accommodation under Section 504 of the Rehabilitation Act.

The selection of a particular assistive technology solution requires unique child-care and classroom considerations (Table 2-2). In addition to outlining the types and examples of assistive technology for young children according to the goal to be accomplished (e.g., written communication, access to toys), unique classroom considerations are included. If assistive technology is to be provided by the school, it should be clearly indicated as part of a preschool child's IFSP or the school-aged student's individualized educational plan (IEP).

The range of assistive technology used at school to promote FAPE under IDEA or as a needed accommodation under Section 504 of the Rehabilitation Act is summarized in Table 2-3. This table is based, in part, on Sarah Blackstone's analysis[7] of assistive technology in classrooms.

## *Assistive Technology at Work*

Most adults spend 8 hours or more each day at work, in paid employment, managing a household, volunteering, or parenting. Adults' value is often defined by the work they

*Text continued on p. 27*

# TABLE 2-2
## *Assistive Technology in Day-Care and Preschool Settings*

| APPLICATION/GOALS | EXAMPLES OF TECHNOLOGY | CLASSROOM/EDUCATIONAL CONSIDERATIONS |
|---|---|---|
| *Communication*<br>Independent and effective means of engaging in play and social interaction with peers, participation in instructional interactions with adults | Language boards, voice output communication devices, assistive listening devices | Staff, children, and family members may need training on the use, updating and maintenance of devices; therefore start early. Ensure vocabulary that facilitates play and socialization. |
| *Telephone Communication*<br>Communication with friends and family across distance, emergency notification | Telephone amplifiers, dialing aids (e.g., memory features, picture keys), telecommunication device for the deaf (TDD/TTY) | Staff, children, and family members may need initial training on use of devices. |
| *Written Communication*<br>Development of preliteracy skills and graphic expression | Unadapted computer and printer with regular or specialized software, adapted computer and printer with regular or specialized software, pencil holders, fat pencils, slant boards | For computer use, staff, children, and family members require training. Structure collaborative learning opportunities around computer use. All classroom software should support access. |
| *Access to Television/Videos*<br>Enhancement and/or interpretation of educational and recreational media content | Open/closed captioning, audio-description | TV must have chip for closed captioning, check for captioning when renting/purchasing videos. |
| *Drawing*<br>Development of self-expression and participation in recreation and socialization activities | Computer with color/monitor/printer and drawing software, fat crayons, paint brushes with adapted handles, alternatives to paint brushes (e.g., bingo markers), switch-adapted spin art | For computer use, staff and children will need training. Allow for multiple channels for graphic expression. |
| *Mobility*<br>Independent movement, exploration, social interaction, and learning | Cooper car, adapted/specialized tricycles/bikes, child-sized walkers (for stability, carrying, and walking), manual or powered wheelchairs | Building and classroom needs to be accessible and have adequate room for assisted mobility. Allow for multiple means and experiences with independent movement. |

*Continued*

# TABLE 2-2—cont'd
## Assistive Technology in Day-Care and Preschool Settings

| APPLICATION/GOALS | EXAMPLES OF TECHNOLOGY | CLASSROOM/EDUCATIONAL CONSIDERATIONS |
|---|---|---|
| **Access to Books**<br>Develop of literacy skills, access to text-based information, socialization contexts | Voice/sound-output storybooks, commercially available tape/storybooks, books on tape or disk, scanners/reading machines, CCTV, automatic page turners, book holders, adaptations for page turning | Initial training of staff, children, and family is needed, lower shelves for book/tape access. |
| **Access to Toys**<br>Fun! Cognitive, linguistic, motor, and social development | Switch-adapted toys, handles on puzzles, play tray or Velcro, game adaptations (e.g., beeping balls or Frisbees) | Consider optimal positioning for effective use of adapted toys, switch-adapted toys may need to be made or specially purchased. |
| **Seating and Positioning**<br>Facilitate access and maximize function | Corner chairs, standers, adjustable chair (e.g., Rifton), mats, wedges, beanbag chairs, customized wheelchair seating systems | Adequate classroom space is needed, allow for multiple means of positioning depending on activity. |
| **Environmental Access**<br>Effective control of the environment without assistance from people | Remote control/large key or adapted remote, touch lamps, lowered light switches, power link | Initial training as indicated on some remote control systems, classroom modifications such as lowered light switch may be needed. |
| **Self-Care**<br>Development of independence and sense of mastery | Built-up or adapted handles or utensils, Velcro closures on clothing, loops on zippers | Classroom modifications may be needed to ensure sinks, toilets, etc. are safe and barrier free. |
| **Access to Playground**<br>Movement and participation in natural contexts with peers | Specialized slides/swings or other equipment, accessibility to playground areas | Accessibility of playground is essential for optimal free-time participation. |

*CCTV, closed-circuit television.*

TABLE 2-3
*Assistive Technology in Classroom Settings*

| APPLICATION/GOALS | EXAMPLES OF TECHNOLOGY | CLASSROOM CONSIDERATIONS |
|---|---|---|
| *Positioning*<br>Increased function and participation through stable and comfortable positioning | Sidelying frames, walkers, floor sitters, chair inserts, wheelchairs, standing aids, straps, trays, beanbag chairs | Students should be upright and midline, forward facing, and have maximal distal function through proximal stability. Positioning should include student's position in relation to peers, teacher, and materials, with multiple systems considered. |
| *Access*<br>Enhancement of speed, accuracy, endurance, independence | Input devices (e.g., switch, expanded keyboard, mouse, trackball, touch window, speech recognition), head pointers, keyguards, key latches, keyboard emulators | Access technologies are key to efficient use of devices. Optimization of control requires delineation of input device (e.g., joy stick, single switch), selection technique (scanning), and rate enhancement (e.g., coding, prediction). Integration of systems (e.g., mobility, augmentative communication, computer) needed to maximize independence and participation. |
| *Environmental Control*<br>Effective control of the environment without assistance from other people | Switch connections for battery operated items, control units for appliances, remote control units, robotics | Environmental controls are used to turn student's computers, and wheelchairs, devices on/off. Use remote control to eliminate wires and optimize independent use of technology. |
| *Communication*<br>Independent and effective means of communicating (e.g., writing, speaking, drawing) | Electronic communication devices with or without speech, language boards, Etrans, regular/adapted computers with regular/specialized software, CAD programs, Internet, fax | Start early. Set up classroom for communication. Use communication boards projected on overhead, language mater cards with messages/symbols, conversational boards/ wallets near activity areas, speech output devices, computer with communication software, and telecommunications, including Internet. Student and partners need training. |
| *Assistive Listening Aids*<br>Appropriate signal to noise (s/n) frequency so that students with hearing disabilities have access to auditory information (e.g., speech, music, auditory alarms) | Hearing aids, personal FM systems, sound field FM systems, telephone amplifiers, captioning, TTD/TTY | Hearing core event leading to speaking, reading instruction. Hearing aids should be checked daily, listener should be seated close to source of sound, supplement with visual information should be provided, listening skills should be taught with appropriate assistive listening devices. |

*Continued*

TABLE 2-3—cont'd
*Assistive Technology in Classroom Settings*

| APPLICATION/GOALS | EXAMPLES OF TECHNOLOGY | CLASSROOM CONSIDERATIONS |
|---|---|---|
| *Visual Aids*<br>Enhancement or interpretation of visual/print information | Screen readers, reading machines, screen enlarger, Brailler, light boxes, high contrast materials, scanners with speech synthesizer, CCTV, audio tapes | Vision is a major learning model. Increase contrast, enlarge stimuli, make careful use of tactile and auditory modes. Monitor responses. For high-tech, student/teacher training needed. |
| *Mobility*<br>Independent movement, exploration, social interaction, and learning | Self-propelled (walkers) or powered recreational (bikes) and mobility aids (e.g., wheelchairs, scooters), recreational devices should not be used as substitutes for mobility devices | Mobility aids are important for independence, socialization, communication, and control. Children as young as 15 months can use powered mobility with good training/supervision. Building/classroom must be wheelchair accessible. |
| *Computer-Assisted Learning*<br>Achievement of educational or vocational goals | Regular or adapted computers with regular or specialized software and speech synthesizer, computer work stations, Internet/World Wide Web, CD-ROM (e.g., reference materials, textbooks) | Computer-assisted learning expands strategies for learning: instructional (drill/practice), revelatory (discovery), conjectural (learner builds own world) and emancipational (strips away barriers to learning). Require training in use. |
| *Recreation, Leisure, Play*<br>Access to materials/activities facilitating peer interaction/relations, hobby development, enjoyable use of free time | Outdoor adaptations (e.g., slides, swings), computer games, adapted board games (e.g., rolling dice), adapted play materials (e.g., Velcro, trays, spin art), books on tape | Consider accessible listening and viewing activities, group games, including computer games and graphics, dramatic play, adapted games and puzzles. |
| *Self-Care*<br>Independent self-care activities | Electronic feeders and page turners, adapted utensils, toilet seats, aids for tooth brushing, washing, dressing, grooming, food preparation, robotics | Incorporate self-care activities/adaptations as they occur naturally in activities of eating, dressing, hygiene, and meal preparation. |
| *Classroom Modifications*<br>Enable entrance, movement, and participation within the classroom | Widened doorways, ramps and elevators, lowered shelves and light switches, accessible bathrooms, adapted work stations, Braille signage, adequate space for wheelchairs | Removal of architectural and structural barriers in the school building, classroom, and playground enable students who use assistive technology to more fully participate. |

Modified from Blackstone S: *Assistive technologies in classroom, Augmentative Communication News 3:3, 1990.*

do. Despite the importance of work the national employment statistics for people with disabilities are discouraging. Figures from the 1990 U.S. Census estimate that of the 14.8 million people with significant disabilities, more than 76% (11.3 million) are unemployed.[8] According to Michael Williams, who spoke with the co-chairperson of the President's Committee on the Employment of People with Disabilities in 1994, the unemployment rate among all people with disabilities has been increasing over the past 5 years despite passage of the ADA.

The reasons so few people with disabilities are employed are many and complex. First and perhaps most important are low expectations that individuals with disabilities have; they believe they cannot or should not work because of their disabilities. Another reason so many people with developmental and other disabilities are not employed is public policy. Approximately 90 cents of every federal dollar and 80 cents of every state dollar spent on individuals with disabilities are spent on keeping them in segregated, nonproductive settings.

Investment in facility-based, segregated employment is not decreasing.[9-11] Work disincentives, the fear of losing public-sponsored health insurance, and the need for reliable and accessible public transportation are other barriers to employment for people with disabilities.[12,13] Finally, despite passage of the ADA, provision of reasonable accommodations on the job, including work site modifications and other assistive technologies, is still far from routine.

Assistive technology solutions and other work-site accommodations enable many individuals with disabilities to be productive employers, employees, and co-workers (Table 2-4). State offices of vocational rehabilitation may pay for an individual's assistive technology devices and services if they are needed to gain or retain employment and are designated as part of the person's individualized plan for employment (IPE). In addition as a "reasonable accommodation" under Title I of the ADA, the employer may pay for work-related technology and work-site modifications. Although many employers fear the high cost of providing accommodations on the job, according to the job accommodation network, the average cost of accommodation for a worker with a disability ranges from nothing to $500. Furthermore, according to the Harris poll survey (1994), employers reported that people with disabilities do the following:

- Work as hard or harder than other workers
- Are as reliable and punctual
- Produce as well or better
- Demonstrate average or better-than-average leadership
- Are *not* more costly or difficult to supervise

## *Assistive Technology in the Community and the Americans with Disabilities Act*

Whether the disabled individual is a young child in school, a working adult, or a retired senior, the community provides many opportunities for recreation and leisure, for purchasing needed goods and services, and for socializing. Fortunately, with passage of the ADA in 1990, some of the barriers to inclusion and participation in community life have been removed for many people with disabilities. Curb cuts are more routinely found on city streets, and access to public accommodations, including stores, movie theaters, restaurants and bars, hotels, and medical and dental offices, has increased as a result of implementation of the ADA.

Additionally, with the increased removal of architectural, structural, and programmatic barriers under Title II of the ADA, access to government buildings and services, parks, and libraries has increased. Under Title IV of the ADA, telephone companies must provide telecommunications relay services for people who have hearing or speech disabilities or people who are deaf. Telecommunications is now more accessible for most individuals with disabilities. Although transportation continues to be a major barrier for many people who use mobility aids (especially powered wheelchairs and scooters), pub-

TABLE 2-4
*Assistive Technology at Work*

| APPLICATION/GOALS | EXAMPLES OF TECHNOLOGY | WORK CONSIDERATIONS |
| --- | --- | --- |
| *Positioning*<br>Increased function and productivity through stable and comfortable positioning of the individual and materials | Wheelchairs, standing aids, straps, trays, materials placed within reach, adjustment of table/desk | Work with employee and employer to determine how positioning of the individual and his/her materials will lead to optimal independence and productivity. Multiple systems may be needed. |
| *Access*<br>Enhancement of speed, accuracy, endurance, independence, productivity | Input devices (e.g., switch, expanded keyboard, mouse, trackball, touch window, speech recognition), head pointers, keyguards, key latches, keyboard emulators, reachers/grabbers | Access technologies are key to independence/productivity. Optimization of control requires delineation of input device (e.g., joy stick, single switch), selection technique (scanning), and rate enhancement (e.g., coding, prediction). Integration of systems (e.g., mobility, augmentative communication, computer) needed to maximize independence and productivity. |
| *Environmental Control*<br>Effective control of the environment without assistance from other people | Switch connections for battery operated items, control units for appliances/utilities, remote control units, robotics | Environmental controls used to turn works computers, wheelchairs, and devices on/off. Use remote control to eliminate wires and optimize independent use of technology. |
| *Communication*<br>Independent and effective means of communicating (e.g., writing, conversation, public speaking and presentations, telephone/telecommunication use) | Electronic communication devices with or without speech, language boards, regular/adapted computers with regular/specialized software, CAD programs, Internet, fax, speaker phone | Communication is necessary for most jobs, whether with supervisor, co-worker, or customers. Communication technology, whether specialized (e.g., electronic communication device) or generic (speaker phone) may be necessary. Employee, supervisor, and co-workers may need training. |
| *Assistive Listening Aids*<br>Access to auditory information (e.g., speech, auditory alarms) needed for effective communication, independence, productivity | Hearing aids, personal FM systems, sound field FM systems, telephone amplifiers, captioning, TTD/TTY | Hearing is a core means for oral communication with supervisor, co-workers, and customers. Hearing aids should be checked daily by user, listener should be seated close to source of sound and sign language interpreter may be needed. |

| | | |
|---|---|---|
| *Visual Aids*<br>Enhancement or interpretation of visual/print information for independence, productivity | Screen readers, reading machines, screen enlarger, Brailler, large print, high contrast materials, scanners with speech synthesizer, CCTV, audio tapes | Access to printed material is often needed on the job. Increase contrast, enlarge stimuli. Bypassing print through use of scanners and reading machines may be needed. Computers should be accessible under Section 508 of Rehabilitation Act. |
| *Mobility*<br>Movement within the work environment for maximal independence and productivity | Manual walkers or wheelchairs or powered mobility aids (e.g., wheelchairs, scooters), desk chairs on wheels | Mobility aids are important for independence, productivity, socialization, communication, and control. Worksite must be wheelchair accessible. |
| *Computer-Generated Products*<br>Independent production of documents, including reports, brochures, graphs, and graphics, independent access to the information superhighway | Regular or adapted computers with regular or specialized software and speech synthesizer, computer work stations, Internet/World Wide Web, CD-ROM (e.g., reference materials, textbooks), CAD, LAN | Computers can be powerful tools for increasing the productivity and independence of an employee. It can also be a barrier if computers used by employee and co-workers are not accessible and compatible. Computer purchases should take into account accessibility issues (see Section 508 of Rehabilitation Act). Training will also need to be provided. |
| *Self-Care*<br>Independent self-care activities while at work | Electronic feeders and page turners, adapted utensils, adapted toilet seats, robotics | Self-care at work is critical for routine health and hygiene. Most can be accomplished by removal of architectural/structural barriers at the work site. |
| *Worksite Modifications*<br>Enable entrance, movement, and participation within the workplace | Widened doorways, ramps and elevators, lowered shelves and light switches, accessible bathrooms and cafeterias, adapted work stations, Braille signage, adequate space for wheelchairs | Removal of architectural/structural barriers at the workplace is key to removing employment barriers for many employees with disabilities. Worksite accommodations can be as simple as raising a desk or rearranging materials. |

lic transportation, including buses and light, rapid, and commuter rail systems, is slowly improving.

With passage of the ADA and with increased access to assistive technologies, people with disabilities are much more visible in the community. Businesses are becoming more aware that people with disabilities are good customers. Finally, people with disabilities are much more active in the community as neighbors, volunteers, students, employees, and employers.

The promise of the ADA and of assistive technologies supporting full community inclusion and participation of children and adults with disabilities must integrate the individual's lifestyle (routine visits to the doctor, avid golfer), the community setting (rural versus urban), and the particular assistive technology solution (Table 2-5).

## Assistive Technology in Recreation, Sports, and Leisure

Advances in assistive technologies have occurred that help individuals enjoy recreation, sports, and leisure. Adapted or specialized wheelchairs allow many individuals to compete in sports such as racing, basketball, or tennis and to move on the beach. Adapted skiing, including the use of a sit ski, enables many people with physical disabilities to enjoy winter sports. Bowling, golf, and Frisbee can be adapted for people who are blind or have physical disabilities. When open or closed captioning and audio description become more readily available, attending movies, plays, and even the opera can become more accessible for people who have sensory disabilities.

The information superhighway also has opened the worldwide community for many people with disabilities who have access to a computer and a modem. Through e-mail, the Internet, listservs, and the World Wide Web (WWW), people can communicate with friends, pen pals, or colleagues around the world. They can obtain information about almost any topic, from information specific to their disabilities or piece of assistive technology to general topics such as the local weather. Joining electronic discussion groups on almost any issue or interest increases access to information and reduces social isolation.[14] "Traveling" to an art museum in Minnesota or "visiting" a foreign city such as La Plata, Argentina is possible through the WWW. The advances made in informational technologies and the assistive technologies that ensure access to these developments have opened the world to exploration by everyone.

## Principles of the Selection and Implementation of Assistive Technology Solutions

Selection and implementation of assistive technology solutions are typically influenced by the knowledge of the professional practitioner or provider and the accepted practices in the profession. These principles are often based on knowledge of body mechanics and typical function and development. Thus, for example, principles regarding physical alignment influence decisions in selecting seating and positioning systems. In addition, function, comfort, and consumer choice are just as important in making the decisions regarding what kind, when, where, and even whether to use assistive devices and services.

Whatever the assistive technology type and whatever the education and experience of the provider, the following is a set of considerations and questions providers and consumers can use to guide the decisions they make.

- *Assistive technology is a means, not an end.* Technology for technology's sake is a waste of money, time, and energy. Procurement or use of a device is not the goal. Most frequently, use of the device follows if it succeeds in helping a user accomplish a meaningful task or activity more effectively and efficiently. The best technology is the technology that works well for the individual. Consider also that assistive devices are similar to fertilizer—more is not necessarily better.

What is it that technology can help the consumer do, cannot do or cannot do well, comfortably, or without great effort?

- *The consumer knows best.* Intended users may not know the specifics about what is needed or all the available options but they probably know what they want to be able to do. Start with a good definition of the function with which a user needs assistance. Base this definition on what they want to do and how, when, where, and with whom they want or need to perform the task.

What should the consumer do? Where does the consumer usually do this? With whom? When?

- *The device is only part of the equation.* Consider the device's characteristics, the user, the task, and the environment and the interactions among these components. For example, learn about the power source by asking the following questions: How long can the device run on batteries? How long will the batteries last? Are they easily replaced or does replacement require the device to be serviced by the manufacturer? Can the device be used while it's recharging? Can the device be used in a manual mode if neither battery nor regular current is available? How does lighting affect the use of the device? Is the screen legible in daylight and under fluorescent light? What is jeopardized if the device malfunctions during use and how can that eventuality be anticipated? What will happen when the rooftop carrier gets iced up and the passenger is stuck in the car on the turnpike? Can a scooter fit in or on your two-door sedan?

Can the devices under consideration present new barriers for the provider and consumer? What are the barriers and how can they be addressed? Can the device facilitate inclusion and interaction?

- *Everything is not a "nail."* A wise man once said that if the only tool a person has is a hammer, everything looks like a nail. Competent, responsible assistive technology service providers are familiar with a range of literal and figurative tools to avoid making recommendations based on their own familiarity with only a limited range of options. Share the advantages and disadvantages of appropriate options with the consumer.

Have all reasonable alternatives for the provider been described and considered?

- *The best is not all "high tech."* Consider and present a range of possible alternatives, along with the advantages and realities of each. Include high-tech, soft-tech or light-tech, and no-tech modifications and alternatives such as the use of personal assistance services or service animals as appropriate.

How does this assistive technology fit in with soft-tech, no-tech task modifications and the use of personal assistance services for the consumer and provider?

- *The decision is not necessarily "either/or."* People use a variety of ways to communicate, such as speaking face-to-face or over the telephone, writing by pencil, chalk, or computer, and using gestures and head movements. They use various ways to move between points in their environment such as by foot, bike, car, plane, or rollerblades. Some of these means involve aids or tools and some do not. Decisions in assistive technology also should provide for flexibility, with solutions matched to functions and environments. Additionally, assistive technology interventions can easily coexist with therapeutic strategies designed to develop natural skills. Introducing augmentative communication approaches does not necessitate abandonment of traditional efforts to improve speech when meaningful progress is occurring.

# TABLE 2-5

*Assistive Technology in the Community and the ADA*

| APPLICATION/GOAL | STORES, RESTAURANTS, HOTELS, GOVERNMENT BUILDINGS |
|---|---|
| **Mobility**<br>Independent access to and participation within community settings | Individual mobility aids should be sturdy/rugged enough to handle the knocks and bumps. ADA Titles II and III require wheelchair access. |
| **Communication**<br>Independent participation and increased control in shopping, banking, recreation, dining out, handling public services, and access to medical and dental care | Individual should use a portable communication device that is understandable to unfamiliar employees and the general public. Reasonable accommodations under ADA Titles II and III exist. Employees should take the time to listen to an augmented communicator. |
| **Telecommunications**<br>Independent and private communication via the telephone whether at home, at a hotel, or with physician or dentist | Individual should have TTY/TTD, telephone amplifier, or speaker phone at home to contact hotel, restaurant, or government by phone. ADA Titles II and III may require same of businesses and government offices. |
| **Access to Auditory Information**<br>Participation and enjoyment at the movies, theater, or cultural events, access to information at community meetings | Individual may bring personal assistive listening device. ADA Titles II and III require reasonable accommodations (e.g., assistive listening devices or sign language interpreter) for public meetings/forums, movies, and theaters. |
| **Access to Print/Visual Information**<br>Independent access to menus and programs, applications, public informational brochures, flyers, and reports | Individual may bring magnifier to enlarge printed materials. ADA Titles II and III require printed materials be provided in alternative formats (e.g., Braille, enlarged print, screen reader or, personal assistance in reading printed information). |
| **Self-Care**<br>Independent self-care (e.g., bathing, personal hygiene, eating) when in the community | Individual should bring any personal adapted utensils or devices. ADA Titles II and III require that bathrooms and public eating facilities should be accessible if readily achievable. |
| **Recreation/Leisure**<br>Participation in sport events as participant or spectator, use of public libraries, movies, theaters, fitness centers, etc. | ADA Title III requires that stores, bars, hotels, theaters, and museums should be barrier free if readily achievable. |

| PARKS, LIBRARIES, RECREATIONAL FACILITIES | MEDICAL/DENTAL OFFICES |
|---|---|
| Individual mobility aids should be rugged enough to handle outdoor recreation. Sports/recreational wheelchairs may be considered. ADA Titles II and III require wheelchair access. | Individual mobility aids should be sturdy/rugged enough to handle the knocks and bumps. ADA Title III requires wheelchair access to building and medical equipment (e.g., dental chairs, mammograms). |
| Same considerations as for stores, restaurants, hotels, and government buildings exist. | Individual should use a portable communication device that is understandable to unfamiliar employees and the general public. Reasonable accommodations under ADA Title III exist. Employees should take the time to listen to an augmented communicator or provide a sign language interpreter for a deaf patient. |
| Individual should have TTY/TTD, telephone amplifier, or speaker phone to contact libraries and recreational facilities. ADA Titles II and III may require same of parks and recreational facilities and libraries. | Individual should have TTY/TTD, telephone amplifier, or speaker phone to contact physician or dentist. ADA Title III may require same of doctor or dentist. |
| Individual may bring personal assistive listening device. ADA Titles II and III require reasonable accommodations (e.g., assistive listening devices or sign language interpreter) for public meetings/forums held at libraries and park/recreational facilities. | Individual may bring personal assistive listening device. ADA Title III requires reasonable accommodations (e.g., assistive listening devices or sign langauge interpreter) for patients with hearing disabilities. |
| Same considerations as for stores, restaurants, hotels, and government buildings exist. | Individual may bring magnifier to enlarge printed materials. ADA Title III requires printed materials be provided in alternative formats (e.g., Braille, enlarged print, screen reader, or personal assistance in reading printed information). |
| Same considerations as for stores, restaurants, hotels, and government buildings exist. | Same considerations as for stores, restaurants, hotels, and government buildings exist. |
| Individual assistive technology for sports include adapted skis, golf, sailing, etc. Many parks/recreational sites have special adapted areas. ADA Titles II and III require wheelchair access when readily achievable. | ADA Title III requires that health or fitness centers be accessible to people with disabilities if readily achievable. |

What is the total picture of available support, including assistive technology devices and services, for the consumer and provider?

- *Knowledge is power.* Empower the intended users in the decision-making process with adequate information. For some types of technology, giving them the opportunity to talk with users of the technology that is being considered and/or those affected by the technology (e.g., teachers, employers, friends, caregivers) is helpful. Similarly, they may want to obtain references from those who have received services from an evaluator, therapist, vendor, or other assistive technology provider.

Has the consumer been involved in this decision? Does the consumer understand the choices?

- *One does not need to earn the right to assistive technology.* Use decision-making models that are based on prerequisites with caution. Most could not ride a bicycle until a bike is acquired on which to learn.

Has the consumer and provider had realistic trial opportunities and other experiences with the assistive technology in question? Have the consumer and provider been careful to not rule out assistive technology without a thorough evaluation of these experiences? Has the support for successful use been provided so that neither the consumer's disability nor the technology is blamed if use of the technology is not successful?

- *Assistive technology should not be a last resort.* Assistive technology can be a facilitator of development and/or an interim solution to a temporary condition. Research indicates that introducing assistive technology does not impede the development of walking or talking when those capacities exist. Waiting until successive failures occur or deferring implementation of assistive technology until all else has been tried may deprive users of their right to experience independent communication, mobility, or other activities or functions.

Can assistive technology provide a means to address a needed function now while the consumer and provider continue to develop natural function or unaided compensatory strategies (if appropriate)?

- *Assistive technology is not a luxury.* Concern because a device is expensive and the possibility that a person is not be able to procure funding for the device does not permit the provider to withhold information regarding its availability. The provider has an ethical and moral responsibility to present the options and to assist the intended user in efforts to obtain the devices and services of choice.

Has the provider advised the intended user of all options, including assistive technology devices and services? Has the provider given guidance in acquisition of the device and/or service, including writing appropriate justifications to third-party funding sources and assisting with appeals (if necessary)?

## Assistive Technology Solutions in Real-Life Contexts

The following stories are presented to highlight the real-life use of assistive technology. Although the vignettes about three people with disabilities do not provide exhaustive information regarding all the assistive technology they use, their stories illustrate the use of high-tech and low-tech, specialized, and generic devices and services. They also illustrate the way assistive technology solutions can be integrated into the lives of individuals with disabilities.

## CASE STUDIES

### CASE 1

M.J. gets up in plenty of time for school. His dad assists him into the shower chair, and he rolls into the roll-in shower. With a typical young teen's increasing attention to hygiene, he is sure to do a good job brushing his teeth with his electric toothbrush, and dad assists him in rinsing with a cutout cup. After 5 minutes of indecision about what to wear, he is dressed and in his power wheelchair. After breakfast, he gets into the van by using a wheelchair lift and is at the middle school within minutes.

Entering the newly ramped building, M.J. takes the elevator to his homeroom. During first period, he uses the computer in the library to prepare his term paper by conducting research via CD-ROM and the Internet. When he needs to take notes from a conventional book, a tabletop easel props it open to the page he needs. To accommodate his wheelchair, the computer is located at an adjustable workstation so that the height can be changed. As he works on his initial draft, M.J. speaks his input, which the DragonDictate software converts to text. In class, he tape-records the teacher's lesson so that he can review the information at home. In addition, M.J.'s friend always makes him an extra copy of his notes. In gym, he uses a personal voice amplification system so that he can be heard above the noise as he referees the volleyball game.

After school, his mom picks him up and takes him for his horseback riding lesson, and soon he is riding high in the saddle, grabbing on to the saddle bar that replaces the conventional horn on the Western saddle. At home, M.J. hurries to the phone, puts on the telephone headset, checks his messages, and spends the next hour talking with his friends. Then it is time for homework.

### CASE 2

J.O. cannot do things as well as she used to—at least that is the way her world would be without her special gadgets. She has discovered the world of microwave oven cooking; therefore she does not have to worry about bending down to put things in the oven or holding hot baking dishes. In addition, as forgetful as she is sometimes, she knows that with the microwave she does not have to worry about starting a fire, which could happen with a kettle boiling on the stove. She loves the special cutting board her son made her; it has a nail that can hold the item she is peeling or cutting. A variety of jar lid poppers and bottle openers and the electric can opener she got for Christmas allow her to open all the ingredients she needs with only her one good hand.

To watch television without disturbing the neighbors, J.O. uses a special listening system with a headset so that it can be as loud as she needs. She bought a remote control with large buttons and loves that her favorite television listings come in large print. Her friend from the senior center told her about a telephone that helps make sounds clearer, and she was able to obtain one through a free program run by the state.

J.O. had her son put up some grab bars in the bathroom, and he was even able to find one in white to match her fixtures instead of ugly chrome. She bought a device at a local electronics store so that she can just turn her lamps on and off by touching the lampshade. When her son takes her to the grocery store, she always uses the courtesy scooter and is thinking about buying a used one.

### CASE 3

At first, D.Z. thought his life was over when he lost most of his vision at age 21 as a result of diabetes. Trained as a social worker, he began to use his network of contacts to discover what might help him keep his job and independence. He contacted a center for independent living, the diabetes support groups in his area, the state vocational rehabilitation agency, and his state's project under the Assistive Technology Act.

After evaluation for assistive technology and training on some of the more high-tech devices, D.Z. can do almost anything he could do before, except drive. He uses a voice-output glucometer and voice-output syringe guide to gauge and prepare his insulin. At home, he keeps up with his correspondence and bills with a voice-output reading machine, although he has found that he prefers tape recordings for books (e.g., books on tape from the Library of Congress "Library for the Blind and Physically Handicapped"). He just recently decided to purchase a new stereo TV and VCR that include a second audio program feature to receive descriptive video, which enable him to continue to enjoy his favorite TV, features, and films.

At the office, D.Z. has worked hard to overcome his initial "technophobia" and now readily uses a computer for reading and writing with a scanner and screen-reading programs. He uses a voice-activated tape recorder for memos and lists and uses special plastic tape to create raised numbers and letters to stick onto anything with keys or a keypad. He has decided not to learn to use Braille, at least for now.

## Conclusion

Technology is a growing influence in all peoples' lives. Rehabilitation professionals, educators, employers, and others who work, learn, and live with people with disabilities have the opportunity to link technology with people who can benefit from it. For assistive technology's potential to be realized, efforts need to be made in the following areas.

The general public must become aware of the scope and benefit of assistive technology. Disability is almost certain to touch all peoples' lives. This can occur through the birth of a child with a disability, an accident that leaves a best friend unable to walk independently, the disease that damages a spouse's sight, or the inevitable losses of function that occur in old age. When people know about assistive technology, they can ask the question, "Is a device or service available that can help perform this task"?

Similarly, people with disabilities need to have an increased awareness about the scope and benefits of assistive technology devices and services. Further, these users of assistive technology need to know what their choices are and where to go for more information. They need to know whom to ask about what using a particular device is really like or about obtaining services from a certain provider. Finally, they need ways to determine whether the devices and/or services are right for their needs.

Users need to be able to share with researchers, manufacturers, service providers, and other people their first-hand knowledge of what works or does not work. People with disabilities need to influence the development and availability of technology, including (1) the use and/or adaptation of technology designed for the convenience and efficiency of the general market, (2) the applications of technology designed for other specialized (nondisability) purposes, (3) adaptation and improvements to existing specialized technology, and (4) the development of new specialized technology.

Once the technology has been identified, resources and mechanisms for obtaining the devices or services must be available. Although the need for resources for acquiring expensive assistive technology (computers, environmental control systems, vehicle modifications, etc.) is obvious, the cost of even inexpensive items can be prohibitive for individuals with fixed or lower incomes. Providers should have pertinent information regarding access to public and private sources (including cash and equipment loans) and they should work in partnership with people with disabilities to make sure that access to needed assistive technology is possible and timely.

The increasing availability of technology has resulted in an increased (and as yet unmet) demand for qualified professionals in every part of the service system. This includes professionals who know enough to ask the initial questions regarding assistive technology as a potential strategy, those who can provide quality assessments, those who can customize devices and adapt environments, those who can teach people the way to use their devices, and those who can develop new technologies.

# References

1. Williams B: Testimony before the House Education and Labor subcommittee on Select Education, Sante Fe, NM, 1991.
2. Public Law 105-394: Assistive Technology Act of 1998.
3. Enders A: *Assistive technology sourcebook,* Washington, DC, 1990, RESNA Press.
4. Public Law 103-218: Technology-related Assistance for Individuals with Disabilities Act Amendments of 1994.
5. National Council on Disability: *Study on the financing of assistive technology devices and services for individuals with disabilities: a report to the president and the congress of the United States,* Washington, DC, 1993, National Council on Disability.
6. Phillips B, Zhao H: Predictors of assistive technology abandonment, *Assistive Technol* 5:36 45, 1993.
7. Blackstone S: Assistive technologies in classrooms, *Augmentative Communication News,* 3:3, 1990.
8. Wright ML, Goldman AS: Assistive technology. In Kurtz LA et al, editors: *Handbook of developmental disabilities: resources for interdisciplinary care,* Gaithersburg, Md, 1996, Aspen.
9. Report of the President's Committee on Employment of People with Disabilities: *Operation people first: toward a national disability policy,* Washington, DC, 1994, President's Committee on Employment of People with Disabilities.
10. Mank D: The underachievement of supported employment: a call for reinventment, *J Disabil Policy Studies* 2:1-24, 1994.
11. Williams B: Developmental disabilities: availability of financial assistance for projects of national significance for fiscal year 1995, *Fed Reg* 60 (117):32056, 1995.
12. National Association of Developmental Disabilities Councils: *The 1990 reports: forging a new era,* Washington, DC, 1990, National Association of Developmental Disabilities.
13. Leslie J: *The employment of persons with severe disabilities: the need for infrastructure.* Pittsburgh employment conference: proceedings of the 1st annual conference, Pittsburgh, 1993, SHOUT Press.
14. Williams MB: The Internet and AAC, *Alternatively Speaking* 3:1-7, 1995.

# Resources

*Assistive Technology Resources for Children*
Assistive Technology Funding & Systems Change Project, United Cerebral Palsy Associations, Washington, DC, and National Assistive Technology Advocacy Project, Neighborhood Legal Services, Inc., Buffalo, NY, 1999. Funding of Assistive Technology: The Public School's Special Education System as a Funding Source: The cutting edge.

*Assistive Technology Resources at School*
Council for Exceptional Children
1920 Association Dr.
Reston, VA 20901
Telephone: (703) 820-4940

Higher Education and Adult Training for People with Disabilities (HEATH), National Clearinghouse on Post-Secondary Education for Individuals with Disabilities
One Dupont Circle NW
Suite 800
Washington, DC 20036
Telephone: (800) 544-3284

*Assistive Technology at Home*
Home Automation: Home Controls for All Abilities, Home Tech, Seaside Education Associates, Inc.
PO Box 6341
Lincoln Center, MA 01773
Telephone: (800) 886-3050 (V), (617) 899-3804 (TT)
E-mail: info@seaside.org
Website: http://www.seaside.org

*Assistive Technology in the Workplace*
Job Accommodation Network (JAN)
809 Allen Hall
West Virginia University
Morgantown, WV 26506
Telephone: (800) 526-7234 (V/TT)

Mid-Atlantic Disability and Business Technical Assistance Center
451 Hungerford Dr.
Sixth Floor
Rockville, MD
Telephone: (800) 949-4232

*Resources about the Internet*
Peterson T, Moss F: *Internet for kids!: a beginner's guide to surfing the net,* 1995, Price Stern Sloan, $8.95 USA.

Cagnon E: *What's on the web,* fall/winter, 1995/1996, Internet Media, $23.95 USA.

ACOLUG: Augmentative Communication On-Line Users Group
(to subscribe, send an e-mail message to listserv@listserv.temple.edu; leave the subject blank. In the message, type "subscribe acolug yourfirstname yourlastname." On seeing the message under the subject "command confirmation request," use the reply function. Leave the same subject and in the body of the message type the word "OK.") For additional assistance, contact or visit the following:
E-mail: kcohen@nimbus.temple.edu
The ACOLUG website: http://nimbus.ocis.temple.edu/~kcohen/acolug.html

*Newsletters and Magazines*
ADVANCE for. . . Merion Publications
650 Park Ave.
Box 61556
King of Prussia, PA 19406-0956
Telephone: (800) 355-1088
E-mail: advance@merion.com

Merion Publications offers a series of ADVANCE magazines, including biweeklies for occupational therapists, physical therapists, speech-language pathologists and audiologists, and directors in rehabilitation. These free publications include features that may relate to assistive technology devices and services, have calendars of training events, and often highlight "new products." Specify the topic of interest to subscribe to (e.g., Advances for Speech-Language Pathologists).

Alternatively Speaking, Augmentative Communication, Inc.
1 Surf Way
Suite 237
Monterey, CA 93940
Telephone: (408) 649-3050
E-mail: sarahblack@aol.com

*Alternatively Speaking,* a quarterly, 8-page publication, is the only independent, consumer-authored publication in the field of AAC. It is written by Michael B. Williams and presents vital issues of concern to AAC users and professionals.

*Augmentative Communication News,* Augmentative Communication, Inc.
1 Surf Way
Suite 237
Monterey, CA 93940
Telephone: (408) 649-3050
E-mail: sarahblack@aol.com

*Augmentative Communication News* is a bimonthly, 8-page news report that covers clinical news, equipment, university and research, consumer, and governmental topics in each issue. It provides a synopsis of what AAC experts around the world are doing and thinking.

Exceptional Parent
120 State St.
Hackensack, NJ 07601

Twelve issues of this magazine, *Exceptional Parent,* are available for about $24. Articles are aimed at families and frequently highlight resources for specific assistive technology devices and services.

Mainstream
PO Box 370598
San Diego, CA 92137-9894

*Mainstream* is a monthly magazine, with 10 issues available for about $24. Each issue typically features a product resource guide to one particular aspect or category of assistive technology. Many articles include first-person stories related to assistive technology and other issues of importance to people with disabilities.

New Mobility
PO Box 15518
North Hollywood, CA 91615-5518

Twelve issues of *New Mobility* are available for approximately $28.00. Features discuss disability lifestyle, culture, and resources, including assistive technology. Articles appear to be focused on the needs and interests of adults with acquired disabilities (especially spinal cord injury).

PALAESTRA
Attention: Circulation Department
PO Box 508
Macomb, IL 61455
Telephone: (309) 833-1902

Four issues of *PALAESTRA,* the forum of sports, physical education, and recreation for people with disabilities, are available for $18.00 per year. This magazine features articles on the challenges and achievements experienced by students and athletes with disabilities and the implications for professionals who work with them.

REHAB Management
21645 St. Paul, MN 55121-0645

*REHAB Management* is a bimonthly glossy magazine that is available at no cost. Although it is "pitched" mostly at rehabilitation professionals rather than consumers, the magazine contains interesting articles related to technology, funding, current trends (e.g., managed care), etc.

*SHHH Journal*
Self-Help for Hard of Hearing People, Inc.
7910 Woodmont Ave.
Suite 1200
Bethesda, MD 20814

Individual membership in Self-Help for Hard of Hearing People, Inc. ($20 per year) provides clinicians with a subscription to the *SHHH Journal* and other membership benefits. This magazine provides information relevant to the needs of individuals with hearing impairments, including assistive technology (hearing aids, text telephones, amplifiers, personal listening devices, etc.).

*Spokes 'n Sports*
Paralyzed Veterans of America
2111 East Highland Ave.
Suite 180
Phoenix, AZ 85016-4202
Telephone: (602) 224-0500
Fax: (602) 224-0507

*Spokes 'n Sports* covers wheelchair competitive sports and recreation, primarily for those with spinal cord injury, spina bifida, amputation, and some congenital disabilities (6 issues for $18.00). Articles about wheelchair sports, recreation, equipment, sports personalities, and related topics are featured.

*Voices*
Hear Our Voices
Unit 301
55 Hanover Circle
Birmingham, AL 35205-1718
Telephone: (205) 930-9025

*Voices* is the newsletter of Hear Our Voices, a nonprofit membership and advocacy organization governed by persons who rely on AAC (membership and subscription cost not available).

*General Resources*
Association of Tech Act Projects
1 West Old State Capitol Plaza
Suite 100
Springfield, IL 62701
Telephone: (217) 522-7985 (V), (217) 522-9966 (TTY)
Fax: (217)-522-8067

National Rehabilitation Information Center (NARIC)
1010 Wayne Avenue
Suite 800
Silver Spring, MD 20910-5633
Telephone: (800) 346-2742

RESNA
1700 N Moore St.
Suite 1540
Arlington, VA 22209-1903
Telephone: (703) 524-6686

# CHAPTER 3

## Human Factors and Environmental Access

*Michael L. Jones*

Human factors play an important role in the design of supportive products and environments. *Human factors* are defined as systematic approaches to improving the fit between the user and the environment. They include indepth knowledge of human functioning in the performance of particular tasks and use of problem-solving strategies to develop environmental conditions that best accommodate performance of these tasks.

Human factors are most often applied to the design of products and environments that enhance the functioning of nondisabled individuals in highly specialized tasks in which user health or safety may be at risk from inappropriate, repeated, or extended use of the product or environment or under extreme environmental conditions. Examples of such products and one such environment include surgical instruments, an ergonomically designed chair used for extended periods of sitting, and the space shuttle environment. Human factors may also be used to enhance the functioning of people with disabilities using *normal* products and environments such as in the design of an automatic teller machine. Human factors can make everyday products and environments more usable by everyone. This concept is called *universal design.*

The concept of universal design is not new. It was first promoted in the early 1980s and was touted as a common-sense idea to help eliminate some of the extra cost and stigma associated with special or assistive products and facilities for people with disabilities. Many of the special features in these products and facilities were found to be helpful to people without disabilities. Because almost everyone experiences some type of disability during a lifetime, whether it is a temporary condition or a natural consequence of aging, making such helpful features attractive and marketable to everyone seems reasonable.

Although few products or environments are truly usable by everyone, certain designs are more usable than others in identifiable ways. Levered door handles, for example, are generally easier for more people to operate than traditional doorknobs; an automatic door opener is usable by anyone able to approach a doorway, making it a more universal solution. Light switches installed lower on the wall are more usable by everyone; a rocker-type switch is easier to use by more people than a toggle-type switch, and a motion detecting sensor that automatically turns lights on when someone enters the room is even more universally usable (Figure 3-1).

Universal design solutions may differ from accessible solutions in two important respects. First, universal design solutions do not segregate users. For example, a separate wheelchair entrance is an accessible solution but not a universal design solution because it means that wheelchair users must take a different route that is often longer and less direct. Second, in making a product or environment more usable by people with disabilities universal design solutions do not become less usable and therefore less desirable by those who are not disabled. For example, requiring everyone to take a longer and less direct route to enter a building is not efficient. Universal design approaches are preferred by all users and thus more widely marketable than existing designs.

This chapter provides an overview of environmental access issues and the role of human factors in achieving more universally usable products and environments. It highlights the growing demand for environmental access and presents important design concepts and principles for creating or modifying environments to enhance accessibility.

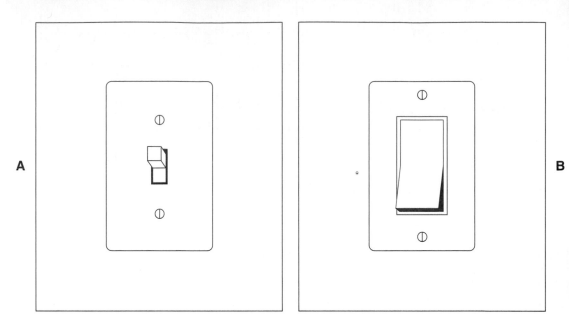

**Fig. 3-1 A,** The standard toggle switch may be difficult to use by people without fine motor control. **B,** The rocker-type switch is a more usable replacement and can be easily operated with a closed fist or an elbow. The motion sensor is more usable still and automatically turns on the lights in a darkened room when someone enters.

## The Growing Market for Accessibility

American society is undergoing sweeping social changes that lend support to a more universal approach to design of products and environments. Among these changes is the growing prevalence of disability in our society. Two major trends account for the rise of disability: decreasing mortality rates for a variety of disabling conditions and aging of the U.S. population.

Medical advances in trauma, intensive care, and neonatal care have resulted in a dramatic increase in the survival rate after severe disability. This means that more infants with congenital disabilities survive, more children and adults who sustain traumatic injury such as brain injury survive, and more older people who experience catastrophic health problems such as a heart attack or stroke survive. Although they survive, they often have severe limitations in functioning. As a result of improved health care, more people with severe disabilities are living longer and more independently.

Because of the increased prevalence of illnesses and injuries with disabling consequences, several facts are known:

- As many as 43 million Americans experience significant limitations in functioning in one way or another.
- Some 7.5 million individuals have disabilities that result in significant impairments in mobility and require the use of an assistive device (e.g., wheelchair, walker) or modifications to the environment. About 1.5 million individuals use wheelchairs on a regular basis.
- An estimated 31 million Americans experience significant limitations in dexterity because of arthritis and other orthopedic disabilities.
- Over 20 million individuals have significant hearing loss.

Disability aside, the largest demographic segment of our population is the baby boomer generation. This market segment includes individuals whose ages range from mid-30s to late 40s. In 10 years, this group will include a significant number of individuals with diminished functioning resulting from age. Baby boomers also comprise the most sophisticated consumer group to date. This group prefers function over form and is a prime market for products and environments that are universal in design.

Moreover, many in this generation are beginning to experience the phenomenon of the *sandwich family.* They are learning the everyday effects of dealing with the dependence of young children and aging parents in a world designed for neither. The baby boomer generation also is on the verge of becoming the aging parent generation. Throughout most of history, only 1 in 10 people lived past 65. Now nearly 80% do. The number of people aged 65 and older has grown from 20.1 million in 1970 to 28.9 million in 1990. This number is expected to grow to 34.9 million in 2000 and 39.3 million in 2010 as the baby boomer generation enters old age. Although this age group accounted for less than 10% of the population in 1970, nearly 1 in every 4 Americans will be aged 65 or over by the year 2020.

Added to this broad and expanding market is the legal mandate for accessibility. Two landmark federal laws now require that most new construction must be built to accommodate diverse user needs. The two laws—the Fair Housing Amendment Act of 1988 and the Americans with Disabilities Act of 1990—make it illegal to design or construct multifamily housing and most commercial properties that do not meet minimum standards of accessibility. Universal design is incorporated into the accessibility requirements of both laws and offers a cost-effective method of achieving desired levels of accessibility without sacrificing aesthetics or marketability.

## Human Factors: Building a Better Interface Between User and Environment

Human factors encompass a broad range of approaches for achieving a better fit between user and environment. Human factors comprise two primary fields of inquiry: anthropometrics and ergonomics. Anthropometrics is concerned with the "measurement of man." This is literally the size and proportions of the human body, including normative standards such as average height and weight of the adult male and ranges of variance in the population such as the range of heights within which 90% of the adult male population falls.

### Anthropometrics

The need for and importance of anthropometric data was first recognized during World War I. Because of Henry Ford's development of the assembly line, mass production played a significant role in this country's efforts to prepare for the war. For the first time, mass production of equipment, supplies, and uniforms was possible. Before this, virtually all clothing was custom-fit, and standard sizes did not exist. Therefore to mass produce uniforms, the military needed data on the standard size of its troops. Body measurements were collected for all military recruits, resulting in the first anthropometric database. These data were then used to establish standard uniform sizes that would accommodate all but the largest and smallest soldiers.

These early data are noteworthy in another respect, as well. Over the years, most anthropometric data have been collected by the military and describe the anthropometric characteristics of young adult men. To this day, design standards reflect this bias. Most consumer products and public environments continue to be designed for the average adult man body size and physical characteristics.

### Ergonomics

Ergonomics is the "study of work" or, more specifically, the analysis of work tasks to identify ways to maximize efficiency and safety. Ergonomics is concerned with three principal elements of work. The first are the workers and their level of skill and effort. Next is the work, the particular task or tasks to be performed, and the level of physical and mental exertion, number of movements or steps, and amount of time required to complete the task. The last element is the workplace, including the space, work surfaces, equipment, tools, and materials needed to complete the task. Using a variety of empirical analysis tools, the objective in ergonomics is to reengineer the work and workplace to reduce or eliminate the worker's physical and mental fatigue.

Ergonomics also has its origin in the industrial revolution. Early time and motion studies were conducted in manufacturing settings to fine-tune assembly tasks and increase productivity. One of the first documented time studies analyzed the time involved in shoveling coal into a steam furnace. The study was used to determine the optimal size of a coal shovel to achieve the highest volume of coal shoveled per hour. Another early ergonomics study used motion analysis to standardize bricklaying. The study found that the average brick mason used up to 18 separate motions to lay a brick. Through careful analysis, the task was reduced to 5 standard motions. As a result, productivity was increased from a highly variable average of 120 bricks per hour to a consistent average of 350 bricks per hour.

Time and motion studies continue to serve as the foundation of extensive human factors methodology for analyzing user-environment fit. Over the years, this methodology has contributed a number of conceptual models to assist in user-environment analyses. For example, the user-machine feedback loop offers a useful conceptual model for analyzing display and control functions in machine and product design. Displays provide the user with important information about the status of operations, and controls allow the user to adjust and control machine operations. Displays may be quickened to facilitate the user's response to important information. For example, most automobiles now include a low-fuel indicator light in addition to a fuel gauge to facilitate the user's response. Controls may be *aided* because the machine helps that part of the control process. Power-assisted brake and steering systems are good examples of aided systems. They do not eliminate but instead assist the user's control of the machine. Principles of display and control design have been established through empirical analysis of normal users. For example, principles of control design specify the location, size, shape, direction of movement, resistance, and reaction time that should be programmed for various types of controls.

Anthropometrics and ergonomics are important to the pursuit of environmental access in at least two aspects. First, the analysis methods and conceptual frameworks derived from these fields are extremely useful for examining user-environment interface issues for people with disabilities. More than nondisabled users, people with disabilities may have significant interface problems, requiring a more careful analysis of user-environment fit. Second, a primary objective in promoting environmental access should be to extend the range of normal anthropometric and ergonomic data beyond the 90th percentile—that is, to include considerations for people with disabilities as part of the design of everyday products and environments.

## Applications of Human Factors to Problems of Environmental Access

Human factors tools and strategies can be useful in promoting environmental access. Several of the following tools are of particular interest and can easily be adapted by rehabilitation professionals attempting to address environmental access issues:

1. The "Enabler" is a useful system for conceptualizing user impairments and corresponding problems the user may encounter when interacting with the environment.
2. The concept of "accessible route" is useful in assessing an environment to identify access and interface problems.
3. Principles of universal design have been proposed as a means of guiding the design process, encouraging creative rather than prescriptive solutions to common accessibility problems.[1] Additional information about their use, including applications to specific access problems in home, work, and play environments, is provided in future chapters.

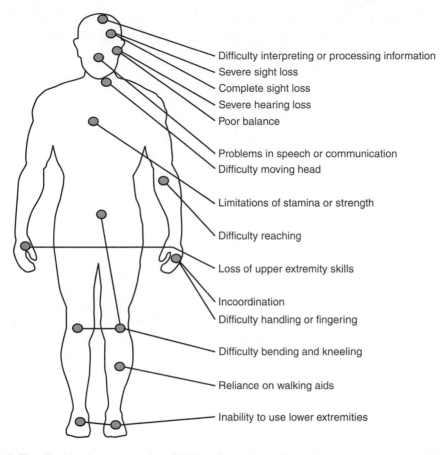

Difficulty interpreting or processing information
Severe sight loss
Complete sight loss
Severe hearing loss
Poor balance

Problems in speech or communication
Difficulty moving head

Limitations of stamina or strength

Difficulty reaching

Loss of upper extremity skills

Incoordination
Difficulty handling or fingering

Difficulty bending and kneeling

Reliance on walking aids

Inability to use lower extremities

**Fig. 3-2** The Enabler represents the abilities of people as they relate to environmental design. It illustrates 15 different functional impairments related to mental functioning, sensory functioning, internal body regulation, and motor functioning. The Enabler diagram is intended as a prompt for the designer to consider the effect of different aspects of the environment on functioning for individuals with different types of impairment. (Modified from Steinfeld et al: *Access to the built environment: a review of literature,* Washington, DC, 1979, US Government Printing Office.)

## The Enabler Model

A variety of taxonomies exist for the classification of impairment and disability. People with disabilities may be classified according to diagnosis (e.g., ICD-9 codes), by age (e.g., developmental disabilities), or by functional impairment (e.g., nonambulatory), but these classifications offer limited insight into a person's particular environmental access requirements. Steinfeld and others[2] developed the Enabler as a visualization of the important functional characteristics of an individual. The Enabler is useful for identifying areas of impaired functioning and their associated design implications (Figure 3-2).

To illustrate use of the Enabler, the functional limitations associated with the normal aging process among persons aged 75 and older should be considered. In the absence of any specific impairment the typical older person might be expected to have the limitations noted in the Enabler illustration in Figure 3-3. The design implications of these common limitations, and features that should be incorporated into an environment frequented by older people, are also included as follows:

1. Reduction in background noise level
2. Warning signals use lower frequency
3. Redundant cueing using visual and auditory media and perhaps touch
4. Supports for maintaining balance and avoiding falls
5. Early warning of emergencies or hazards

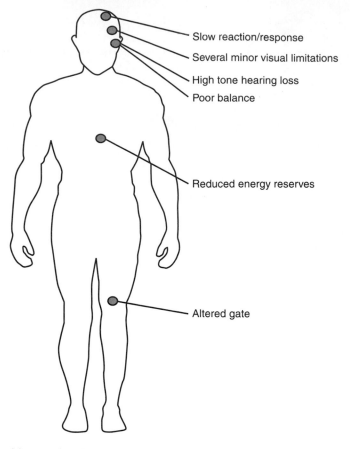

**Fig. 3-3** The Enabler used in the analysis of the environments' effect on functioning of an older person and performance limitations. See text for design implications. (Modified from Steinfeld et al: *Access to the built environment: a review of literature,* Washington, DC, 1979, US Government Printing Office.)

6. Reduction of glare, greater quantities of light, and gradual changes from dark to light and vice versa
7. High visible signage

Because of high-tone hearing loss among older people, auditory signals such as doorbells, phones, and smoke detectors should have lower frequencies. In addition, because of poor balance, reduced energy reserves, alterations in gait, and vision limitations, walkways and especially stairs should be equipped with supports so that a person can maintain balance and avoid falls. Of course, these same design elements would result in safer and more usable environments for all (see Chapter 23 for an example of the Enabler's use to identify and document limitations presented by a particular user).

## Accessible Route

The term *accessible route* has a formal definition in most accessibility standards (e.g., the Americans with Disabilities Act Accessibility Guidelines, or ADAAG), referring to an unobstructed route of travel into and through the public use areas of a facility.[3] The concept of accessible route is useful for assessing an environment and documenting access problems; for example, follow the typical path of travel for users of an environment (Box 3-1). Begin with the initial approach from parking or pedestrian entrances, through public receiving areas, and into common function areas. Note any problems along the way. By taking these actions, the evaluator can envision just how accessible or inaccessible the setting may be for users with disabilities.

BOX **3-1**

*Elements of an Accessible Route*

1. An accessible route should be provided from public transportation stops, accessible parking and passenger loading zones, and public streets or sidewalks to the accessible building entrance. This route should coincide with the route for the general public (i.e., not a back or secondary entrance).
2. An accessible route should connect all accessible buildings and facilities on the same site.
3. An accessible route should have a minimum clear width of 36 inches. If less than 6 feet wide, the route must have (60 x 60 inch) spaces for passing at 200 foot or less intervals.
4. The route should have clear head room of at least 80 inches (6' 8").
5. The route should have a slope no greater than 1/20 (no more than 1 foot in grade change for 20 feet of "run") and a cross-slope no greater than 1/50. Slopes of 1/12 are acceptable but must include handrails if greater than 1/20.
6. The surface of an accessible route should be stable, firm, and slip resistant. If the surface is carpeted, a low-pile, level loop carpeting with minimal padding should be used.
7. If an accessible route has changes in level greater than ½ inch, then a curb ramp, ramp, elevator, or platform lift must be provided. An accessible route does not include stairs, steps, or elevators.
8. Doors along an accessible route should have a minimum of 32 inches clearance in the doorway (this usually requires a 34-inch wide door). Doors should have at least 18 inches of clearance on the latch or strike-side of the door to provide space to open the door from a wheelchair. Doors should have levered handles or automatic openers. When two doors are positioned in sequence with a vestibule in between, a minimum of 48 inches is needed between the *swing* of the doors.

*From The Center for Universal Design, Raleigh, NC, 1996, NC State University.*

In Box 3-1, elements that comprise an accessible route are summarized. These elements are general guidelines for accessibility in public environments. All elements are not relevant for all people with disabilities and do not apply to all environments. An example of the use of this approach is provided in Chapter 26.

## Principles of Universal Design

Universal design solutions are shown in a growing number of products and environments. Additional examples include single lever faucets in the kitchen and bathroom, which can be easily operated by someone with limited gripping ability (e.g., somone with severe arthritis, someone whose hands are full of dishes). The volume control on a public telephone is another good example. It allows people with impaired hearing to use the phone and it makes it easier for everyone to make a call from a noisy airport. A full-length sidelight window at the front door is a good example in housing design. The window allows anyone (a child, adult, or wheelchair user) to see who is at the front door without using the peephole.

Universal design is usually described by using examples and by recognizing good designs that demonstrate the concept. The principles of universal design reflect efforts to create a common language of universal design so that a closer agreement occurs as to what the term means, when it should be applied, and how to accomplish universal design (Box 3-2). Each one has specific guidelines detailing how to implement the principle in design. The principles and related guidelines are intended for use in three ways. The first is to evaluate existing products and environments to determine how universally usable they are. The second is to guide the design of new products and environments that are more universally usable. And finally, the third is to educate designers and consumers about what makes for more usable products and environments.

BOX 3-2

*Principles of Universal Design*

*Principle One: Equitable Use*
The design does not disadvantage or stigmatize any group of users.
*Guidelines*
1a. Provide the same means of use for all users (identical whenever possible, equivalent when not).
1b. Avoid segregation of users.
1c. Provisions for privacy and security should be equally available to all users.

*Principle Two: Flexibility in Use*
The design accommodates a wide range of individual preferences and abilities.
*Guidelines*
2a. Provide choice in methods of use.
2b. Accommodate right-handed or left-handed access and use.
2c. Facilitate the user's accuracy and precision.
2d. Provide adaptability to the user's pace.

*Principle Three: Simple and Intuitive Use*
Use of the design is easy to understand, regardless of the user's experience, knowledge, language skills, or current concentration level.
*Guidelines*
3a. Eliminate unnecessary complexity.
3b. Be consistent with user expectations and intuition.
3c. Accommodate a wide range of literacy and language skills.
3d. Arrange information consistent with its importance.
3e. Provide effective prompting for sequential actions.
3f. Provide timely feedback during and after task completion.

*Principle Four: Perceptible Information*
The design communicates necessary information effectively to the user, regardless of ambient conditions or the user's sensory abilities.
*Guidelines*
4a. Use different modes (e.g., pictorial, verbal, tactile) for redundant presentation of essential information.
4b. Provide adequate contrast between essential information and its surroundings.
4c. Maximize "legibility" of essential information in all sensory modalities.
4d. Differentiate elements in ways that can be described (i.e., make giving instructions or directions easy).
4e. Provide compatibility with a variety of techniques or devices used by people with sensory limitations.

*Principle Five: Tolerance for Error*
The design minimizes hazards and the adverse consequences of accidental or unintended actions.
*Guidelines*
5a. Arrange elements to minimize hazards and errors (most used elements, most accessible; hazardous elements eliminated, isolated, or shielded).
5b. Provide warnings of hazards and errors.
5c. Provide fail-safe features.
5d. Discourage unconscious action in tasks that require vigilance.

*Principle Six: Low Physical Effort*
The design can be used efficiently and comfortably and with minimal fatigue.
*Guidelines*
6a. Allow user to maintain a neutral body position.
6b. Use reasonable operating forces.
6c. Minimize repetitive actions.
6d. Minimize sustained physical effort.

*Principle Seven: Size and Space for Approach and Use*
Appropriate size and space is provided for approach, reach, manipulation, and use regardless of the user's body size, posture, or mobility.
*Guidelines*
7a. Provide a clear line of sight to important elements for any seated or standing user.
7b. Make reach to all components comfortable for any seated or standing user.
7c. Accommodate variations in hand and grip size.
7d. Provide adequate space for the use of assistive devices or personal assistance.

*From The Center for Universal Design, Raleigh, NC, 1996, NC State University.*

## Examples of Universal Design

### Drafting Lamp

The common drafting lamp has one minor design change that makes it much more usable by people who have limited finger dexterity. The manufacturer has modified a small knob at the top of the lamp to include a larger, decorative knob, which is easily operated without the need of a precise finger-thumb grasp (Figure 3-4).

### Bridge and Berm Entrance

Most houses have a few steps up that lead to the main entrance. When wheelchair access is required, usually an unattractive ramp, often constructed of treated lumber, is added to the front of the house. The ramp greatly detracts from the appearance of the home and also stigmatizes the home by signifying that someone who is different lives there. An alternative is the bridge and berm entrance that creates an attractive entrance usable by anyone (Figure 3-5). The entrance is created by berming up the front yard and bridging over to the house. This eliminates any potential drainage problems at the front door and provides an excellent location for landscaping.

### Raised Planter Bed

For the family gardeners, a raised planter bed makes it easy to tend plantings without having to kneel or stoop over (Figure 3-6). The sides of the planter can also be used for seating, which add to the versatility of this design.

### Wet Area Shower

The roll-in or wet area shower is a great example of how universal design can be functional and attractive. The shower has no curb or edge to step or roll over, making it more usable by wheelchair users and those who may have difficulty stepping up and over the curb (Figure 3-7). Instead, the floor slope is sufficient to ensure water drains adequately. The wet area shower is also a convenient location to water large houseplants, or give the dog a bath. The hand-held shower is good for spraying the kids on a hot summer day.

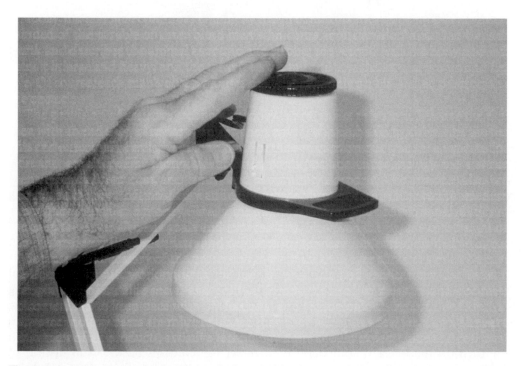

**Fig. 3-4** A drafting lamp that has been designed with a larger switch, making it more operable by persons with limited fine motor control.

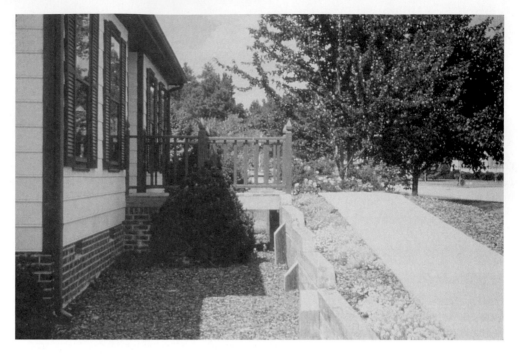

**Fig. 3-5** An earth berm and bridge used to create an accessible entrance to an existing home.

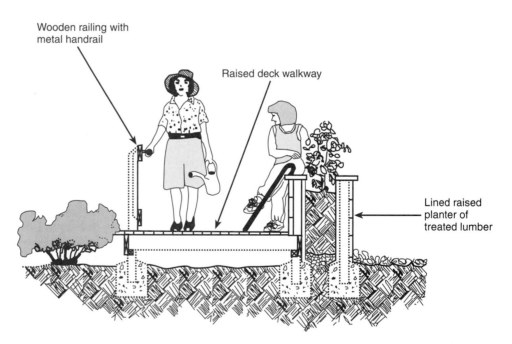

**Fig. 3-6** Raised planter bed makes gardening easier for everyone by eliminating kneeling and bending.

### Offset Tub Controls

The offset controls illustrate that universal design is often no more than thoughtful design (Figure 3-8). By offsetting the standard mixer valve for a tub and shower, turning the water on and off without getting into the tub becomes easier. This is a relief for those who have difficulty bending over or for young children. It positions the controls in a more usable position for wheelchair users as well. Users also will not get soaked when they turn on the water if someone forgot to set the controls back to tub instead of shower.

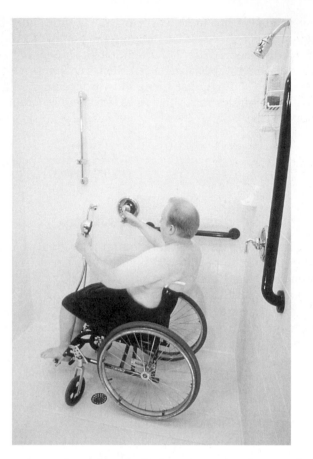

**Fig. 3-7** This wet area shower is equipped with two shower heads, one of which is hand-held and mounted on a slide bar so that the height can be adjusted. Note also the single-lever water controls.

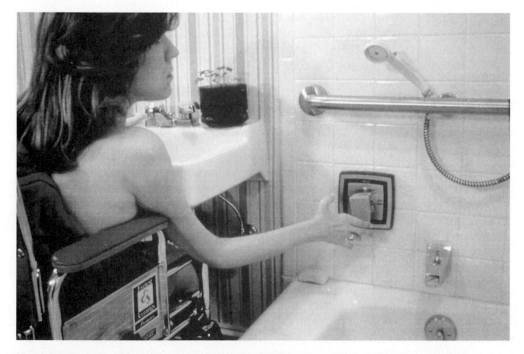

**Fig. 3-8** Offset water control can be easily adjusted from outside of the tub or shower.

Although these principles are intended primarily to guide the design of everyday products and environments, they are also useful in the design of products and environments intended for individualized use. This might include designing a customized workspace, for example. People with specialized needs such as patients who require the design of a rehabilitation clinic also might use them. Most work-site modifications to accommodate people with disabilities make the work environment more user-friendly for everyone (see Chapter 23).

## Additional Considerations in Environmental Access

### Customized Versus Universal Design Solutions

Universal design solutions are intended to be more generally usable and affordable but do not necessarily work for someone with highly specialized needs. For example, the commonly recommended 5 x 5 feet turning area in kitchens and bathrooms may not be sufficient for someone who uses a reclining powered chair. In an individual home, to increase the turning area to a size that is workable would make sense. However, in many public settings such as apartments and hotel rooms the expense of increasing the standard turning area beyond the recommended 5 x 5 feet may be prohibitive.

If the environment is intended primarily for personal rather than public use such as a home or individual work site the space may be customized to meet the individual user's needs. The space may be tailored to the exact anthropometric specifications and ergonomic requirements of the user. But when others such as family members or co-workers also use the space, it should not be so customized that it is not usable or desirable by others. Potential problems with a highly customized environment are that it generally works well only for the intended user, it may involve considerably greater expense to achieve, and it may lose in market value, or at the least it may be difficult to recover the added expense of customization.

Therefore even in cases in which a considerable degree of customization is desired, universal design should be the default design. Those elements that do not need to be customized should adhere to principles of universal design. Universal design may eliminate the need for or the degree of customization required, making the environment more usable and attractive to other users. As a result, creating a usable environment requires less expense and its market value is likely to be retained.

### Integrated Versus Renovated Solutions

*Integrated solutions* refers to accessible elements that are incorporated into the original design of a product or environment. *Renovated solutions* refers to modifications made after production to make the product or environment more usable. The closed captioning circuit included in all new television sets is an integrated solution, whereas the addition of a decoder box to access closed captioning is a renovated solution. In most instances, integrated solutions are preferred over renovated solutions. When accessibility is planned from the beginning and built in, the result is usually more usable and attractive because it is integrated with the overall design. In most cases, integrating accessibility with the original design is also significantly less expensive.

Renovated solutions are inevitable because most of the built environment was created before much thought was given to accessibility. In housing particularly, most new construction remains inaccessible, with steps at the entry. Housing is also an area in which the decision to modify an existing home for accessibility warrants careful consideration. Most older homes are multistory or a ranch-style design. Multistory homes have obvious limitations regarding wheelchair access. Most older ranch-style houses also have small bathrooms. A 5 x 7 feet bathroom was the norm throughout the 1950s and 1960s. Most floor plans with three bedrooms and two bathrooms were designed with the bathrooms adjacent to each other. The only way to create an accessible bathroom within the existing space is to combine the two bathrooms into one larger one. However, because the house now has one bathroom not two, its market value will be negatively effected. The addition of a new bathroom rather than the renovation of two existing ones may be the best choice. Even though the initial cost may be higher, the market value of the home is retained if not increased.

## Structural Versus Nonstructural Solutions

Some access problems may be addressed with the addition of devices or fixtures that do not require extensive effort or expense. For example, the cost of a motion-sensor light switch is about $25.00. A somewhat skilled person can replace the existing light switch with a motion-sensor switch in less than an hour. No clear advantage is associated with structural or nonstructural solutions to the same problem except that many nonstructural features can be installed without professional builder or remodeler assistance.

## Important Outcomes of Environmental Access

Successful efforts to improve environmental access should yield three desirable and easily verifiable outcomes: increased independent functioning, increased choice and control in activities and in the venues where they are performed, and enhanced safety and use for all users. As with most assistive technology interventions, improved environmental access should result in increased independence among users with disabilities and, consequently, reduced need for assistance from others in the completion of everyday activities.

Increased accessibility to home, work, play, and other community environments also means greater choice and control in the selection of activities and the power to decide the settings to pursue these activities. For example, housing that is accessible to people with disabilities can minimize physical and emotional stress, reduce home-care needs and costs, and offer people increased safety and satisfaction in accomplishing daily activities. Accessible housing that is available in all communities allows people with disabilities the same level of freedom as other citizens to pursue educational, employment, and personal goals.

## References

1. Stay MF: Maximizing usability: the principles of universal design, *Assistive Technol* 10 (1): 4-12, 1998.
2. Steinfeld E et al: *Access to the built environment: a review of literature,* Washington, DC, 1979, US Government Printing Office.
3. Americans with Disabilities Act Accessibility Guidelines: Architectural and Transportation Barriers Compliance Board, 36CFR Part 1191: Americans with Disabilities Act Accessibility Guidelines for Buildings and Facilities, *Fed Reg* 56 (1440), 35408-35453, 1991.

CHAPTER 4

# Service Delivery in Assistive Technology

*Jean L. Minkel*

According to Cook and Hussey,[1] assistive technology refers to a broad range of devices and services that are conceived and applied to improve the problems faced by persons with disabilities. In U.S. Public Law 100-407 the Technology-Related Assistance for Individuals with Disabilities Act, an assistive technology device is defined as any item, piece of equipment, or product system, whether acquired commercially off-the-shelf, modified, or customized, that is used to increase or improve functional capabilities of individuals with disabilities. The same public law defines assistive technology service as any service that directly assists an individual with a disability in the selection, acquisition, or use of an assistive technology device.

## Assistive Technology Service Delivery: What Is Involved?

For many people who have not had previous experience or training (e.g., those with disabilities and health care professionals), exploration and application of assistive technology is overwhelming. In the following sections, I will discuss the steps involved,[2] the roles of different players and the settings, or models, in which many of theses service delivery activities occur (Box 4-1).

## Critical Considerations in Assistive Technology Service Provision

### Needs Assessment: Mutually Understood Goals

Acknowledgement of need is the first step in the service delivery process. Initial identification of need may be done by a number of different people: the potential user, advocates, family members, social workers, case managers, or any other team member. Situations may arise when the needs identified by someone other than the potential users are not identified or acknowledged by the users. In such situations, careful consideration should be taken before proceeding with the rest of the process. This is necessary because technology abandonment can result when technology resources are applied and the intended user does not identify or acknowledge the need.

The first step in a technology assessment is the determination of mutually understood goals between the potential assistive technology user and the person or team with whom the consumer is working. The following questions should be asked:

- What does the user want to accomplish as a result of applying technology resources?
- In what environments will these activities take place?
- How will the consumer and the team know whether they are making progress and when the goal has been achieved?

The amount of experience people have with their disabilities has a tremendous effect on their involvement in the assessment process. People who have recently

## BOX 4-1

*Steps in the Service Delivery Process*

> Needs assessment of mutually understood goals
> Assessment of functional capability and environments
> Development of an intervention strategy
> Implementation of intervention
> Determination of outcome

acquired a disability may not have sufficient experience living with the disability to be an active, articulate participant in the process. The team working with this type of client must listen and facilitate involvement by the individual before making any recommendations. Conversely, those persons who have a great deal of experience living with their disabilities may have incredible amounts of insight and information about what works and what does not work in their life context. Again, the team must listen and integrate this insight and information when working with the user to develop an intervention strategy. Quite often careful listening to the potential user can lead directly to an effective solution, thus avoiding extended trials of other unsuccessful options.

### Assessment of Functional Capability and Environments

To facilitate the accomplishment of mutually understood goals an assessment of the user's functional abilities and limitations needs to be completed. A full assessment is completed when a person with a disability is exploring a technology for the first time. On repeat purchases the complete assessment is not always needed unless a change occurs in the user's physical functioning, environment, or desired outcome.

A holistic assessment (e.g., physical, sensory, cognitive, environmental, etc.) often requires the input of many team members. Gathering previous evaluations and direct communication with providers of related services can often provide the framework for this holistic assessment. Depending on the technology application being explored, a need may arise for indepth, specific assessments (e.g., hearing, visual and language testing for augmentative communication applications, postural alignment and skin inspection for seating interventions, and work site assessment and transportation assessment for job accommodation). Although no *one* service provider is expected to safely and competently perform all of these evaluations, recognizing the need for and facilitating the collection of information is the overall responsibility of *each* assistive technology service provider.

In addition to understanding the functional capabilities of the individual, having an understanding of the environment in which the individual wants to accomplish the task is critical. In some cases the environment is specific such as modification of a job site to allow access and operation of a machine or tool. In other cases the environment is variable and changing—using a manual wheelchair at home, on the bus, at work or during leisure activities. An assessment of functional capability without information about the environment in which the tasks are to be performed provides only half the information needed.

### Development of an Intervention Strategy

The technology service provider, working in collaboration with other team members, needs to synthesize the information gathered during the assessment, including the mutually agreed goals, and develop an intervention strategy. The intervention strategy may include trial use of potential technology devices that the individual may want to evaluate. Just as often the solution may be to teach the person a different strategy, using existing resources to accomplish the task. Intervention strategies do not always involve specific device identification. In most instances the solution is a combination of identifying useful technologies, the strategies needed to use a device, and the personal services needed for successful implementation of the technology into the individual's environment.

Bounding each potential solution is the cost associated with implementation. The person with a disability needs to be informed of all the options: those that involve the least out-of-pocket expense, perhaps through the involvement of a third-party payer, and those options that involve the greatest out-of-pocket expense such as those solutions that may not be covered by the third-party payer. Teams need to be certain not to make purchasing decisions for the individual based on their knowledge of what the payer routinely approves or rejects for payment.

Once identified, all the options should be shared with the potential user and all involved team members. Feedback from the person who uses the proposed options forms the foundation of an implementation strategy. The user can then make a purchasing decision and choose which option to pursue first.

Depending on the nature of the intervention, device trials are arranged, training sessions are scheduled, and, if needed, further funding is pursued to cover the cost of the desired intervention. If a device is part of the solution, actual use before purchase is often critical in the decision process. Whenever possible the device trials should be conducted in the environment in which it is used on a regular basis.

## Intervention Implementation

When one strategy is deemed most likely to succeed, a procurement process is initiated. If a specific device is identified as part of the solution, the recommendation should also include any related set up, delivery or training services that need to accompany the device delivery, to ensure optimal use of the device. Next, product specifications are drafted, the type and amount of related services that are needed are identified, and funding is sought. The service delivery models, several of which involve a third-party payer, each have a different approval or authorization process. Regardless of the method, authorization to purchase is a critical step in the process. Once authorizations are received, then products and services are purchased.

Delivery of a device may only be the first step in the implementation phase. Fully integrated use of the device by the individual in a variety of environments may require training for the person with a disability and others functioning in the person's environment. This training may be self-directed for experienced technology users. The new user, however, may need extensive, guided instruction to develop strategies that facilitate maximal functional use of the device.

## Determination of Outcome

Service providers in assistive technology need to actively inquire whether the mutually agreed goals have actually been accomplished. Attainment of the desired outcome may occur well after the delivery of the device and conclusion of training. Determination of goal achievement is much easier when the original goal is expressed in measurable terms. For example, a user may have sought adaptation for a computer to improve efficiency at work. Without a clearer definition of "efficiency at work," the goal would be hard to measure 6 months later. For example, if the original goal is expressed as "able to produce five pages of written text in an hour," as opposed to the current rate of producing one page of text in an hour, then a phone-call inquiry 6 months after delivery can determine if the desired outcome of five pages an hour has been achieved. If the intervention is serving the intended purpose, then the desired outcome or goal has become the actual outcome. If not, careful follow up is needed to identify the factors that led to a different outcome.

## Service Providers as an Expert Source of Information: An Interactive Model

Underlying each of the outlined steps in service provision is the foundation information that the service provider brings to the process regarding available technologies, possible strategies for use, related services, funding, and a network of other service providers with whom to collaborate, if required.

An underlying philosophy of assistive technology service delivery is a team approach, but who the team members are and what roles they play in the assistive technology service delivery process are questionable. All too often in multiprofessional teams, the most important team member, the potential assistive technology user, is left out of the decision-making process. The reasons for this all-too-common flaw in assistive technology service delivery are many. Often, the professionals involved in an assessment have been trained in the traditional practice of an expert model. Therapists, counselors, teachers, and physicians are trained to be the experts and provide their expert advice to those who enlist their services.

Effective assistive technology service delivery, however, requires that the service provider shift from the expert model to an interactive model. As described by Scott,[4] the interactive model recognizes potential assistive technology users as the only team members who possess the intuitive, personal knowledge about their own capabilities, needs, environments, and anticipated expectations from using technology. The other team members have information about potential technology applications, strategies, and supports that may be able to meet these needs and expectations. Only through the interaction between these two parties can an effective solution be identified. The interactive model embodies the philosophy of consumer responsiveness: to be responsive to the consumer's input and participation during an assessment and in all decision making.

## Who Are the Team Members in Assistive Technology Service Provision?

### The Person with a Disability: New or Experienced Assistive Technology User

The primary member of the team is the potential assistive technology user. As noted earlier, establishing whether the person with a disability has acknowledged the need or desire to explore technology is important. Once the need is acknowledged and the individual has used initial solutions, the person matures not only as an assistive technology user but also as an informed team member. For many satisfied assistive technology users, the support of advocates, family and/or caregivers is a critical component to achieving the best functional use of the technology. With support and experience in using the technology in pertinent environments, the user becomes more articulate about capabilities, needs, and expectations. To gain this experience, however, a person with a disability may have often experimented using trial and error or taken a guided journey working with a team of people familiar with technology applications. Although experimentation teaches invaluable lessons and the eventual outcomes are often successful, the toll is high in terms of time and resources spent. The guided tour, while not inexpensive, often smoothes and shortens the learning curve for many potential users. The team members who can provide the guided tour will be described in detail later in this section.

### The Payer: The Person with a Disability or a Third Party?

Another pivotal team member is the payer. If the potential assistive technology user is purchasing the solution using personal resources, then the payer and user are one. If, however, an insurance company, school district, or government agency has been approached to fund the solution, then the payer is a third party. The third-party payer becomes the decision maker regarding the allocation of resources to meet the user's need. The potential assistive technology user is no longer a consumer, in the sense of payer and user. Rather, the potential assistive technology user is now a client trying to access technology through allocation of resources by a particular system. Many different types of third-party payers are involved in assistive technology service delivery. Each is described in more detail in the models of service delivery section.

## The Practitioner: Therapist, Physician, Teacher, or Counselor

Initially, when people have little or no experience with their disability or with particular technology applications, they will seek out or work with professionals who can assist in identifying and articulating their capabilities and needs related to technology applications. These professionals have varied backgrounds that often relate to the setting in which they work and the type of technology being explored. Primarily, they include occupational therapists, physicians, physical therapists, speech pathologists and audiologists, special educators and vocational evaluators, and counselors, just to name a few. In many cases, these professionals have made an additional investment, beyond their professional training, to learn about assistive technology options and when technology applications may enhance an individual's functional independence. In addition to assisting individuals in assessing their capabilities and potential technology solutions, these professionals are often uniquely qualified to assist with training. Mastering a task may involve individualized training on the use of a particular technology or may involve training others in how individuals use the device to complete a task.

## The Supplier

If the needs of the individual can be met through the use of a commercially available device, then the device is often purchased through a supplier. Suppliers have detailed information on available options and specific product specifications. In many areas of assistive technology application, especially when the need requires a complex solution, it is the supplier who is able to translate the generic device features identified by the practitioner and consumer into currently available product options. Many suppliers provide demonstration equipment and make it available before a purchase.

Once the user has selected a specific device, the supplier details the product specifications including cost information to be submitted for funding. After authorization, provided either by the consumer or a third-party payer, the supplier orders, configures, assembles, and adjusts the device to meet the user's needs. In addition, after a purchase the suppliers have the information and expertise on device maintenance and repair.

## The Engineer

When the readily available commercial options do not meet the need, a rehabilitation engineer may be included in the team process. The engineer offers solutions that may be available through a different market, may provide substantial modifications to existing products or designs, or may also fabricate custom solutions that would be suitable in a particular application. The engineer is uniquely qualified to assess the safety considerations associated with any substantial modification or custom fabrication that might be needed as part of the solution.

In many situations, all three service providers work together to provide a user with all the components needed for an optimal solution. In addition to these technology team members, many potential assistive technology users also have teams providing personal care and therapeutic services. Ideally, all those involved meet together, share information, and develop a solution. Time and resource allocations often make this same location, total team assessment impossible. Therefore communication among all team members is critical. Through the effective communication and the combined expertise of all the team members, however, the most effective solution can still be identified.

## Credentialing of Service Providers by the Rehabilitation Engineering and Assistive Technology Society of North America (RESNA)

RESNA has acknowledged the multiple participants in assistive technology service delivery. The association's members spent several years defining and verifying the knowledge base these assistive technology providers need to obtain, in addition to their basic training, to offer safe and effective service to persons with disabilities interested in technology applications. RESNA's credentialing program offers a voluntary, entry-level certification to professionals who demonstrate mastery of the foundation knowledge by taking and passing a written examination. The topic areas that have been identified in the entry–level knowledge–base areas are outlined in Box 4-2.

Any service provider who has experience in direct, hands-on client service and wants to demonstrate competence in this knowledge base may apply to take the written examinations. Currently, two designations are available for candidates who successfully pass the multisection exam. The candidates indicate which designation they are applying for and must pass those sections of the exam. The following is a description of each designation:

- The assistive technology supplier's credential is for the professional primarily involved in the sale and service of commercially available assistive technology devices.
- The assistive technology practitioner credential is for those professionals primarily responsible for identification of the client's functional abilities and limitations and the potential technology applications to meet those needs. If needed, the practitioner is also actively involved in providing individualized instruction on a particular device to meet the user's needs.

The background training of the assistive technology supplier, assistive technology practitioner and rehabilitation engineers, and the specific technology applications with which they are most familiar varies and often depends on the type of service delivery model in which the professional is practicing. Regardless of the model, effective service delivery relies on the professional's understanding of the user's capabilities and needs, the tasks to be accomplished, and the environments in which the tasks are performed. To effectively match a productive solution to the needs and environments, many people must give their input, which emphasizes the need for the team approach.

## BOX **4-2**

*Content Topics in Assistive Technology Service Provider's Knowledge Base*

*Foundation Knowledge*
1. Psychology and sociology
2. Principles of learning and teaching
3. Human anatomy and physiology
4. Kinesiology and biomechanics
5. Disability studies

*Application/Practice Specific Knowledge*
1. Assessment procedures
2. Assistive technology product knowledge
3. Principles of design and product development
4. Integration of person, technology, and the environment

*Profession: Specific Knowledge*
1. Service delivery systems and funding
2. Professional conduct

## Points of Entry: Where Services Are Delivered

Because assistive technology has broad-based applications in the lives of potential users, a variety of payers exist, including the consumer. These payers include medical insurers, individual school districts that are part of state educational systems, and vocational rehabilitation agencies. Potential users may need to access several different payer agencies to meet all their functional needs. Each of these payers has a different fiscal responsibility to the person with a disability and the agency workplace. This results in several different service delivery models from which potential users may receive their device and related services. Four models exist: medical, educational, vocational rehabilitation, and consumer direct.[3]

The first three models, medical, educational and vocational rehabilitation, are examples of service delivery models that involve a third-party payer. Understanding the perspective of the third-party payer provides insight into the service delivery systems that have developed around each payer. Each agency has a different obligation in meeting the needs of a person with a disability. As each of the service delivery models is described, the obligations of that payer, the types of technologies most often procured through that system, and the backgrounds of the service providers are explained (Table 4-1).

In the fourth model, consumer direct, the assistive technology user is the payer. As the payer, the consumer makes decisions about resource allocation. For many consumers, the experience gained from using a particular technology that was first procured through a third-party system provides the background and insights to be an active participant in the consumer-direct model of service delivery.

### Medical Model

Health insurance is the source of private or government funding in the medical model. These insurance programs have the obligation to provide "medically necessary" equipment to a person with a disability. Coverage of assistive technology in this model is dependent on the insurer's interpretation of medical necessity. Regardless of the payer's particular interpretation, approval for coverage and payment always requires physician documentation of medical need.

For the experienced, articulate consumer who is using medical insurance to fund a repeat purchase, the process may be as easy as bringing the necessary paperwork to the

## TABLE 4-1

*Service Delivery Models*

| MODEL ASSISTIVE TECHNOLOGY | USER REFERENCE | SCOPE OF OBLIGATION | SOURCE OF FUNDS | EXAMPLES OF ASSISTIVE TECHNOLOGY PURCHASED |
|---|---|---|---|---|
| Medical | Patient | Medically necessary items: physician's prescription | Medical insurance, policy specific | Durable medical equipment: braces, wheelchairs, communication and hearing aids |
| Educational | Student | Free and appropriate education: documented need in IEP | State and local school budgets | Writing aids, adapted desks and chairs, computer access equipment |
| Vocational rehabilitation | Client | Assistance to enter, remain in, or return to work: documented need in IWRP | Federal and state funds | Driving controls, work-site modifications, adapted machinery |
| Consumer-direct | Consumer | Personal decision | Personal funds | Recreational equipment, environmental control units, vans, computers |

physician for signature, submitting it to the insurance company, and ordering the product when funding has been approved.

For the new or less-experienced technology user the process is often more complex. Many physicians work with other health care professionals when determining the needs and solutions for first-time or inexperienced technology users. The type of health care professional worked with often depends on the type of technology the person needs. These professionals may include audiologists, orthotists and prosthetists, speech and language pathologists, and occupational, physical, respiratory, and recreation therapists. When an individual has multiple needs a social worker or medical case manager may oversee the procurement process to be sure it is coordinated in a timely and cost-effective manner.

Assistive technology devices that are usually covered under medical insurance include hearing aids, artificial limbs, braces, wheelchairs, seat cushions, back supports, and devices that assist in expressive communication (augmentative communication systems). Interpretation of medical necessity is often limited, omitting items such as bathing aids (e.g., tub bench or hand-held shower head) and environmental control devices that are considered convenience items and therefore not routinely included in medical insurance policies.

Each of the following is an example of a medical insurance that may cover medically necessary assistive technology devices:

- Government insurance programs such as Medicaid, Medicare, and the Veteran's Administration
- Private insurance programs, including traditional fee-for-service policies such as Blue Cross/Blue Shield and managed care policies such as Kaiser Permanente

Each government program and private insurance policy has its own assistive technology coverage policy in which assistive technology is often referred to as "durable medical equipment." In addition to a wide variety of coverage policies, a broad difference in procurement procedures also exists. An individual may have multiple insurers, all of which could be approached for funding, often in a particular sequence. Often, the person with a disability or their advocates knows which sources (e.g., Medicare and Medicaid or two private insurance policies—one primary, the other secondary) are available and comprehends the authorization procedure that is required by each source to obtain funding. If the service provider and the person involved are unsure of the funding options or procedures, the supplier, social worker, representative from an area independent living center, or funding specialist from the state Technology Assistance (Tech Act) Program can often help.

## Educational Model

In 1975, the Education for all Handicapped Children Act (PL 94-142) established the right of all children to a free and appropriate education, regardless of their disability. Under the requirements of this law an individual educational plan (IEP) must be written for each child. The IEP outlines the measurable objectives for each child's educational program and then describes the services and supports needed to achieve those objectives. Once agreed on by the parents and the school district personnel, the services and supports must be provided.

For many children, properly supported assistive technology devices allow for significantly increased participation in school. For many students, use of effective assistive devices and strategies allow for participation in a less-restrictive educational environment. Full integration of the students and their technologies require substantial effort and team work of all involved: the students, families, teachers, therapists, and administrators.

In 1991, PL 94-142 was reauthorized and renamed *the Individuals with Disabilities Education Act (IDEA)*. This act includes the assistive technology definitions in the Tech Act legislation, PL 100-407. IDEA mandates that if assistive technology is instrumental to the child's education, then the local school district is responsible for providing those devices and related services that directly relate to the child's educational program. For children who need assistive technology as part of their educational program the devices and related services must be part of the IEP. Once devices and services become part of the IEP, the local district becomes the third-party payer.

The team members involved in the educational model include the student, parents or advocates, the classroom teacher, related services personnel, and the school district administrators. Depending on the child's needs, related services personnel may include a classroom aide, school nurse, occupational therapist, physical therapist, and/or speech and language pathologist. The classroom teacher may have a general education background or specialty training in special education. In a given school district, several of these team members may have developed expertise in assistive technology applications in an educational setting. In other school districts, none of the team members may have this expertise. Because of the different levels and varieties of expertise available, the mechanisms for technology assessments are often quite different among states and districts.

Ease of availability of assistive technology through the school district is often related to the availability of funds in that district. A technology evaluation may be available within the school or district, if the expertise is locally available. An evaluation, outside of any educational or district setting, may be also requested. Results of the evaluation and the recommendations regarding particular devices and related services need to be written into the IEP. The parents and the school team, including the school and district administrators, must agree to the IEP. This process is often time consuming and frequently needs to be initiated at least 1 year before the anticipated need in the classroom.

Many districts have technology resource centers available to the teachers and families within that district, and many schools have technology resource rooms. The special education district director can provide information about the resource structure and availability within a particular district. In addition, the families of other children with disabilities who are using assistive technology in the school or district are invaluable sources of information.

The technologies procured through the educational model must have an effect on the child's educational needs. Several examples of services and devices include the following:

- Adaptations made to pens and pencils
- In-class occupational therapy services to assist the child in developing fine motor skills for writing, including penmanship and number formation
- Services of a speech and language pathologist and a classroom teacher to integrate the use of a laptop computer for all classroom activities for a nonverbal child
- Sign interpreter for a hearing-impaired student or a Braille writer and screen reader for a child with visual impairments

As noted earlier, the most functional outcome for any child is the full, integrated use of any technology in classroom activities that occur each day. To achieve this goal, significant technology training must be available for the individual technology user, the classroom teachers, the family, and the related service personnel working with the child. Especially in the educational setting, procurement and delivery of a device is not the end of the process but very often just the beginning.

## *Vocational Model*

Just as the IDEA legislation mentioned earlier provides the framework to meet the educational needs of children with disabilities, The Rehabilitation Act of 1973 provides the foundation to meet the vocational needs of disabled workers. This act was reauthorized in 1992 with specific mention of rehabilitation and assistive technologies. Each state has a vocational rehabilitation agency to administer programs to assist individuals with disabilities to enter, remain in, or return to employment. Employment may be competitive, supported, or sheltered, which offers wide-ranging employment opportunities to a large number of people with disabilities.

An individualized written rehabilitation work plan (IWRP) must be written for each eligible person with a disability as part of the vocational planning process. In this system the individual meets with a rehabilitation counselor to formulate the work plan. The counselor develops the plan that assists the person with a disability in securing employment. An assistive technology evaluation may need to be part of this development process. If the person's ability to obtain or sustain a job would be enhanced through the use of an assistive technology device, then the device and the related services become part of the IWRP and are funded by the state agency.

Devices most commonly associated with vocational funding include modifications to job sites, including adaptations for computer access, driver controls for vans or automobiles, assisted listening devices, and lifts or ramps to allow access to work and transportation. Job accommodations may involve custom and specific modifications for a particular worker such as handle adaptations, which allow operation of a machine with an upper-extremity prosthesis, or a more generalized accommodation such as an automatic door, which every employee uses during the day.

Vocational rehabilitation agencies are accustomed to cost sharing. Often the IWRP outlines a plan that involves several payers. As an example, a powered wheelchair might be funded through medical insurance, a van might be purchased with personal funds, and adaptations to the van, including driver controls and a lift, might be funded by the vocational rehabilitation agency so that the person can get to work independently. The vocational rehabilitation agency would also fund supportive services such as driver's training so that a driver's license could be obtained.

In the vocational model the counselor or the person and the person's advocates may initiate assistive technology services. The awareness of technology options and availability of services may vary widely among states and even offices within a state agency. In addition to the rehabilitation counselor and the vocational rehabilitation evaluator, occupational therapists and rehabilitation engineers may also perform work-site assessments. As part of the IWRP, many other related services may be needed, including physical, occupational, or speech therapy. For cases in which skill acquisition is needed, vocational rehabilitation agencies even fund the job training or advanced education (beyond secondary school) that the person with a disability may need to qualify for a particular job.

For a person with a disability, employment can be a complex issue. This is especially true when loss or decrease of health benefits may be a consequence of securing a job and having increased income. For those persons motivated to enter or return to the work force, however, accessing the vocational rehabilitation agency can facilitate the removal of barriers and make full employment achievable.

For many persons with disabilities the first step toward personal and economic independence is the opportunity to live independently. Independent living centers (ILCs) are available in each state to assist persons with disabilities to live in independent environments. Each of these centers is directed and operated by people with disabilities. The ILCs offer peer assistance with many issues, including personal assistance services, recycled or resale of equipment, and accessible housing locations. ILCs may be community-based organizations or may be closely associated with a state's vocational rehabilitation agency. In most instances the ILC does not provide the funding directly for technology services or devices, rather its staff partners with a potential user in accessing the service delivery model most appropriate to meet the individual's need. Because the ILC is directed and operated by persons with disabilities, each center offers tremendous grass roots information and a network of experienced consumers.

## Consumer-Direct Model

When the assistive technology user is an experienced consumer, perhaps a repeat buyer of a particular type of technology, and is using personal resources to purchase a device, the delivery of services is similar to any other commercial transaction. The user may purchase the device from a catalogue or a retail store or directly from the manufacturer. The consumer already knows which device and features to buy because of personal experience. A repeat purchase indicates that the user has been sufficiently satisfied with the functioning of the particular device to purchase another one. The consumer, as the payer, is able to evaluate the usefulness of the technology and the cost of the device and then makes an independent purchasing decision.

In making their own purchasing decisions, consumers need to determine the availability of technical support in their personal networks. The consumer or someone in the immediate environment who is technically capable and physically able can perform all needed maintenance and repair. Such skills and abilities may potentially save a significant amount of money. If, however, a consumer needs to rely on outside resources for maintenance and repair services, the availability of these services may be related to the method of purchase. Although items available through a mail-order service are less expensive, they do not have the same set up, maintenance, and repair services that a supplier or retail store has.

For those consumers who have limited incomes and receive government disability benefits the Social Security Administration (SSA) manages a program called the *Plan for Achieving Self-Sufficiency (PASS)*. This program allows a person with a disability to develop a plan for saving money to be used to purchase equipment or services that allows the individual to achieve a vocational goal. The plan details the amount of money needed and a timetable during which the funds are saved. During this time the SSA does not count the saved funds as income in determining monthly benefits. The individual can then use the designated funds to purchase items not routinely covered by other agencies, but which are necessary for the individual to gain employment. Such a program allows people to participate in the consumer-direct model, even when they are not *technically* spending their own funds.

## Summary

The range of options in assistive technology devices, services, and payers leads to multiple points of entry into the service delivery system. Several models of service delivery have been described, including the medical, educational, vocational rehabilitation, and consumer-direct models. For those persons with disabilities who are accessing the service delivery system for the first time, relying on available credentialed professionals (assistive technology suppliers or assistive technology practitioners) may ease the confusion of initial entry. Each credentialed professional is able to guide an individual to the most appropriate service delivery program and team. Regardless of the model, each person with a disability who is interested in exploring technology is a valued team member and is actively involved in the assessment and decision-making phases of the process. Technology improvements and continued growth in the field of assistive technology is completely dependent on open communication among all team members within and across service delivery models.

## References

1. Cook A, Hussey S: *Assistive technologies: principles and practice,* St Louis, 1995, Mosby.
2. RESNA: *Guidelines for basic knowledge and skill for assistive technology service provision,* Arlington, Va, April 1996, RESNA.
3. Warren CG, Norgaard N: *Assurance of quality in assistive technology service delivery grant national institute on disability-related research,* ref # 133A30038-95, Arlington, Va, 1993, RESNA.
4. Scott R: *Legal aspects of documenting patient care,* p 127, Gaithersburg, Md, 1994, Aspen.

# CHAPTER 5

## Outcomes and Performance Monitoring

*Frank DeRuyter*

People have long recognized the correlation between the delivery of goods and services and the resulting outcomes. Many examples throughout the past century have existed in which the manufacturing and service delivery sectors have strongly promoted the use of various objective measures to enhance the delivery of goods and services. Over the past decade the increasing importance that society has placed on accountability and personal responsibility has led to an even greater emphasis being required in people monitoring service delivery practices, including a close examination of the relating outcomes. This emphasis has placed new challenges on the assistive technology service delivery sector because evaluating the services is more difficult than examining the goods. Just as persons cannot "kick the tires" before providing services, persons "returning services" to complaint departments is equally difficult. Various stakeholders within the assistive technology community have begun to realize the validity of this statement, not to mention the difficulties in developing performance monitoring and accountability systems.

## Overview

For the current generation, the demand for assistive technology services has grown at a rapid pace, despite costs for assistive technology being a significant and frequently a lifelong expense. In the United States during the past decade the clinical service delivery sector has observed several significant events that have demanded performance monitoring. The more significant events of the decade have included the following:

1. Public policy realignment from a social-ethical agenda in which consumers had access to goods and services irrespective of cost toward an economic agenda in which the access to goods and services is gradually becoming rationed through a pricing paradigm
2. The reversal of a significant national budget deficit
3. Dramatic changes to the global economy
4. An explosion within the information technology field that has led to the initiation of dynamic service delivery, collaborative, and e-commerce environments
5. The inclusion of universal design features in everyday technologies

As a result, the assistive technology community is trying to determine whether it can deliver its current level of goods and services in the future and whether the current method of delivering those goods and services is the most efficient and effective.

All stakeholders within the assistive technology community must constantly strive to identify alternative and more efficient ways of providing goods and services and continue developing performance-monitoring systems to make a higher degree of accountability obvious. Providers should be able to exhibit positive outcomes of high value at a reasonable price and must accept whether the expenses associated with assistive technology justify the benefits gained. Accountability today reduces the denial of goods and services tomorrow.

## Quality and Accountability

### *The Mandate*

The declaration for quality and accountability is not a recent phenomenon. Quality is subjective and is therefore a perception. However, providers should recognize that perceptions form expectations that become realities. Providers of goods and services must measure and manage those perceptions to demonstrate accountability.

During the past century the manufacturing sector has suggested numerous objective measures to improve the delivery of various products. Clinicians most widely credit Florence Nightingale with incorporating the first scientific approach to evaluating quality. Only in the past 3 decades, however, have providers placed a greater significance on accountability and performance monitoring as they relate to clinical activities. During the monitoring, they have focused on measuring the quality of care they have provided, although recently they have shifted their emphasis toward measuring functional and cost outcomes and quality of life. Ironically, the assistive technology community exhibited reluctance toward the quality and accountability mandate until recently, which is surprising because several assistive technology stakeholders (i.e., manufacturing and providers) derive from sectors that have embraced performance monitoring for many years.

Activities that began in the late 1960s have controlled much of the present day quality and accountability directive. Health care and education adopted these initial quality measurement efforts that were retrospective use plans. These activities led to the development of professional standards review organizations in the 1970s, which attempted to evaluate the quality of service provided. These efforts rapidly led to the development of peer review organizations and eventually quality assurance programming designed to monitor the quality of services they provided. However, they typically only focused on chart audits and client satisfaction surveys designed to ascertain people's complaints and/or problems. Clinical service providers articulated great concern during this period because they alleged they were being asked to participate in a process that in reality could never be assured. Despite the quality decrees of the 1970s and 1980s, providers had few compelling reasons to be accountable or to measure and demonstrate quality. Consequently, performance monitoring was typically ignored because few incentives existed to account for "doing the right thing" or examining the effectiveness of the clinical services that providers delivered. As a result, quality was acclaimed as an idealistic goal that was too difficult to measure or define; thus accountability remained an esoteric concept.

Around 1986, the attitude toward quality and accountability began to change. Many service sectors witnessed economic difficulties associated with the national deficit spending crisis. The result was a period of fewer resources within the healthcare, education, and manufacturing sectors. As the policy changes and budget cuts began to affect these sectors, quality was severely affected. However, the relaxed attitudes toward quality during the 1970s and 1980s meant that only minimal, often anecdotal, data existed to support this debate. Consequently, the incentives to survive overshadowed doing the right thing. The result to the clinical sector was devastating for consumers and providers, evidenced through widespread organizational reengineering, denied or limited access to services, poorer quality, and in some instances the outright elimination of specific services.

By the late 1980s, consumers realized the effect of what was occurring. The result was a major public outcry, marking another period of major change. For clinical service providers the change was often referred to as a *paradigm shift*. Providers therefore had many specific new requirements, including program monitoring. For the first time, they not only had to monitor their program activities but also accountability of specific clinical providers. This requirement was eventually referred to as *quality assessment and improvement*. More recently, this has been referred to as *performance monitoring*. Today, the clinical service delivery sector has to continually manage and evaluate the care it provides to minimize the associated costs and to maximize the desired outcomes. Furthermore, clinical service provider agencies and facilities must now include providers *and* consumers as active participants throughout the entire evaluation, training, and education process.

As providers of goods and services, the assistive technology community must be included in the measuring and managing of perceptions to demonstrate accountability. All stakeholders must accept accountability in all aspects of delivery of assistive technology goods and services.

## The Mandate within Assistive Technology

Accountability and performance monitoring within the assistive technology community should provide qualitative and quantitative data that evaluates the comprehensiveness, effectiveness, and efficacy of the goods and services they provide. This information should specifically ascertain the value and best practices of practitioners, services, products, and programs. The evaluation process must at least manage the outcome. Specifically, it must measure and establish a baseline of what works, identify how well and for whom it works, and determine at what level of economic efficiency it works. The process whereby the assistive technology community selects data to answer these questions requires them to gather information from several performance monitoring dimensions. This process, which is commonly referred to as *outcomes management,* may include any number of dimensions. In the clinical service delivery sector, dimensions they frequently use may include clinical status and results, functional status, quality of life, satisfaction, and cost.[1]

The assistive technology community frequently conducts accountability, performance monitoring, and outcomes management within a framework whereby they correlate data with specific processes or systems that they may modify. This management enhances the effectiveness and efficiency of service delivery and ultimately improves the outcome. During the past decade, this process has been referred to as *continuous quality improvement (CQI)* and *total quality management (TQM).* Irrespective of the terminology, the assistive technology community measuring performance and outcomes provides the greatest indication that process or system changes are improving quality levels. During the past several years, numerous clinical service delivery environments have clearly demonstrated that these initiatives have actually improved patient and client outcomes and have decreased the variations in clinical practice. Despite the conventional wisdom that better quality costs more, good care usually costs less than poor care over time. Several leading practitioners claim that the best way for providers to reduce costs is to improve quality.

The assistive technology community did not fully participate in performance monitoring and accountability for several years. People have debated whether this has been an asset or a liability to the assistive technology community. Irrespective of the merits of the arguments, some specific aspects of the scope of assistive technology service delivery practice have had a profound influence over the ability to effectively participate in the performance monitoring and accountability agenda or agree on the need for quality. By not having adequately developed performance-monitoring systems, people raised serious questions regarding the effectiveness and efficiency of the assistive technology service delivery system and the efficacy of the provision of these services.

Many within the assistive technology community simply assumed that they could derive accountability and improved outcomes through better technologic solutions. As a result, they sought technologic solutions for improved outcomes without any corresponding data to support the assumption. This view is rather myopic because users are likely to abandon almost one third of all devices,[2] and the prevalence of device disuse ranges from 8% to 75% for particular devices.[3] Although abandonment or disuse may not be a genuine indicator of user discontent and because the community looks forward to high-tech solutions moderating, they are renewing an emphasis on performance monitoring that examines the validity and benefits of the technologic solutions. During the past few years, numerous conference presentations and several publications have addressed performance monitoring as it relates to assistive technology. Although a paucity of information exists, the assistive technology community has not entirely been void of performance monitoring activities.

At a system level, several articles have addressed the need for the assistive technology community to establish accountability, including areas that are service specific (access, augmentative and alternative communication [AAC], seating/positioning and mobility, etc.), institutional specific (pediatric rehabilitation), organizational specific (RESNA), and agency specific (NIDRR).[4-14] All of these efforts, however, began after a legislated mandate occurred to provide services and equipment. Consequently, the assistive technology service delivery community has been "in the position of having to deal with the cart being before the horse."[14]

At a person-served level, people within the assistive technology community have written a number of small-sample study reports or single-case study reports, including the following:

- A follow-up survey of prototype vocational aids for the blind[15]
- A follow-up survey of various devices used 16 weeks after device delivery[16]
- A retrospective study of client satisfaction with device function and comfort 5 years after delivery[17]
- A telephone survey of device use 2 weeks after delivery[18]
- A study of device use and quality of life[19]
- A follow-up study on device use in rural areas[20]
- A study on the differences between high-tech users and nonusers[21]
- A national survey on technology abandonment[22]
- A study of post-discharge device use in relation to functional status[23]

The greatest shortcoming of most of these reports is that they have consisted of retrospective reviews rather than prospective studies. As a result, these informative studies have provided little insight into the way for providers to change the manner in which they deliver services or they way to improve the quality of services.

To date, little long-term prospective studies have occurred. These long-term, prospective, performance-monitoring studies affect positive changes in the delivery of assistive technology clinical services. The following studies have focused on various aspects of performance monitoring and are important to the assistive technology community in that they have influenced and changed the way that they provide services:

- The use of augmentative and alternative communication systems over a 1-year period by 50 individuals who were nonspeaking as the result of traumatic brain injury and stroke[24-25]
- User feedback as it related to assistive technology user satisfaction and device performance across five different service delivery centers[26]
- Post-discharge device use of 47 individuals in relation to functional status that documented perception discrepancies between therapists and consumers regarding utility, aesthetic aspects, and strategies to maximize appropriate device use[23]
- A study that followed over 100 children and adolescents for a 2-year period, examining use and appropriateness and underlying and contributing elements that ultimately influenced the outcomes[27]

Finally, at the organizational level, the assistive technology community has witnessed several broad-based efforts to address the quality mandate. The first was the 1994 amended reauthorization of the State Tech Act legislation (PL 103-218), which was subsequently followed by the 1999 Assistive Technology Act legislation. This enabling legislation required that recipients of these discretionary grants conduct annual assessments of their program initiatives. The American Medical Association developed *Guidelines for the Use of Assistive Technology: Evaluation Referral Prescription* in 1994, which was a major milestone for validating the provision of assistive technology services in the healthcare arena. These guidelines eventually led to the inclusion of assistive technology services in the standards of the Commission on Accreditation of Rehabilitation Facilities (CARF). CARF, a major healthcare accreditation organization, uses customer-focused standards to help organizations measure and improve the quality, value, and optimum outcomes of persons they help.

Other initiatives at the local, statewide, and professional organizational levels have begun to address the need for accountability and performance monitoring. The result has been an emergence of stakeholders within the assistive technology community being held to a new level of accountability and performance monitoring. Despite all of these efforts, however, no single measure or system exists that clearly satisfies all objectives and dimensions of the mandates.[7]

## Outcomes and Performance Monitoring in Assistive Technology

For some time, many providers within the assistive technology community worked from the assumption that better outcomes were derived simply through improved technologic solutions such as smaller, newer, faster, more portable, and more sophisticated systems. Consequently, they sought technologic solutions for improving outcomes without data to support the assumption. However, many stakeholders typically provide assistive technology services using a multidisciplinary service delivery model. These stakeholders include a wide range of individuals who may come from an extremely diverse group of service delivery environments, such as medical clinic, healthcare, educational, academic, or vocational settings, manufacturer and vendor showrooms, independent living centers, research labs, personal homes, and private practices. Furthermore, the array of stakeholders involved is as diverse as the service delivery settings. Stakeholders typically include the consumer (primary and secondary), occupational and physical therapists, speech pathologists, rehabilitation engineers, manufacturers, vendors, payers, researchers, policy makers, and numerous others.

Because the multidisciplinary service delivery model that specialists use is complex and the array of stakeholders involved in delivering the services is vast, the assistive technology service delivery model is therefore complicated. To be accountable, the service delivery system and its various stakeholders must respond to several performance monitoring dimensions (clinical status and results, functional status, quality of life, satisfaction, and cost) each having variant significance to each of the different stakeholders, agencies, and sectors. Although all stakeholders seek a successful outcome, not all of them want the same outcome. What may be a successful outcome to one stakeholder group may be an ambivalent outcome to another stakeholder group.

Deciding on which outcomes to measure and which tools or instruments to use is probably the most problematic aspect of performance monitoring within the field of assistive technology. As the field continues to emerge, a hierarchy in terms of complexity of outcomes becomes apparent.[28] Although several general-purpose instruments exist in the field of rehabilitation such as the Functional Independence Measure (FIM), the Patient Evaluation Conference System (PECS), and the Level of Rehabilitation Scale (LORS), these are limited in value to the field of assistive technology because they were not developed with assistive devices in mind.

More recently, the emergence and enhancement of the following tools has occurred. Two instruments that report to examine aspects of quality of life or more accurately measures of psychologic well being include the Psychological Impact of Assistive Devices Scale (PIAD)[29] and the Matching Persons and Technology (MPT).[30] A user-centered instrument designed to assess satisfaction is the Quebec User Evaluation of Satisfaction with Assistive Technology (QUEST).[31] An instrument that assesses cost-effective and cost-utility methods to determine the provision of assistive technologies is known as the *Cost Effective Rehabilitation Technology through Appropriate Indicators (CERTAIN)* project.[32] Each of these instruments is promising and relevant with potential pitfalls as they create new directions in outcomes and performance monitoring in assistive technology.

## What Lies Ahead

A fundamental truth in the history of the development of assistive technology, its scope of practice, and the makeup of its community is an appreciation of the diversity of the components and entities of this service delivery sector. Confounding this diversity is the premise that within the assistive technology arena an integration of the components and entities must occur to be successful. Although this assumption is debatable, little objective assessment of the assumption has occurred, and numerous anecdotal reports appear to support the validity of the premise. As a result, the practice of assistive technology has evolved into a complicated service delivery model that requires diligence in managing its outcomes and monitoring performance.

Today performance monitoring and accountability within assistive technology has undoubtedly become the norm. The mandate is more than a fad. Consumer pressure within the disability community has motivated the performance monitoring and accountability agenda. Although practitioners used to be able to control the clinical service delivery and payments systems for many years, policymakers, payers, and consumers are managing today's systems.

Two obvious aspects as they relate to performance monitoring are in the future. A further delineation and clarification of the roles of the assistive technology community stakeholders will occur. Improved methodologies and strategies for reporting performance monitoring and outcomes will also occur.

In terms of delineating the role of the stakeholder, many believe that only the individual in need of clinical services is the customer and consumer of assistive technology goods and services. This myopic view warrants reconsideration, as all stakeholders involved in assistive technology are consumers. The importance of this distinction is what impels the future of outcomes and performance monitoring. The recipients of a service typically have little interest in the issues that concern or relate to the providers of the service. As such, performance is largely measured intuitively.

Conversely, those who deliver the service are more concerned about the qualitative and quantitative aspects of what they delivered. Although performance monitoring and accountability are important to all stakeholders, their significance depend on the role of the stakeholder. However, in the field of assistive technology, stakeholders are frequently a consumer and a provider of services. To illustrate, a clinician interfaces with a client while conducting a training session and concurrently interfaces with a manufacturer and vendor who are providing a specific device for the clinician to use. The clinician as a stakeholder suddenly is confronted with monitoring performance in capacities that are diametrically opposed to each other. Therefore in the future, the roles of the various stakeholders need further clarification and delineation to define capacities that require monitoring and accountability. This ultimately enhances the quality of service the providers offer as they develop new outcomes and performance monitoring ideas in assistive technology.

Despite the rising popularity with providers ranking lists and quality report cards to improve methodologies and strategies for reporting performance monitoring and outcomes, only a minimal or marginal effect on consumer choice appears to occur.[33] Characteristics such as program prestige and size play a greater role in consumer choice. Obviously neither of these characteristics accurately predict quality of care or outcome. However, improved quality measures and the potential use of the Internet are promising in the production of better-leveraged consumer reports for empowering consumer choice and keeping performance monitoring concerns foremost among providers.

Consumers continue to become more educated and demand information, which encourage clinical service delivery sector not only to define quality and outcomes but also to describe them in performance terms. Although manufacturing has embraced this widely for many years, the assistive technology community will continue to accept it over the next few years. Accountability, performance monitoring, and the evaluation of outcomes is the expected norm in assistive technology. Probably the most difficult challenge for the assistive technology community is going to be assessing and answering whether what it does is indeed the right thing to do and whether they did it efficiently. As the field moves further into delivering services through technologies developed in the area of telemedicine and delivering goods through e-business, society will have to determine whether the assistive technology community provided services responsibly. According to Tom Peters, "Each day, each product or service is getting relatively better or relatively worse, but it never stands still."

# References

1. DeRuyter F: The importance of outcome measures for assistive technology service delivery systems, *Technol Disabil* 6:89-104, 1997.
2. Phillips B: Technology abandonment, *RESNA News* 4:1-4, 1992.
3. Scherer MJ: Assistive device utilization and quality-of-life in adults with spinal cord injuries or cerebral palsy, *J Appl Rehab Counsel* 19:21-30, 1988.
4. DeRuyter F: *The importance of outcomes and cost benefit analysis in AAC,* Augmentative and Alternative Communication Intervention Consensus Validation Conference Resource Papers, Washington, DC, 1992a, NIDRR.
5. DeRuyter F: *Evaluating outcomes in AAC service delivery programs,* ISAAC Research Symposium Proceedings, McKee City, NJ, 1992b, CTA Inc.
6. DeRuyter F: Evaluating outcomes in assistive technology: do we understand the commitment, *Assistive Technol* 7:3-16, 1995.
7. Fuhrer MJ: *Assistive technology outcomes research: impressions of an interested newcomer,* Keynote presentation at the International Conference on Outcome Assessment in Assistive Technology, Oslo, Norway, 1999.
8. Jutai J et al: Outcomes measurement of assistive technologies: an institutional case study, *Assistive Technol* 8:110-120, 1996.
9. Jutai J: Quality of life impact of assistive technology, *Rehab Engineer* 14 (1):2-7, 1999.
10. NIDRR RESNA: *Technical assistance ad hoc working group on performance guidelines,* Arlington, Va, 1994.
11. Smith RO: The science of occupational therapy assessment, *Occup Ther J Res* 12:3-15, 1992.
12. Smith RO: Measuring the outcomes of assistive technology: challenge and innovation, *Assistive Technol* 8:71-81, 1996.
13. Warren CG: Criteria for and outcomes of assistive technology interventions, *RESNA News* 4:6-7, 1992.
14. Warren CG: Cost effectiveness and efficiency in assistive technology service delivery, *Assistive Technol* 5:61-65, 1993.
15. Brabyn LA: *A follow-up survey of prototype vocational aids for the blind,* San Francisco, 1981, Smith Kettlewell Institute for Visual Services.
16. Caudrey DJ, Seeger BR: Rehabilitation engineering service evaluation: a follow-up survey of device effectiveness and patient acceptance, *Rehab Lit* 44:80-84, 1983.
17. Kohn JG et al: Provision of assistive equipment for handicapped persons, *Arch Phys Med Rehab* 64:378-381, 1983.
18. McGrath PJ et al: Assistive devices: utilization by children, *Arch Phys Med Rehab* 66:430-432, 1985.
19. Scherer MJ: Assistive device utilization and quality-of-life in adults with spinal cord injuries or cerebral palsy, *J Appl Rehab Counsel* 19:21-30, 1988.
20. Willkomm T: *The application of rural rehabilitation technologies, a community based approach,* Easter Seal Society of Iowa, 1988, Farm Family Rehab Management Program, Final.
21. Scherer MJ, McKee B: High-tech communication devices: what separates users from non-users? *Augmentative and Alternative Communication* 6:99, 1990.
22. Phillips B, Zhao H: Predictors of assistive technology abandonment, *Assistive Technol* 5:36-45, 1993.
23. Cushman LA, Scherer MJ: Measuring the relationship of assistive technology use, functional status over time, and consumer-therapist perceptions of ATs, *Assistive Technol* 8:103-109, 1996.
24. DeRuyter F, Kennedy MR: *Augmentative communication following traumatic brain injury: communication disorders following traumatic brain injury,* Austin, 1990, Pro-Ed Publishing.
25. DeRuyter F, Kennedy MR, Doyle M: *Augmentative communication and stroke rehabilitation: who is doing what and do the data tell the whole story?* Boston, 1990, The National Stroke Rehabilitation Conference.
26. Kohn JG, LeBlanc M, Mortola P: Measuring quality and performance of technology: results of a prospective monitoring program, *Assistive Technol* 6:120-125, 1994.
27. DeRuyter F: The importance of outcome measures for assistive technology service delivery systems, *Technol Disabil* 6:89-104, 1997.
28. Smith RO: *Accountability in assistive technology interventions: measuring outcomes: resource guide for assistive technology outcomes-measurement tools,* Arlington, Va, 1998, RESNA Publications.
29. Day H, Jutai J: Measuring the psychological impact of assistive devices: The PIADS, *Can J Psychol* 9 (2):159-168, 1996.
30. Scherer MJ: Assistive device utilization and quality-of-life in adults with spinal cord injuries or cerebral palsy, *J Appl Rehab Counsel* 19:21-30, 1988.

31. Demers L, Lambron RW, Ska, B: Development of the Quebec user evaluation of satisfaction with assistive technology (quest), *Assistive Technol* 8:3-13, 1996.
32. Andrich J, Ferrario M, Moi M: A model of cost-outcome analysis for assistive technology, *Disabil Rehabil* 20 (1):1-24, 1998.
33. Murkamel M: *J Qual Improv,* Jan 2001.

# CHAPTER 6

## Funding and Public Policy

*Kathleen Gradel*

This chapter reviews current funding streams that reflect today's overarching public policy affecting the acquisition of assistive technology. These funding streams also shape evolving practice patterns in terms of their distribution and access. This chapter also presents action strategies for dealing with assistive technology funding obstacles and focuses on the visible anchors to somewhat elusive policy trends.

From the most pragmatic perspective, these funding alternatives facilitate access for some people, some of the time, in some locales. However, challenges to existing entitlements and options under today's funding streams may make all or part of this chapter's information obscure in the near future. The reader should stay current through interaction with colleagues, vendors, providers, funders, policy makers, and others and by participating in training, reading publications, and connecting with local, regional, and national assistive technology resources.

Many misconceptions exist about access to and funding for assistive technology. For example, some think that the Assistive Technology Act, formerly called *the Technology-Related Assistance for Individuals with Disabilities Act (Tech Act)*, guarantees individual entitlements to assistive technology for children, youth, and adults with disabilities, which is wrong.[1] Some have heard that the Individuals with Disabilities Education Act (IDEA) is a guarantee that technology is available for students of all ages with disabilities and for families too, which is also incorrect.[2] Misconceptions also exist about Section 508 of the Rehabilitation Act ensuring that accessible technology is available to all people with disabilities in the workplace, which only occurs occasionally.[3] The Americans with Disabilities Act (ADA) being the cornerstone for making the world accessible including using technology has also been a mistaken belief.[4] Lastly, private insurance, Medicaid, Medicare, and now managed care do not always pay for technology that is essential to people's well being and health.

Many public and private funding streams, in addition to the individual's own finances, pay for assistive technology and related services. However, once funding options are reviewed, users realize that they have to pay for augmentative communication devices, for example, obtain an environmental control unit for home use, or even purchase a keyboard to use with the computer at school or work. Reality today represents a unique blend of public policy, state and local implementation of policies and regulations across several distinct but sometimes overlapping funding streams, and case-by-case eligibility and approval considerations.

At the time of passage of the ADA, more than 43 million individuals with disabilities were estimated to live in the United States. More than 2.5 million people have been projected to need assistive technology devices that they do not have, largely because of cost and inadequate funding mechanisms to support these costs.[5,6] Reasons for this include the following:

- Rules of public and private funding sources (e.g., eligibility criteria)[7-9]
- Inability of purchasers with disabilities to obtain loans from lending institutions (e.g., banks)[9]
- Insufficient personal resources and low income levels of many individuals with disabilities who need the equipment[10]
- Cost of the technology[11]
- Inconsistency in service availability[12]

- Failure of much mainstream technology to be designed to be usable by people with disabilities

## Policy Foundation for Current Authorizations and Opportunities

The assortment of funding possibilities that currently make assistive technology a reality in the lives of individuals with disabilities and their families has been shaped by legislative, social, political, economic change, and in some measure the country's recent desire for technology. A brief summary of the foundations for today's policy and practice capsulizes—and perhaps oversimplifies—policy, practice, and philosophy orientations that have had a direct effect on current orientation for assistive technology (Box 6-1).[13-16]

Profound attitudinal change is thought to have occurred over the past 25 years. This change can be witnessed in the following ways: (1) rise of the disability rights movement, (2) enactment of major civil rights laws such as the ADA,[4] (3) greater consciousness of disability and people with disabilities in the planning and activities of many institutions, and (4) greater visibility of people with disabilities in many sectors of society.

### BOX 6-1

#### The Foundation for Today's Policy and Practice

*Disability* is now viewed as a fully encompassing term and includes people who have the full range of physical, mental, cognitive, and emotional disabilities. For most legal and jurisdictional purposes including the ADA disability is defined principally in terms of a physical or mental impairment that substantially limits one or more major life activities. Such a limitation goes well beyond medical issues and makes everyone aware of educational, social, and vocational concerns.

The curative or medical model of rehabilitation is being replaced by an individualized, functional, capacity-building approach to service delivery.

A changing mix of values, expectations, and opportunities exists for individuals with disabilities (e.g., inclusion versus institutionalization and segregation, self-direction and self-determination versus caregiver models, and the overarching view of the productivity and capacity of individuals with disabilities).

Disability is no longer viewed as the cause of diminished access, unemployment, or other life problems. Rather, systems are now perceived to have major roles in generating rather than removing barriers.

Less reliance on an artificial continuum of services exists, with continuing pressure to divest emphasis in prerequisites for entering or leaving service systems.

Greater inclusion of the end user (people with disabilities and their family members) and their advocates in planning, implementing, and evaluating services for themselves and for broader groups and systems (i.e., consumer-responsive language and practice) exists.

Increased use of technology-related definitions and terms in legislation, policy statements, practice guidelines, and decisions, as well as greater cross-referencing between public documents exists.

Increased recognition exists that as important as case-by-case solution building is, the critical need is for system-wide change and solution generation.

Definitions for, attention to, and incentives for outcomes related to service provision are expanding.

Increased civil rights mandates as an overarching approach to securing services and ensuring equality.

Technology is becoming a solution and a necessity for mainstream America. Today's foundation is based on what has been learned from the early 1900s approaches to rehabilitation, shaped by collective experiences. Berkowitz[13] characterizes this history as an unorganized and conflicting set of definitions, outcomes, approaches, and incentives, and Mendelsohn[17] provides additional perspective.

What these changes have meant in terms of quality of life and the way these changes have improved access to education, employment, and economic and social equality are still being debated. High levels of unemployment among those with disabilities still exist. The income of individuals with disabilities still lags behind the incomes of their nondisabled peers. The media still stereotypes individuals with disabilities. A backlash against the gains made by those with disabilities can be seen in congressional attempts to roll back rights and services through ADA[4] and IDEA.[2]

## Federal and State Agency Programs and Authorizations

### Individuals with Disabilities Education Act

In its regulation and statutory provisions, IDEA provides guarantees for access to technology by children and youth who need it to benefit from a free, appropriate public education.[2] Schools must ensure access but do not necessarily directly pay for assistive technology that is identified as necessary for students, unless the technology is specified in the student's individualized education plan (IEP), in which case the school system must provide it. Part C (formerly part H) of IDEA focuses on the youngest potential technology customers: infants and toddlers with disabilities. Part B applies to school-aged children and youth aged 3 through 21.

The original passage of Public Law 94-142 in 1975 did not cite assistive technology as a special-education, related, or supplementary service.[18] The express recognition of technology under IDEA dates from the IDEA amendments of 1986.[19] Although the amendments were best known for creating early intervention programs for infants and toddlers, they also provided funding and authorization for the development of specialized formats and media, for expanded use of captioning, and for a number of technology-oriented personnel preparation initiatives.[20] In addition, these amendments created an entitlement for infants and toddlers up to age 3 along with their families to secure assistive technology through early intervention services.

The 1990 reauthorization, PL 101-476, included the act's name change to IDEA and increased clarity regarding assistive technology emerged and has supplied the current framework for providing technology in public schools. The 1990 amendments continued the process of incorporating technology into the special education process by adopting "assistive technology devices" and "assistive technology services" as authorized activities in appropriate cases. In addition, they defined these terms as they were defined in the Tech Act.[1] For the next few years the terms were also defined in other major federal programs.

Currently, IDEA sets standards for special education programs to be administered through local school districts. The IEP guides each school-aged student's program and services. Individualized family service plans (IFSPs) are for infants, toddlers, and their families. In IDEA, "assistive technology devices" and "assistive technology services" are closely related under the broader definition of "related or supplementary services." The free, appropriate public education mandate in IDEA prohibits consideration of cost when an IEP or IFSP is developed and requires that educational services be delivered in the least restrictive environment. In reality, fear of excessive cost underlies much of today's debate about getting technology into students' education plans and programs and often has an effect on technology's use in the least restrictive settings. Evaluations that are part of the IEP process should be designed to identify the student's assistive technology needs.

Federal law does not specify when a particular student should be provided with assistive technology. That is a function of the needs identified in the IEP planning process for each student. What IDEA does require is that technology be *considered* in the student's evaluation. Complementary training, maintenance, and other support needed by the student, staff, and family to ensure that the equipment is used effectively must also be planned and implemented as part of the student's overall educational program.

However, faculty and staff cannot be required to take courses or otherwise significantly modify their regularly assigned activities under the authority of an individual student's IEP only.

## *Rehabilitation Act*

Vocational rehabilitation is the federal-state program that has a historic mandate to assist individuals with disabilities in securing and maintaining employment and living independently.[21] Vocational rehabilitation programs funded since 1918 (under the Vocational Rehabilitation Act of 1918) have mirrored policy and societal trends on disability with an ever-evolving expansion of allowable services. Current law (PL 105-220) requires state rehabilitation agencies to delineate how a range of technology services is provided at all stages of the rehabilitation process, how related training is delivered to vocational rehabilitation professionals, and how assistive technology devices and services provided for under a service recipient's IPE is provided.[3] Recent amendments are significant because they refer to disability as a natural part of human experience, set a tone for redirection from the medical and curative rehabilitation models of the past (i.e., by presuming an ability to work, cross-referencing to the ADA and the Tech Act of 1988 for technology-related definitions), and incorporate concepts such as *informed choice, self-determination, inclusion, full participation,* and *person-family involvement* in the rehabilitation process.

Vocational rehabilitation is not an entitlement program; however, an individual eligible for services has the right to it and will receive services governed by an IPE, formerly called an *individualized written rehabilitation program (IWRP)*. Similar to the IEP in special education, the IPE is the document that *describes* the service plan for an individual who is receiving vocational rehabilitation services and it can be the means for guiding technology service delivery. Under a 1990 rehabilitation services administration policy directive,[22] vocational rehabilitation agencies must do the following:

- Identify whether technology support would affect the client's potential for employment.
- Make rehabilitation engineering support available during evaluation and the annual review and as a part of postemployment services.
- Provide rehabilitation engineering services regardless of whether similar services and benefits are available under other programs. (Note: rehabilitation engineering services include technology methods, approaches, or devices that help individuals with disabilities overcome barriers to education, rehabilitation, employment, transportation, independent living, and recreation.)

In the vocational rehabilitation system, decisions about technology, training, and acquisition are typically made after the agency conducts an evaluation. Where appropriate, technology also is required for use in the evaluation process. Choosing assistive technology equipment in this case is likely to be part of the overall rehabilitation process and paid for by the vocational rehabilitation agency. Initial training may be provided by the agency, especially if it has been recognized as necessary in the IPE. However, once the designated equipment is secured and installed, additional training or other needs related to its use may become an issue. In cases in which a vocational rehabilitation agency and the client agree that devices should be included in the IPE, care should be taken to ensure that the necessary services and support arc also included. State Client Assistance Programs (CAPs) offer advocacy aid to individuals who are having difficulty securing assistance through the vocational rehabilitation system and work to resolve disputes between the agency and those receiving services.

The issues surrounding financial responsibility for the funding of assistive technology needed by individual job seckers and programmatic responsibility for the provision of assessment, training, and other assistive technology services have become considerably more complicated as a result of recent statutory developments. The Federal Rehabilitation Act amendments of 1998 were enacted as Title IV of the Workforce Investment Act.[3] This legislation, which essentially revamped the entire framework for federal participation in the employment training and job development sectors, created the "one-stop centers" as the entities through which most people would seek and receive employment services. The law clearly envisions a high degree of cooperation between these mainstream centers and the specialized vocational rehabilitation system. The new law, as it relates to potentially costly assistive technology and to access to those employment resources and opportunities technology makes available, is less than clear about how the benefits of the mainstream system and the specialized resources of the vocational rehabilitation (VR) system are coordinated and combined on behalf of job seekers with disabilities.

Further complexity and uncertainty may result from enactment of the Ticket to Work and Work Incentives Improvement Act (TWWIIA) of 1999 (PL 106-170). Among other things, TWIIA provides for the creation of what is in effect a voucher system through which Social Security disability insurance (SSDI) and supplementary security income (SSI) recipients can purchase vocational services from "employment networks" of their choice. Such employment networks are compensated on the basis of participant milestones or outcomes over a 60-month period. State VR agencies are eligible to participate in such employment networks. The concern from the standpoint of assistive technology is again whether under this system of per capita reimbursement employment networks are prepared to seek or accept customers with substantial assistive technology needs.

The Rehabilitation Act also has had an effect on the rights of many persons who are not recipients of vocational rehabilitation services. First enacted as part of the Rehabilitation Act Amendments of 1986,[23] Section 508 was substantially revised and its provisions made mandatory by the 1998 amendments.[24] This provision requires that "electronic and information technology" purchased by the government for its own use or for use by the public, be *accessible* to persons with disabilities, except when certain exceptions including undue burden apply.

Section 504 of the Rehabilitation Act established the right of people with disabilities to seek redress when they are discriminated against in programs including employment operated by the federal government or by other recipients of federal financial assistance.[25] Section 504 is the first major federal disability civil rights statute that has provided the model for subsequent laws. Furthermore, the recent amendments to Section 508 make Section 504 the procedural vehicle through which complaints of violation of Section 508 are to be brought. This makes Section 504 an important tool for achieving equal access to technology and information.

## Americans with Disabilities Act

The Americans with Disabilities Act of 1990 provides critical civil rights protection to individuals with disabilities in the workplace ranging from the questions that an employer can ask in a job interview to the right to reasonable accommodation on the job. It also covers state and local governmental services and public accommodations. Significant changes in awareness, conscience, and the practices of business and government have been documented in polls and surveys.[26] However, as enforcement challenges continue the ADA's long-term effects are still not known. The ADA is not a direct source of funding or provision of assistive technology devices and services, but because of what it mandates employers, government agencies, and public accommodations to do, assistive technology is often the mechanism for ensuring adherence to the ADA. Mendelsohn[27] said the following:

> The ADA nowhere mentions the words "assistive technology," but it does require employers to provide "reasonable accommodations" to workers or job-seekers with disabilities; it requires government agencies to make their programs and services "accessible"; and it requires public accommodations (that is, private firms and others who do business with the public) to provide reasonable accommodations and "auxiliary aids and services," as well as to remove barriers, among its other provisions.

None of these requirements necessarily implicates assistive technology, but as a practical matter, technology may represent the most effective and the least costly path to compliance in many instances.

The adage for assistive technology under the ADA is "reasonable accommodations," that is, change in practices, procedures, and/or equipment that enable an individual who is otherwise qualified for a job to perform the essential functions of that job. The right to reasonable accommodation is significant for those who need or use assistive technology, but no simple standards exist for defining a reasonable accommodation. Mendelsohn[17] also said, "Sometimes technology will be one of several available accommodations, along with job restructuring or other approaches. Other times, it will be the only reasonable accommodation available."

In those cases where it does not impose an undue financial hardship on the employer, where it does not fundamentally alter the nature of the activities in businesses or other organizations, and where it poses no danger to anyone, the law requires that appropriate assistive technology be provided. Many questions about enforcement and violations of the ADA continue to be decided individually.

## Assistive Technology Act

With the passage and subsequent reauthorization of the Technology-Related Assistance for Individuals with Disabilities Act (PL 100-407) in 1988 and 1994, which has been amended and renamed the *Assistive Technology Act of 1998,* states have been given funding to develop, expand, and coordinate statewide customer-responsive, or consumer-responsive, technology programs for individuals of all ages with disabilities. In 1988, Congress recognized that the following was fundamental to the passage of the act[1]:

> Provision of assistive technology devices and assistive technology services enables some individuals with disabilities to: (a) have greater control over their own lives; (b) participate in and contribute more fully to activities in their home, school, and work environments, and in the communities; (c) interact to a greater extent with non-disabled individuals; and (d) otherwise benefit from opportunities that are taken for granted by individuals who do not have disabilities.

The initial Tech Act defined assistive technology devices and services and authorized states to develop and implement statewide programs to meet the technology-related needs of individuals with disabilities. Core purposes of the Tech Act include (1) grant support to states for implementation of statewide, comprehensive, and consumer-responsive programs of technology-related assistance, (2) reduction of federal barriers to financing technology, and (3) improvement in the federal capacity to deliver technical assistance and other capacity-building support to states. State grants were awarded to expand technology services in local communities. Subject to a number of refinements, this basic structure remains in effect as states are nearing the likely end of the program.

Through the efforts of state Tech Act projects, individual devices and services have been made available to people with disabilities, but individual solutions have never been the primary mandate. In its 1994 reauthorization,[28] the Tech Act was amended to focus greater effort on systems change and advocacy activities. A key element of this refinement was the creation of the Protection & Advocacy for Assistive Technology (PAAT) Program, which required the state assistive technology projects to coordinate their activities and share some funding with their state P&A programs. The 1998 amendments, while continuing the emphasis on advocacy, severed the financial connection between the AT Act and P&A projects, providing a separate funding stream for each. Through increasing focus on work-scope inclusion of advocacy, accountability, and systems change, state implementation efforts are increasingly involving collaborations of lead Tech Act agencies with the full range of traditional and less traditional partners. An overarching commitment exists to direct involvement in the process by end users, individuals with disabilities and their families, of these services. Generically, the AT Act projects now have a primary mission of "systems change"—getting systems such as education to undertake new initiatives targeted for increasing compliance with requirements or eliminating practices or policies that are barriers to compliance.

## Telecommunications Act

The Telecommunications Act of 1996, which substantially revised the structure for regulation of media and electronic communications in this country, also included important civil rights provisions for people with disabilities.[29] Section 255 of the act requires that telecommunications equipment and telecommunications services be accessible to individuals with disabilities when such accessibility is "readily achievable." Some of the key issues addressed by the Access Board and the Federal Communications Commission (FCC) in the development of guidelines implementing Section 255 included the definition of "readily achievable," the allocation of responsibility for accessibility features among numerous manufacturers and service providers involved in the creation of complex systems, and explanation of the extent to which product developers should be expected to document their accessibility design efforts.

Section 255, similar to Section 508, is an example of a universal design or accessible design approach. Such approaches have two major implications for assistive technology. First, insofar as people with disabilities can access and use mainstream devices, the need for assistive technology is reduced. Second, to the degree that the costs of accessibility are spread among all the customers for mainstream technology the financial burden on end users with disabilities and on specialized funding streams is also reduced.

## Other Indirect and Direct Funding Options

In addition to the funding streams previously described, several other federal and federal-state programs may provide assistive technology. These programs range from the AgrAbility program administered by the Department of Agriculture to help farmers with disabilities access the rehabilitation services provided by the Department of Veterans Affairs.

### Veterans Administration Services

Established in 1930, the Veterans Administration is the largest single medical care system in the country and one of the most consistent federal purchasers of all types of assistive technology. Funded to administer veteran benefits, just some of the many Veterans Administration programs include pensions, disability compensation, vocational rehabilitation, employment aid, medical care, and home adaptation.

### Social Security Administration Services

For individuals with disabilities who are receiving supplemental security income, the Social Security Administration has various programs that can fund or aid in funding assistive technology. These and other programs have been sources of funding for a variety of equipment, including augmentative communication devices, home modifications, prostheses and orthoses, work-site modifications, assistive listening devices, vision aids, and vehicle modifications. Two of the frequently used programs are the Impairment-Related Work Expense Program, which allows the purchase of assistive technology and allows the cost of that technology to be deducted from the recipients' income after determining how much they made and the Plan for Achieving Self-Support Program, which allows disabled people to set aside income and/or resources that they need to meet an occupational objective.

Other programs including Headstart, programs under the Older Americans Act, and the current national and community service program authorize funds to accommodate participants with disabilities, which may include funds for assistive technology. Although assistive technology has become common in many programs and statutes and for many practitioners, many programs still never mention assistive technology by name. Mendelsohn[30] cited two primary obstacles to using mainstream programs to meet assistive technology needs.

In some cases the funding statute may specify that assistive technology be included as a service; however, the ways in which technology should be addressed by the program may not be specified. In other cases the law does not address assistive technology but it can be inferred in other program features or regulations that mandate equal access by everyone eligible. Most federally funded programs that are not specifically targeted to individuals with disabilities have little to no experience with or knowledge of assistive technology. These should serve as reminders of the collective need to be vigilant as funding and systems change opportunities are sought.

## Federal, State, and Private Insurance Programs

The following sections address key federal, state, and private insurance programs that can sometimes fund (with the right wording, right prescriptions, right personal eligibility, etc.) various assistive technology devices and services. The following should be remembered: (1) the world is in flux and thus these programs and plans may change in terms of current authorizations and (2) various programs purchase devices and services through assorted mechanisms. For example, managed care as a health services option can be bought and paid for by different programs and funding sources, not limited to one means (i.e., a person can be in managed care if receiving Medicaid or if private insurance is paid for by the employer). Different rules, funding options, and appeal strategies may be superimposed on the individual not only by the funding stream but also by the provider or source of the actual health, medical, rehabilitation, or assistive technology service.

### Medicaid

Medicaid is a health insurance program for the poor, paid for with federal funds and requiring state matching funds. It is available to people with disabilities who meet its low income and other eligibility criteria. In 39 states, it is automatically available to recipients of SSI. Medicaid defines the scope of services and the purpose of the services. These services are broad categories of treatment (e.g., prosthetic devices), not discretely defined equipment or interventions. These definitions are used to determine covered versus services not covered. Medicaid is available to people of all ages but with more generous income eligibility standards applicable for certain services provided to children. Medicaid services are available to people living at home and to those residing in institutions; however, the specific services available differ with residential status, and many critics of the current system believe that the Medicaid program favors institutionalization over community-based care.

Federal guidelines establish the program's parameters, with each state developing and implementing its own regulations. However, certain services (required or mandatory) are required as part of each state's Medicaid program. States may choose to offer additional or optional services beyond the mandatory services. Categories of Medicaid-reimbursable equipment and services have no uniform definition.

The reference in Medicaid to "covered" services is a limitation on Medicaid's scope. Generally, Medicaid is not required to and may not provide *all* treatment services a person may need. For people who are eligible for Medicaid, "not covered" is the most general reason Medicaid can offer for declining a request for a specific treatment service. The denial is not based on any facts specific to the individual. Rather, the sole basis of the denial is Medicaid's claim that it is not required to provide the requested treatment service. The key is to explore what services are or must be covered by each state to determine whether a specific individual's needed treatment services must be provided.

Although multiple categories have been used to secure funding under Medicaid, one of the most functional from the disability advocate's perspective has been durable medical equipment. Reimbursements for equipment have also been supported through Medicaid's Inpatient Hospital Care Program and its Community-Based Waiver programs. Medicaid-reimbursed equipment has included prostheses and orthoses, hearing and vision aids, wheelchairs and other mobility aids, daily living aids, and in some states, augmentative communication devices. In addition, assistive technology services (e.g., physical, speech, or occupational therapy, equipment fabrication) are reimbursed. In theory, Medicaid must fund all three components related to securing and using equipment, including evaluations, equipment acquisition, and follow up (e.g., setup and installation, customization, and training). This requirement stems from the provision of the federal Medicaid statute that all services must be sufficient in "amount, duration, and scope" to meet the medical need for which they were prescribed. In reality, however, states do have broad latitude to define services narrowly and to make fairly arbitrary decisions among optional services as to which is provided and which is excluded from coverage.

## Medicaid's Early and Periodic Screening Diagnosis and Treatment (EPSDT) Program

Expanded in 1990, EPSDT is a health benefits program for children and youths under age 21.[31] Traditionally, it has emphasized preventive care and required states to cover regular examinations and then deliver any medically necessary services covered under Medicaid. The EPSDT Program has special applicability to younger, potential technology users. It serves as a funding source for evaluating assistive technology needs of youngsters and for funding services and equipment that may have been excluded previously or that are still not covered in the state's regular Medicaid program. In the broader Medicaid program, states may choose to fund only mandated services. In the EPSDT Program, states do not have this choice because they must cover all mandatory and optional services a particular child needs. Funded equipment remains the property of the individual for whom it is funded, although the equipment may be leased by Medicaid. The program has been used to fund most types of equipment with the exception of environmental controls, vehicle modifications, and computer applications.[32]

## *Medicare*

Medicare, also a federal grant insurance program, is likewise administered by the Social Security Administration and the Health Care Financing Administration. Individuals, who are age 65 or older, those who are blind, or who have total or permanent disabilities and have received Social Security disability income for at least 24 months and individuals in renal failure are eligible. Medicare can fund assistive technology when it is deemed a covered service that is medically necessary. Typically funded equipment includes wheelchairs and mobility aids, seating and positioning equipment, and prostheses and orthoses. Rarely funded items include equipment used in the bathroom such as grab bars, which are considered convenience rather than medical items, and vehicle modifications.

## *Buy-In Programs*

To help cope with the work disincentives associated with the risk of benefit loss if people with disabilities enter employment, several recent legislative changes (most notably TWWIIA) make it possible for people to earn more income without forfeiting the health insurance benefits associated with the SSI and SSDI programs. Although income still results in reduction or cessation of cash benefits, states now have discretion to raise the income eligibility cutoff points for Medicaid recipients who return to work. Similarly, the Social Security Administration has been granted new authority to experimentally waive or modify those provisions that imperil the continued availability of Medicare coverage for SSDI recipients who reenter the workforce.

## Private Health Insurance

Private health care is an increasingly important resource for assistive technology funding, especially because of the current predicted changes in the Medicaid program. Private health insurance is often a part of wage and benefit packages provided by employers to their employees and their families. It may also be secured through professional or other organizations (e.g., labor unions) or enrolled in directly by individuals. Significant variation in the scope of coverage is permitted in private health care. The following four common types of health insurance programs are available to people who get insurance through an employer, through an association, or by individually purchasing them (Medicare and Medicaid also fit in these categories):

1. Indemnity programs allow free choice of health care providers, who are then reimbursed on a fee-for-service basis.
2. Preferred provider organization plans encourage participants to use providers who contract with the plan; the providers are paid on a discounted fee-for-service basis. The plans require lower co-payments (out-of-pocket expenses) to meet part of the cost of the service. Use of other providers is permitted, but at higher cost.
3. Point-of-service plans provide participants with a primary care physician, who arranges referrals to specialist care. Inherent in these plans are financial incentives to use providers who contract with the plan.
4. Health maintenance organizations require enrollees to use only providers who contract with the plan.

The freedom to choose a health care provider is different in each of these programs and can ultimately affect an individual's ability to secure assistive technology services through the particular plan. Health insurance and benefits plans have been and will probably continue to be a major assistive technology provider. This includes coverage for augmentative communication devices, bath safety equipment (e.g., shower and bath chairs, lifts), hospital beds, environmental control devices, hearing aids, individual lifts, mobility devices (e.g., walkers, manual wheelchairs, and scooters), and seating and positioning devices (e.g., custom seating systems, standing frames, seat-lift chairs).[33] Services such as durable medical equipment, prosthetic devices, and rehabilitative therapy services (e.g., occupational or physical therapies, speech and language pathology services, and rehabilitative services) may be covered in health insurance policies or benefit plans. If these services are covered by the policy or benefits plan, they can be a basis for funding assistive technology devices. However, despite these possibilities, significant challenges exist to securing assistive technology funding in the private health care arena. According to Golinker,[33] these challenges include the following:

- No mandate for universal coverage exists, either for people or for services.
- No common benefits list exists that applies to all insurance policies or health benefits plans. People must review and understand their own health care coverage policies, specifically in terms of (1) where and how technology-related terms are defined in the covered and excluded services of the plans and (2) the decision-making rules on which interpretations are based, including definitions of various covered services and terms (e.g., medical need, coverage limitations, and exclusions).

## Alternative Funding Options

### Private Funding Sources

Private funding sources have historically supplemented (and in some cases supplanted) public funding sources for assistive technology. These diverse sources apply variable eligibility requirements, restrictions on reimbursements, and more. They include community groups (e.g., Lions Club, Kiwanis, Rotary, Sertoma, Elks, Knights of Columbus, Optimist Club), special-interest groups (e.g., sororities and fraternities), and nonprofit service organizations (e.g., the Muscular Dystrophy Associations). "Wish" groups or foundations also have recently entered the funding mainstream, with a special focus on particular illnesses and attention typically given to children. No general rules apply; each organization requires individual contact, with applications and written requests dictated by the program's own requirements and its mission. The full range of assistive technology is potentially fundable, depending on the mission, funding levels, and need of the sponsoring organizations. Also in the category of private assistive technology funding is employer or business funding as a strategy to meet "reasonable accommodation" standards.

### *Credit Financing*

Wallace[32] said, "Credit financing is an alternative of vast potential for individuals with disabilities that may provide creative payment opportunities using the substantial resources of the credit industry for the purchase of assistive technology." Credit financing is viewed by some as a highly promising strategy to help funding assistive technology for individuals who are not eligible for other third-party programs. Reeb[34] has cited multiple examples of corporate-nonprofit partnerships resulting in the purchase of high-cost devices. One of the most common approaches in this evolving field has been the use of loan guarantees as an incentive to potential lenders. Such programs typically provide for longer payment terms and/or reduced interest rates. Many currently funded state Tech Act projects and collaborators are piloting or extending the activities of loan programs. These efforts further test the viability of this funding alternative.

A major infusion of federal funds into the assistive technology loan sector occurred with the funding of seven programs during 2000, pursuant to the first-ever appropriation of monies under Title III of the Assistive Technology Act. Title III requires the establishment of Alternative Funding Programs (AFP) and for the establishment of an Alternative Funding Technical Assistance Program (AFTAP). Including required state matching funds, the program could generate around 7 million dollars in capital for assistive technology loan programs in its first year.

## Advocacy in the Assistive Technology Funding and Policy Arena

People who have attempted to receive funding for a device even once or twice or get support for someone to learn using a new device know that advocacy is a critical component of assistive technology funding. Even when statutes are written, policy directives are clarified, and responsibility is assigned, implementation and enforcement are not automatic. As systems change, efforts continue at the grass roots, state, and national levels and ongoing advocacy becomes a necessary ingredient for obtaining assistive technology. Federal funds have been designated for advocacy efforts in various systems or funding streams to ensure the rights of individuals with disabilities.

Most notable among such advocacy systems or services are state P&A programs established under the Developmental Disabilities Bill of Rights Act and CAP operating as part of the vocational rehabilitation system. Other formal and informal advocacy support exists in local communities and states and regionally and nationally. For example, Parent Training Information Centers often support person-to-person or lay advocacy among families of children, youth, and adults with disabilities. The Family Center on Technology and Disability Program operated by a consortium of organizations led by UCP, Inc. (Washington DC, www.ucp.org/fctd) also provides a variety of important technology-related informational resources and important linkages in this area. Similarly, many local and nationally affiliated nonprofit organizations offer a range of advocacy outreach, direct assistance, mentoring alternatives, and connections to others facing similar challenges. In addition, more generic ombudsman services may be brought to bear on assistive technology issues. Such services are available through specific funding streams (e.g., Offices on Aging, Departments of Mental Health, Mental Retardation, Developmental Disabilities, etc.) and through local and state offices of individuals with disabilities. Others can be found in disability services in colleges and universities and through services targeted to specific audiences (e.g., individuals who are homeless, battered, aging, receiving welfare benefits, etc.).

No one advocacy strategy works with each and every funding stream, and idiosyncrasies in policy, procedure, and practice are to be expected even within a single funding stream. Several strategies are helpful in securing funding under specific streams (Box 6-2). Four basic strategies are important to approaching any and all funding streams as follows:

1. Be vigilant to the potential of assistive technology as a solution and the possibility that the program may provide or use technology.
2. Know what each funding stream funds, then use the language, documentation, and rationale that match those policies, procedures, and practices. Find out whether expenditures for assistive technology are allowable—either explicitly or by inference—to meet the goals of a program and/or to meet a program's antidiscrimination requirements.
3. Know and document what is needed and the way assistive technology equipment and/or services affect the customer with a disability. Document technology-related needs in the context of complementary service needs and/or within the routine application to a program or request for services.

## BOX 6-2

### *Strategies for Securing Funds under Specific Streams*

Know the contents of the law, policy, or procedural rules that are applicable to the particular funding situation and need. This means becoming familiar with such phrases as *reasonable accommodation, undue hardship,* and *qualified individual with a disability.*

Ensure that any program plan addresses assistive technology equipment and service needs, including Individual Program Plans, IEPs, and IPEs. Be sure to also include requirements for evaluations and service and support.

Ensure that requests for assistive devices and services are written into placement or service identification meeting minutes or proceedings.

Use policy letters issued by the federal sources (e.g., Office of Special Education Programs, Rehabilitation Services Administration), state bodies, and other policy-making groups in (1) individual cases to remove a barrier and enable access to technology and (2) broad systems change efforts that can lead to legislative changes.

Become involved in the budget and planning process for services (e.g., Special Education Advisory Panels, school boards, special-interest support groups, task forces, consortium efforts planning state block grant and implementation).

Identify model programs and success stories from other systems, other programs, and other locales and use this information to promote adoption of best practices.

Join or help initiate task force groups that include individuals with disabilities, family members, providers, and advocates to develop compliance guidelines on assistive technology access issues.

Secure and/or work with others to develop guidelines to serve as standards for compliance of providers. Knowing these standards, learn how services are evaluated and use these findings to guide individual and system advocacy efforts.

Ask vendors (those companies that develop, manufacture, and sell technology products) to help secure funding and make connections to other individuals who have been successful in securing funding solutions.

Talk to legislators and other policy makers about needs; they may be willing to investigate the budgeting of state or federal funds, address needs in the budget, or change laws or regulations.

Take responsibility for advising and educating employers, co-workers, students, and others about what is needed.

Practice effective communication skills to clearly and consistently articulate what is needed.

4. Be persistent and document all requests. Modify requests or applications as needed based on experience with rejections; use appropriate due process procedures or equivalent strategies.

## Conclusion

As a caveat to the advocacy strategies cited in the previous section, Mendelsohn[17] said that in this rapid state of flux, the following should be done: (1) select issues and advocacy forums wisely; concentrate on making decisions on issues in which the greatest effect can be achieved and resources can be most effectively leveraged; (2) ensure that any and all approaches involve concrete education and inclusion of end users—individuals with disabilities and family members—in the importance of the issues and in strategies used to influence decisions and make change; and (3) propose strategies that "hold promise of breaking down barriers in ways that do not create resentment or equity issues in connection with the new responsibilities or new costs involved."[17]

At the beginning of this chapter, several partially misleading questions were posed, followed by a review of funding streams and strategies. If the locale, agency, state, or own case is the primary referent—and if the case is a positive one—some may believe that assistive technology systems change is fairly straightforward and slow. In the context of special education, Golden[35] said, "Nothing could be further from the truth. After 20 years of special education case law decisions, there are more fuzzy, unresolved questions than ever, and assistive technology questions are adding to the pool of already complex issues."

Access issues continue to be determined over time through administrative and court decisions, policy interpretations, and implementation practices and guidelines. Golden[35] also said, "In the interim, states should view the lack of clarity as an opportunity to fill in the gaps with policies and interpretations that support access to assistive technology."

Perhaps the best departure from this challenging topic is to quote Mendelsohn,[17] who has attempted to put the future into perspective with the past and present:

> The past cannot predict the future. The challenges faced by advocates in the coming years will be unlike any met before. Meeting these challenges will require strategy, community mobilization, and expertise in a broad range of subject areas and technologies. History may reveal that successful systems change efforts display a number of common elements. However, it will be up to the advocates of our day to determine how to apply those lessons in their advocacy and work.

## References

1. The Assistive Technology Act of 1998: PL 105-394, codified at Title 29 of the United States Code at Section 3001 and following (29 USC Sec. 3001 et seq.), amending PL 103-218 (1994) and PL 100-407 (1988).
2. Individuals with Disabilities Education Act of 1997: PL 105-17 (20 USC Sec. 1400 et seq.).
3. Rehabilitation Act Amendments of 1998: PL 105-220, Sec. 508, 29 USC Sec. 794d.
4. Americans with Disabilities Act of 1990: PL 101-336 Title 42 USC 12101 et seq.
5. LaPlante M, Hendershot G, Moss A: *Assistive technology devices and home accessibility features: prevalence, payment, need, and trends,* Washington, DC, 1992, National Center for Health Statistics.
6. McGuiness K: *Stalking the elusive buck,* Boston, 1982, Environments Center, Massachusetts College of Art.
7. Ward C: *Subsidy programs for assistive devices,* Washington, DC, 1989, Electronics Industries Foundation.
8. US Congress, Office of Technology Assessment: *Technology and handicapped people,* Washington, DC, 1982, US Government Printing Office.
9. Reeb K: *Revolving loan funds: expanding equipment credit financing opportunities for persons with disabilities,* Washington, DC, 1987, Electronics Industries Foundation.
10. Hemp R et al: *Financing assistive technology: an annotated bibliography,* Chicago, 1991, University of Illinois, Assistive Technology Financing Project.

11. Hoffman A: Funding: how you can make it work? In Costor CA, editor: *Planning and implementing augmentative communication services delivery,* Washington, DC, 1988, RESNA Press.
12. Morris MW, Golinker L: *Assistive technology: a funding workbook,* Washington, DC, 1991, RESNA Press.
13. Berkowitz E: *Disabled policy: America's programs for the handicapped,* New York, 1987, Cambridge University Press.
14. Enders A: Funding for assistive technology and related services: an annotated bibliography, *Phys Occup Ther Pediatr* 10 (2):147-173, 1989.
15. Haber L: Trends and demographic studies on programs for disabled persons. In Perlman LG, Austin GF, editors: *Social influences in rehabilitation planning: blueprint for the 21st century,* pp 20-23, Arlington, Va, 1985, National Rehabilitation Association.
16. Wallace JF et al: Legislative foundation of assistive technology policy in the United States. In Flippo, Inge KJ, Barcus JM, editors: *Assistive technology: a resource for school, work, and community,* pp 3-21, Baltimore, 1994, Paul Brookes.
17. Mendelsohn S: *New strategies for systems change,* United Cerebral Palsy Associations, Inc. Assistive Technology Funding & Systems Change Project, Washington, DC, 1996, Tech Express.
18. Education for All Handicapped Children Act of 1975: PL 94-142.
19. Education of the Handicapped Act Amendments of 1986: PL 99-457.
20. Behrmann MM, Morrissette SK, McCallen MH: *Assistive technology issues for Virginia schools,* Richmond, Va, 1992, State Special Education Advisory Committee.
21. Vocational Rehabilitation Act of 1918: PL 65-178, (16 USC 486A-486W).
22. US Department of Education Office of Special Education and Rehabilitative Services: *Policy directive,* Washington, DC, Nov 16, 1990, Rehabilitation Services Administration. *See also* RSA Technical Assistance Circular 98-04, September 1998.
23. PL 99-506, Sec. 509, 1986.
24. 29 USC Sec. 794d.
25. 29 USC Sec. 794.
26. United Cerebral Palsy Associations: New ADA snapshot on America shows changes in lives of Americans with disabilities, Washington Watch 2 (22):2-n-3.
27. Mendelsohn S: The ADA and assistive technology, United Cerebral Palsy Associations, Inc., Assistive Technology Funding & Systems Change Project, *AT Funding News, 1995.*
28. 29, USC Sec. 2201 et seq: Superseded and repealed by 29 USC Sec. 3001 et seq.
29. Communications Act of 1996: PL 104-104, especially Sec. 255 (47 USC Sec. 255). See also Title 36 Code of Federal Regulations Part 1191 (36 CFR 1191).
30. Mendelsohn S: Accessibility in the federal workplace, United Cerebral Palsy Associations, Inc., Assistive Technology Funding & Systems Change Project, *Tech Express,* January 1995.
31. Medicaid Early and Periodic Screening, Diagnosis, and Treatment Amendments of 1989: PL 101-239 (*see* generally 42 USC Sec. 1396 et seq.).
32. Wallace JF: Creative financing of assistive technology. In Flippo, Inge KJ, Barcus JM, editors: *Assistive technology: a resource for school, work, and community,* pp 245-268, Baltimore, 1994, Paul Brookes.
33. Golinker L: Assistive technology funding by private health care reimbursement sources, United Cerebral Palsy Associations, Inc., Assistive Technology Funding & Systems Change Project, *Tech Express,* late Fall 1995.
34. Reeb K: *Assistive financing for assistive devices: loan guarantees for purchase of products by persons with disabilities,* Washington, DC, 1989, Electronics Industries Foundation.
35. Golden DC: Special education systems change: Missouri style, United Cerebral Palsy Associations, Inc., Assistive Technology Funding & Systems Change Project, *Tech Express* February 1995.

*Special Thanks to Steve Mendelsohn for his updates to this content.*

# PART 2

........................................................................................................

## Technologies for Information, Communication, and Access

........................................................................................................

*Peggy Barker*

Technologies for information, communication, and access incorporate the latest electronic and computer technologies. Because these technologies are so new and still evolving, they change and offer more options and opportunities for all people with disabilities.

The evaluation process is therefore crucial and should result in technology features required to meet a particular person's abilities and goals in the environments that the assistive technologies are used. The features should then be matched to the available technology. Each device or system needs to be evaluated with the user to ensure that it is practical and functional. This process is dependent on being able to get current information regarding the latest developments in technology and strategies to implement the technology.

In Chapter 7, Computer Access, computer applications, components, and access tools and strategies are reviewed. Functionality, user competence, trustworthiness and longevity, and the goals identified in this chapter are applicable to all the technology addressed in Part 2. Longevity is defined in this chapter as it relates to the skills of the user. Technology changes quickly, and upgrading the systems that are recommended on a regular basis is expected. One of the most valuable contributions that a clinician can make is to support the user in the development of skills that can be generalized and applied to future technologies.

The chapter on Information Technologies, Chapter 8, focuses on the need to have access to information available with a variety of technologies including computers, telephones, television, and public electronic kiosks (e.g., ATMs). These technologies are used by the mainstream and are changing faster than any of the assistive technologies.

In Chapter 9, Augmentative and Alternative Communication, intervention strategies are identified and matched to diagnosis and characteristics of a diagnosis. Strategies are presented to identify goals for intervention that incorporate AAC devices and to identify features of systems. High-tech and low-tech components of an individual's communication system are discussed. Finally, a variety of implementation and training strategies and resources are listed.

Chapter 10, Integrated Systems, describes the integration of systems, the way a system is put together, or more specifically, the way all the components are interconnected electronically and mechanically. Too often the devices that a person uses are selected in isolation from the other devices that a person is using or wants to use. Selection of devices that are not compatible can make integration difficult and can increase cost. A well thought-out integrated system can ensure independence, optimize productivity, and contain costs.

Sensory aids have been considered for vision and hearing. In Chapter 11, Sensory Aids: Vision, low, high and no technology are considered for people with visual impairments that include blindness, low vision, and functional vision impairments. The tools and strategies are applicable to and incorporate the other technologies addressed in this part for AAC, computer access, and information systems. This chapter also emphasizes the need to continually address what the outcome should be and to choose tools and strategies to obtain it.

Chapter 12, Sensory Aids: Hearing, describes assistive listening aids and signaling devices that need to be considered to improve communication when traditional hear-

........................................................................................................

ing aids are not sufficient. Careful evaluation of a person's situations and needs as well as training and counseling in the use of the device are essential for successful implementation.

The formidable challenge is to stay knowledgeable about these technologies and the upcoming new ones and implement them intelligently for persons with disabilities.

CHAPTER 7

# Computer Access

*Jutta Treviranus*
*Linda Petty*

## Application and Goal

Computers are becoming an essential tool in education, vocation, and recreation. Today, computer literacy is frequently considered a mandatory skill. Throughout the day, computers are used for writing, drawing, preparing taxes, banking, shopping, playing, learning new concepts, joining discussion groups, and searching for recipes. For someone with a disability, computers can play several roles. Computer access is needed for universal things such as word processing, sending e-mail, and playing computer games. Computers may also provide alternative methods of performing tasks that are difficult to do the standard way, for instance banking by computer for someone with limited mobility or speech. Last, computer systems can augment or act as substitutes for impaired sensory, motor, or cognitive abilities (e.g., reading machines, electric wheelchairs, cochlear implants, augmentative communication devices, and wayfinding systems). This chapter discusses the use of assistive technology to access standard computers.

Selecting a computer access system for a person with a disability may entail choosing the assistive technology as well as the computer and all its components, or simply choosing the assistive technology that is compatible with the person's existing system. Whatever the scenario, four overarching goals exist for an accessible personal computer system.

### Functionality

Functionality seems a somewhat obvious goal, but frequently computers are chosen for their own sake rather than the functions they are intended to fulfill. An essential part of choosing a computer system is to carefully delineate exactly what the primary user wants to do with the computer. The computer system should allow that person to perform the desired tasks as efficiently as possible.

### User Competence

The user should feel competent using the system. A careful match of the user's skills with the skills required to control the system should be made. This may not mean that the system that is easiest to use is selected. Frequently, a more complex system is needed to perform targeted tasks. However, the user should receive sufficient training in system use to gain expertise. This entails mastery of the alternative access method or the primary application and proficiency of all tasks related to use of the computer system and the peripherals. The assistive technology should be carefully integrated and customized to allow efficient control of application programs, easy transitions between computer applications, manipulation of the desktop, and control of all relevant peripherals.

An important prerequisite to achieving user confidence is teaching the user to diagnose the sources of errors such as a software bug, poor software design, or a personal error. A sure sign of a user not feeling competent in using a system is generalizing that either the computer causes all errors or the user must cause everything. Competence does not mean the absence of user errors; however, competence is supported if error correction is set up to be an easy, foolproof procedure.

## Trustworthiness

The user should be able to trust the system. The system should be reliable. Frequently the individual components of a system are reliable but they are not compatible with each other, which may cause system breakdown. Thus set up and thorough testing of the entire system are essential. Setting up an alternative computer access system also entails setting up a maintenance support plan. This involves a series of contingencies including help lines, accessible experts, and vendor warranty procedures.

## Longevity

Longevity encompasses not only a particular set of hardware and software but also the skills learned by the user. Significant time and energy are invested in mastering a computer system. The skills and approaches should not be treated as disposable. An access approach that meets the user's needs for an extended period should be chosen, which can be achieved by selecting a system that is flexible and extendible. Consequently, as the user's requirements change, the system can be modified to address the changes without requiring command of a whole new system.

## Function and Ability

To control a computer, the user must be able to achieve the equivalent of controlling a mouse, typing on a keyboard, reading a display, and listening to auditory system cues. The user must also be able to interpret and determine the appropriate response to the computer user interface. Accordingly, access to the computer demands visual, auditory, perceptual, motor, and cognitive skills.

Users who can benefit from alternative computer access systems include those who have the following characteristics:

- Have difficulty or cannot control a keyboard
- Find controlling a mouse difficult
- Have repetitive strain injuries
- Have difficulty seeing or are unable to see the display
- Are unable to hear auditory cues
- Have a learning disability that makes writing or reading text difficult
- Require simplified interfaces because of cognitive impairments

## Keyboard Control

Control of standard computer keyboards requires that the user have range and resolution required to accurately target the keys, strength required to depress keys, ability to hold down several keys at once, coordination to avoid hitting unwanted keys, and timing required to release keys before inadvertently repeating keys.

## Keyboard Adaptations

Keyboard adaptations have several benefits. They remove the need to hold several keys at once, provide stabilization and isolate keys to prevent inadvertent activation of keys, and slow the repeat rate to avoid unwanted repeats.

## Alternative Keyboards

Alternative keyboards can vary the spacing, size, layout, and activation force of keys, thereby accommodating variations in range, resolution, and strength. They also accommodate pointing with other body parts.

## Voice Recognition Systems

Voice recognition systems allow input using continuous or noncontinuous speech. Keyboard replacements or switch input devices eliminate the need to point or target. This is replaced with the prerequisite skills of timing switch activation, timing the duration of switch activation, or entering a sequence of long and short switch activations that form a code.

## Mouse Control

Mouse control requires the following subskills:

1. Moving the pointer to the target, including the following:
   a. Holding or making controlled contact with the mouse or pointing device
   b. Moving and stopping the pointer at the desired location
2. Selecting the desired target, involving the following:
   a. Maintaining the pointer on the target while activating a button
   b. Activating the button at the appropriate time
3. Dragging, which involves the previous subskills and the following:
   a. Maintaining hold on the button while moving the pointer to a new location
   b. Releasing the button at the appropriate time while maintaining the pointer on the second target
4. Moving between use of the keyboard or keyboard emulator and the mouse or pointing device

## Mouse Alternatives or Replacements

Mouse alternatives or replacements can eliminate the need to hold the mouse, vary the movements required to point the mouse pointer, replace the button with switches that can be activated with alternative actions, and allow pointing with alternative body parts and movement of the mouse in incremental steps using discrete keys.

## Computer Displays

Standard computer display methods require that the user be able to read text, decipher graphics or icons, and locate and follow a small mouse cursor. Good figure-ground perception is required. Color and texture are used to communicate function and must be distinguished by the user.

## Alternative and Adapted Displays

Adapted displays enlarge portions of the display and vary color and contrast. Alternative display methods read the text on the display using a text-to-speech synthesizer or by displaying the *text* on a refreshable Braille display, thereby replacing visual information with auditory or tactile information. With the transition from the command line interface to the graphical user interface (GUI), the task of accessing the computer using a screen reader (and to some extent screen magnifier and Braille display) became much more difficult. Screen readers display small chunks of information, one at a time. Although this is well suited to the disk operating system (DOS) interface, the GUI interface presents information in no discernible sequential order, presents information simultaneously, and uses graphic images and non–text-based graphic conventions to communicate structure and function.

Consequently, a new set of strategies is frequently required to complete a task. Strategies are required to visualize the layout of the screen, to orient, to navigate the interface, to become aware of visual events occurring elsewhere on the screen, and to find alternative methods of accessing information presented graphically or to make up for the information gaps this causes. Screen readers are slowly becoming more GUI savvy, thereby making it easier for the user. However, successful use of a screen reader involves a large initial learning load.

Screen readers designed for individuals with learning disabilities highlight the text as it is being read, providing auditory and visual supports for reading. These may also be paired with other computer-based tools such as spell checkers, grammar checkers, and outliners.

### Simplified Interfaces

Concept keyboards can be adapted to simplify and routinize the input choices for people with cognitive impairments. In a GUI, many times material gets "lost" by the user inadvertently choosing or moving desktop components. Desktops can contain a confusing array of objects to choose from. Utilities exist that mask the standard desktop and replace it with a simplified desktop.

## Considerations, Options, and Technology

When configuring a system that best meets a user's needs, a person must make a number of interrelated choices. These include choices related to the assistive technology, the computer system, and the set up, training, and support mechanisms that allow the system to become a functional tool for the user. When the user's skills, needs, and the desired functionality are clearly defined, the choices become fairly straightforward.

### General Considerations

#### Comprehensive Needs Survey

Computer technology can be the interface to many functions. Any needs assessment to determine an optimal computer system should encompass all of the client's needs, roles, and environments.[1] The chosen computer and access system should be sufficiently extensible to accommodate these varied needs. An access system that is optimal for one function may not be optimal for another function, requiring a more flexible interface or several interface alternatives. If the client uses dedicated assistive technology, allowing communication between the computer and the dedicated device is frequently desirable.

#### Potential for Change

Consideration must be given to the individual's prognosis and potential changes in living situations and work or school environments so that the recommended equipment can accommodate anticipated changes in need or physical status. Sometimes, choosing equipment that has capabilities such as memory and speech capacity that can be expanded can accommodate these changes. In other situations, leasing or borrowing equipment rather than purchasing it can accommodate change.

#### Integrated Control of Multiple Functions

At times, having the user access several types of assistive technology with the same interface is desirable or essential. This may be because only one reliable access site exists, which is also the optimal access method for each assistive device or because the user prefers integrated controls for personal reasons. Integrating environmental controls or augmentative communication aids with the computer system may be preferable if all systems need to be portable, or cost or space constraints exist that prohibit overlapping or duplicate stand-alone systems.[2]

## Portable Versus Stationary Technologies

Portability is required if the computer access system must be used in several environments. Portability can be achieved by using a portable system or by using systems that have modular components that can be detached from the stationary system. With portability, issues of wear and tear on devices and prevention of theft or damage need to be considered. Mounting of the device and the access interface need to be addressed carefully and systematically to ensure that function, safety, independence, and cosmesis are not compromised.

## Cost

Although prices for standard systems have decreased significantly with the increased numbers in use, the same economies of scale do not apply to assistive technologies. In fact, the cost of assistive peripherals or software frequently exceeds the cost of the computer system. Occasionally, the same functionality can be achieved using either general market software and hardware or using software and hardware specifically designed for users with disabilities (e.g., document scanning and optical character recognition). General market software and hardware solutions have the advantage of being less costly and receiving local support. Specialized software or hardware solutions accommodate the specific needs of the user with a disability but cannot be serviced by standard computer repair services.

## Availability of Maintenance, Training, and Support

Ideally, local vendors should be available to support the basic computer system and the access technology. In reality, equipment choice may be constrained by limitations on vendor availability or technical support in the user's geographic area, work, school, or home environment. Computer users should identify and collaborate with people who are identified as technical experts or support staff in their environments to ensure adequate expertise is available. Having and training a committed support team in the maintenance of the system and the operational needs of the user and system is essential. Funding or clinical time for training may be limited, yet adequate training and follow up are crucial to successfully implementing the technology.

## User and Support Team Acceptance of Technology and Access Method

The effect of technology on the users and others in their environment can be intrusive. The effect of the technology on daily routines, communication patterns, and use of space and time need to be anticipated, clearly communicated, and approved by the user and others in their environment before implementation. The expediency of using a less cosmetic or uncommon access method such as switching input by head or foot movement or using an unusual interface needs to be clearly understood and accepted by the user and support team to prevent equipment abandonment or under use.

## Anticipated Changes in Technology

Computer technology is changing rapidly. Unfortunately, computer access technology is usually lagging, sometimes leaving the user with access to older operating systems or software applications. Meeting current user needs is usually advisable rather than waiting for the next generation device, as new versions and upgrades are often promised long before delivery. If existing technology meets all of a person's needs, replacement with newer technology is not necessary, unless upgrades can bring benefits in speed or functionality that justify the change. Computer access tools should not be expected to last more than 5 years, resulting from changes in computer technology. A hardware or software interface older than 5 years eventually has conflicts or incompatibilities with the newer operating systems, software applications, or hardware.

## Configuring the Alternative Access System

When choosing an optimal access system, the clinician should first assess the client's skills and derive a list of abstract requirements for the access technology that can then be matched to existing technologies rather than "trying on" available devices. The latter is a limiting process that results in asking the client to adapt to the technology rather than optimizing the technology to the skills and needs of the client. Frequently, a number of access technology products exist that accommodate the user's optimal access method. With some exceptions, a system should be chosen that provides transparent access to the desktop and all application software the user may wish to control and allowing optimization for specific applications (see Optimization of Alternative Access System on p. 99).

Because not all application programs and desktop controls have keyboard equivalents for all mouse actions, the access system should include a method of emulating mouse actions. However, because mouse emulation is frequently a tedious, unintuitive method of controlling the desktop, more direct methods of manipulating it should be provided. These might include macros or buttons for resizing windows, calling up specific applications, moving windows, and minimizing or maximizing windows.

## Low-Tech or No-Tech Options for Computer Access

Computer access may be improved by simply repositioning the user or the computer system. This can be accomplished by using height adjustable chairs, computer tables, keyboard trays, or monitor arms. Providing additional stabilizers or supports may improve control and reduce the risk of repetitive strain injuries. Available supports include wrist rests, movable forearm supports (e.g., Ergo Arm), and keyguards.

Users who are unable to access a keyboard using their hands or arms but who have good head, neck, and upper torso control may be able to type on the keyboard using a mouthstick or head/chin pointer.

## High-Tech Options for Computer Access

High-tech computer access systems perform one of the following three functions:

1. Translate or enhance the display
2. Replace or enhance the method of controlling the computer
3. Reorganize or enhance the application content

The access system comes in the form of built in or shareware/freeware software modifications or adding sophisticated hardware and/or software packages. The options described next are usually available for either Apple or Windows compatible systems and are listed in order of increasing complexity.

### Enhancements to the Visual Display

A number of adjustments can be made to the visual display using built-in system controls or free software. These adjustments provide higher contrast and can enlarge icons, display fonts, and mouse cursors.

If this is not adequate, a large number of screen magnification or screen enhancement programs are available. The following features should be considered:

1. Quality and degree of font smoothing at higher magnifications
2. Types of viewing windows available for viewing magnified text (line, window, box, etc.)
3. Options for scrolling or moving to desired areas of the screen
4. Options for tracking the cursor, the insertion point, alert boxes, focus, etc.
5. Choices of text and background color
6. Integration with screen reading
7. Ability to extract text and reformat text for easier viewing

8. Quality of image magnification
9. Complexity of keyboard or mouse commands required to control the magnifier

For those who have difficulty reading or writing because of a learning disability or emerging literacy, talking word processors and add-ons are available that highlight words or phrases as they are being read. They allow reading in chunks such as by syllable, word, or sentence. These programs also support writing by echoing what is being typed.

### Alternative Displays

Alternatives to the visual display include screen readers that speak the text displayed on the screen and refreshable Braille displays that translate the text to Braille.

A number of screen readers are available. Screen readers that are compatible with Windows or the MacOS have various approaches to dealing with the GUI. Some require that the user visualize the desktop and use its layout as a referent in navigating. Others reorganize the desktop in a two-dimensional hierarchy. The approach best suited to the users depends on the person's previous experiences and skills in grasping inherently spatial models. In setting up a screen-reading access system, control of the interface without use of a mouse must also be considered. Many actions can be performed with keyboard equivalents, but the user is required to learn these. Input alternatives must be found for actions that have no keyboard equivalents such as macros.

Considerations in choosing a screen reader include the following:

1. Completeness and cohesiveness of the display model presented
2. Methods available to navigate to desired sections of the display or interface
3. Differentiation of insertion point and exploration cursor so that users can look around without losing their places
4. Supports to assist in orienting to status and location (answering the questions "Where am I?" and "What is happening?")
5. Options available for echoing what is typed (e.g., letter, word, phoneme)
6. Options available for reading text (present, next, previous word, line, sentence, etc.)
7. Pronunciation dictionaries and speech options (e.g., rate, pitch, volume, prosody, modulation, voice, voice change tied to different functions)
8. Strategies available for getting information about nontext items (e.g., reading tool tips)
9. Strategies for controlling interface controls that do not have a keyboard equivalent
10. Compatibility with the software applications the user prefers

Braille displays vary in the number of cells that are displayed (usually either 40 or 80), the method of navigating on the display, the status information that can be displayed, and the available quick reference keys or short-cut keys available. Some Braille displays are designed to be compatible with screen readers.

### Enhancements and Alternatives to the Auditory Display

For individuals who cannot hear or fail to attend to auditory system cues such as alert sounds, system software (ShowBeeps) can be used to provide visual cues in place of auditory cues. Captioning is just beginning to be explored for audio streams or audio tracks of videos. CD manufacturers, in response to ADA legislation and educational buyers, are starting to provide text transcripts or captioning for audio. World wide web authors are becoming aware of the need to develop caption and file formats that accommodate a captioning track. Caption authoring packages are available to add multimedia, overlay captioning to computer-based video.

### Rate Enhancement or Literacy Supports

Major word processors have a variety of features that may enhance the user's input. For instance, abbreviation-expansion and spelling and grammar aids are a standard feature. Macros and templates are available, which allow the automation of tasks and keystroke input. Word prediction, word-completion predication and abbreviation-expansion software, with or without auditory feedback, help users who have slow keyboard input or difficulties with spelling.

### Mouse Alternatives and Replacements

Trackballs, joysticks, and various forms of tablets are frequently easier to control than a mouse. The mouse pointer may also be controlled using head movement, which is tracked with infrared or ultrasound technology. Buttons on many alternative-pointing devices can be programmed to perform a double click or to lock down the mouse button for a drag. Mouse buttons can be replaced with puff-sip switches and foot-pedal switches or with software that performs the mouse click, double click, and drag by lingering on a target for a predetermined time and then moving the mouse cursor in one of four directions.

The mouse pointer can be controlled using keys on the numeric keypad or on an onscreen keyboard. Mouse emulators exist for single switch users and users of voice recognition systems. These employ vector scanning strategies or grid systems to quickly focus on the target.

### Keyboard Modifications and Alternative

Free software or operating system modifications allow changes to be made to keyboard response by slowing response time, eliminating or slowing key repeat rate, and holding keys used in multiple key depressions when selected sequentially. Standard keyboards are also available with onboard memory for text or command macros. Mainstream keyboard alternatives include keyboards that are smaller, more ergonomically shaped, provide alternative keyboard layouts (e.g., DVORAK versus QWERTY), and have built-in trackballs or other mouse alternatives.

Specialized keyboards have been developed to accommodate a variety of individual needs. Miniaturized keyboards accommodate those with limited range of movement or strength. These may have mouse emulation as a built-in feature. Enlarged keyboards are more suited to those with poor motor control but with adequate range of movement. Programmable keyboards allow for customization of the keyboard layout (key content, key size) with individualized overlays depicting the key contents for the user. Keys may also be programmed with mouse emulation functions.

Numerous onscreen keyboard software programs allow the user to select keystrokes (letters, words, commands, phrases) using a mouse or mouse emulation. Word prediction is often available as a keyboard option to support literacy, limit fatigue, or improve speed.

### Switch Input

Switch input is also used to emulate keyboard and mouse functions. Single, dual, or three-switch input of Morse code can be translated by a hardware and/or software interface into keyboard and mouse input to the computer. Onscreen keyboards support a number of scanning strategies including the following:

1. Stop and continuous automatic scanning
2. Inverse scanning (in which a person holds a switch down to move the cursor, releases when the target is reached, and hits a second switch or waits to select)
3. Step scanning
4. Directed scanning (in which a person directs cursor movement by holding one of four directional switches)

Considerations when choosing a scanning onscreen keyboard include the presence of the following:

1. Strategies for controlling the desktop and manipulating windows
2. Methods of emulating the mouse
3. User-definable keyboard layouts
4. Integration of acceleration strategies such as abbreviation-expansion or word completion prediction

5. Context-sensitive keyboard layouts
6. Control of scan speed, initial delay, debounce time, and switch configurations

### Voice Recognition

Voice recognition of commands or text input is available with some operating systems. Voice recognition software is able to provide text input, mouse control, and software application control, including optional levels of vocabulary and macros for various professions or specialty groups.

Dictation systems have advanced to allow recognition of continuous speech rather than discrete recognition of one word at a time. Although voice models in the system allow the recognition of words without explicit training, users have their own voice model file that must be carefully "trained" to allow optimal recognition. Proper maintenance of the voice model requires vigilance to errors made by users and the system and proper correction of the errors. Most voice dictation systems have large dictionaries, but users must add proper names and specialized vocabulary. Several dictation systems rely on mouse control to control the desktop and dictation functions.

### Optimization of Alternative Access System

The alternative access system should be optimized to improve efficiency and to simplify control of application software. This is done by providing customized layouts for onscreen keyboards or alternative keyboards, supplying simple voice commands that perform frequently used functions for voice recognition systems, setting up a screen reader to automatically announce status or alert information when it appears, or similar customization routines.

## Configuring the General Computer System

When researching, evaluating, and choosing the computer system, the list of available features, model types, processor types, operating systems, and peripherals on the market may seem overwhelming. Remember to follow the user's needs and the desired functionality as a guide in making these decisions. Availability of compatible, chosen access systems is also an important consideration.

## Application Software

The list of desired functionality determines what application software is required. The user's cognitive skills and developmental level narrow the selection. Software should be chosen that is "access system friendly." This means that the software can be easily controlled by an alternative access system and makes available the information the access system needs. This is achieved by adhering to the following standard interface guidelines:

1. Presence of keyboard equivalents to perform all mouse actions
2. Ability to tab through controls in a dialog box in a consistent manner
3. Use of standard system controls rather than bitmapped images for dialog boxes, toolbars, and palettes.

The best way to determine whether a program is access system friendly is to thoroughly test all functions on that user's intended access system.

## Memory

The memory requirements are determined by the application software and access system. Software that involves the manipulation of graphic or audio files frequently requires large amounts of memory, as do recognition programs such as voice recognition systems and optical character recognition systems. More memory is also required if several applications are running simultaneously.

## Operating System

Presently available operating systems include the MacOS, Windows 98, Windows 2000 or ME, Windows NT, Linux, and Unix. The operating system chosen is partly determined by the alternative access system and the application programs selected. Because access system development lags behind the general market, the largest selection of alternative access systems are compatible with Windows 2000 and the MacOS, with Windows NT compatible access tools quickly catching up. The choice of operating system is also influenced by the systems most commonly available in the user's work, school, or home environment.

## Storage

In addition to the hard disk drive that should be large enough to accommodate all the application programs and user files required, a number of other storage mediums should be considered. Internal or external drives are needed to swap files between computers, install programs, and access reference material and backup material. The choices may include floppy disk drives, CD-ROM drives, tape drives, optical drives, and cartridge drives.

## Peripherals and Ports

Peripherals (i.e., printers, scanners) that are easy to manipulate and can be controlled primarily through software should be chosen. Automatic sheet feeding is preferable to manual sheet feeding if the client can scan materials independently or has large numbers of pages to scan at once.

The peripherals and access systems to be used determine the number and type of available ports required. These include parallel, serial, USB, and SCSI. The number of ports specified for the system is frequently not the number of available ports. For instance, serial ports could be already assigned to the mouse or an internal hard drive and would therefore not be available for a voice synthesizer.

## Display

If portability is not required, the bigger the display the better within the constraints of work surface space and budget. A larger display reduces the need to scroll windows, especially when using screen magnification. It also allows several applications or utilities to share the desktop, which is critical when using an onscreen keyboard. The faster the refresh rate, the easier finding the mouse cursor. For clarity and legibility, a higher resolution should be chosen.

## Networking and the Web

Frequently, computer systems are networked within a school or office environment to share files, access common resources, and use the Internet. The network determines the type of network interface in existence at the user's work place or school. Compatibility problems frequently arise among access system software and network software and hardware; therefore careful testing and configuration are required. The access system developer should be contacted for known incompatibilities and possible fixes.

For home systems, modem and communication software should be considered. The number of services and information resources available on the World Wide Web is growing. The advantages for people with disabilities are numerous. The Internet can be used to socialize, shop, bank, search for and publish information, request services, troubleshoot the computer system, take courses, and play games. Accessing these services through the Web removes the restrictions of time and place. Information over the Internet is also in electronic form and can therefore be magnified, spoken through text to speech, paged through, and printed in Braille much more easily than material on paper.

Choosing the fastest modem available is important because baud rate requirements are constantly increasing. The faster the baud rate, the shorter the online time and the lower the online costs. In addition to a modem and a communication software package, an Internet service provider (ISP) must be chosen. Local community guides exist that compare Internet service providers available in a local dialing area. If proprietary communication software is provided by the ISP, compatibility with the access system software and hardware should be carefully tested and the access system software should be optimized to control the software efficiently.

A helpful resource in choosing web browsing and authoring tools is the Web Accessibility Initiative, which produces guideline documents on Web access. The URL is http://www.w3.org/WAI.

## Central Processing Unit

The Central Processing Unit (CPU) chosen is largely determined by the Operating System (OS), the application software, the alternative access system, the peripherals, the display, the storage medium, the network hardware and software, and the memory requirements. Purchasing an established brand name system is best. Access and application hardware and software is frequently beta-tested only with the most common brand-name computers. The faster the processor speed, the better. If a slower processor speed is chosen because of cost, it should be upgradable to a faster processing speed when this becomes affordable or essential. The computer should have sufficient expansion bays, expansion slots, and memory sockets to allow upgrading as the user's needs change.

## Outcome and Social Validation

Generally, computer access technology improves the quality of life of users by enabling them to participate in normal educational, vocational, and recreational opportunities that would otherwise be precluded or limited by physical disabilities. The functional status of users is improved as they can become independent in performing common tasks such as writing, communicating via e-mail, researching, reading, etc. The costs of computer access technology are slowly decreasing, although the need for upgrades and modifications to suit changing needs result in ongoing equipment expenses. If the technology is applied successfully, the costs are easily justified by comparing them with the costs of paid assistance or long-term costs to society of an individual unable to obtain an education and employment. For employed people who acquire a disability, them being able to continue working using assistive technology is generally far more gratifying and far less costly to the employer than providing sick leave, disability pensions, and training for new employees.

Although many examples exist in clinical settings of users who improved their quality of life and functional status through computer access technology, limited documentation of outcomes exists in a way that is acceptable to increasingly business-oriented medical and funding agencies. Pressure is increasing to assess the outcomes of applying computer access technology to prove efficacy to third-party payers, service delivery funding agencies, consumers, and other payers.[3] A number of factors have made gathering objective data difficult. These include the lack of quantitative, non–laboratory-based measurement tools, the variance in the user population and environmental contexts, the variance in service delivery, and the multiple strategies and approaches to intervention used in assistive technology.[4] Published research has focused on more easily defined tasks such as comparing features of available commercial computer access technology or comparing tests by users without disabilities.[5,6]

User needs and impairments are individual, however, performance variables with computer input methods can be measured in terms of rate of text input and number of errors made in completing set tasks. Clinicians can compare input methods objectively using these measurements. These can be paired with observations and user reports of fatigue, discomfort, etc. Performance with the assistive technology of choice can then be compared with the use of an unadapted system in providing a rationale for funding agencies. These comparisons must take into consideration the learning curve that is required after introducing any new tool. The initial assessment can also incorporate user rated performance and satisfaction scores such as those used in the Canadian Occupational Performance Measure.[7] These can then be compared with scores obtained during subsequent reassessments. Compiling data on changes in user satisfaction/performance scores can support program evaluation. This can be supported by changes in objective data such as speed and accuracy and completeness of control of a computer system using the access technology. Consumer satisfaction questionnaires can also be used to support or improve programs.

The increasing use of technology in society, education, and the work force raises the acceptance of computer access technology by users, support teams, and environments. The increased use of computers in early education, for example, makes having equipment allocated and modified to support students with disabilities who need computer access technology easier. Technical changes enabling computer access tools to be developed as less expensive software modifications rather than as specialized hardware devices make them more affordable and practical to modify. This makes keeping up with corresponding changes in computer technology almost possible.

## CASE STUDIES

### CASE STUDY 1

#### Goal

S.H. was a humanities professor at a large urban university. At age 48, he was diagnosed with amyotrophic lateral sclerosis (ALS). His goals for computer access were to continue to teach, mark assignments, council students, exchange information with fellow academics and his department members, prepare and modify his lectures, and conduct research as long as possible. The goals for the computer access system were adaptation to his changing condition and to not have a substantial initial learning curve.

#### Functions, Abilities, Considerations, and Options

In response to his changing skills and goals, the computer access system was modified during a 2½-year period. Throughout the process, access system components were chosen that would require skills that could be transferred to access systems used at later stages.

When initially assessed, S.H. identified his major problems as difficulty controlling a mouse, poor control of a pen, difficulty handling books and papers, and fatigue when working at the computer for extended periods. Finger and wrist movement was well controlled, and larger arm movements were more difficult. Holding or gripping objects caused fatigue. A trackball that required primarily finger and wrist movement was used to replace the mouse. S.H. was taught keyboard shortcuts for several mouse actions. He was also tutored in more efficient control of the desktop and the most frequently used computer applications. A macro, abbreviation-expansion package was prescribed. His mailer was upgraded to a more efficient one that performed a number of the tasks automatically. He was also provided with a wrist rest, document holder, and book holder.

In anticipation of challenges in the future, a number of changes were made to his job tasks. Books or papers on the computer do not need to be handled, can be easily searched, can be read by a voice synthesizer, and can be annotated. S.H. was made aware of sources of electronic reference and research materials and electronic catalog tools. He was also referred to an electronic-text transcription service. The majority of his students had computers or access to computers and many also had access to e-mail. Instructions were prepared so that students could submit papers and assignments on disk or by e-mail. With assistance from academic computing staff and network staff at the university, a listserv was established for exchanging information between S.H. and his students and between the students themselves. This was later used to conduct tutorials.

Approximately 6 months later, his endurance and accuracy in using the standard keyboard had greatly deteriorated. He was loaned a miniature keyboard that required a reduced range of movement, reduced the pressure required to activate the keys, and optimized the keyboard layout to decrease the movement required between keys. The volume of his voice had declined, making delivery of lectures difficult. His lecture hall was modified to include a microphone and a computer projection panel. He was taught to prepare overheads and slides to clarify his lectures using an application called *Power Point.*

During the next phase, the range of movement of his wrist was further reduced as was his finger control. He was able to control an analog miniature joystick accurately with his index finger when modified with a thimble-like top. However, he was unable to keep the cursor over a target and activate a switch. Therefore targets were selected using a method called *dwell select,* in which the user holds the cursor over the intended target until a time threshold is reached. He was prescribed an onscreen keyboard with a keyboard layout that matched the miniature keyboard. He also purchased a portable computer with a voice synthesizer and voice utility to clarify his speech and converse with strangers.

During the next academic year, he reduced his job tasks to teaching one graduate course that did not require lectures. He also supervised thesis students and completed final editing of a book and two articles. He now had difficulty in targeting keys with the analog joystick. However, he was able to control the four directions of a miniature gated joystick with a similar thimble top. The selection method used with the onscreen keyboard was therefore changed to a quartering technique, whereby the keyboard was divided into four quarters, each of the quarters into four quarters, and each of these quarters into four quarters (Figure 7-1). S.H. would select a key by choosing the overall

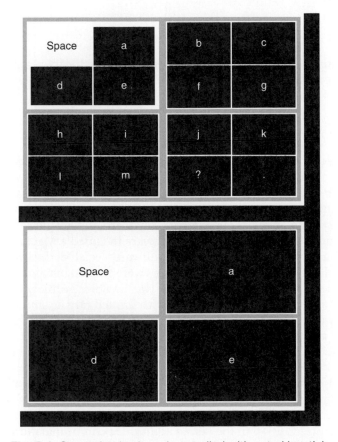

**Fig. 7-1** Quartering keyboard controlled with gated joystick.

quarter, then the subquarter, and then the sub-subquarter, using the four positions of the joystick. Word completion prediction was also added to the onscreen keyboard.

During the last 4 months before his death, S.H. could no longer control his index finger. His remaining voluntary movement was jaw opening and closing. He used automatic single switch scanning (and the same onscreen keyboard) to finish his writing, to communicate through e-mail, and to converse face-to-face with unfamiliar listeners.

## OUTCOME AND SOCIAL VALIDATION

As much as possible, new skills were introduced early when S.H.'s energy was least compromised. Tools requiring skills that could not be transferred to the next phase were avoided. He mastered each of the access systems introduced within a single teaching session and made steady gains in speed and accuracy until his physical condition deteriorated. With the introduction of each new access modification, his endurance and productivity improved in the short term.

Equipment that was required for a shorter time was loaned (i.e., the miniature keyboard, the wrist rest, the track ball). Despite his rapidly changing skills and needs, additions to S.H.'s computer were limited to the onscreen keyboard, two joysticks, one chin switch, and the mounting system. The most costly item was the portable computer with voice synthesizer.

With the assistance of alternative computer access, computer-mediated instruction, and computer-based text, S.H. was able to continue teaching until shortly before his death. He found that he conversed with more of his students using e-mail and the listserv than he had previously face-to-face. S.H. also felt that discussions were livelier, involving a greater proportion of the class. However, he found conversing with the voice synthesizer frustrating. He was not able to interject or claim his turn in academic debates. Conversing by e-mail or the listserv removed the time constraints of face-to-face communication, thereby allowing him to converse on a level playing field.

## CASE STUDY 2

### Goal

The problem addressed by this application was to provide flexible computer access and equipment to meet the developing physical skills and educational, literacy, and communication needs of a young child with the congenital condition called *cerebral palsy*.

### Function and Ability

C.O. was initially assessed for technology access at age 4. Computer access recommendations were given to his community team for single switch programs to develop motor control and letter recognition. Further assessment and equipment trials after 4 months of training resulted in the lease of a Macintosh LC II computer system with Ke:nx, several single switches and an expanded Unicorn keyboard and keyguard, and an Apple IIe emulator card and disk drive (Figure 7-2). Software included a Macintosh talking word processor, Intellitalk, Apple IIe early learning software (e.g., Charlie Brown's ABCs, First Letter Fun, etc.). His family and support workers were trained in running the system and programming overlays. The computer access was flexible, promoting concrete, direct upper extremity targeting for some software with limited targets, and training scanning skills with hand targeting of single switches for other software packages. Fluctuating muscle tone and reflexes affected C.O.'s motor control. The flexible access promoted development of motor control while operating fun, age-appropriate and educational software programs.

Other technology recommendations at that time were improved seating and a power wheelchair training program for the following summer, using a DU-it Armslot switch for power chair access with limited upper extremity control, which resulted in a power chair and seating prescription in the fall. In addition, a communication book with a variety of large targets that were spaced out for clarity of indicating choices and a low-tech

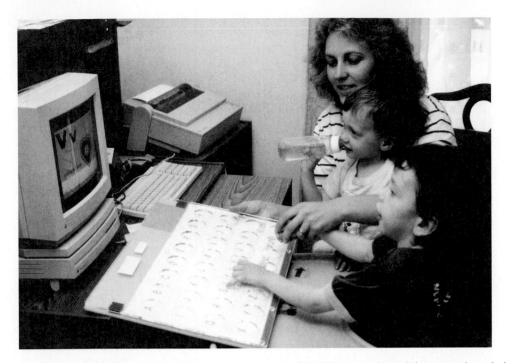

**Fig. 7-2** C.O. at 4½ years old. New Macintosh system with Unicorn keyboard, key guard, and alphabet overlay, with Mom and younger sibling.

switch-operated signaling aid for telling jokes, passing on news from nursery school, and greetings were suggested. For first grade the following fall, the use of a similar Macintosh system with a CD-ROM was also suggested.

Reassessment of physical access after 1 year indicated increased muscle tone after a growth spurt, increased prominence of an asymmetric tonic neck reflex, and increased athetosis that affected active movement patterns. Quantified computer access trials shown to C.O.'s parents and the support team demonstrated the greater effectiveness of using a switch accessed with head rotation for critically timed access needs such as scanning for face-to-face communication and letter input to the computer system. A Zygo lever switch and mount was added to his computer access set up, and his computer was upgraded to a Macintosh Performa 580CD to give adequate RAM and CD-ROM access for educational and reading programs. ClickIt software was added to the use of Ke:nx for single switch access to CD-ROMs, using programmable "hot spots" (Figure 7-3).

Other technology recommendations included the use of a portable Apple Powerbook system with Speaking Dynamically, Boardmaker, ClickIt, Ke:nx and a talking word processor, and Intellitalk for use at school for face-to-face and written communication. This system was accessed with the lever switch to obtain the best possible speed and accuracy needed for scanning. As he used the larger Armslot switch on his tray for driving, the Powerbook system was secured in its place on his tray for in-class or in-home sessions only, rather than always being available. C.O. continued to use his communication book and eye gaze for immediate communication needs.

By the following year, C.O. was demonstrating improved physical control, particularly of his right upper extremity. This was attributed to extensive driving practice with the arm-slot switch, maturation, excellent seating, and therapy. A gated, center-mounted joystick was introduced for driving, and after a training period, it was substituted for the Armslot switch. The new power chair access allowed for flexibility in mounting the portable computer system and new options for computer access using the joystick. Trials were next completed with Direct Point computer access technology, in which an interface allows the user to "drive" the computer cursor using the wheelchair control with a remote selection switch. This was successful, offering faster, more immediate access to face-to-face communication displays and an onscreen keyboard for computer access.

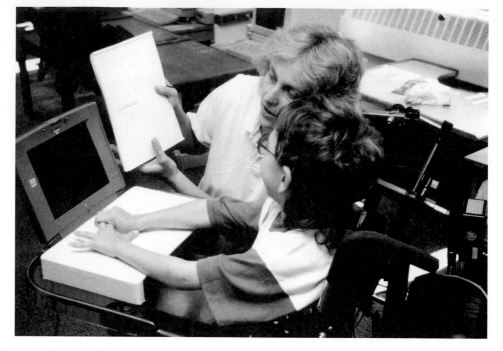

**Fig. 7-3** C.O. at 6 years old. Mounted head switch for scanning "hot spots" on reading CD-ROMs.

The head switch was still used for selecting targets once the mouse pointer dwelled over them, as this was faster and more accurate than selecting with a timed dwell setting (Figure 7-4). Because the Armslot switch was no longer positioned on the wheelchair tray, his portable computer system could be mounted with a modular bar and bracket to give him multiple work surfaces and improved ready access to his portable system. The Direct Point was used to access his stationary system for dedicated writing and literacy activities, and the portable system was used for face-to-face communication and portable writing needs.

## Considerations, Options, and Technology

Technology is available to support even young children with multiple disabilities; however, the funding and support systems need to be flexible to allow regular reassessments and changes of equipment to suit changes in physical status and educational and communication needs. Integration, compatibility, and overlap of training with systems used for communication and education need to be considered and promoted in choosing equipment.

## Outcome and Social Validation

The computer access equipment described supported this child through crucial formative years of development (from ages 4 to 8) and from nursery school to second grade in educational and communication content. The cost of the original computer system and access technology was approximately $3,000.00 (U.S. dollars); however, as he had rapidly changing needs, he was able to use a Province of Ontario leasing program. This provided flexibility and recycling of equipment as his needs for physical access and educational and communication material changed. As technology was also changing throughout this time, it supported the transition between the early use of Apple IIe software to Macintosh educational CD-ROMs 2 years later. The cost of his later system, the DirectPoint, Performa 5800, and so on was approximately $3500.00 (U.S. dollars). The access hardware was shared between the stationary and portable system. The changes in hardware, software, and access methods were justified by assessments that clearly demonstrated gains in speed and accuracy.

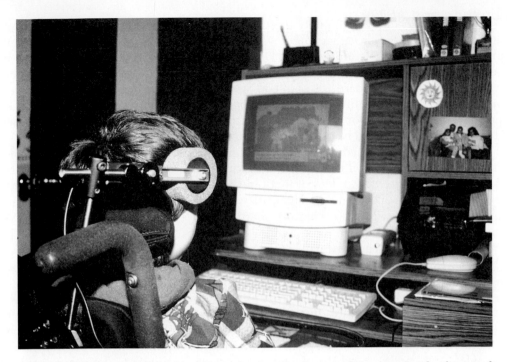

**Fig. 7-4** C.O. at 5½ years old. New Powerbook with single switch scanning for face-to-face communication and writing at school. Wood cover protects Powerbook keypad from food and abuse, giving him a place to rest his hand.

Changes were also made in response to the compatibility and computer input requirements of the school environment. This made the requests acceptable to the funding and leasing agency. The changes were accomplished through thorough discussion and consultation with the family, school staff, and support team, with documented rationale, resulting in full support by all concerned. The changes were also introduced sequentially to prevent overwhelming the user and support system with new technology for computer, mobility, and communication all at once.

C.O. was able to access technology for age-appropriate and grade-appropriate, written and face-to-face communication with minimal frustration because of his physical limitations.

The uncounted costs of not providing this progressive access technology and support would have been behavioral problems resulting from frustration, limited literacy and communication skills, and increasing dependence for any educational programming. In contrast, this child attends a regular school independently, with some teaching assistance support for his equipment and full opportunities to participate in classroom and home-learning opportunities. Although the equipment could not eliminate the limitations of severe physical impairments, his family members were pleased to have equipment available that minimized the limitations in mobility, communication, and writing and maximized his participation and learning opportunities.

## CASE STUDY 3

### *Goal*

D.L. was a high school student with an acquired long-term disability of C4 quadriplegia. He required a computer access system suitable for completing school work in high school and a postsecondary educational setting and writing at home. D.L. used Peach Tree controls for power mobility and supportive seating. Macintosh computers were available in the high school resource room and drafting classes; however, he and his family were technically adept in the use and support of IBM compatible systems.

## Function and Ability

The initial assessment in January 1990 was for access to a 386 IBM compatible system running WordPerfect 5.1 for home use. D.L. had good control of head and neck movement and speech. As voice recognition was financially unfeasible and limited in performance, a miniature keyboard with built-in Sticky Keys, the Bloorview Mini Keyboard, was prescribed for use with a mouth stick (Figure 7-5). This keyboard was a modified Sharp 360 pocket calculator and plugged into the keyboard port of the 386. It provided mouse emulation or could be used in conjunction with a trackball.

In 1991, this teenager had returned to a full high school program and found a voice-activated tape recorder ineffective for note taking. Reassessment indicated that a notebook computer, a new technology at that time, would have a small enough keyboard to be effective for note taking and in-class work with a mouth stick or could be paired with the use of a Bloorview Mini Keyboard. A Sharp PC 6641(40 MB hard drive, 4 MB RAM) was prescribed with a custom mount and wheelchair battery adapter (Figure 7-6). The notebook system lasted approximately 5 years. Recommendations were given to the high school staff who provided a Bloorview Mini and trackball for use with the Macintosh systems for drafting and other graphics needs.

D.L. enrolled in a large urban university after high school and was able to obtain Vocational Rehabilitation Services financial support for computer equipment at home to support his studies. At the onset of the migration from DOS to Microsoft Windows, he was able to upgrade his home system to Microsoft Windows 3.1, accessed with the Bloorview Mini and a trackball. When the Bloorview Mini was no longer available, a SpaceSaver keyboard was found as a replacement.

By 1996, D.L. was able to upgrade his home computer system to a Pentium running Windows 95 and accessed using Dragon Dictate voice recognition and/or the SpaceSaver keyboard and trackball (Figure 7-7). Use of voice recognition improved his speed of text input for writing and eased the demand on neck musculature, which was heavily used for driving and mouth stick access. A 21-inch monitor also decreased the need for accessing scroll bars and provided additional screen space for running multiple applications. At the university, a Pentium system was made available with Dragon Dictate for

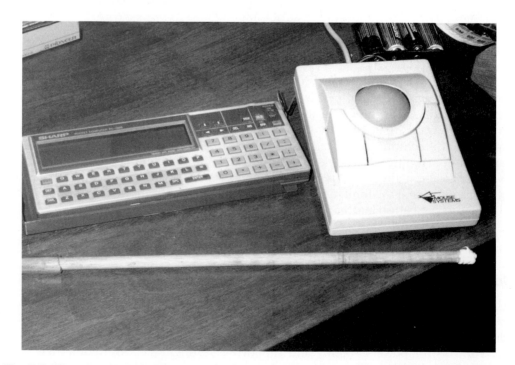

**Fig. 7-5** Bloorview Mini Keyboard, trackball, and mouth stick—client's original stationary computer access technology.

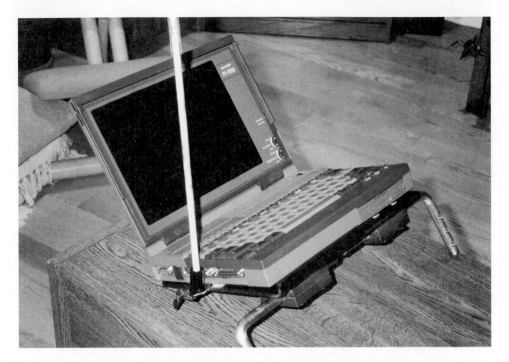

**Fig. 7-6** Sharp notebook computer with custom mount for access from power chair and mouth stick dock.

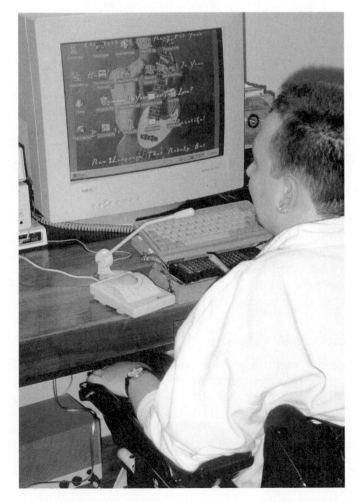

**Fig. 7-7** D.L. operating Pentium system with a mouth stick, using the trackball and SpaceSaver keyboard.

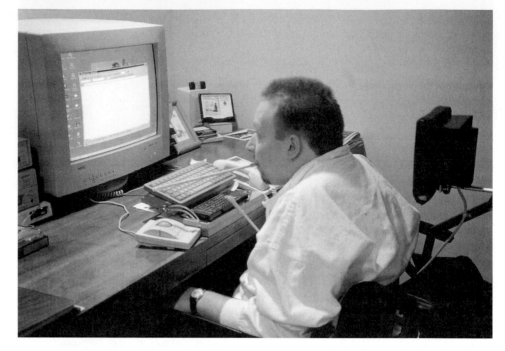

**Fig. 7-8** Tabletop microphone for text and mouse emulation using voice.

exam writing and onsite writing needs (Figure 7-8). The library was also modified to improve wheelchair access to the computer systems and to offer sticky keys and mouse control via the system keyboards.

## Considerations, Options, and Technology

Commercial and access technologies are changing rapidly. Addressing immediate needs with existing but state-of-the-art technology, while recognizing that it is not a permanent solution is important. Coordination with educational facilities and other areas of the user's environment is crucial to maximize the person's functioning in various environments and prevent the unrealistic expectation that one piece of technology meets all needs in all settings. Technical access solutions in the late 1980s and early 1990s often required custom fabrication of equipment such as mounting devices, battery adapters, or modification of commercially available products such as the Bloorview Mini. Current access technology can frequently be found in mainstream product lines or companies that produce a commercial product such as Dragon Dictate marketed to the mainstream and rehabilitation or disability markets.

## Outcome and Social Validation

Each technical solution met this person's existing needs; however, each solution eventually became inadequate as newer technology offered greater speed of access or compatibility with current software. The cost of the original Mini keyboard was $250.00 (U.S. dollars); the notebook system was $3,000.00 (U.S. dollars); and the custom mounting and power supply totaled $800.00 (U.S. dollars). The user's system in 1996 was a powerful, state-of-the-art Pentium with a large monitor and 32 megabytes of RAM, retailing at approximately $3500.00 (U.S. dollars). The classic edition of Dragon Dictate was obtained for $500.00 (U.S. dollars) and the Space Saver keyboard for $125.00 (U.S. dollars). The user was able to receive funding through provincial Ministry of Health equipment programs and Vocational Rehabilitation Services to support the equipment purchases over time.

Improvements in performance with each system were simple to document, as each system offered improved speed of text input and system control over the previous one or enabled D.L. to fulfill the normal scholastic demands that had previously been unmet. Successful outcomes could also be verified by surveying staff members at his educational facilities about his ability to complete standard course load requirements.

## References

1. Law M et al: The person-environment-occupation model: a transactive approach to occupational performance, *Can J Occup Ther* 63 (1):9-23, 1996.
2. Guerette P, Sumi E: Integrating control of multiple assistive devices: a retrospective review, *Assistive Technol* 6 (1):67-76, 1994.
3. DeRuyter F: Evaluating outcomes in assistive technology: do we understand the commitment? *Assistive Technol* 7 (1):3-8, 1995.
4. Smith R: Measuring the outcomes of assistive technology: challenge and innovation, *Assistive Technol* 8 (2):71-81, 1996.
5. Novak M, Klund J: If word prediction can help, which program do you choose? *Closing The Gap, Microcomputer Technology For People With Special Needs* 15 (3), August/September 1996.
6. Higginbothom DJ: The evaluation of keystroke efficiency for five augmentative and alternative communication technologies, *Augment Alternative Communication* 8 (4):258-272, 1992.
7. Law M et al: *Canadian occupational performance measure manual,* ed 2, Toronto, 1994, CAOT Publications ACE.

## Resources

*Case 2*
Ke:nx, single switches: alternative access interface for the Macintosh from Don Johnson, Inc.
1000 N. Rand Rd., Bldg. 115
PO Box 639
Wauconda, IL 60084-0639
Telephone: (800) 999-4660 (United States and Canada; (847) 526-2682 (United States and Global)
E-mail: djde@mcs.net
Website: http://www.donjohnston.com

Unicorn keyboard, Intellitalk, ClickIt software: expanded keyboard and software
IntelliTools, Inc.
55 Leveroni Ct., Suite 9
Novato, CA 94949
Telephone: (415) 382-5959 or (800) 899-6687
Fax: (415) 382-5950
Email: info@intellitools.com
Website: http://www.intellitools.com

Armslot switch controller
APT Technology, Inc.
DU-IT CSG, Inc.
236A N. Main St.
Shreve, OH 44676
Telephone: (330) 567-2001
Fax: (330) 567-3073
E-mail: apt2duit@valkyrie.net
Website: http://www.apt-technology.com

Zygo lever switch
Zygo Industries, Inc.
PO Box 1008
Portland, OR 97207-1008
Telephone: (800) 234-6006
E-mail: zygo@zygo-usa.com
Website: http://www.zygo-usa.com/

Zygo switch mounting
David Cooper
Sunnyhill Health Centre for Children
3644 Slocan St.
Vancouver, BC, V5M 3E8, CANADA
Telephone: (604) 436-6527

Boardmaker speaking dynamically
Mayer-Johnson Co.
PO Box 1579
Solana Beach, CA 92075-1579
Telephone: (619) 550-0084
E-mail: MayerJ@aol.com
Website: http://Mayer-Johnson.com/

Direct Point
Jerzy Antczak
Bloorview MacMillan Centre
350 Rumsey Rd.
Toronto, ON M4G 1R8, CANADA
Telephone: (416) 425-6220
E-mail: ortcja@oise.utoronto.ca
Website: http://www.oise.utoronto.ca/~ortcklt/products.htm

## Resources

*Case 3*
SpaceSaver keyboard
Datalux Corporation
155 Aviation Drive
Winchester, VA 22602
Telephone: 1-800-datalux; (540) 662-1500
Fax: (540) 662-1682
E-mail: sales@datalux.com
Website: http://www.datalux.com/keyboards.html

Dragon Dictate, Classic Edition
Dragon Systems, Inc.
320 Nevada Street
Newton, MA 02160
Telephone: (800) talk type; (617) 965-5200
Fax: (617) 527-0372
E-mail: info@dragonsys.com
Website: http://www.dragonsys.com

## General Resources for Computer Access Products and Information

Abledata, a searchable database of assistive technology products and disability-related resources
Website: http://www.abledata.com/index.htm

The Adaptive Technology Resource Centre at the University of Toronto, Canada
Website: http://www.utoronto.ca/atrc/
This site includes a listing of computer access equipment.
Website: http://www.utoronto.ca/atrc/tech/techgloss.html

A resource for outcome measures in assistive technology is also supported by the ATRC at:

The Alliance for Technology Access (ATA), a network of community-based resource centers dedicated to providing information and support services to children and adults with disabilities and increasing their use of standard, assistive, and information technologies. Information on assistive technology and service providers in the United States can be found on their site.
Website: http://www.ataccess.org/

Apple Computer has a listing of access features, software to download, and third-party hardware and software for Macintosh computers
Website: http://www.apple.com/disability/welcome.html

Microsoft lists assistive technology products available for Windows environments
Website: http://www.microsoft.com/enable

Sun has a resource page on Java and Unix access
Website: http://www.sun.com/access

Trace Research and Development Center at the University of Wisconsin
Website: http://trace.wisc.edu/
Their site includes a computer access program with information on freeware and shareware
Website: http://trace.wisc.edu/world/computer_access/multi/sharewar.html
"Typing Injury FAQ: Alternative Keyboards & Accessories" by K.S. Wright and D.S. Wallach (1997) has sources and images of a variety of keyboards and pointing devices
Website: http://www.tifaq.org/

RESNA's Special Interest Group on Computer access has a website and listserv information
Website: http://www.resna.org/sigs/sig11/resourc.htm
WebABLE! includes a web directory for disability-related Internet resources and a searchable accessibility database
Website: http://www.webable.com

Web Accessibility Initiative. The World Wide Web Consortium initiative to promote an accessible Web
Website: http://www.w3.org/WAI

# CHAPTER 8

# Information Technologies

*Peggy Barker*

## Application and Goal

Information technologies are significantly changing lives. New technologies, devices, machines, and services that make dealing with more information than ever before possible surround everyone. Information networks and services are available that can connect everyone and provide new opportunities for productivity, learning, and entertainment. The technologies include accessing information through computers, the Internet, telephones, pagers, cellular phones, television sets, and public electronic kiosks.

These information technologies include electronic methods of communicating and accessing databases that allow us to bank, shop, pay bills, get books to read, and make travel plans and arrangements from home. They make telecommuting possible and provide more options for running a business from home. Many job functions can be easily performed when access to needed information resources and telecommunication services are provided. Access to multimedia educational materials on CD-ROM or the World Wide Web (WWW) give students experiences that were never possible before and are available by using a computer anywhere. Courses and degree programs are also offered electronically and make it possible for people to participate without having to leave their homes or communities. These information technologies are also a great source of entertainment such as "surfing the web" to learn and share more about hobbies, places, and people and playing the latest multimedia games.

Importantly, these technologies have the potential to serve all people. Information technologies are flexible and have the potential to be accessible to anyone who can understand their use. People with vision, hearing, physical, and cognitive limitations should be able to use information technologies. This is most often achieved with adaptive hardware, software, and services that can be added to personal and public equipment such as telephones, computers, and kiosks. The designers of information technologies should also address the needs and abilities of people with disabilities by adding features that facilitate accessibility. This can be achieved through more widespread use of universal design in which as many people as possible including people with disabilities use these specially designed products. Currently, universal design is being incorporated into the design of many but not all Web pages and into the design of publicly accessed equipment such as electronic kiosks.

Information technologies are also affecting how services to people with disabilities are provided. Programs, databases, and electronic text on CD-ROM and the Internet are valuable resources for becoming more aware of the technology that is available and how it is being used. Consumers and service providers can use the Internet to brainstorm their assistive technology questions and problems with others around the world and can obtain current information from manufacturers.

## Function and Ability

People with disabilities need to be supported in manipulating data and related information resources to take advantage of the wide variety of functional opportunities offered by information technologies.[1] Because they are computer-based and electronic devices, they offer a great deal of flexibility for the human/technology interface, the processor, environmental interface, and activity output. Because of the many possible combinations of these assistive technology components, the needs of many different consumers can be met.[2]

For people with physical disabilities, the physical aspects of writing, turning pages, or picking up the phone handset can be eliminated with information in an electronic form. Alternative input or control devices for the keyboard, mouse, and/or telephone functions need to be addressed, as should input strategies such as onscreen keyboards and word prediction that can increase the effectiveness of the input devices.

People with vision impairments are not able to take advantage of the visual feedback provided by screens on personal computers and electronic information kiosks (e.g., ATMs). Individuals with blindness can use synthesized speech and refreshable Braille. For people with low vision, enlarged text and high contrast displays can be useful. For phone use, messages retrieved from voice mail are definitely preferred to handwritten messages.

People with hearing impairments are functionally limited when information is presented auditorily. This becomes a problem with telecommunication equipment. Telephone devices for the deaf (TDDs), amplification devices, handwritten communications, typing to others using a computer, e-mail, language interpreters, American sign language, and fax are the alternatives.

For people with cognitive impairments, the content may be the barrier and may need to be presented differently. Printed material can be read or spoken or presented as symbols or graphics. Personal web pages can be individualized to show less information at a time or may be used with a browser that allows the user to scroll through the links.

## Considerations, Options, and Technology

### Clinical Considerations

One of our greatest responsibilities for clinicians is to ensure consumer education regarding not only the technology but also the skills needed to find personally useful or relevant information. Consumers must be involved in the process of determining which technology is the most useful and best addresses their abilities, goals, and environments. Through information technologies, access to a proliferation of electronic data is now possible. People are accustomed to using the telephone to get information but are not necessarily familiar with the opportunities to get and organize information using electronic mail (e-mail), online news services, and databases. Many people are not aware of the options for telephone access and use and fewer still understand Internet access and applications.

Principles that apply to the implementation of other assistive technologies also apply to information technologies. Some include the following:

- Identifying and providing the appropriate tools and strategies to accommodate people's abilities and goals is fundamental to achieving accessibility.
- The adaptive technology and information technologies should be tried before purchase. Buying a computer or an adaptive device because it worked for someone else does not justify the purchase.
- Training often needs to include not only the operation of the adaptive equipment but also the strategies and skills required to effectively use the information technologies.

Access to information technology throughout a person's day can greatly enhance productivity, independence, and quality of life. The environment people are in and the equipment they are relying on for position (i.e., sitting, lying, standing) needs to be considered. This can have a great effect on the ability of people and reduces some of the dependency on caretakers. For example, a person who spends a great deal of time in bed and in a wheelchair should have input devices and strategies for both of these positions so that access to these technologies occurs from the wheelchair and the bed. Many people get a head start on the day working from bed or continue to work, communicate, or be entertained into the night using telecommunication equipment and information technologies.

## *Technology*

### Access to the Phone

TDDs, often referred to as *teletypewriters (TTYs)*, are frequently thought of for people with hearing impairments to access the telephone (see Chapter 12). Many people with speech impairments also use them. Most TDDs are operated with a keyboard, with the user typing each message letter by letter and reading a text message on a screen.

Many other alternatives are available that include telephone services and features better addressing the abilities of people with vision, physical, cognitive, and speech impairments (Table 8-1).[3] For example, several options exist for answering, hanging up, and dialing the telephone for people with physical impairments. The most basic solution is a speakerphone adapted with a single switch. The user answers the phone by pressing the switch when the phone rings and can dial out by talking to an operator who then connects the user with the receiving party. A more sophisticated system addressing the needs of a person with physical (manipulation) and speech impairments might include features to dial phone numbers, speed dialing, an introductory message, and speech feedback for scanning through each of these functions.

Equipment distribution and loan programs and telephone services are available in each state of the United States to ensure that consumers have access to the telephone.[4] In addition to the regular services available to telephone company customers, relay services are available for use by people with disabilities. People with hearing and/or speech impairments who use devices that provide information in an electronic format such as a TDD or a computer with modem can communicate to people without TDDs through relay services. Relay operators, equipped with TDDs and computers, relay the typed and spoken messages in the appropriate mode to the sending and receiving parties.

Speech-to-speech relay services are available in some states for people with speech that is difficult to understand or who use speech output from an augmentative communication device or computer.[5] Trained operators translate speech that is difficult to understand by unfamiliar listeners or provide a real voice for someone that relies on synthesized speech. Many people attempting to use synthesized speech to initiate a telephone conversation have reported that unfamiliar receivers hang up on them either because of the time delay required to create a message or the receiver's lack of tolerance of a machine voice. Speech-to-speech relay services address this problem but are often not used by people primarily because many of these individuals are not accustomed to telephone communication. People with speech impairments have not had tools to use the phone and therefore have not relied on its use or developed the skills associated with using the telephone. When implementing adaptive tools for telephone use, as with many other AT devices, training in the functional use must be included.

Other relay options are available.[3] Voice carry over (VCO) is an option for people with a significant hearing loss and is used with a telephone with a text screen. The user is able to talk to the other person. When the other person talks, an operator types back the words that are being said. Another option is hearing carry over (HCO) for people with speech impairments. The user types messages using a TTY, also known as a *TDD*, which are relayed by the operator. The user is able to listen to the other person.

### Wireless Phones

Wireless, cellular, or mobile telephones facilitate mobile or remote access to telecommunication networks. For people with disabilities, wireless phones can contribute to inde-

## TABLE 8-1

*Telephone Features and Services for People with Impairments*

| IMPAIRMENT | FEATURES† | SERVICES |
|---|---|---|
| Physical: mobility | Speakerphone<br>Remote access (i.e., wireless) from another device (i.e., electronic aid for daily living) | |
| Physical: manipulation | Telephone headset or speakerphone for hands-free calls<br>Cordless phone<br>Remote speakerphone<br>Speech dialing<br>Redial the last number dialed<br>Access from another device (e.g., computer, augmentative communication device)<br>Single switch access including:<br>  Speakerphone<br>  Independent dialing for all keys including * and #<br>  Quick access to a "help" phone number<br>  Redial of last phone number<br>  Dial prestored phone numbers<br>  Phone number storage with additional numbers (password or social security number)<br>  Visual display of choices<br>  Auditory beep with scan<br>  Auditory presentation of choices (choices spoken)<br>  Adjustable scan speed | |
| Vision | Large button phone<br>Cordless or speakerphone<br>Speed dialing/prestored numbers | |
| Hearing: hard of hearing | Volume control/amplification<br>Loud telephone ring<br>Flashing light for telephone ringing | |
| Hearing: deaf | TDD<br>VCO telephones<br>Flashing light for telephone ringing | Telephone relay service<br>VCO |
| Speech | Speech amplifier<br>Artificial larynx<br>TDD | Speech-to-speech<br>Three-way calling with assistance from a familiar third party<br>HCO |
| Cognitive | Memory dialing<br>Speech dialing<br>Speakerphone with visual display of numbers dialed | Three-way calling with assistance from a familiar third party |

*Based on Maryland Relay Brochure: Thousands keep in touch through Maryland, 1999, The Deaf and Disabled Telecommunications Program, http://www.mdrealy.org/graphic_htm/General.html. TDD, telephone devices for the deaf; VCO, voice carry over; HCO, hearing carry over.*
*†Other features that should be considered include battery backup and support for other phone company services (i.e., call waiting, message indicator).*

pendence and safety. Several models have features that meet or can be adapted to meet the needs of users with disabilities, including the following[6-9]:

- Tactile feedback from buttons
- Nibs on "5" key for centering hand
- One-touch dialing for prestored phone numbers
- Large programmable memory for numbers, prestored messages, and incoming messages
- Auto answer-to-answer calls without having to press the send button (after a few rings the phone automatically connects with the caller)
- Audio cues for functions
- Uniquely shaped keys for touch identification of functions
- Larger keypad buttons
- Headset jack for external audio output using a speaker or headset with microphone and personal speaker enabling hands free conversation
- Bright and backlit displays to enhance visibility
- Visual displays to indicate phone functions in use
- Oversize display screen to support larger visual display of information as well as features including zoom displays (to change size of text and amount of text displayed)
- Vibrating ringer (instead of ring to announce incoming caller)
- Hearing aid compatibility
- Send and receive text messages
- Wireless modem that can be used to send and receive email messages from the cellular phone as well as an attached laptop computer
- TTY (TDD) compatible

Basically, of the two general types of cellular telephones, analog and digital, the digital phones are the newer technology and offer better quality sound but are not available in as many locations. Some cellular phones may not be compatible with hearing aides; some digital phones may cause a buzz when held close to some hearing aides. Multiple digital technologies are available, so a person with a hearing impairment should try each to determine which format works best. Other features that may be useful include volume control and a built–in t–coil coupling capability that works with telecoil-equipped hearing aids.

## Pagers

The traditional pagers receive phone numbers or numeric messages originating from a telephone. However, pagers are available with many more features that may be useful to people with disabilities, including the following[7-11]:

- Two-way paging
- Text messages
- One-touch call back to press one button or key to respond to a page
- Message origination from not only a phone call but also from faxes, Internet e-mail, and telephone dispatch service (a person who receives or hears the message over the telephone and sends the text to the pager)
- Computer interface (i.e., RS-232, IR data port) for message construction and downloading messages

A pager with two-way alphanumeric messaging can be considered for individuals not able to use a cellular phone because of a hearing, physical, cognitive, and /or speech impairment. For example, an individual who is not able to use the pager keyboard or read the display could use a laptop computer or an augmentative communication device (with RS-232) with appropriate accommodations (e.g., screen reading, alternate input tools and techniques) interfaced to a two–way, text–messaging pager with a computer interface for mobile communication.

## The Internet

The Internet, also known as the *World Wide Web (WWW)*, is made up of thousands of interconnected computer systems around the world. People using the Internet can exchange mail and files created with a computer and are able to search for information and use a variety services. E-mail (electronic mail) is a basic Internet function, in which an Internet account is needed to exchange text messages with anyone else with an Internet account. Files can be sent with or attached to an e-mail message and then opened with an appropriate application (i.e., word processor, spreadsheet, or database). The other primary Internet function is interacting with computers on the Internet to search for information or use one of the many available services (Table 8-2). Browser software (e.g., Microsoft Explorer, Netscape Navigator, Opera) is used to interact with websites that contain text, pictures, movies, sound, files, and an overwhelming amount of information.

## Connecting to the Internet

Typically, a personal computer, a modem, an account with an Internet service provider (ISP), and Internet software is needed to use the Internet. When users are planning to only use e-mail, almost any computer works. Appliances also are used just to send and receive e-mail.[12]

More people are discovering that the WWW is an extremely useful tool and provides a great deal of entertainment. However, computers that process data fast and have sufficient memory (RAM) and hard disk space are required.[14] The computer using a Windows operating system should have at least a 486 processing chip. If the computer is a Macintosh, it should have a 68040 processing chip or better. Processing speeds of 100 MHz or better is desirable. A bare minimum of 16 MB RAM is needed to use most of the graphics and sound on the WWW. At least 5 MB of hard disk space is needed for the software. More hard disk space is needed if the user is planning to save retrieved items from the Internet. These guidelines are minimal. Many resources available on the WWW are requiring more speed and memory.

The modem connects the computer to the Internet using a phone line. Modems can either be packaged as an internal component of the computer or can be offered in an external box that plugs into one of the serial ports on the computer. The speed of the modem should be 56 Kbps (Kilobytes per second) although older modems with speeds of 14.4 Kbps and 28.8 Kbps work. These modems are used with standard dial up (modem dials a phone number, preferably local, to connect to the Internet) analog (standard telephone transmission method) services to connect to the Internet.

Many phone companies and other ISPs are offering integrated services digital network (ISDN) and digital subscriber line (DSL) services using standard telephone lines that allow for transmission rates of 128 Kbps and 384 Kbps to 1.5 Mbps (i.e., 10 to 50 times faster than a standard analog service), respectively. ISDN, a dial-up service, requires an ISDN service using the phone lines, an ISDN modem, and an ISP that accepts ISDN. DSL requires a DSL service using the phone lines to make a permanent connection to the ISP and a DSL modem. The DSL Internet connection is always on so that no need exists to dial into the service as with an analog or ISDN service. ISDN and DSL should be considered when a person is spending a great deal of time searching for and/or downloading information from the Internet because these are faster and more efficient. DSL should only be considered if Internet access is from one location only. The Internet connections at universities or commercial locations are often much faster because they use a connection that does not rely on telephone lines.

An ISP provides a connection to the Internet and a variety of services. The most basic services are access to e-mail only. E-mail services can be found that are free. Most ISPs provide several services including e-mail, transferring files, database searching, and browsing the WWW. They also provide space to store web pages. The cost of a connection to the Internet depends on the available services, time connected to the Internet, and geographic location. A telephone number (for analog and ISDN services) is needed when using the Internet. To avoid long-distance calls, use an ISP that offers local tele-

## TABLE 8-2

*Internet Application and Location*

| INTERNET APPLICATION | WHERE TO FIND THE INFORMATION |
|---|---|
| Banking: check balances, check cleared checks, transfer funds between accounts, bills paid electronically | Work with local bank to determine Internet access availability. Bank should provide an Internet address and a password to access the account. |
| Travel: find places that are wheelchair accessible, travel agents that specialize in travel packages, or tours for people with disabilities, airplane flights. Make reservations for air travel, hotels, cars, etc. | Travel agencies, airlines, and other travel services have websites, found with a search engine. |
| News | Available in online newspapers (request news in only areas of interest) |
| Borrowed assistive technology equipment from a loan library | Available on "Check it Out" websites (e.g., http://www.check-it-out.org) |
| Trial or sample software program | Available from software manufacturers. See sites that list links to manufacturers |
| Taxes | Complete electronically available tax forms available from the IRS website. Use tax software to help through the process of filling out the tax forms and then submit them electronically. Ask the IRS about tax laws. |
| Shopping | Electronic shopping malls and many companies selling almost anything have an electronic storefront (i.e., website) |
| Grocery shopping | Local food chains offer online services to select items that can be delivered to a home. |
| Movie reviews, local movie listings and times | Search for websites with the name of the movie or the distributor of the movie. |
| City information including services and latest city council meeting minutes | Specific city websites |
| Local school information including lunch menus, homework assignments and school calendars | Specific school websites |
| Weather | Newspaper and the National Weather Service's websites |
| Send electronic cards that are animated | Internet card companies may provide this service free. |
| Job searches | Company information and classified ads |
| Learn to effectively use the internet | ISP websites |

*Adapted from Trace Research and Development Center: Access to current and next-generation information systems by people with disabilities, 1997, http://www.trace.wisc.edu/docs/access_info_ss/full_doc.html. ISP, Internet service provider.*

phone numbers. Some ISPs, often referred to as *commercial providers,* offer an 800 number or local phone numbers for a wide range of geographic locations and service packages that include their own software.

Internet software is needed to connect to the ISP, to get online, and to have access to the resources. ISPs often provide software that is configured to work with their services. Many companies that offer connection to the Internet require software for e-mail and for using the WWW. The basic programs are often free but for more features, programs are available from software distributors.

The software has the greatest effect on whether a service is usable to a person with a disability. E-mail is text based and can be read with a screen reader or can be copied and pasted into a word processor that has voice output.

The software used to access the WWW is referred to as a *browser*. Browsers are used to display files created in hypertext. Hypertext files include tags used to format the document and links. A *link* is a line or a graphic that connects with another section of a document or with an entirely different document. Hypertext is used because browsers in all platforms including Unix, MacOS and Windows can read it. Many browsers are available.[15] A few text-based browsers exist such as Lynx[13,16] but most including the popular Netscape Navigator and Microsoft Internet Explorer are used with graphical user interfaces (GUIs) such as MacOS and Windows. The GUI-based browsers typically require a person to point and click with a mouse to the desired selections or links.

Tools used for mouse control are used to make selections with a browser (see Chapter 7). User preferences can be set with many of the browsers. These can include changing the font and font size, the color of the text and/or background, whether images download automatically, whether the toolbars show, and which website or page the browser loads on startup. The most recently introduced browsers for GUIs are including keyboard equivalents for the operation of a browser. This makes using many of the available computer access tools possible, in which the user can make selections using input devices including alternate keyboards, a single switch with scanning, voice recognition, and Morse code.

The WWW is being designed as a multimedia tool depending on browsers that can incorporate graphics, sound, and video. For people with visual impairments, screen magnification and screen-reading software can be useful. Screen-reading programs are most effective with Web pages that have been provided in a text-only alternative version. Many screen readers cannot interpret the graphics on a standard web page unless the author of the page has created "Alt" tags with descriptions of the graphics and the user has set the browser preferences so that the images are not downloaded. Several recently introduced browsers provide auditory access to web pages while leaving the graphics intact. This is useful not only to people with vision impairments but also those who have difficulty reading.

For people with learning disabilities who would benefit from having the text read, screen readers are useful. Again, the graphics can be difficult for screen readers to interpret, but several of the newer screen reading systems can read a web page leaving the graphics intact. The user can also copy the text from the browser and paste it into word processors with built-in speech output.

Several browsers with adaptive features can facilitate accessibility.[17] Internet Explorer has built-in hooks that work with Windows 95-based screen readers. A talking Internet browser, pwWebSpeak, provides speech and enlarged video output, which is useful to individuals with visual impairments, those with learning disabilities who find reading text difficult, and those with physical impairments using alternative input devices to scan and select the links. It does not require a separate screen-reader program for the speech output. Users can scan through the pages by word, sentence, paragraph, or links.

Several products are being developed with an external standard connector than can be used to connect alternate displays and/or alternate input devices. For example, many devices include an infrared receiver and/or transmitter that can be operated with a remote control. Other devices such as the TV Internet terminal made by Philips Magnavox and Sony that are used to access the Internet with TV and telephone lines (without a computer), can be operated using devices plugged into its standard keyboard jack. Any adaptive keyboards designed for use with a computer with a PS/2-type connector can be used to operate these TV Internet terminals. Keyboard equivalents for all functions are available using a remote control that comes with the TV Internet terminal.

## Using E-mail, Listservs, and Newsgroups

E-mail is an efficient communication tool and eliminates many of the difficulties associated with trying to reach people by telephone. E-mail can also be used to send the same message to a group of people on a list. A *listserv* is a server with a mailing list whose members are interested in the same topics. Professional, service, and educational organizations have listservs. The listserv is subject-interest or group-interest oriented. The University of Toronto's Assistive Technology Resource Centre's website has an excellent list of listservs related to assistive technology and rehabilitation. *Newsgroups* are bulletin boards to which e-mail can be sent and posted. Other Internet users can then go to the bulletin board to read the posted messages. These are being incorporated into many websites. People ask questions and then anyone visiting the website can make a comment or suggestion.

## Electronic Text

Books and other written materials have been made available in "electronic text" (e-text). E-text can be found as hypertext, ASCII (e.g., files ending in .txt), as compressed binary files (e.g., files ending in .zip) at several websites, or are available on disk or CD-ROM. Scanners with optical character recognition (OCR) software can be used to convert regular text into e-text. The e-text in ASCII or compressed files can be opened in a word processor to be read. This eliminates the need to turn pages. It can also be opened in a program that speaks the text with either a talking word processor such as Write Out:loud and Intellitalk or opened in a word processor with a screen-reading program such as JAWS or Outspoken (see Chapter 7).

Hypertext is a strategy for presenting information in small amounts that are then connected to more information. Hypertext transport protocol (HTTP) is the language used with hypertext so that the files created for the web are cross platform (i.e., a browser can read them). Instead of reading text in rigid, linear structure (such as a book) with files in hypertext, users can easily skip from one point to another, get more information, go back, jump to other topics, and navigate according to current interest.

The e-text files are downloaded to a computer from the computer with the stored files. Files are generally found in ASCII or they are compressed. If they are compressed, a program is needed to decompress them. Electronic text is available for several resources on the Internet including the Project Gutenberg Library (http://www.promo.net/pg/). This particular resource includes the following on its website:

- Light literature such as *Alice in Wonderland, Peter Pan,* or *Aesop's Fables*
- Heavy literature such as the *Bible* and other religious documents, works by Shakespeare, *Moby Dick,* and *Paradise Lost*
- References such as Roget's thesaurus, almanac, encyclopedia sets, and dictionaries
- Links to other sites with e-text

Operation manuals for technology are notoriously difficult to understand. Use of electronic formatted material on disk, CD-ROM, or the Internet can address this issue. Searching for information is difficult when the material cannot be read because of visual or cognitive impairments or when pages cannot be turned because of physical impairments. Documentation in an electronic format can be easier to use as long as a computer is available and accessible. The electronic formatted material, preferably in ASCII, can be used across platforms more readily and converted to Braille, large print, or speech output. It is also much easier to search for information when it is in an electronic form rather than hard copy.

## Electronic Kiosks

Electronic kiosks are public information systems used to get information, find places, make purchases, and/or perform transactions.[1,18] ATMs, maintained by banks and other financial organizations, facilitate financial transactions including depositing and withdrawing funds, paying bills, and transferring funds between accounts. Many people have become dependent on the always-available ATMs and never go into a bank. Kiosks are being used in different places including airports, hotels, shopping malls, buildings, and universities for a variety of other applications. They provide all kinds of information and services. Many of the kiosks include a touch screen and GUIs that are designed to be user friendly but pose many access issues for people with disabilities. They tend to be difficult to use by people with visual or motor impairments and often are not accessible by wheelchair users. Kiosk design is being addressed so that they are more universally accessible. A kiosk is currently being evaluated in the Mall of America in Minneapolis, which has input options available for people with visual and physical impairments.

## Outcome and Social Validation

Implementation of information technologies and the appropriate accommodation tools promote communication and productivity and ensure access to needed information. Increased interaction, access to information, and independence in the activities can be measured.

In education, students are able to independently use more reading materials and reference materials, are able to exchange information with other students and experts around the world, have access to information about the world and what is occurring, and are more prepared to participate in the global economy that has developed because of the information technologies.

To address daily living needs, information technologies are instrumental in getting more information and providing a means for doing activities independently such as shopping for groceries or gifts, banking, filling out and filing tax forms, and making travel plans. Independence in these activities is cost effective.

In the work environment, as most companies have discovered, communication with co-workers and customers is enhanced with the use of the Internet and internal intranets or networks. Access to all kinds of information for all employees is essential. The information technologies also make working from home possible. Working from home everyday may not be desirable, but those days that are spent working from home can reduce the costs associated with employees having to get to work and function in that environment. These technologies also increase opportunities for home-based businesses.

## CASE STUDIES

### CASE 1

### *Student with Speech and Physical Disabilities*

#### APPLICATION AND GOAL

A 17-year-old student with cerebral palsy had spent the first 12 years of his life at home and then attended a segregated school until he turned 16. At 16, he began taking adult education classes in academics and computer applications. One of the needs identified by the student and his educational team was to become more familiar with the world outside of his home and school. One of the major concerns was that his concept of the world was too limited and therefore limited his perceived personal options.

#### FUNCTION

The student used an augmentative communication device (ACD) (Prentke Romich Company Liberator with Word Strategy and MIKE), a keyboard emulator to connect the ACD to a computer (Prentke Romich Company T-TAM), and a computer with a CD-ROM. These tools facilitated writing and mouse emulation. Using the Liberator keyboard, the student was able to navigate a GUI without being able to use a mouse. He was using the system for face-to-face communication and writing.

The student used the Liberator for 4 years and learned word strategy quickly then developed literacy skills that facilitated spelling, reading, and writing. He wrote a book about his experience of moving to the United States from Mexico.

## CONSIDERATIONS AND TECHNOLOGY
At the time of this writing, the school that he attends is not yet wired for the Internet but one of the classrooms has a telephone. A free e-mail account was acquired for this student and the Internet account at the school was made available to him.

## OUTCOME AND SOCIAL VALIDATION
The student began to communicate with others on a listserv of other augmentative communication users and uses e-mail to maintain contact with pen pals. He was also able to use CD-ROM on the computer system for reading and reference materials. He uses the WWW to explore the world and learn more about local resources.

## CASE 2

### *Single Switch User*
## APPLICATION AND GOAL
The user was successfully using a single switch with a communication device and a computer system. She was able to use the switch with only one of these devices at a time. The following needs were identified:

- Independent and efficient computer use for writing and Internet access
- Independent control of TV/cable, VCR, garage door, telephone, and house lights
- Integration of equipment to optimize use of a single switch for independence in using all systems

The components of the existing system did not have features that facilitated integration for the use of a single switch.

## FUNCTION
Two issues were addressed with information technologies. The first was that the service provider used the Internet to discover whether any products were available that could be used with the single switch to select and operate the several devices needed by the user.

The other issue was access to the telephone and to the Internet with a single switch.

## CONSIDERATIONS AND TECHNOLOGY
Abledata and other assistive technology databases were searched to find the desired switch output selector and to determine which manufacturers might make similar products. An available product was not identified but several manufacturers were identified that produced similar products. The manufacturer's representatives were contacted by e-mail and telephone to identify a product with the desired features. E-mail describing the problem was sent to the RESNA rehabilitation engineering professional specialty group listserv and the inquiry was sent to a service on a website in North Carolina that addresses assistive technology implementation strategies on the Internet. From these resources, several people responded with different strategies to modify available equipment and a product that had most of the desired features. Internet and telephone access were achieved through use of a personal computer with scanning of the keyboard and mouse functions. An onscreen keyboard with the functions to operate the browser and keys with pictures representing favorite sites were scanned with the single switch.

## OUTCOMES
By using a strategy of efficient offering of ideas using the Internet with service providers and manufacturers, a satisfactory solution was developed. The user was able to select which tools she uses independently, allowing her care providers to do other things while

she is using her environmental control system and her computer and telephone systems for entertainment and while she communicates with friends and does her homework.

## References

1. Trace Research and Development Center: *Access to current and next-generation information systems by people with disabilities*, 1997, http://www.trace.wisc.edu/docs/access_info_ss/full_doc.html.
2. Cook A, Hussey S: *Assistive technologies: principles and practice*, St Louis, 1995, Mosby.
3. Maryland Relay Brochure: *Thousands keep in touch through Maryland*, 2001, The Deaf and Disabled Telecommunications Program, http://www.mdrelay.org/main/about/mdrelayoverview.htm.
4. The Deaf and Disabled Telecommunications Program, 2001, http://www.ddtp.org.
5. Segalman R: *A full description of speech-to-speech*, 1998, http://www.interwork.sdsu.edu/ablenet/sts2.html.
6. Cellular Telecommunications Industry Association: *WOW-COM's world of wireless communications*, http://www.wow-com.com/consumer/access_wireless/.
7. Motorola, Inc: *Motorola's commitment to telecommunications access for people with disabilities*, 2001, http://www.commerce.motorola.com/consumer/QWtml/accessibility.html.
8. Nokia: *Accessibility solutions*, 2001, http://www.nokiausa.com/accessibility/.
9. Stephanidis C: Excerpt from *Everyone interfaces*, 1999, reprinted at Trace Research and Development Center Website, http://www.trace.wisc.edu/docs/phones/tcrd1/summary/index.htm.
10. Motorola, Inc: *Motorola consumer catalog – pagers*, 1999, http://www.commerce.motorola.com/consumer/QWhtml/pager_cat.html.
11. Direct Network Access: *The DSL center*, 2001, http://www.dslcenter.com.
12. DCP Communications, Inc: *Appliance.com consumer connection*, Internet Appliances, 2001,http://www.appliance.com/cc/office/html/body_internet.html.
13. Koblas D: *DosLynx v0.8 alpha release information*, 1990, University of Kansas, http://www.ftp2.cc.ukans.edu/pub/DosLynx/readme.htm.
14. Perry B: Got what it takes to get online? *Exceptional Parent* 26 (11):38-41, 1996.
15. Nasby G: *List of web browsers*, 2001, includes a list of browsers designed for use by people with disabilities, http://www.browserlist.browser.org.
16. Grewal S: *Extremely lynx*, 2001, http://www.trill_home.com/lynx.html.
17. Bosher P, Brewer J: *Alternative web browsing*, 2000, W3C, Web Accessibility Initiative http://www.w3.org/WAI/References/Browsing.
18. The Productivity Works, Inc: *pwKiosk*, 2000, software for an FCC and ADA compliant information and service Kiosk, http://www.prodworks.com/homecontent/pr_0706200.htm.

# CHAPTER 9

## Augmentative and Alternative Communication

*Judy Henderson*
*Molly Doyle*

### Application and Goal

#### Augmentative and Alternative Communication Intervention

Augmentative and alternative communication (AAC) intervention enhances daily interactions of persons with severe communication disabilities. AAC intervention is used to improve quality of life, to improve personal relationships by increasing interaction with others, to increase independence, and to satisfy basic needs. People who are temporarily, permanently, or developmentally at risk for spoken or written language at any time in their lives and cannot meet their communication needs through standard modes can benefit from an AAC system.

An AAC system is "an integrated group of components, including symbols, aids, strategies and techniques used by individuals to enhance communication."[1] Symbols are representations of vocabulary or messages such as line drawings or printed words. Aids are devices used to transmit or receive messages and include manual communication boards and electronic devices. The way messages are transmitted such as through scanning or natural gestures are called *techniques*.[2] Strategies are the ways symbols, aids, and techniques are used to maximize communication.[3] Retrieving preprogrammed social phrases or typing only relevant portions of a message to speed communication are examples of strategies.

AAC intervention is appropriate for persons who have the intent, need, and desire to communicate but cannot do so through standard means (i.e., speech or traditional writing). Some individuals with cerebral palsy whose speech is slightly slurred or dysarthric can rely on speech to meet all communication needs and may rely on techniques such as repeating, rephrasing, spelling, or giving a topic to enhance understanding. For others with less speech intelligibility, an alphabet board or a communication device may be effective. Individuals with severe cognitive and language delays may be using idiosyncratic signals or less conventional modes to communicate information (e.g., yelling or withdrawing to indicate "don't want," "stop," or "go away") that are not understood by untrained and unfamiliar partners. Through AAC intervention, these behaviors may be shaped or replaced by more iconic or readable modes (e.g., pointing to symbol to communicate "stop"). The AAC methods people use change as they learn new skills, participate in new activities, or enter new environments.

### Function and Ability

#### AAC Intervention with Different Populations

Individuals with different types of disabilities can benefit from AAC intervention (Table 9-1).

## TABLE 9-1

*Key Issues for AAC Application Among Disability Groups*

| Diagnosis | Characteristics | AAC Intervention Strategies |
|---|---|---|
| **Congenital** | | |
| Cerebral palsy | Developmental neuromotor involvement exists. | Oral motor training and speech therapy indicated for young children to develop word approximations. |
| | Type is characterized by motor impairment (e.g., spastic, athetoid). | Early intervention to train various motor sites should occur. |
| | | Primary site (i.e., eye point) may be used for communication while switch and light beam are in training. |
| | Associated problems of developmental delay, seizure activity, visual and auditory perception, and acuity exist. | Use AAC to improve communication and enhance language development. |
| | | Systems including devices change as skills improve and environmental demands change. |
| | | Emphasize literacy skill development. May use prediction, Minspeak[6] or dynamic display to increase speed of message transmission. |
| Autism | Social interaction skills are delayed or impaired. | Pragmatics need to be supplemented and trained. |
| | | Voice output may help with pragmatics to decrease frustration. |
| | Receptive language may be age appropriate. | May use visual and spatial skills to advantage with an icon or words-based system. |
| | May be ambulatory with fine motor problems. | Portability is an issue. |
| | Verbal expression delays prevalent. | |
| | Structure and routine assists in training. | Teach use of AAC during routines. Can use a symbol-based calendar to anticipate new events. |
| | | Consider use of simple signs or gestures. Use environmental and visual cues to structure and promote early communication. |
| | | Use AAC to improve communication and language development. |
| Speech/oral apraxia | Receptive language may be age appropriate. | Use AAC to improve communication and language development. |
| | Fine motor problems may interfere with traditional sign language. | Teach gestural or modified manual sign language to the extent possible with motor planning. |
| | May see increased verbalizations as use of AAC lessens effort on communication. | Consider multiple portable components. |
| Cognitive limitations | Communication and language skills are delayed. | Use multimodal approach. Train in natural environment. |
| **Acquired** | | |
| TBI | Majority of recovery occurs 6-9 months after injury. | Improve functional communication, teach family strategies, use flexible system, and use AAC to facilitate cognition and language recovery. |
| | Recovery of speech usually occurs within 12 months but may continue to improve several years postsurgery. | Ensure user has insight and judgment before device purchase. Provide extensive trials before purchase. Educate family about the benefits of AAC; they may see AAC interfering with recovery of speech. |
| | Cognitive, behavioral, and motor control problems occur. | |
| | Memory deficits and difficulties with new learning exist. | |

*TBI, traumatic brain injury; CVA, cerebrovascular accident; ALS, amyotrophic lateral sclerosis.*

TABLE 9-1—cont'd

## Key Issues for AAC Application Among Disability Groups

| Diagnosis | Characteristics | AAC Intervention Strategies |
|---|---|---|
| *Acquired—cont'd* | | |
| CVA | Left CVA, nonfluent or Broca's are candidates. | Provide trials before purchasing. |
| | Language deficits primarily influence AAC use. | |
| | Majority of recovery is 6 months postonset, with gradual gains in speech and language processes several years postonset. | |
| | May be resistant to voice output. | Begin with manual components. |
| | | May benefit from voice output in specific situations. |
| | Reading and spelling skills may be impaired. | Consider communication notebook with lists of names and blank paper for writing or drawing. |
| | May be able to recognize a written word. | May use voice output to practice verbalizing words or phrases. |
| | Visual cues (icons or words) may help word retrieval and verbal expression. | Teach to use a phone book, map, or catalog to retrieve information. |
| | Older populations want to talk about past events and experiences. | Use vocabulary to promote social closeness and sharing of information. Interview family about past history. |
| | Ability to use telephone is needed. | Voice output can be used for specific situations. |
| Brainstem | Recovery patterns are variable. | Establish alternative "yes" and "no" responses. |
| | May be called *locked-in syndrome*. | Eye-gaze boards may be used for interactions with nursing and caregivers. |
| | Visual perceptual and integration deficits may be present. | |
| | Generally, one reliable motor access site exists. | Integrate technologies. |
| Spinal cord injury | Level of injury influences Intervention. | Speaking valves, voice amplifiers, and electrolarynges may be indicated. |
| | If complete injury, expect no spontaneous return. | Provide individual and family time to accept and cope with disability. |
| | Cognition and language usually intact. | Take time to explore various technologies. |
| | Patient may fatigue easily. | Monitor fatigue and task "loads." |
| *Progressive* | | |
| ALS, or Lou Gehrig's disease | Different manifestations occur, generally rapid decline. | Provide flexible system. |
| | | Intervene as mobility, motor control, or communication needs change. |
| | Usually no change in cognition occurs. | Use alphabet-based and text-based techniques. |
| | Patient may be resistant to further adaptations in technology as it indicates further loss of function. | Introduce new components as the need arises. |
| | | Capitalize on residual skills. |
| | | Maintain communication until death. |
| Multiple sclerosis | Manifestations differ; some symptoms are temporary. | Provide new components as symptoms arise. |
| | Progress is usually slower than ALS. | Use technologies for longer periods. |
| | Cognitive and visual perceptual deficits may be present. | Font size and complexity of visual display are important to monitor. |
| Parkinson's disease | Slow progression occurs. | Consider voice amplifiers. |
| | Hand tremors may influence motor access. | Manual systems and strategies may supplement speech (e.g., alphabet and initial letter cueing). |
| | Cognitive and language deficits may be present at end stages. | Icons may be useful. |

Children with congenital disabilities use AAC solutions to assist in language development and to augment spoken language until the time that speech may develop sufficiently to closely match their receptive language. Using speech output is motivating to users and aids in language growth and development by providing a visual or auditory representation of expanded language.[4] For instance, if a student selects a cell with the picture of a drink, a full sentence, "I want a drink now," may be seen and heard on a display. Early intervention and speech output for children at risk may help them avoid communication failure and passivity by empowering them in their environment.

Young children may be trained using parent intervention and environmental modifications. Intervention may be used to develop consistent motor access sites and compensate for difficulties in timing and motor planning.[5] Some young children with motor impairments may show actual improvements or changes in motor functioning. Techniques and technology are used in demonstrating the power of communication and are modified as new skills emerge. These children need to have their AAC intervention plan modified as they progress.

The nature of an individual's medical diagnosis and resulting symptoms may influence key AAC intervention issues. Persons with acquired injuries such as traumatic brain injury (TBI) and left cerebrovascular accident (LCVA) often show improvements in cognitive, language, and motor skills in the first 6 to 8 months after the injury. AAC techniques and strategies are modified as the individual improves. For example, an individual with TBI may rely on "yes" and "no" responses and simple gestures to communicate basic needs immediately after the injury. As attention and memory improve, along with changes in motor control, more complex AAC technologies are introduced such as an alphabet board, a small typewriter, or a communication device. AAC solutions are flexible—they may be frequently changed to accommodate and facilitate changes in functional communication skills. This situation may be the first time the family has experienced an insufficient ability to communicate. They are often competent communicators who simply need to learn background in AAC.

AAC intervention for individuals with progressive disabilities is similar to acquired injuries in that techniques and strategies are modified to accommodate changes in function. However, rather than showing improvement in function, as with TBI and LCVA, persons with progressive disabilities such as amyotrophic lateral sclerosis (ALS) or Parkinson's disease demonstrate loss in various abilities associated with functional, independent communication. The nature and rate of progression varies depending on the type of disability. In addition, variability in symptoms and rate or progression is not uncommon among persons with the same diagnosis. For this reason, recommended communication systems must have the ability to accommodate different input methods (e.g., direct selection, scanning) as motor skills change. Slowly introducing technology and strategies may also be necessary to enable the individual to gradually accept limitations. Ongoing follow up with this population is critical to ensure AAC technologies are modified to meet the individual's needs.

### Goals

People receiving AAC services typically have goals for functional use of their system in a variety of situations with different communication partners. Goals need to reflect a time line, they need to be accurate, and they should specify the person responsible for measurement. For a goal's outcome to be significant, it needs to be measurable. Determining the prompt hierarchy used by the communication partner to validate the independence of the communication may also be important. For students, some goals are geared for the educational environment. People in the workforce have goals centered on their work environment or community participation. Goals should be sought from all team members as different communication partners have different goals and desire different outcomes. Indicating the communication partner (trained, untrained, familiar, or unfamiliar) also clarifies the specific goal. Baselines can be taken in expressive language (vocabulary or communicative intents), in the number of different communication partners, in the number of times communication is independently and appropriately initiated, or in device-use accuracy. The following are a few examples of possible goals:

In _____ months, _____ will make comments from a choice of 10 different messages _____ times throughout the day independently and appropriately initiated using the communication device.

In _____ months, _____ will use the manual board to ask questions of unfamiliar partners (e.g., store clerk, school secretary) with 90% accuracy and intermittent cueing, given $\frac{3}{5}$ opportunities.

In _____ months, _____ will expand the topic of conversation with peer or staff by retrieving the appropriate message on the device or communication book with 80% accuracy and occasional cueing, given $\frac{3}{5}$ opportunities.

## Considerations, Options, and Technology

This section includes issues and procedures related to assessment, selection, and design of an AAC system, as well as the training of people and their support systems in the use of AAC. Informal screening protocols, which service providers may use when conducting assessments, are also included. Using standardized tests is often difficult because of the lack of oral speech and the motoric involvement of these individuals. However, determining the receptive language functioning of an individual is still important so that a proper device match can be made.

### Evaluation Using the Features/Characteristics Approach

A thorough evaluation of an individual's needs and abilities and knowledge of the different features/characteristics of AAC devices and techniques are critical in identifying optimal AAC solutions. The feature approach entails identifying features/characteristics required, needed, and desired in an AAC system, based on an individual's needs, abilities, and preferences. The purpose of the AAC assessment is to identify AAC techniques and strategies that promote functional and independent communication. Techniques and strategies are determined after analyzing the individual's needs and goals, after evaluating specific skills related to functional communication, and after providing trials with a variety of AAC techniques and features/characteristics. During assessment and trial training, techniques and strategies are identified that facilitate active participation in those activities or environments that are important to the individual, the family, and other communication partners such as teachers or peers.

These techniques, strategies, needs, and abilities are then matched to specific features/ characteristics contained in devices, or software or manual components of a communication system to determine a communication device match. Techniques or devices that have these features are then provided for trial. Speech output, portability, and picture-based are examples of features. If these were indicated as needs during the evaluation, products that have these characteristics would be provided for trial. Generally, several features are specified before proceeding to device trials. After trials with different techniques, pros and cons of the different options are discussed. Rarely does one product have all the desired features. The device is one component in addition to the manual aspects, techniques, and strategies that make up the individual's AAC system.

Several benefits exist for the feature approach. The individual's needs and abilities are held primary and the design of the system (techniques and technology) becomes the base, rather than fitting the individual to the device. Through this process, the individual and the support team realize that technology is a tool rather than a magical solution. The need for compromise is modeled, and multiple components and techniques are reinforced.

The *Guide to Augmentative and Alternative Communication* (GAAC), developed by the Rehabilitation Engineering Research Center on AAC (University of Delaware, 1996), is an example of a chart that provides a comprehensive list of commercially available AAC products and their features/characteristics (Box 9-1). Newer products have been introduced, but this guide is good for examining features and helps clinicians select an appropriate device after the features/characteristics that an individual needs have been identified.

BOX **9-1**

*Features/Characteristics Category Examples*

*Output* (what type of output helps user interact with communication partners):
   Auditory: digitized or synthesized
   Visual/written

*Feedback* (what type of feedback helps user prepare or retrieve messages most effectively):
   Auditory
   Visual
   Tactile

*Input Method* (motorically, what is the most efficient way to access messages):
   Direct selection
   Scanning: single, multiswitch, directed

*Symbol Size* (what size, in inches, of symbol is easiest to see and physically access)

*Symbol Type or Item Representation* (what type of symbol does user understand):
   Photograph, colored, black/white, Minspeak, etc.

*Language Access/Message Storage and Retrieval* (what strategy is optimal for retrieving messages):
   Levels
   Encoding (color, letter, icon)
   Prediction

*Flexibility* (user may need product that is flexible to accommodate changes in physical status, communication needs, etc.):
   Print size can be altered
   Accommodates scanning and direct selection

*Portability:*
   Weight and mounting

*Durability:*
   Exposure to weather or dropping

*Cost/Warranty:*
   Extended warranty

*Manufacturer Support:*
   Toll-free number and hours of operation

*Integration and Compatibility with Other Assistive Devices* (to include environmental controls, power wheelchairs, and computers)

## Critical Issues and Principles in the Assessment Process

Several issues critical to the assessment process for AAC include the following:

- A thorough assessment of those skills related to AAC use before providing trials with techniques or devices
- Use of criterion-based assessment protocols
- Attention to levels of exertion or "loads"
- Use of a team approach to improve delivery of services
- Inclusion of the individual's support system and appropriate professionals
- Consideration of long-term and short-term needs and goals

Device trials to evaluate features/characteristics are conducted after the analysis of communication needs and abilities, the identification of goals, the assessment of skills, and the delineation of features (Table 9-2). The use of criterion-based assessment involves measuring the level of performance on a series of cognitive, language, motor, or visual tasks sufficient to allow the user to use or benefit from a given approach. Modifications within activity or environment are often necessary, along with modifications to the AAC techniques to ensure that communication and participation are maximized.

During the evaluation and subsequent training, balancing the level of exertion or "load" of the area to be examined with other areas of difficulty is necessary. For a person with multiple challenges, exertion such as pointing with a finger to make a selection may interfere with listening to oral directions. "Loads" range from light to heavy and easy to difficult (see Table 9-2).

If a high level or difficult task is required, "unloading" the other areas not being assessed by placing an easier load on those areas is necessary. For instance, requiring someone to initiate a topic in a rapid conversation (respond quickly) and to use a finger point without keyguard support may make the task harder than the motivation required to interact. In training, if a child who normally yells to gain attention has to walk across the room and point to a symbol, the task requirement is higher than the motivation and the chances of the child accomplishing this mode substitution are decreased.

Along with observing and analyzing activities and environments, assessing the way individuals in a particular activity or environment interact and participate is often beneficial.[2] Participation plans delineate which strategies and technology are used during specific environments and time periods within a school day.

For example, Melissa uses a voice output communication device, manual communication boards, and sign language to communicate. In her special education class, she relies on sign language and to a lesser extent on her communication device to socialize and complete schoolwork. In her regular science class, the teachers and peers are unfamiliar with sign language and therefore need Melissa to use the communication device along with activity-specific communication boards. The communication boards contain vocabulary specific to the science lessons (e.g., names of dinosaurs). Academic vocabulary and social phrases such as "Did you do the homework?" and "I like your outfit" are preprogrammed in her device. The custom boards and stored vocabulary help her participate in classroom discussions, learn the curriculum, and socialize.

## TABLE 9-2

### Communicative Load

| | Easy | Difficult |
|---|---|---|
| Communicative intent | Respond | Clarify |
| Symbolic representation | Object | Read word |
| Expressive language | One word | Complex sentence |
| Receptive language | Noun | Modifier |
| Physical response | Eye point | One finger point |
| Switch use | Cause/effect | Scanning |

Long-term and short-term considerations are critical because of the changes in the individual's cognitive and academic growth, in technology, and in progression of a disability. Communication devices are replaced over an individual's lifetime. The application should be functional and provide for growth or change (see Case Studies). Individuals are expected to be able to use the devices, not grow into them in a few years. Flexibility is a major features/characteristic for this consideration.

## Decision-Making Sequence and Assessment Strategies

A thorough evaluation of a person's skills and needs is critical before recommending an AAC system. Evaluating the needs and abilities of an individual before matching the person to device characteristics is the preferred method to select an AAC system (Box 9-2).

The analysis of needs and abilities and the identification of goals can be completed through interviews, intake forms, or team interaction. A team format for the establishment of this information has the benefit of the inclusion of team members and fosters understanding among them. In particular, examining team member's expectations of technology highlights any misconceptions concerning its use. By focusing the team's efforts in the beginning stages, the evaluation becomes more efficient.

## BOX 9-2

### Decision-Making Feature Approach Sequence

Analyze communication needs and abilities and identify goals.
List the environments where individual spends time and needs to communicate.
Survey partners and identify communication goals.
Identify current communication techniques and effectiveness (see Table 9-3).
Identify goals and expectations of technology.

Assess skills.
Identify optimal positioning of body and materials (e.g., device/display).
Determine optimal motor access site.
Assess vision and hearing (acuity, perception, and processing).
Determine language and communication functioning (see Boxes 9-3 and 9-4).
Assess cognitive and memory skills as they relate to AAC (assess symbols use type, field).

Delineate critical and desired AAC features (see Box 9-1).
Match needs and abilities to device features (see Table 9-4).
Match anatomic sites to input devices.
Configure displays with appropriate symbols.

Provide trials with techniques.
Evaluate features through initial trials.
Chart accuracy, speed, and overall effectiveness.
Discuss preferences.

Modify equipment and set up as needed.

Discuss pros and cons of different techniques.
Reassess features and prioritize.
List compromises.

Provide extended trials with techniques with data collection.
Collect data regarding functional use for funding justification.

Make recommendation and justification for AAC system.
Provide written report with vendor and prices.
Include functional goals related to system use.
Indicate training needs and follow-up plan.

## Communication Mode Checklist

For those challenged by little or limited ability to write and/or talk, the modes, channels, or forms used in their communications are different than those of a talking person, but vary (Table 9-3). Some individuals with severe cognitive abilities may scream to communicate removal from an activity or person. These individuals and their behaviors may be mislabeled or misinterpreted as noncommunicative. During intervention, these behaviors can be changed to alternate modes that are more functional or conventional.

Modes may differ according to the environment, the expertise and familiarity of the partner, or the contexts. Those areas need to be supplemented by AAC techniques, strategies, and technology. The mode checklist in Table 9-3 can be used as a baseline to measure current function and as a follow up to measure change.

Assess language functioning by consulting the speech pathology evaluation report, individual education plan (IEP), and/or psychoeducational evaluation. These reports can provide background information on language comprehension. Consult with appropriate professionals regarding what skills to expect given the individual's chronologic age, medical diagnosis, and deficit areas. Criterion-based evaluations may involve using language developmental charts for receptive and expressive language. Standardized tests can be adapted to the individual's communication method. Informal screening of language function can be done in addition to a speech and language assessment. Be sure to pro-

## TABLE 9-3

*Communication Mode Checklist*

|  | Home | School/Work | Community |
| --- | --- | --- | --- |
| *Communication Modes* | | | |
| **Speech** | | | |
| Understandability % | | | |
| Word approximations | | | |
| Vocalizations, crying, laughing | | | |
| Inflection, volume | | | |
| **Gestural** | | | |
| Modified signs | | | |
| Natural gestures (pointing, waving) | | | |
| Eye gaze to object | | | |
| Facial expression | | | |
| Head movements (for "yes" and "no") | | | |
| Body tone change | | | |
| **Proximal** | | | |
| Take partner to object | | | |
| Stand near partner | | | |
| **Writing** | | | |
| Typing | | | |
| **Manual components** | | | |
| Alphabet boards | | | |
| Symbol boards, books | | | |
| Eye-gaze charts | | | |
| **AAC devices (see Table 9-4)** | | | |
| **AAC strategies (partner and user)** | | | |
| "Yes" and "no" to questions | | | |
| Present choices | | | |
| Partner-assisted auditory scan (choices are listed out loud, user indicated when choice is reached) | | | |
| Point to pictures and objects in the environment | | | |
| First letter cueing (point to the first letter of a word as it is spoken) | | | |
| Topic cue (point to a category word or icon) | | | |

*Fill in N, needs; H, has.*

vide a sufficient number of trials. Individuals with memory deficits may answer a question incorrectly because they are not able to recall the information not because they have an inability to process and comprehend the question. In addition, as questions get longer and vocabulary becomes more complex, the individual may need more time to process the information. Therefore timing the processing to establish a baseline is helpful.

## Functions of Communication

Just as speech is used for a variety of intents or pragmatic functions, AAC technology and strategies are used for a full range of communicative functions (Box 9-3). These functions are important to consider in AAC evaluation and training to ensure that all areas that benefit the user are included. This can also be used for baseline and follow-up data and may be used with individuals as a teaching tool to demonstrate communicative functions using their techniques, strategies, and technology.

## Language Comprehension Screening

Screening tools can be used to gain information about language processing when a standardized test is not possible because of a person's limited or lack of speech or motor control to point to answers (Box 9-4). Information about receptive language functioning is critical to the evaluation of AAC.

## Device Characteristics and Client Needs and Abilities

Selected device features/characteristics can be listed and matched with specific clients needs and abilities (Table 9-4). For example, digitized speech, a type of auditory output, may be an appropriate AAC component or features/characteristics for an individual who

## BOX 9-3

*Functions of Communication*

> ***Give Information*** ("Come back for me in an hour.")
>     Protest ("No!" "Stop!")
>     Confirm/deny ("That's right.")
>
> ***Receive Information***
>
> ***Describe Events***
>     Present/past ("We had a party at school yesterday.")
>
> ***Persuade Partner***
>     Request action ("Please get me a glass of water, I'm so thirsty.")
>     Opinions ("The reason I don't agree is. . .  ")
>     Feeling ("I'm really angry.")
>
> ***Indicate Desire for Further Communication*** ("I have another thought.")
>     Gain attention ("Excuse me, could you help me?")
>
> ***Entertainment***
>     Jokes/tease ("I gotcha.")
>     Secrets ("Bob called me last night.")
>
> ***Interaction***
>     Social closeness ("That's great!")
>     Clarification and repair ("That's not what I meant.")
>     Greetings, comments, and conversational fillers ("Hi, I'm fine, thanks," "Wow, that's great!")

does not spell, has predictable needs, and/or has unmet needs in specific situations. Although the features/characteristics in Table 9-4 are similar to those used in the GAAC, not all features/characteristics were included. The table is merely a guide that shows the way results of a few components of assessment may help determine device features/characteristics. Additional information is needed before determining what AAC system is optimal.

## BOX 9-4

*Language Comprehension Screening*

### 1. Answers Questions

The individual has the ability to give consistent, accurate "yes" and "no" responses when asked questions of varying complexity and answers simple questions pertaining to here and now or personal information (e.g., "Are you at home?" "Is your roommate here?" "Are you wearing a jacket?"). The individual also answers complex and abstract questions (e.g., "Do you plan to go out for lunch after your appointment today?"). The practitioner should describe a "yes" and "no" response system and indicate strategies that help the individual answer questions accurately and reliably. Strategies can include the following:

Repeat the question.
Vary stress or intonation.
Simplify the question.
Provide visual cues (e.g., point to or show item talked about or use gestures).
Provide choices (present items or choices and ask, "Do you want _____ or _____?").

### 2. Understands Directions

The individual has the ability to consistently understand directions of varying complexity. (Directions given are within one's motor capabilities. Keep instructions short and simple, give one direction at a time, and provide visual cues if needed.) The individual does the following:

Follows 1-step directions (e.g., "Close your eyes." "Touch my hand.")
Follows 2-step directions (e.g., Turn your head to the left and hit the switch 2 times.")
Follows complex directions (e.g., Go to the front lobby, get a glass of water, and then come back and give the water to your brother.")

### 3. Understands Conversation

Attention and memory may influence the complexity of vocabulary used in conversation. The individual does the following:

Recalls details from story or conversation.
Describes components of activity that was described by evaluator.

### 4. Understands Visual Information Through Symbol Assessment

This determines the symbol system to use with the AAC device or strategy. Visual acuity and perception influences performance. Provide sufficient number of trials with each task. Word knowledge and experience also have an effect. Determine number and size of items in the choice field. The individual does the following:

Recognizes objects used as a referent (e.g., points to an object to request, may use eye point or hand/arm point).
Discriminates and uses colored line drawings to represent desired objects or activities.
Discriminates and uses black and white line drawings to represent desired objects (i.e., people and activities).[7]
Matches words to pictures.
Reads at sentence or paragraph level (specify grade equivalent).
Spells at word, sentence level (specify grade level).
Categorizes icons.
Sequences pictures.
Associates several meanings or concepts to icons (e.g., "sun" icon = hot, yellow, round, outside, etc.).
Sequences two to three multimeaning icons to generate messages (e.g., exit sign + apple = "Let's go out to eat.").

## TABLE 9-4

*Device Characteristics and Client Abilities and Needs*

| Features/Characteristics | Ability/Required Skill | Client Needs |
| --- | --- | --- |
| **Communication Output** | | |
| Auditory output digitized | Ability to hear and process spoken messages, spelling nonfunctional or just emerging | Has predictable needs, unmet needs in specific situations (may be used to supplement other AAC components), music/song output |
| Synthesized | Spelling functional or uses icon sequencing or dynamic display to communicate | Needs device as primary mode of communication, conveys complex, unique information by spelling and requires text to speech |
| Message display | Able to read at single word or phrase level, visually discriminate text on display, self monitors, makes corrections | Assists with message preparation, helps communication partner anticipate or predict message, backs up speech output in noisy environments, allows user to cue listener to speech |
| **Written Output** | | |
| Printer (internal or external) | Spelling functional to supplement speech<br>Identifies key words in message | Needs visual clarification of the voice output<br>Prefers to use own speech with written back up, needs to prepare assignments or lists, uses for letter writing, allows client to prepare messages in advance, allows interaction with hearing-impaired partners, permits interaction in quiet environments, requires partners to be literate at fourth to sixth grade and to have adequate vision |
| **Language Features**<br>Item Representation | | |
| Alphabet | Spells at fourth to sixth grade level, able to generate short phrases, spelling errors phonetic and approximate target | Allows generation of novel utterances and nonreliance on preprogrammed phrases |
| Whole word | Recognizes written words, uses words functionally to convey ideas | Allows more adult appearance than icons, faster retrieval of a word than spelling, word recognition may be stronger than spelling |
| Photo, picture, or icon, Dynasyms, Mayer-Johnson Minspeak | Understands label or referent symbolized in picture form, associates minimum of one concept to picture | Needs to expand communication system |
| Object | Recognizes preferred items and objects, may use simple gestures or idiosyncratic signals | Has preferences and dislikes, needs to learn cause and effect of communication |

## AAC Design and Vocabulary Selection

The design of the AAC manual and electronic components of the system follow the same guidelines. The parameters (e.g., size of symbol/text, choice field/number of selections, placement of cells, type of device) of the input display are largely determined during the evaluation and refined during a person's training in different environments. Certain

## TABLE 9-4—cont'd

### *Device Characteristics and Client Abilities and Needs*

| Features/Characteristics | Ability/Required Skill | Client Needs |
| --- | --- | --- |
| *Language Storage and Retrieval* | | |
| Level organization | Categorizes symbols by activity or function, scans message options, sequences minimum of two or three steps to move between displays, understands categories, recalls location of messages across displays (specify number), may need concrete symbols to communicate | Conveys information in different situations or activities |
| Letter encoding | Understands initials or abbreviations, assigns logical codes to messages, retains codes, identifies key words in messages | Some needs are predictable and recurring (e.g., social greetings) |
| Word prediction | Reading skills higher than spelling, able to shift visual focus between keyboard and display and screen, inputs slowly or fatigues | Increase speech of message transmission used to increase literacy skill, minimizing key strokes may increase message preparation |
| Icon encoding | Associates multiple concepts to icon (abstract reasoning), categorizes, sequences, recalls codes (memory for new information) | Increased speed of message transmission, one overlay/display |
| *Physical Interface* | | |
| Direct selection | Requires motor accuracy and range | Concrete form of selection, fastest input method |
| Encoded input (Morse code) | Requires consistent motor response, sequencing, and memory with use of one or two switches | |
| Scanning | Requires timing and accuracy of response, requires understanding and motor ability to "wait" for selection | Has one repeatable, accurate motor response pattern, as scanning patterns vary, meets needs for fastest form of message transmission |
| Dual switches | More abstract than single switch, as each has a different purpose, requires two motor response patterns that are timed and sequenced | |
| Multiswitch | Ability to accurately use several switches | |
| Directed (joystick) | Need spatial ability and planning, may be more concrete than dual or multiswitch, has motor abilities to move joystick | |

considerations including type of symbol, use of color, or sequencing of cells may also be adapted.

Vocabulary must be sufficient to express a wide range of communicative intents. A vocabulary of 500 to 600 words is comparable to that of a talking 2-½ to 3-year-old child. Care must be taken that within the restricted vocabulary many ideas can be expressed. Requests, comments, and general conversation are powerful intents to use in the initial design of vocabulary for a device or manual display.

One method of determining vocabulary to use in the AAC system is to survey the environments in which the user spends time and list the motivating actions, people, items, and intents in that environment. Yorkston[8] provides a question/answer format for interviewing significant others to obtain vocabulary information that is relevant for adults who have had TBI. Goossens and others[9] describe a system of obtaining vocabulary for "vocabulary sets." Beukelman[10] has vocabulary listed by age groups, used for "small talk" or chatting.

Once vocabulary is determined, it is matched to picture icons or words and organized into the AAC system. Vocabulary can be organized in several ways depending on the users' abilities, needs, and goals. The situation or environment also influences whether this vocabulary is arranged by topic or activity, category, or syntax. If topic or activity specific, the overlay, page, or screen has messages (i.e., words, icons, phrases, or complete sentences) pertaining to that topic or activity. For example, an overlay for McDonald's restaurant would include the following:

Cheeseburger, large, small, thank you, and I'm ready to order.

If organized by category, clothing, food or drink, people or location, items may be on one page. A main group of vocabulary may contain basic needs and vocabulary that occurs across contexts. The user would then move to more specific vocabulary organized elsewhere. When vocabulary is organized syntactically, nouns, pronouns, verbs, modifiers, and nouns are presented in color-coded lists moving from left to right (Figure 9-1). This arrangement prompts the user to point or indicate symbols or words in each column to formulate a message such as the following

I + want + salted + French fries.

Color coding assists in visual scanning of the material to locate words. Sequencing of words assists in learning syntax and grammar. This arrangement can assist in producing a wide variety of sentences. This arrangement requires the user to make several selections per message. For fast message retrieval of time-sensitive vocabulary (i.e., I need to use the bathroom), a phrase is contained within one selection rather than requiring a series of word and symbol selections.

Another arrangement shows groups of words or pictures that are meaningful to the user (Figure 9-2). Vocabulary may be categorized by language function. Social phrases, questions, and things to do may all be grouped in one area of the communication display.

Users can also retrieve prestored phrases, words, and letters through multimeaning icons. Icons are assigned a variety of meanings (e.g., sun = hot, summer, yellow) and then sequenced to retrieve messages. Because users have determined the associations of the icons, their memory for sequencing a set of icons is enhanced.

Dynamic displays present a main menu or group of vocabulary from which other displays are reached by linking or branching to another page. For instance, when a category or topic is selected, the display changes and is replaced by vocabulary pertaining to that

| I want | to eat a | Small | cheeseburger | coke |
|--------|----------|-------|--------------|------|
| You | to order a | Medium | chickenburger | milkshake |
| My friend | to read | Large | fries | root beer |
| My teacher | to thank | Vanilla | hamburger | 7-Up |
| | | Strawberry | ice cream | |
| | | Chocolate | | menu |
| NO | | | PLEASE | YES |

**Fig. 9-1** Language board or overlay arrangement with Fitzgerald key used in miniboard or topic board format. Columns can be color-coded. Words or picture symbols can be used. Modified from Fitzgerald E: *Sign language for the deaf,* Washington, DC, 1976, Alexander G. Bell Association for the Deaf.

topic or category. Organizing vocabulary in a logical way is important for users. Color coding of cells and consistency of page design is helpful in the mapping process. Within this system, vocabulary can be organized according to topic, category, or communicative function.

Displays are also organized according to user access ability. Frequently used vocabulary is placed on the display where it is easiest and quickest to access. This has implications for individuals who scan. Frequently used time-sensitive vocabulary such as "I'm fine, thank you" would be programmed into the upper left quadrant. Because this configuration changes for different types of scanning, careful observation of the timing of positions precedes programming vocabulary.

For individuals who spell, a variety of letter arrangements are available. Alphabets can also be organized on displays for ease of access, QWERTY (typewriter or computer keyboard layout), or ABC format. Children who are beginning to learn the alphabet may use the ABC format. Users who have limited hand access can have a keyboard rearranged so that the most frequently used letters are within the easiest range. Individuals who use single switch scanning benefit from letters arranged by frequency of use.

## AAC Training

AAC training and implementation includes setting up the AAC system, instructing the user and support team the way to use a variety of AAC methods, and teaching strategies on the way to incorporate AAC into everyday functional activities. The support team consists of professionals and family or caregivers working with the client.

Using a team approach in AAC evaluation and training helps ensure that the system is properly set up and implemented to maximize functional communication. Teams are particularly important for children and adults with multiple disabilities. For example, a physical therapist and occupational therapist can provide valuable ideas on seating, mobility, motor control, and vision and the positioning of the device and input tools. All of these may directly influence the selection, design, and successful implementation of an AAC system for an individual with severe motor involvement. Other team members such as

| Hi, how are you? | Fine, thanks | Not so great | What have you been up to lately? | What did you do this weekend? | Bye, see you later. |
|---|---|---|---|---|---|
| You look nice today. | Is that a new shirt? | I saw a great movie this weekend. | | | |
| I need a tissue. | It's in my backpack. | I need my communication binder. | Would someone help me with my homework? | Something is wrong with my wheelchair. | Help me use the restroom. |
| I'll start to spell. It begins with the letter: | A B C D | | E F G H I J | | |
| | K L M N | | O P Q R S T | | |
| | T U V W | | X Y Z . ? | | |
| I'm talking Try again | about a You go it. | Person That's not quite what I wanted to say. | Place I didn't understand you. | Thing Please repeat that. | Event |
| Who? NO | What? PLEASE | When? | Where? | Which one? THANKS | YES |

**Fig. 9-2** Communicative functions arranged in groups.

teachers, job coaches, and parents ensure the AAC system meets the user's needs in school, work, and home activities. They may help select vocabulary, program the AAC device, and assist in teaching the person with disabilities how to use a variety of AAC strategies.

Team collaboration benefits the AAC user and team members. For the user, team collaboration increases the consistency of the training approach and increases likelihood that training is functionally based. Teaming fosters advocacy training and a chance for everyone involved to offer comments and to summarize thoughts during meetings. The family and caregiver benefit because communication among professionals is enhanced and requires less time. They also learn new information in the process of listening to professionals interact and have the opportunity to ask questions. Team meetings offer the family and caregiver participation in a process that enhances their advocacy skills. The professionals benefit in the efficiency of communication, receive a global view of the family and caregiver and AAC user, and share the responsibility of AAC system design and training. A team evaluation form is available in a book by Johnson and others.[12]

### Fundamental AAC Training Strategies

Several of the following fundamental training strategies have proved valuable in establishing independent and effective communication through the use of AAC:

- Provide user with instruction in all four areas related to functional AAC use, including basic operational skills (e.g., turning on/off, programming, retrieving messages), language skills (e.g., teaching vocabulary, syntax, or the use of language to maximize communication), social skills (e.g., establishing topic, maintaining eye contact, giving listener feedback), and strategies (e.g., using the most effective communication method, giving listeners feedback, shortening messages to make communication faster).[13]
- Monitor "loads" during initial training to increase probability of success.
- Introduce new vocabulary and symbols gradually, providing immediate opportunities to use new vocabulary in functional context. Minimize drill and practice.
- Conduct inservice for caregivers on system set up and maintenance, including ongoing vocabulary modification.
- Teach caregivers how to solve simple device problems and consider providing written instructions ("cheat sheets").

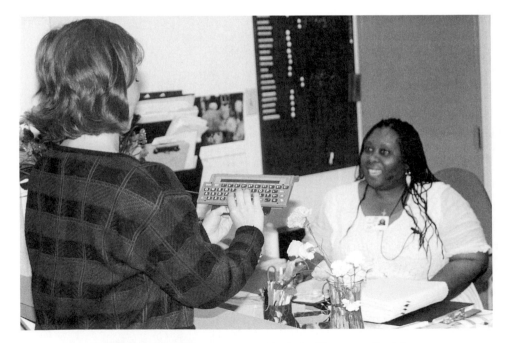

**Fig. 9-3** An AAC user communicates with a receptionist.

- Use scripts (e.g., telephone conversation is a natural script) to teach the user new vocabulary or the way to recognize and interpret cues from communication partners.
- Provide practice with specific communication intents (user may have little experience in using language to respond to a greeting or to ask questions) (Figure 9-3).
- Teach a sequence of modes to be used during a communication breakdown in specific environments (e.g., a user may use speech with an unfamiliar or untrained partner and then use an AAC device or manual board. For the telephone, the person may begin with a spoken output message and follow that with dysarthric speech).
- Establish concrete and functional goals with the user. Provide regular input on progress towards those goals.

### Strategies for Young Children or Individuals with Severe Developmental Disabilities

Several of the following strategies for young children or individuals with severe developmental disabilities are helpful:

- Train across environments within natural settings.[14]
- Ensure team acknowledges and fades prompting to minimize user's dependence on it.[15-17]
- Model AAC components or strategies to help validate these methods of communication for the user.
- Manipulate the environment to create the need for the user to use the communication system (e.g., leave out an item in an activity, supply the activity and wait for a response).
- Increase the likelihood that AAC components are used by providing easy accessibility to these components in all environments.
- Provide literacy instruction (e.g., writing and reading with symbols). Users may learn to sequence words as a way to communicate novel ideas.
- Label the environment with picture symbols to inundate and reinforce the use of symbols as a communication technique.
- Use symbols to represent the steps of a specific activity or to represent the sequence of activities that occur during a typical day (e.g., circle time, snack, PE). The child uses the symbols to request, comment, or indicate that an activity has been completed.
- Introduce new language through cause and effect training with 100% reinforcement (e.g., when a child indicates the message "jump," the trainer immediately reinforces by jumping).

## Outcomes and Social Validation

Establishing measurable goals for AAC use and monitoring progress towards these goals is one way clinicians can determine whether their intervention was effective (Table 9-5). Special educators use IEPs to measure a student's progress in different academic areas. Services the child receives and goals in the area of AAC can be incorporated. For students transitioning from high school to the community, individual transition plans (ITP) are used to measure progress. Outcomes related to AAC intervention can also be viewed using the World Health Organization (WHO) model.[18] The following five levels are in the revised WHO model:

1. Pathophysiology
2. Impairment
3. Functional limitation
4. Disability
5. Societal limitation

Some clinicians who provide traditional speech language services focus on the impairment level (i.e., reducing deficits in articulation and language) and administer standard-

## TABLE 9-5

*Measuring AAC Interventions*

| Level | Intervention Goals | Measurement Strategy |
|---|---|---|
| Impairment | Improve speech intelligibility | Intelligibility tests count number of times patient has to clarify, compare intelligibility with different partners (familiar versus unfamiliar) |
| | Improve expressive language | Measure type and number of vocabulary expressively produced on system, measure expressive utterance length |
| | Increase use of compensatory strategies to increase understandability of speech | Chart strategies in various environments |
| | Accuracy in operational use | Measure accuracy (i.e., switch activation or recall of symbol sequence), timing and charting |
| Disability (focus is placed on the individual) | Increase modes of communication | Frequency and success with telephone communication using AAC device, communication mode checklist (see Table 9-3) |
| | Increase speed of retrieving and formulating messages | |
| | Increase functions of communication in a conversation | Functions of communication (see Box 9-3) |
| Societal limitations (focus is on the individual in society) | Increase communicative independence | Measure level of prompting dependence on others to interpret |
| | Increased access to curriculum or participation in increased number of situations and contexts | Participation plans satisfaction surveys (survey user, teacher, employer, etc.) |
| | Interaction with additional partners | |

ized tests or informal tasks before and after intervention to measure the individual's progress. Sometimes these tools provide no indication that functional communication has improved. AAC intervention needs to focus on the level of disability and if at all possible, societal limitation.

Satisfaction changes with the user's increased ability to communicate and participate in various environments. Participation plans and satisfaction surveys may be used to measure the effectiveness of AAC intervention. Using an action plan is a mechanism to measure discrete steps in goal attainment and is a tool for including the family members as team members in an organized and informative way. The action plan keeps the AAC user and team members accountable for implementing different aspects of AAC intervention. During team meetings all team members develop strategies to meet the identified goals, assign team members who are responsible for the action, and determine a time for goal accomplishment.[19]

The participation plan also clearly demonstrates changes in implementation in the classroom and community. Models of participation are presented by Buekelman and Mirenda[2] and Bigge[20], in which decisions are made about the amount of participation and integration in the general education classroom. These models are helpful to set the parameters and expectations for the use of technology for communication and academics (see Case 1). Periodic surveys can be used to canvas stakeholders for their input as to progress of the team and intervention.

## Future Trends and Needs

An increased awareness of AAC use in the areas of autism and stroke and the geriatric population in general combined with a more general awareness of technology in the news affects all practitioners. As students are mainstreamed into their home schools, an increased number of speech-language pathologists have AAC users on their caseloads. No AAC coursework is required currently at the national level in the field of speech-language pathology, although some is available through different universities. This has resulted in a shortage of qualified practitioners. AAC evaluation centers, used as resources especially for rural communities, have declined because of the federal decrease in grant funding. As more AAC technology becomes available through vendors, practitioners may feel pressure to make device decisions by bringing in one or two vendors rather than the preferred method of working with device characteristics/features in a team evaluation approach. In addition, the Internet has begun to increase access to information about technology, and video conferencing will eventually increase the availability of long-distance expertise.

## CASE STUDIES

### CASE 1

## Application and Goal

J.M. was a 5-year-old boy student with the diagnosis of cerebral palsy affecting gross motor movements in all limbs and accompanied visual disability (Table 9-6). He attended a general education kindergarten class. He was nonambulatory and had a custom seat insert in his manual wheelchair for stability and to improve function. He had a wooden school chair for the classroom adapted with some positioning components.

Functional vision evaluation recommended symbols to be of high contrast black and white with slight color and 4 inches high when presented at a distance of 12 inches from his eyes. J.M. could grossly point with his right hand, make gross movements with a light beam placed on his head, do some simple gestures (e.g., wave) and activate a switch placed near his head. Receptive language tests presented in a modified format placed J.M. at approximately the 3-year receptive language level.

J.M.'s team consists of family, aides, a special education teacher, a kindergarten teacher, a speech pathologist with specialty in augmentative communication, a speech and language pathologist with specialty in oral motor therapy, an occupational therapist, a physical therapist, a vision therapist, and administrative staff.

## TABLE 9-6

*Specific Applications for Cases 1, 2, and 3*

| Name | Age | Diagnosis |
| --- | --- | --- |
| J.M. | 5 years | Cerebral palsy |
| C.J. | 18 years | Head injury |
| A.P. | 45 years | ALS |

ALS, amyotrophic lateral sclerosis.

## Function and Ability

J.M.'s communication system included word approximations for "more" and vocalizations to call for help, the modified sign for "all done," facial expressions, pointing in directions he wanted to move, body tone changes to indicate apprehension, a smile for "yes/acceptance," and a head shake for "no/denial."

He used a two-fist choice selection that involved a communication partner speaking two choices represented by two fists. He selected his choice by touching the hand represented by the choice he wanted.

J.M. used a whole hand pointing response to large pictures when two are presented in a field. He was unable to isolate a finger to point, and his visual difficulties limited his field to three large pictures. He was able to sequence two picture symbols to represent agent + action (dog walks) and modifier + agent (red cow), by pointing to two picture symbols.

## Considerations, Options, and Technology

### FEATURE MATCH

J.M.'s team members wanted him to develop independent responses in any or a variety of modes so that they could understand what he was attempting to communicate. Another need was to have equipment delineated for the use in the classroom. Positioning equipment for his wheelchair was recommended by his occupational therapist. His general communication goals included the following:

- Using multimodalities to expand expressive language
- Increasing the number of symbols, words, and gestures used for expressive communication
- Increasing his receptive and expressive vocabulary used for basic concepts
- Developing preliteracy skills
- Increasing his scanning skills with the use of a single switch for a response indicator
- Increasing his articulation of "t" and "d" sounds through improved respiratory and oral motor functioning

## Feature Match and Intervention Plan

J.M. could move his head from side to side. Initially, switches were placed at his head for single switch access. Gradually, switches were placed at right and left sides of his head mounted to his wheelchair and were adjustable and removable. He was then trained to activate cause and effect computer programs with each head switch to determine if two-switch site would be functional. He also used a digitized speech device with one switch (Tash VoiceMate).[21] Messages were recorded to be used with each of the two switches, and J.M. was learning the motor planning to use both switches through cause and effect language ("let's go" and "stop a minute"). The switches were used functionally in classroom literacy activities in which he was assigned a line in the story that is prerecorded in the VoiceMate. When time for that line to be spoken occurred, he activated his switch that produced the story line. Manual auditory scanning by pointing to pictures while naming them was in the training phase. J.M. had difficulty with scanning on the computer and specifically manual auditory scanning because of motor planning issues. He was able to give a "yes" indication to single questions where timing was not involved.

Because he demonstrated some controllable head movement, J.M. was given a light beam with custom head strapping to secure it in place and was given a sequence of light–beam motor–training activities. He engaged in cause and effect training by shining his light on the blackboard. Fellow students followed the light with chalk and produced a "drawing." As he advanced in his control, he could shine his light on photographs of classroom peers that were mounted on a wall, again in a cause and effect format.

A speech and language pathologist with specialty in AAC gave ongoing equipment training in operational strategies to school personnel. Specialists modeling new strategies and introducing technology gradually conducted team training throughout the year. Summer training sessions were planned for new staff before the beginning of the

## TABLE 9-7

*Participation Plan for J.M.*

| Activity | Goal | Tech Used | Strategy Used | Facilitator |
|---|---|---|---|---|
| Snack | Choices | Two switch/TVM | Two picture symbols | Aide |
| | Comments | One switch/TVM | One picture symbol | Teacher |
| Literature | Repetitive phrase | Two switch/TVM | Two picture symbol | SLP teacher SE teacher |
| | Respond to "who" and "what" questions | | Arm point to person or thing symbol | SLP |
| | Expressive noun and verb | | Two symbol, ask to point to noun and verb | SLP |
| Computer | Independent single switch scanning | Computer, Discover switch, one-switch software | Cause and effect scanning followed by "wait" for choice | SLP SE teacher aide |
| Light beam | Drawing | Light beam, custom head strap, dimly lit classroom | Cause and effect use, peers follow light with chalk or crayon | SLP, OT, aide, peers |

*TVM, tash voice mate; SLP, speech and language pathologist; SE, special education; OT, occupational therapist.*

school term. In addition, team meetings were held at 2-month intervals throughout the kindergarten year. All team members gave verbal or written input. A small notebook was carried in J.M.'s backpack to provide increased communication among professionals.

To organize the classroom activity time to integrate training, a participation plan was used (Table 9-7).

## Outcomes

As a result of the team intervention, J.M. gained increased competence in all areas, except the use of the light beam. Because of restricted training time, the light beam was used sporadically during the year. He gained the most motor control in the use of two head switches when used together to "speak" two different messages. He increased his concentration from 3 minutes to 15 minutes in the back of the classroom when working with two peers on switch or literacy activities. Because he could participate in reading books, his excitement about storytelling increased as demonstrated by overflow activity and increased vocalization during the activity. His speech approximations increased through the addition of five new words. The family expressed excitement at the length of time (up to 30 minutes) that J.M. could work independently at the computer, verbalizing to the teacher when he wanted the software program changed. The school administration was pleased that J.M. could adjust to the kindergarten curriculum, and the general education classroom teacher was relieved to find support in integrating this student.

## CASE 2

## Application and Goal

C.J. was an 18-year-old boy who was unable to speak because of a TBI sustained in a motor vehicle accident approximately 4 years before assessment. He communicated by vocalizing, answering "yes" and "no" questions, gesturing, and spelling out messages on a communication board. The board was his primary means of communication. Although C.J. hoped his speech would improve, he recognized his difficulties communicating with teachers, peers, and people in the community. The board was slow and tedious, particularly for unfamiliar listeners and in-group interactions.

## Function and Ability

C.J. was enrolled in special education at his local high school. He had a left hemiplegia. He had a manual wheelchair that he propelled with his right hand and foot. Despite limited vision in the left eye, he was able to see standard-sized print. Physically, he could directly select keys on standard and minikeyboards using his right index finger. He was also able to approximate "one-handed" signs with his right hand.

His reading comprehension and written language approximated the sixth grade level. He required cues to use a combination of words and spelling on his communication board. At times he spelled words that were already written on the board. C.J.'s math skills approximated the third grade level. He had a mild deficit in memory and new learning. He also had limited insight into his deficits. Problem solving and safety judgment was impaired. C.J.'s social interaction skills, specifically topic selection and maintenance, were impaired. At times, his comments and questions were inappropriate to the situation. His teachers reported that he had behavior problems and would sometimes act out in class. They attributed this in part to his difficulties with communication. C.J.'s speech was severely dysarthric, and no functional improvements in speech production had been noted in the last 2 years.

## Considerations, Options, and Technology

### FEATURE MATCH

C.J. was evaluated to determine the features needed. He was able to type simple messages using text-to-speech voice output. His resulting "spoken" messages were often difficult to understand because of his cognitive deficits that caused him to omit letters and words. With cues, he reviewed his message as he typed and made appropriate corrections. In these instances, the spoken messages were easy to interpret. A visual display with large letters helped him review and correct his messages. He successfully used letter encoding to recall stored messages when written cue cards were available to aid his memory and recall. Word prediction was not a useful strategy because the cognitive demands of reviewing a list of words slowed typing. Initially, he was resistant to voice output but recognized the benefit when he saw how quickly listeners understood his message and responded favorably. He had the motor ability to move a device out of the way to transfer from his chair.

C.J. needed a device that was portable, accessible from his wheelchair, and easy to move out of the way to allow for independent transfers. The device also needed to be accessed by direct selection with a finger, have ½-inch letters or cells, be alphabet-based, have access to stored messages via letter encoding, and have a visual display and text-to-speech voice output. He was willing to try a communication device, which his team encouraged.

## Intervention Plan

The communication board was modified to include relevant words and phrases. Color was added to highlight phrases for easier visual scanning for information. He was encouraged to scan or review his stored phrases before spelling a message. He was also encouraged to start with carrier phrases such as the following:

I need help with _____. I want to go to _____.

C.J. was taught five new gestures to help him interact with teachers and aides. He was given a 2-month trial with a speech output communication device in the form of a

LightWRITER SL35, which contained the appropriate features for him (e.g., large visual display, letter encoding, small and lightweight).[22]

## Outcomes

He successfully communicated with more people in a greater variety of situations. He was integrated into a music class and was more readily establishing friendships. His previous behavior problems associated with communication had decreased. In the community, he was able to convey his own needs via the LightWRITER and was less dependent on parents and teachers to communicate for him.

## CASE 3

### Application and Goal

A.P. was a 45-year-old man with amyotrophic lateral sclerosis (ALS). He was diagnosed with bulbar ALS within a year of his evaluation; however, he noticed symptoms approximately 18 months before. He lived alone but he had a part-time housekeeper. He worked for many years as a high school math teacher and continued to participate in community activities. Although he was able to walk and get around his home, he used a scooter for longer distances. Walking even short distances was getting progressively worse, so he was considering a wheelchair.

His speech was severely dysarthric. People familiar with him such as his stepson and housekeeper were able to understand him about 50% of the time. The quality of A.P.'s speech fluctuated and tended to be harder to understand when he was tired. A.P. supplemented his speech with gesturing, writing on a dry erase board, and typing on an electric typewriter. The extent to which a particular method was used depended on the quality of his speech, to whom he was talking, and what he was talking about. He was becoming more dependent on writing and typing as his speech deteriorated. A.P. also used the typewriter to write letters, make "to do" lists, and prepare messages in advance. He relied on his stepson or housekeeper to make telephone calls. His swallowing was also becoming progressively worse. He ate soft foods and thickened liquids. A gastrostomy feeding tube was being considered.

### Function and Ability

With prescription glasses, A.P. was able to see standard sized text. He wrote legibly but slowly with his right hand, producing one to two sentences before fatiguing or feeling cramps in his hand. He could use his right hand to directly select or type on standard or minikeyboards. Typing was less fatiguing than writing.

A.P.'s cognition and language skills were within functional limits. He readily used strategies to enhance communication such as writing messages ahead of time and shortening messages or using abbreviations when he wrote.

### Considerations, Options, and Technology

FEATURE MATCH

A.P. wanted to be as independent as possible and remain active in the local community. Evaluation results indicated that his communication system should have the following features or characteristics:

- Portable and accessible in a variety of situations (e.g., home, community)
- Alphabet-based to allow for novel message production
- Access to acceleration features such as letter encoding and word prediction, to assist with retrieval of frequently used messages and the generation of novel messages
- Expandable to multiswitch or single-switch input to accommodate changes in motor control

- Have text-to-speech voice output given the severity of his speech, his need to communicate over the telephone, his desire to interact with a wide audience, and the complexity of his messages

## Intervention Plan

Continued writing using short messages and abbreviations was recommended for interaction with familiar partners, particularly when partners misunderstood only portions of the utterance. This mode was the most efficient for "quick" conversational exchanges.

The local telephone company was contacted for a telecommunication device for the deaf (TTD) for phone communication. This was provided on long-term loan and was free.

He acquired a DynaVox communication device after a 4-week trial because it had the critical features he needed and he demonstrated initial proficiency.[23]

## Outcomes

A.P. had independent communication using the telephone with the TTD or the DynaVox. He had increased communication in the community with less familiar partners. He felt less isolated and increased his participation in community activities and maintained his quality friendships.

## References

1. American Speech-Language-Hearing Association: Competencies for speech-language pathologists providing services in augmentative communication, *ASHA* 31:107-110, 1989.
2. Beukelman D, Mirenda P: *Augmentative and alternative communication*, Baltimore, 1998, Brooks.
3. Cottier C, Doyle M, Gilworth K: *Functional AAC intervention: a team approach*, Bisbee, Ariz, 1997, Imaginart.
4. Blackstone S: What is language? How do children who use AAC learn it? *Augmentative Communication News* 5 (4), 1992.
5. Goossens C: *AAC Augmentative and alternative communication, aided communication intervention before assessment: a case study of a child with cerebral palsy*, pp 14-26, 1989, Williams & Wilkins.
6. Prentke Romich, Wooster, Ohio.
7. Mayer-Johnson, Solana Beach, Calif.
8. Yorkston K: *Augmentative communication in the medical setting*, Tucson, 1992, Communication Skill Builders.
9. Goossens C, Crain S, Elder P: *Engineering the preschool environment for interactive symbolic communication*, Birmingham, Ala, 1994, Southeast Augmentative Communication.
10. Beukelman D: AAC Journal Home Web Page, 1996, University of Nebraska.
11. Fitzgerald E: *Sign language for the deaf*, Washington, DC, 1976, Alexander G. Bell Association for the Deaf.
12. Johnson J et al: *Augmentation basic communication in natural contexts*, Baltimore, 1996, Paul Brooks.
13. Light J: Towards a definition of communicative competence for individuals using augmentative and alternative communication systems, *Augmentative and Alternative Communication* 5 (2):137-144, 1989.
14. Calculator S, Jorgensen C: Integrating AAC instruction into regular education settings: expounding on best practices *Augmentative and Alternative Communication* 7:204-211, 1991.
15. Reichle J, York J, Sigafoos J: *Implementing augmentative and alternative communication*, Baltimore, 1991, Brooks.
16. Hart B, Risley T: *How to use incidental teaching for elaborating language*, Bellevue, Wash, 1982, Edmark.
17. Musselwhite C: *Adaptive play for special needs children*, San Diego, 1986, College-Hill Press.
18. Blackstone S: *Augmentative Communication News* 8 (1):3, 1995; Disability in America: toward a national agenda for prevention, Washington DC, 1991, Institutes of Medicine, National Academy Press.
19. Henderson J: *Preschool AAC checklist*, Solana Beach, Calif, 1992, Mayer-Johnson.

20. Bigge J: *Teaching individuals with physical and multiple disabilities,* ed 3, New York, 1991, Macmillan.
21. TASH, Ontario, Canada.
22. ZYGO Industries, Portland.
23. DynaVox Systems Technology, Pittsburgh.

## Resources

American Speech-Language-Hearing Association: Report: augmentative and alternative communication, *ASHA* 33 (suppl 5): 9-12, 1991.

Glennen S, DeCoste D: *Handbook of augmentative and alternative communication,* San Diego, 1997, Singular.

Light J, Collier B, Parnes P: Communication interaction between young nonspeaking physically disabled children and their primary caregivers, part II, *Augmentative and Alternative Communication* 1:98-107, 1985.

Loyd L, Fuller D, Arvidson H: *Augmentative and alternative communication: a handbook of principles and practices, specifically "vocabulary selection,"* Boston, 1997, Allyn and Bacon.

Rehabilitation Engineering Research Center: *The guide to augmentative & alternative communication devices,* 1996, University of Delaware.

Sieget-Causey and Guess: *Enhancing nonsymbolic communication interactions among learners with severe disabilities,* Baltimore, 1989, Brooks.

# CHAPTER 10

## Integrated Systems

*Kevin Caves*

## Application and Goal

Using the input device or access method of one assistive technology to control other technologies a user may have is now possible. An *integrated control system (ICS)* is defined as using a single input device or access method of one assistive technology to control other assistive technologies. For instance, a wheelchair controller may be used to also operate a communication device. Using separate input devices or access methods to operate separate pieces of equipment is termed *distributed control (DC)*. Examples include a wheelchair operated by a wheelchair controller, an environmental control operated with a separate remote switch, a computer operated with a different and separate input device, or an access method. Commonly integrated equipment includes augmentative and alternative communication systems (AAC), computer systems, electronic aids for daily living (EADL), and power mobility. Before deciding whether to use either an integrated or distributed control system for a particular user with multiple technology needs, the advantages and disadvantages of an ICS and a distributed control system (DCS) must be measured.

This chapter covers the factors to consider when deciding between an ICS or a DCS. The chapter does not contain technical information regarding the components of integrated wheelchair controllers or other assistive technology, nor all the possible ICSs. Beginners in this area should seek help from professionals with advanced clinical experience and technical expertise. Such professionals include physical and occupational therapists, speech and language pathologists, rehabilitation engineers, and rehabilitation technology suppliers who have worked integrated control systems more extensively.

## Function and Ability

An ICS allows people with severe physical limitations who would not be able to access separate input devices to operate several pieces of equipment through a single input device. This could be users with a high-level spinal injury who use a single input device to drive their power wheelchair and type on a computer or users with cerebral palsy who are severely dysarthric and use a communication device to have conversations and change television channels. Integration is often considered the process of "pulling it all together." It includes deciding which devices, input devices, and access methods are most appropriate and addresses how each device is set up and positioned to facilitate its use.

Careful consideration of equipment positioning and mounting can greatly influence a technology solution's success. A communication device that shares an input device with a power wheelchair is not a useful system if it is mounted to interfere with the individual's ability to drive the chair or interferes with the user's visual field.

ICS technology is being built into systems at a more basic level; for example, an individual being evaluated may have a wheelchair with an ICS and may only need cables or connections between equipment. Newer mobility, AAC, EADL, and computer systems have the ability to link to other technologies or even have those technologies incorporated. More is possible because of improvements in technology and market forces. Similar to everyone else, users of assistive technology want and expect more from the technology they use today.

A technology solution may be only one of many possible solutions. A high technology solution is not inherently better than a low technology or nontechnology solution. Solutions that are the most practical and easiest to implement, use, and maintain should be considered. Possible solutions should be contrasted and compared. Then, if a technology solution seems appropriate, equipment with the delineated features can be researched and identified. Equipment trials should then be provided, along with practice sessions and further performance trials. Comparisons among possible solutions can be made, and pros and cons of different systems can be discussed.

## Considerations, Options, and Technology

### *When to Consider an ICS*

Integration of control of assistive technology has advantages. Integration may provide more technology options for individuals with limited physical control. Using a single input device can facilitate access to multiple technologies and make setup and positioning easier and more straightforward. The use of an ICS may improve the portability and/or aesthetics of a system by reducing its number of components. Another important benefit is that an ICS can bring independence to an individual in operating technology. Integration may be indicated in several situations.

### One Reliable Access Site

An access site is the body location and the action that is used to activate an input device. Positioning several input devices at an access site may be limited by the physical range and strength of the user and by the physical space available for these controls. If the input devices are too close, the user could unintentionally activate one input device while intending to activate another (Figure 10-1). Integrating control simplifies the setup of the entire system without requiring additional switches to be swung away or repositioned by someone else.

### Similar Optimum Input Device and Access Sites

Integrated control should also be considered when the optimum access sites and input devices are the same (e.g., an individual is evaluated for technology for mobility and communication and the optimum input device for mobility and communication is determined to be a joystick). In this case, use of an ICS using the joystick as an input device may be appropriate. For an individual using a sip and puff system to drive the wheelchair and a sip and puff Morse code system for computer input, an integrated system may be appropriate. Measuring the advantages of integrating control against the potential compromise in performance is important.

### Personal Preference

An individual's personal preference should be considered. A person may prefer the integrated controller for perceived performance benefits or for aesthetic reasons. In many cases, a single input device means less equipment and provides a more compact, cleaner system.

### Independence in the Environment

Integrating control can give the user increased independence. An individual may be able to use several input devices or methods, but an integrated solution may allow

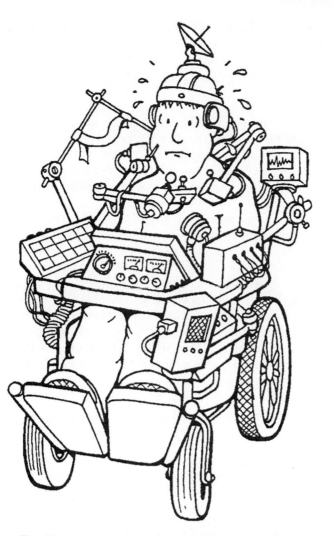

**Fig. 10-1** An individual in need of integrated control.

that person to independently use technology (e.g., an individual is evaluated and can access a computer through directed scanning using a joystick with an onscreen keyboard and can also access a standard keyboard with hands if it is carefully positioned by an attendant). Because the wheelchair joystick can be used to operate the directed scan and that command signal can be sent to the computer wirelessly, using an integrated system can permit access to the computer without requiring additional assistance.

## Technical Abilities of the User's Support System

A desirable feature of an ICS is that daily system setup for the user can be simplified because a single input device exists to position. In some settings in which the user's support system is untrained or inconsistent, having to position only one input device can help ensure that the technology is set up properly.

## *When Integrated Control Is Not Recommended*

Although integration of control of assistive technology has advantages, it is not for everyone. A study comparing integrated with distributed control systems reported that DCSs were recommended almost 4:1 over ICSs for individuals who had multiple technology needs and were seen at that center.[1] Use of an ICS may not be appropriate for an individual for several reasons.

## Potential Compromise in Performance Accessing Different Technologies

When considering integration of assistive technology, substituting a preferred input device or access method for one that the user is less proficient with but that can be integrated is often necessary (e.g., a person is evaluated for mobility and communication). A proportional joystick is identified as providing the best control of the wheelchair, and a switched joystick would be the best input device for the communication device. An integrated system may be indicated.

However, evaluating performance again with the integrated system is important. In this example, the individual can still drive optimally but because of the lack of switch tactile and auditory feedback from the proportional joystick, communication performance is compromised. Because one of the features of an ICS is the ability to use different input devices, a switched joystick could be substituted for the proportional joystick with no compromise in communication access. The ability to drive the chair, however, would likely be compromised by the use of a switched joystick for mobility.

Therefore integration means substituting a less desirable mode of access for one assistive device to integrate the control of all assistive technologies into the same input device is often necessary. Performance with one or many of the devices may thus be poorer with integrated control.

## An ICS May Be Cognitively and/or Visually Demanding

A person using an ICS to operate two or more separate pieces of technology must be able to enter a mode and use the input device, exit that mode and then enter another, and use the input device to operate another device. Therefore the individual must understand the following two points:

1. The input device is capable of operating the different technologies.
2. The input device is able to do this because of control modes.

Using one input device to control other devices is not necessarily logically inferred (Figure 10-2).

In addition, some integrated controllers require the user to interpret visual or auditory cues to switch between modes. This task is more cognitively demanding, requiring memory, organization, problem-solving skills, abstraction, flexibility, and the ability to generalize.

## Technical Limitations

Not all assistive technology can be integrated. For example, no commercially available integrated system exists for an individual whose optimal access to communication is head pointing using a light pen (optical pointer). This is because no wheelchairs are available that can be driven with light pens. Some situations exist in which integration is not physically possible.

## Environment

If an individual needs to use any of the integrated assistive devices from positions other than the power wheelchair (e.g., from bed or a manual chair), then the use of an ICS may be impractical if the control system and the input device are on the power wheelchair. For example, a person who uses an ECS operating the wheelchair joystick when in a power wheelchair may need a separate switch for the manual chair or bed. If this type of duplication is not used the individual could not access the ECS without sitting in the chair.

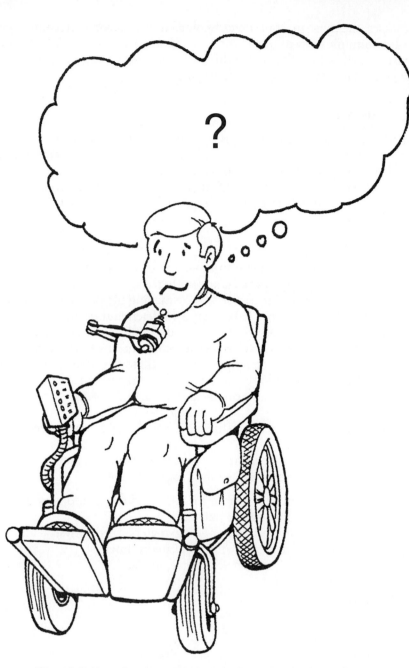

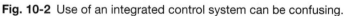

**Fig. 10-2** Use of an integrated control system can be confusing.

## Integrated Control Malfunction

If the device that the system is integrated around requires repairs, the user loses the ability to control all assistive devices that are integrated, unless other input methods have been established. Integration of technologies may necessitate a backup system.

## Cost

An ICS on wheelchairs can be expensive. ICSs can cost up to $3,500 more than a standard power wheelchair. Furthermore, duplicating input devices is sometimes necessary to accommodate different positions or environments or to be prepared in the event of an ICS or wheelchair malfunction.

In some cases, the most appropriate technology may be a completely integrated solution (e.g., a communication device that has computer access capabilities and environmental control capabilities). The cost of this one device may be less than the cost of three separate devices that perform the same functions.

## Personal Preference

Many individuals who are able to use an ICS simply prefer a distributed system. An individual may have used a specific input device successfully in the past and prefers not to change the way different assistive technologies are controlled. One user, a teenage girl, preferred to use a keyboard rather than another means of input required to use an integrated controller to blend in better with other members of her school class.

## *Evaluation Process*

The decision of whether to integrate should be one of the last considerations made in the evaluation process. Although information gathered in the evaluation may indicate a need to integrate, the individual is best served by making the decision to integrate after the evaluations for all technologies have been completed and desired features of those technologies have been identified.

An evaluation for each desired assistive technology such as a wheelchair, an AAC, a computer, and an ECS should be completed independently of other technology evaluations. Each technology area should be examined independently of the others so that the optimal solution for a particular need can be identified. If the decision is made to use an ICS at the beginning of an evaluation and technologies are chosen solely on their ability to be integrated, the solution may not be the most efficient and might even be ineffective for particular needs.

Evaluations for specific assistive technology areas may differ somewhat, but any evaluation should include assessments in the following basic areas:

- Needs and goals (long-term and short-term goals and expectations of possible technology solutions to meet those goals or needs)
- Environments in which the assistive technology will be used (physical and social, including support personnel available within the environments)
- Functional abilities (physical, sensory, cognitive, social, etc.)
- Previous equipment experience
- Personal preferences
- Other equipment to be used
- Any future needs that can be identified

From these assessments, the features of the technology are identified and possible equipment solutions can be delineated for each assistive technology area. For example, an individual may be evaluated for verbal and written communication needs, and the team decides to consider electronic assistive technology in the areas of AAC and computer access. After the communication evaluation, the team identifies features of a solution that best meet the individual's communication needs. After the computer access evaluation, the team identifies features of technology that are the best suitable for the individual's computer writing needs.

The team should then consider integration. A number of the factors listed previously may influence the decision of whether to recommend a distributed system consisting of a dedicated communication device and a dedicated computer or computer-based AAC system. All of the technology needs can then be considered, and compatibility and integration issues with other equipment and the variety of activities the user performs can be discussed.

## Role of Speed, Accuracy, Endurance, and Independence

Each of the technology areas (EADL, communication, computer access, and mobility) has different input requirements related to speed, accuracy, endurance, and independence. For example, EADL access does not need to be immediate. Taking several seconds to turn on a light, change the TV channel, or open a door is adequate for most individuals. Accuracy and endurance are not generally critical requirements for EADL because the user is not continually accessing the device for hours at a time. What is more important is that the user is able to access the EADL independently.

With an AAC device, speed, accuracy, and independent access to input are important to communicate as quickly as possible. Endurance with the input method is less important because the user is usually not accessing the device continually for long periods during a typical conversation.

A person using a computer for writing or entertainment is likely to work for longer periods. Speed, accuracy, and endurance are critical factors. Because most people plan to spend extended periods using a computer, having to take some time to set up or have assistance assistance setting up the work environment is not unreasonable. Any person who works on a computer should take some time to position the keyboard and monitor so that it can be used most comfortably and efficiently. Because users may need some assistance with setup, they sacrifice some independence for increased efficiency and endurance.

Regarding mobility, speed, accuracy, endurance, and independence are all important. A wheelchair driver needs to be able to operate the chair efficiently and independently, sometimes for long distances (Table 10-1).

These general principles need to be remembered when considering use of an ICS. Substituting an input device or access method when using an ICS can affect the ability to operate one or all of the technologies. The ultimate goal in the assistive technology process is to make users are as independent as possible and that they are allowed to perform at as high a level as their abilities and the technology allow.

## Pulling It All Together

After the features of the individual technologies have been matched to the user's needs, all of the technology needs can be considered as a whole and compatibility and integration issues with other equipment and with the variety of activities to be performed can be discussed. This is the time to consider the way all the different technologies work together. The following questions should be asked:

- Can the individual drive, stop, and initiate conversation?
- Can the individual independently answer and use the phone?
- Can the individual request a glass of water?

Technologies cannot be considered in isolation of other equipment to be used and other activities to be performed throughout the day in various environments.[2]

The user needs to know all the considerations of the way the technology works, looks, and is mounted. Knowing the amount of assistance needed from others and the way the

## TABLE 10-1

*Technology and Factors Ratings*

|  | Speed | Accuracy | Endurance | Independence |
|---|---|---|---|---|
| EADL | Not crucial | Not crucial | Not crucial | Important |
| AAC | Important | Important | Less important | Important |
| Computer | Important | Important | Important | Setup OK |
| Mobility | Important | Important | Important | Important |

*EADL, electronic aids for daily living; AA, augmentative and alternative communication.*

equipment may or may not interfere with other activities are also important. Compromises often need to be made. The service provider's responsibility is to consider possible compromises and the pros and cons and to present these to the user and/or family and caregivers. The user must make the final decisions on which compromises, if any, are to be made, provided cost is not prohibitive, as the user is the one who must use the technology daily.

This is also the time to consider the physical integration of all input devices and assistive devices.[3] The service provider should be aware of any special equipment or mounting that is required to integrate or what cables or other connections are available to link input devices and technologies. Several different ways are available to link assistive technologies but the two most basic are direct connection or *hard wiring* and remote connection or *wireless.*

A direct connection is a physical wire that connects the input device to the assistive technology. Two of the most common wireless connections are infrared (IR), which is what a TV remote control is based on, and radio frequency (RF), which is what portable phones and garage remote controls are based on. Both of these transmission technologies employ a transmitter and a receiver to send a signal from one point to another without wires. The only real difference between the two is the signal. IR transmits an invisible light that is directional and does not go through walls or other obstacles. Similar to the TV remote control, the user needs to point the control at the receiver for the remote to work. RF transmits a radio signal that is multidirectional and can travel through walls and obstacles such as a garage door opener.

## The Team Approach

Much has been written about the team approach in assistive technology. Most assistive technology assessment manuals or texts include sections on the importance of the team approach, which is absolutely essential when considering integration of multiple technologies. The use of one technology, access method, or input device could affect the choice and use of all other technologies. All of the technologies and their potential effect on other technologies and activities must be considered together.

Members of the team typically include clinicians such as occupational, physical, or speech therapists who perform the evaluations and assessments for features needed for different technologies. Other members such as rehabilitation engineers assist with the evaluations and provide technical knowledge and expertise regarding positioning and integration of different technologies. Finally, rehabilitation technology suppliers provide technical information on possibilities, specific components, and ordering information. The user is the primary team member and essentially leads the team. The user is the one who applies the technology in daily life and is the one who should make the final decisions regarding the various pros and cons of possible technology solutions.

## Documentation and Funding

Maintaining documentation of what was done during the evaluation and equipment trial sessions is important. Because integrated systems are often more technologically complicated, careful recording of equipment tested, settings, cabling, and switch positions can help in the report writing, justification, and delivery stages of the assessment.

Documentation should detail the specific equipment and components necessary for integration of the assistive technologies and should include justification for the integration. Components necessary to integrate control through the wheelchair controller are often easier to obtain as part of the wheelchair order. Cabling or software necessary for interfacing AAC, computer, or an ECS should be specified in the documentation for those technologies.

Components needed for integration cost from a few dollars for cables and several hundred for wireless technology to connect one device to another, to thousands for integrated wheelchair controllers and components. If a user is paying with private funds, any device or combination of equipment desired can be obtained. In this situation, the service provider is helping the user make an educated choice. When a third-party payer is funding equipment, the service provider is not only helping the user make an educated choice but also must justify this choice to the payer.

The service provider is required to make some judgment of the value of a particular solution if the payer is a third party. In other words, the following question should be answered: Does the benefit of this solution justify its expense over other less-expensive possible solutions? Conflicts may result if a service provider cannot justify the particular solution a user might want. This does not mean that a user wants the most expensive solution. Users are usually well aware of the need to compare value among possible solutions, regardless of funding origination, especially when they are funding the equipment.

With respect to an ICS, an integrated solution may be considerably more expensive and may only increase the users performance marginally. As described earlier, it may in fact compromise performance. If two access methods, one being a more-expensive integrated system, allow a user to input text to the computer at the same rate, the reason the more expensive of these access methods is being recommended should be well documented and justified. These reasons may include safety, ease of setup and use, and independence.

Because some medical insurance companies only fund certain types of equipment while the person is an inpatient, therapists may be speculating regarding a patient's possible technology needs. This approach is not ideal because these particular patients are changing physically and cognitively and do not know their potential technology needs. Therapists may be asked to complete a power wheelchair order before the need for an ICS is known. Therefore some determination needs to be made regarding the cost of adding on components that allow for an ICS later. Technologies that are less likely to be funded by medical insurance are best addressed once patients have gone home, determined what they want, and have established a potential need for assistive technologies.

## Training

Training in the use of all assistive technologies is important. Individuals who receive an ICS may need additional training to learn to switch from one assistive technology to another or close one application and then open another. The use of an access method should be as transparent as possible. The use of an ICS should not make a task significantly more complicated to perform, and the user should not have to train for a long time to use the ICS. The amount of training varies, depending on type, complexity and/or sophistication of the technology, and the expertise of the user, family, caregivers, and other support personnel.

## Outcomes and Social Validation

Successful outcomes when considering integration of assistive technology depend on the goal of the technology intervention. A successful outcome is just as likely to come from a system in which integration was not decided. Similarly for the practitioner, successful use of these principles depends on what the goal is for the use of the technology.

Performance can be measured in many different ways: objectively and subjectively. Words per minute can be a measure of typing performance. The ability to express a want or need may be a measure of performance for a communication device. Other examples of performance measures include the ability to independently change a TV channel or to drive the wheelchair from the bedroom to the living room, to answer the door. Performance measures for a technology may be unique to individuals; for example, one person may retrieve a message stored in an AAC device to ask for a drink and another person may use the device to write speeches and participate in conversations forming unique messages. Because the needs are different, the performance measures need to be different. Integration of control of assistive technology may provide more technology options for an individual with limited physical control, and for another person, the trade off in performance may make the decision not to integrate the more successful option.

Factors such as the user's physical, cognitive, and sensory abilities, the user's environment and level of independence, the abilities of the user's support system, and the user's preferences contribute to the decision of whether to use an integrated system. Factors such as performance trade-offs, cost, technical limitations, and malfunctions also need to be considered. All of these factors need to be considered with respect to the user's quality of life, functional status, and the costs of the equipment and any training the user or the support staff needs to be able to use the equipment.

Assistive technology manufacturers are adding features to their devices that facilitate integration. These device enhancements are expected to make the clinician's job to integrate assistive technology easier.

## CASE STUDIES

### CASE 1

J.J. is a 15-year-old young man who is nonverbal with spastic cerebral palsy. He is mainstreamed and is expected to graduate with his class. He has been referred by the school for an evaluation of his writing needs.

### Background

J.J. is an experienced user of assistive technology. He has used a power wheelchair and an AAC device for 8 years. Using a proportional joystick with his right hand, he is able to independently drive his power wheelchair (Figure 10-3). He accesses his communication device through direct selection using his right hand and can accurately select cells on his device's 128-key membrane keyboard.

### Evaluation

Evaluations for mobility and communication identified that his current strategies and assistive technology were meeting his needs. J.J. and his teachers determined that his primary writing need was to be able to generate reports and papers at school. His parents were interested in obtaining equipment for him to use at home. The school was ini-

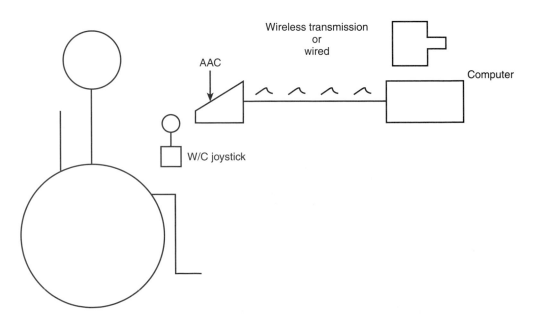

**Fig. 10-3** J.J.'s system includes a distributed mobility/AAC system and integrated AAC/computer access.

tially interested in an integrated laptop-based communication and writing system that would be mounted to the chair so that the equipment would be with him when he needed to type.

## Computer Access Equipment Trials

J.J. could easily select characters from keys on a standard keyboard without fatiguing but his key selection rate was slow. Trials with computer–based rate–enhancing techniques (e.g., word prediction and completion, abbreviation expansion) did help increase his typing speed to acceptable levels.

His communication device used a language strategy to encode language that allowed him to generate unique phrases, and he could enter a mode to spell what he could not generate using the language strategy. His device also had the ability to store custom phrases or commands. The system was capable of sending what the user typed to a computer. Trials using J.J.'s communication device as the input system for the computer were comparable to the direct selection on the computer with the rate-enhancing techniques.

## To Integrate or Not To Integrate

A needs assessment identified that J.J. did not need to write in multiple environments but instead only needed to write in one classroom. A computer was available in the classroom that could be dedicated to his use.

J.J. preferred using his communication device to accessing his computer because he knew his system well. A cost comparison showed that using the communication device to access the computer required less equipment to be purchased. Based on the evaluation, his family purchased a home computer compatible with the computer he used at school that he and the rest of the family could use.

## Recommendations

Because J.J.'s mobility and AAC systems were already meeting his needs, continuing to use them was recommended. His AAC had the capability of being connected to the computer at school and home with an inexpensive cable. The computers required no additional special software to take input from the communication device. He was familiar with his communication system and was able to quickly produce the reports and papers he wanted to write. Information was also provided on a wireless system that would eliminate the need to physically connect the communication device to the computer.

## CASE 2

S.Z. is a 30-year-old woman who was injured 6 months ago and has a complete spinal cord injury at the C1-2 level. She is ventilator dependent. She has a degree in computer science and was employed as a computer programmer for a large software company before her injury. She would like to return to work.

## Background

Switch access evaluation from her wheelchair revealed she could activate pneumatic switches (sip and puff) or a light-touch switch carefully positioned at either side of her jaw. From bed, she could only reliably activate a pneumatic switch.

## Evaluation and Equipment Trials

Evaluations for mobility, computer access, and environmental control from S.Z.'s wheelchair and bed were conducted. From these evaluations, sipping and puffing was determined to be the best access for mobility. For computer access, Morse code using a sip and puff switch was the preferred method. For environmental control, a single switch scanning infrared controller capable of operating her phone, bed, and IR devices using either a pneumatic or light touch switch was deemed best.

### To Integrate or Not To Integrate

The team contemplated integration at this point. Because the optimum input devices for mobility, computer, and ECS were the same (sip and puff), an integrated system was considered. Independence using and switching between mobility, computer, and ECS was also identified as an important need. Equipment trials using the wheelchair's sip and puff switch as the input to the computer system proved successful. Because the wheelchair already contained the integrated control system, all that was needed was to purchase an IR remote transmitter/receiver to send the signal to the computer. The ECS was mounted on S.Z.'s chair and it was directly connected with a wire to the wheelchair's integrated control system. With this setup, she was able to operate her chair, computer, and ECS independently by switching between the wheelchair's driving and accessory modes.

### Other Environments

From bed, S.Z. felt that she did not need access to her computer but did want access to her ECS, a phone, and the controls of her bed. A mount was identified for her scanning IR remote control that would allow her caregivers to transfer it from the chair to the bed. A separate pneumatic switch was mounted so that she could operate the ECS and the phone.

### References

1. Guerette P, Sumi E: Integrating control of multiple assistive devices: a retrospective review, *Assistive Technol* 6:67–76, 1994.
2. Bain BK: Steps in a problem-solving evaluation for assistive technology, *Technology Special Interest Section Newsletter of the American Occupational Therapy Association* 5 (2), June 1995.
3. Lee K, Thomas D: *Control of computer-based technology for people with physical disabilities: an assessment manual,* 1990, University of Toronto Press.

### Recommended Readings

Bain BK: Steps in a problem-solving evaluation for assistive technology, *Technology Special Interest Section Newsletter of the American Occupational Therapy Association* 5 (2), June 1995.

Cook A, Hussey S: *Assistive technologies: principles and practice,* St Louis, 1995, Mosby.

Guerette P, Caves K, Gross K: One switch does it all, *TeamRehab Report* 26–29, Mar/April 1992.

Guerette P, Sumi E: Integrating control of multiple assistive devices: a retrospective review *Assistive Technol* 6: 67–76, 1994.

Lee K, Thomas D: *Control of computer-based technology for people with physical disabilities: an assessment manual,* 1990, University of Toronto Press.

Trefler E, Angelo J: Surveying users of integrated controls: a pilot study, *Proc ARATA* 17–19, Oct 1995.

### Acknowledgments

A portion of the material for this chapter was drawn from a Rehabilitation Engineering and Research Center (RERC) study that focused on integrated controllers. Support for the RERC was provided by National Institute on Disability and Rehabilitation Research, U.S. Department of Education (Grant No. H133E00015).

I wish to acknowledge the staff at the Las Floristas Center for Applied Rehabilitation Technology (CART) at Rancho Los Amigos National Rehabilitation Center.

# CHAPTER 11

## Sensory Aids: Vision

*Diane C. Bristow*
*Gail L. Pickering*

## Application and Goals

The purpose of implementing assistive technology is to enable clients with visual impairments to function to their maximal potentials educationally, vocationally, and socially and in activities of daily living (ADL). In the selection and implementation of assistive technology for people with visual impairments, the ultimate goals and anticipated outcomes must be considered first and throughout the process. Appropriate goals and an effective implementation process can lead to a successful outcome (Figure 11-1). With the focus on the goal to be achieved, the individual can determine necessary steps to reach those goals. If the ultimate intent, for example, is only that the individual be able to independently distinguish among various medicine bottles rather than reading extensive materials at work, the recommended technology and implementation procedures are quite different. If the person has multiple disabilities, the goals and implemented technology may be more extensive and require the integration of various technologies.

Goals should be considered in each of the following areas of the user's life:

1. Education: if the person is enrolled in school or intends to enroll
2. Employment: if the person is employed or is on a career path toward employment
3. Mobility: if the person has difficulty with mobility
4. Communication: if communication is restricted because of a disability
5. Independence: if the level of independence is restricted
6. Recreation and play: for involvement in extracurricular or leisure activities
7. Community: to increase the person's involvement in the community

In identifying the goals, the assistive technology specialist must determine the plans of the individual and the family, teacher, optometrist or ophthalmologist, allied health professional, and/or employer (Box 11-1). Often the goals of each may be quite different. To identify the most appropriate and realistic goals, the assistive technology specialist must act as the facilitator to discuss the various viewpoints.

Implementation of this technology requires an analysis of the person's goals, needs, abilities, and potential capabilities. Through a comprehensive evaluation, the assistive technology specialist selects and matches the most appropriate technology. The assistive technology, however, is only a tool. Once the individual can independently and successfully implement the use of the technology, the technology is effective. This can involve custom modifications, extensive training, and ongoing assessment by a team of individuals who may include the person with a visual impairment, family members, teachers, a vision specialist, an employer, a vocational rehabilitation counselor, an ophthalmologist or optometrist, a rehabilitation engineer, and/or a physician. Additional specialists such as a speech and language pathologist, an occupational therapist, and a physical therapist may be required if the individual has multiple disabilities.

| Appropriate goals | + | Effective implementation | = | Successful outcome |
|---|---|---|---|---|

**Fig. 11-1** Obtaining a successful outcome.

BOX 11-1

*Factors to Consider in Establishing Assistive Technology Goals*

---

*Education*
What does the teacher target as the classroom goals for the year?
What is the adult client's academic major?
What academic skills does the client want or need to acquire?

*Employment*
What vocational skills does the client want or need to acquire?
What are the anticipated vocational opportunities for a person with visual impairments who also has cognitive, speech, or physical limitations?
What are the specific job tasks required for the client's employment position?

*Mobility*
Does the client have difficulty ambulating because of a visual impairment?
Does the client have a visual impairment and a physical impairment that affect mobility?
Does the client want to drive independently?

*Communication*
Do the client's visual impairments affect the ability to read body language and facial expressions?
Do the client's visual impairments inhibit the ability to immediately recognize a familiar person?
Are the communication limitations restricted to unfamiliar listeners?
Do the client's visual limitations affect the use of an augmentative communication device?

*Independence*
Does the visual impairment affect the client's ability to perform ADL such as eating, dressing, hygiene, or cooking?

*Recreation/Play*
What would the client like to do recreationally?
What are the child's or family's favorite type of play and/or recreational activities?

*Community*
Is the client actively involved in community activities?
What community activities would the client enjoy?
Does the client require assistance in transportation within the community?
Do limitations occur in being able to shop?

---

Assistive technology is changing rapidly because of advances in computer technology and equipment design. When recommending or selecting assistive technology, the practitioner must consider availability, features, expandability, effectiveness compared with similar devices, and application for individuals with visual disabilities.[1,8]

## Function and Ability

Visual impairments may include blindness, low vision, and functional vision deficits. The term *blindness* means that a person has no usable vision. Low vision indicates that a person cannot perform visual tasks with conventional optical correction. Functional vision involves the person's ability to identify, interpret, and understand the environment. The primary needs for a person with low vision or functional vision deficits are education and training aimed at maximizing use of the available vision. The selection and use of assistive technology depend on the person's amount and type of visual impairment.

## BOX 11-2

*Visual Impairments*

*Albinism:* A congenital condition characterized by partial or total lack of melanin pigment. The individual is vulnerable to adverse effects of sunlight frequently resulting in photophobia and astigmatism.

*Amblyopia:* Also known as *lazy eye*. Reduced vision in an eye that has not received adequate use during early childhood, often resulting from a misalignment of a child's eyes (e.g., crossed eyes) or when a difference in image quality occurs between the two eyes (i.e., one eye focuses better).

*Astigmatism:* An error in refraction. When light strikes the eye, it is refracted or bent by the eye lens and the cornea, which is the transparent membrane in front of the eyeball. Errors of refraction occur if the lens, cornea, and length of the eyeball are not perfectly balanced, resulting in blurry vision.

*Blindness:* No usable vision. Legal blindness, however, is defined as a person whose central acuity does not exceed 20/200 in the better eye with corrected lenses. This terminology is used for legal purposes to define tax status, insurance, and compensation benefits and other allotments.

*Cataract:* An opaque or clouding of the eye's lens that blocks or changes the passage of light essential for vision. A cataract is most often associated with the normal aging process; however, other factors that may be related are infection, hereditary and congenital influences, chemical or physical injury to the eye, exposure to intense heat or radiation, and certain general diseases such as diabetes.

*Cortical Blindness:* Blindness resulting from a lesion in the visual center of the cerebral cortex of the brain.

*Diabetic Retinopathy:* A disorder in which the small blood vessels nourishing the retina (back layer of the eye) weaken and break down or become blocked. The blood vessels in diabetic retinopathy may begin to bulge (aneurysm), leak fluid, bleed, grow abnormally, or close completely.

*Functional Vision:* Involves the ability to identify, interpret, and understand what one sees. The effective movement, alignment, fixation, and focus of both eyes as a team enhance the interpretation of visual information.

*Glaucoma:* A condition in which increased intraocular pressure develops, causing damage to the optic nerve. Damage begins at the edge of the visual field, affecting only the peripheral vision. If allowed to progress, the glaucoma can cause increasingly narrowed vision and eventually complete blindness.

*Hemianopsia:* A loss of either the right or left half of the visual area. Hemianopsia can occur in stroke and traumatic brain injured.

*Low Vision:* Indicates an inability to perform visual tasks with conventional optical correction. A person who has 20/50 or less vision is considered to have low vision. With 20/50 vision, an individual must be within 20 feet of an object to see it, whereas, an individual with normal vision (20/20) can see the same object at 50 feet.

*Modified from Anderson KN: Mosby's medical dictionary, St Louis, 1994, Mosby.*     *Continued*

Visual impairments may be the result of a disease, abnormalities in the growth pattern, or an accident (Box 11-2). The effective movement, alignment, fixation, and focus of both eyes as a team enhance the interpretation of visual information (Box 11-3). Any person with a visual impairment can benefit from the use of assistive technology. Therefore no specific prerequisite skills exist for the implementation of some assistive technol-

## BOX 11-2

### *Visual Impairments—cont'd*

*Macular Degeneration (Juvenile or Age-Related):* A degenerative disease that affects a small area in the back of the eye called the *macula,* the central part of the retina that is responsible for sight in the center of the field of vision. The peripheral (side) vision is not affected. This disease may be associated with arteriosclerosis, hereditary factors, or eye trauma.

*Retinal Detachment:* A separation of the inner layers of the retina from the pigment layer. Severe trauma to the eye or a penetrating wound may be the proximate cause, but retinal detachment may result from changes in the vitreous chamber associated with aging or inflammation of the interior of the eye.

*Retinits Pigmentosa (RP):* An inherited disease that is characterized by bilateral degeneration of the retina beginning in childhood and progressing to blindness by middle age.

*Hyperopia:* Also called *farsighted.* A condition resulting from an error of refraction in which rays of light entering the eye are brought into focus behind the retina.

*Myopia:* Also called *nearsightedness.* Caused by the elongation of the eyeball or by an error in refraction so that parallel rays are focused in front of the retina.

*Nystagmus:* Involuntary, rhythmic movements of the eyes. The oscillations may be horizontal, vertical, rotary, or mixed.

*Optic Atrophy:* Degeneration of the optic nerve and optic tract. Optic atrophy may be caused by a congenital defect, inflammation, occlusion of the central retinal artery or internal carotid artery, alcohol, arsenic, lead, tobacco, or other toxic substances. Degeneration of the disc may accompany arteriosclerosis, diabetes, glaucoma, hydrocephalus, pernicious anemia, and various neurologic disorders.

*Presbyopia:* Farsightedness resulting from a loss of elasticity of the lens of the eye. The condition commonly develops with advancing age.

*Strabismus:* An abnormal ocular condition in which the eyes are crossed. Both eyes are not simultaneously directed at the same object.

*Modified from Anderson KN: Mosby's medical dictionary, St Louis, 1994, Mosby.*

ogy for this population. However, the selection and use of various low and high technologies can vary greatly, depending on the individual's vision, cognition, language, and physical skills. For instance, people trained in the use of refreshable Braille displays (raised Braille characters that display information stored in files) require the prerequisite skills of reading and writing in Braille. Unfortunately, however, not all children who are blind have learned Braille. Consequently, their written language skills may not be at age level, which can affect the introduction of this technology. Therefore specialists may need initial training in developing new skills such as Braille reading to use the technology.[2]

A specialist may not have previously diagnosed some visual impairments because they are subtle. Teachers or therapists must screen each child to determine if any visual problems exist. Poor academic performance, behavioral problems, or poor social interaction may be because of visual deficits.

## CASE STUDY

P.N. is an adult college student with severe spastic quadriplegia cerebral palsy and undiagnosed visual problems. To plan for employment accommodations, he had an assistive

BOX **11-3**

*Definitions of Visual Skills*

*Binocularity:* Ability to use both eyes together.

*Depth Perception:* Ability to judge relative distances of objects and to see and move accurately in three-dimensional space.

*Distance Acuity:* Ability to clearly see, inspect, identify, and understand an object at a distance.

*Fixation:* Ability to quickly locate and inspect a series of stationary objects, one after the other, with both eyes.

*Focus Change:* Ability to look quickly from far to near and vice versa without momentary blur.

*Maintaining Attention:* Ability to keep doing a particular activity without interfering with the performance of other skills.

*Near Vision Acuity:* Ability to clearly see, inspect, identify, and understand objects at a near distance within arm's length.

*Peripheral Vision:* Ability to monitor and interpret what is going on in the environment while attending to a specific central visual task.

*Tracking:* Ability to follow a moving object with both eyes.

*Visualization:* Ability to form mental images and retain them for future recall.

technology evaluation. P.N. accessed the computer by single-key entry using various fingers. To verify the information typed, his mother read back everything that was on the computer screen. Generally, however, P.N. dictated his written assignments to his mother who then typed it because this was faster and less stressful than using the technique previously described. In addition, P.N. reported that although he read all of his own textbooks, he only accomplished this by isolating himself in his bedroom, kneeling on the floor, with his arms resting on the edge of his bed and with his book positioned in front of his face. Reading a few pages took him hours.

During the evaluation, P.N. did not accurately select the keys on the computer keyboard and was unable to read the monitor without struggling to interpret. During observations while he was typing, his eyes did not act as a team. When asked to read back the typed information, P.N. had difficulty maintaining his place and exhibited constant visual search. He also became frustrated in attempting to complete the task. P.N. confirmed that this was typical of his reading pattern. When the visual contrast (bold black print on a white background) was changed and the size of the print and line spacing was increased, P.N.'s performance improved and his level of frustration decreased. Once the possibility of a visual problem was addressed, P.N.'s mother asked, "Why didn't you ever tell me that you had trouble seeing?" P.N. responded, "I thought that was the way everyone saw."

After this initial evaluation, P.N. was referred to a functional vision optometrist who diagnosed severe functional visual deficits. The doctor also initiated visual training and provided recommendations for visual accommodations. At the time of the evaluation, P.N. had already taken 10 years to complete a bachelor's degree in computer programming. The amount of time it took him to complete assignments was always attributed to his physical limitations rather than any visual problems. If this disability had been diagnosed earlier, his college education would not have been such a struggle.

If people have been visually impaired throughout life, they may not realize they see differently from others. This is especially true for children. Therefore professionals must

BOX **11-4**

*Behavioral Signs of Functional Visual Deficits*

*General Behaviors*
- Excessive physical fatigue or discomfort after doing intense visual activity
- Double vision complaints
- Decreased accuracy after an intensive visual activity
- Decreased speed of access after an intensive visual activity
- Visual suppression (covering one eye while reading or looking at an object)
- Inefficient eye-hand or eye-body coordination
- Increased visual search after an intensive visual activity
- Headaches near the eyes or forehead or at the back of the head
- Increased visual search
- Frequent change of focus
- Increased or decreased muscle tone
- Increased motor stress and frustration
- Back-and-forth moving of the head rather than only the eyes while reading or looking at an object
- Poor attention span or drowsiness after prolonged visual work that is less than an arm's length away
- Blurred vision
- Red-rimmed, encrusted, or swollen eyelids
- Inflamed or red eyes
- Squinted eyes or frowns during visual activity
- Difficulty with adjusting to a dark room
- Sensitivity to light or glare
- Black spots or flashes of light
- Halos or rainbows around light
- Dark spot at center of viewing
- Distorted or wavy vertical lines
- Excess tearing eyes
- Dry eyes with itching or burning
- Spots
- Peripheral vision loss
- Excessive eye rubbing
- Placement loss when moving gaze from desk work to chalkboard

recognize this disability and listen to the complaints or behaviors their clients might be reporting or observe signs that indicate visual difficulties (Box 11-4). When these behaviors are identified, a physician should refer the patient to a behavioral or functional optometrist. Behavioral optometry includes the practices of developmental and functional optometry. It is an expanded area of optometric practice that tests and trains specific visual skills. A behavioral optometrist takes a holistic approach in treating the person to prevent or normalize visual problems and to enhance visual performance (see Appendix B at the end of the chapter).

## Considerations, Options, and Technology

### Technical or Clinical Expertise Needed

Because credentialing is not required and state licensing does not exist, no clear criteria exist to designate someone as an assistive technology specialist in the field of visual aids. Therefore providers of assistive technology must be ethical and should state when they do not have the knowledge or skills to assist a certain population.

## BOX 11-4

*Behavioral Signs of Functional Visual Deficits—cont'd*

### Additional Signs Related to Writing
- Uphill or downhill writing on a flat piece of paper
- Irregular letter or word spacing
- Reversal of letters (e.g., b for d) or words (e.g., saw for was)

### Additional Signs Related to Computer Use
- Slow refocusing when looking from copy to computer monitor or from monitor to distant objects
- Difficulty seeing clearly at a distance after prolonged computer use
- Color perception changes
- Lowered visual efficiency and more frequent errors
- Tension or pain in neck and shoulder
- Strain in eyes from the computer video monitor

### Additional Signs Specifically Related to Reading
- Slow reading
- Difficulty maintaining concentration while reading
- Problems with comprehension of reading
- Skipping words or lines of print while reading
- Blurred distant objects after extended reading
- Double vision while reading
- Floating or moving words appear around the page while reading
- Using a finger or a marker to maintain place while reading
- Rereading words or lines while reading
- Closing or covering one eye when reading
- Tendency to move head closer to or away from the material while reading
- Decreased body alignment when engaging in a visual activity
  - Holding or positioning a book or object close to the eyes
  - Holding the head at an extreme angle while reading or looking at an object
  - Frequently shifting posture when reading or looking at an object

The assistive technology specialist must have knowledge of the specific disabilities and a clear understanding of the way these disabilities affect a person's life. Disabilities manifest in unique ways. Even though the individual with disabilities may appear to resemble someone from a previous case, the underlying conditions and symptoms can be quite different. Many times, subtle differences exist that would not be recognizable to someone who did not understand the disability. Often, a well-meaning person with computer expertise develops a personal and unique system without understanding the functional abilities of the client or systems already commercially available. When this occurs, the user may not get a system with all the features needed and must typically rely on the maker for troubleshooting and repair.

The assistive technology specialist must have an understanding of the various low-assistive and high-assistive technologies that are commercially available for persons with visual impairments. The specialist also should have a clear knowledge of the features the assistive technology must have based on the person's needs and goals. For some people with disabilities, their ability to operate the high-technology systems is not an issue. They may need only low-technology solutions in one environment such as the home. Their use of magnifiers to read labels on cans, cooking directions, or medicine bottle labels may be sufficient. At work, however, they may require a high-technology solution such as a closed-circuit television (CCTV) to increase the size of all printed material, thus strengthening performance and improving accuracy.

When multiple disabilities are present, the assistive technology specialist for the visually impaired needs to know systems available for other populations or should network with other assistive technology specialists. If system integration is needed, the assistive technology specialist must have a clear understanding of the feasibility of integrating the systems and the ways to accomplish integration. Some answers may only be obtained after additional research. In addition to understanding assistive technology, the specialist must have a basic comprehension of current computer technology, including the operating system. An added advantage exists if the assistive technology specialist has a basic understanding of the funding sources available and the way to best secure this funding through well-documented written reports.

During an assistive technology evaluation the specialist should provide the user with the particular equipment being considered to ensure usability and acceptance. Whenever a doubt arises regarding the appropriateness of a particular device, the assistive technology specialist should make arrangements for the user to loan or rent the equipment for an extended time before any final purchase. To accomplish this, the specialist should have a good rapport with the manufacturers and their representatives to facilitate arrangements.

The assistive technology specialist often has to act as a facilitator to discuss and resolve all problems and solutions. When appropriate the specialist should refer the client to other professionals to obtain additional input before recommending any assistive technology. Many family dynamics affect decisions about assistive technology; therefore the specialist must be extremely sensitive. For example, sometimes an individual does not want the technology but the family does. This conflict necessitates extensive discussions among all parties for resolution.

## Problems and Needs Assessments

The assistive technology specialist should first address the specific problems and needs of the person with the visual impairment, itemize the current assistive technology, and determine the efficiency and effectiveness of its use. If the person relates problems with current technology, the specialist must determine the reasons they are occurring. If the technology is currently not being used, the following reasons are common:

1. The individual or family members are not interested in any assistive technology.
2. The specialist did not provide adequate training.
3. The technology did not meet the user's needs and abilities.

In addition, specialists should consider the obsolescence of the technology, which prohibits it from accommodating newer versions of software being used in the school or work environment. Furthermore, specialists should determine whether the technology is broken and whether they can meet the assistive technology needs of their clients by repairing it. Finally, assistive technology specialists should determine whether family members, school personnel, and employment supervisors expect assistive technology to immediately solve various problems the client may have in performing to the highest potential.

Additional considerations exist when an individual has multiple disabilities such as vision and communication impairments, vision and mobility impairments, vision and cognitive impairments, and any combination of these disabilities. Because of multiple disabilities, the individual may be unable to use some technologies or require a combination of assistive technologies to be successful.

Assistive technologies that a person with multiple disabilities may consider are vision aids, hearing and amplification devices, augmentative communication devices, environmental control systems, computer access devices, power wheelchair controls, and workplace or school modifications; integration of these technologies may be necessary. When specialists are determining the most appropriate equipment for someone with multiple disabilities, they should first identify equipment needs to address all disabilities and then

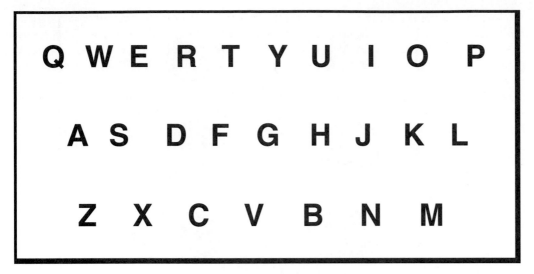

**Fig. 11-2** Qwerty keyboard.

determine integration requirements and feasibility because some of the technologies may need to interface (see Chapter 10).

CASE STUDY

M.M. was diagnosed with Hansen's disease, commonly known as *leprosy.* As a result of Hansen's disease, he was blind, some fingers had atrophied, and he had decreased tactile sensitivity. M.M. was a storyteller—his goal was to write his stories independently. He dictated his stories but was dissatisfied with this method because the transcriber, his wife, frequently edited them. He was unable to use a standard keyboard (Figure 11-2) or Braille keyboard (Figure 11-3). He learned to use Morse code as a child and still recalled many of the letter codes and was able to enter Morse code letters into the computer using a single switch.

Because M.M. also was blind, he needed a screen-reading program and a speech synthesizer to read back the stories he wrote. Screen-reading programs, which are software based, were not compatible with the software-based Morse code systems. Therefore he needed a hardware-based Morse code system that could act as a transparent interface with the computer. In other words, the system needed to send messages to the computer as if a standard computer keyboard was being used. Once the hardware-based system was selected, M.M needed to try it with the screen-reading software to ensure that the hardware was transparent and would work with the screen-reading software. Specialists made arrangements to borrow the various components from the manufacturers to test the system before integrating it. After M.M obtained and tried the equipment, the specialists determined that the systems could be integrated.

## Factors to Consider in Assistive Technology

When selecting assistive technology, specialists must remember some general factors (Box 11-5). First, they should determine the availability of the equipment. If the manufacturer has recently announced a new piece of equipment, it may not be immediately available. Assistive technology specialists also should consider whether currently available equipment will be discontinued soon. Although manufacturers may continue to

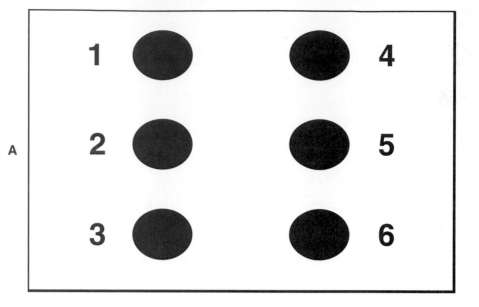

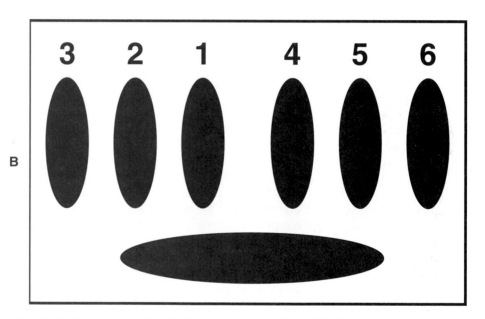

**Fig. 11-3** Displays standard Braille arrangement **(A)** and Braille notetaker/keyboard **(B).**

BOX 11-5

*Assistive Technology Factors*

Availability
Flexibility
Durability
Quality
Dedicated versus nondedicated device
Ease of use
Compatibility with current and proposed equipment
Ability to upgrade
History of the manufacturer
Warranty
Service and support
Cost

support repairs of certain equipment, it may be difficult to obtain parts for discontinued equipment.

Assistive technology must be flexible, especially for visually impaired people. Systems that provide more than one function are desirable. As one visually impaired person stated, "It would be nice not to have to carry around so much stuff." Mobile visually impaired adults may require low-technology and high-technology solutions. After selecting the various technologies, the specialist needs to position them for ease of access and use in different environments.[3] Devices may include a check-writing guide (Figure 11-4), a typoscope to read information more easily by isolating specific text (Figure 11-5), a signature stamp, an electronic dollar bill reader, a talking watch, a tape recorder to take notes, an embossed ruler, magnifiers, bioptic glasses, and a talking calculator. Other equipment may include a laptop computer with a screen-reading program and speech synthesizer and/or a text enlargement program, talking telephone directory, and talking calendar. The use of devices that serve multiple purposes greatly reduces the amount of equipment the visually impaired person must transport. For example, some electronic talking notetakers provide the combined features of an appointment calendar, a talking and Braille clock, notetaker, word processor, a phonebook organizer that stores names, phone numbers, and addresses and dials phone numbers, and a scientific calculator.

Durability and quality are critical components because people use assistive technology continually. If equipment is not durable, it is not cost effective. The quality of the equipment includes how well it is made and how often it needs repairs. The specialist can assess durability and quality by obtaining from the manufacturer their techniques

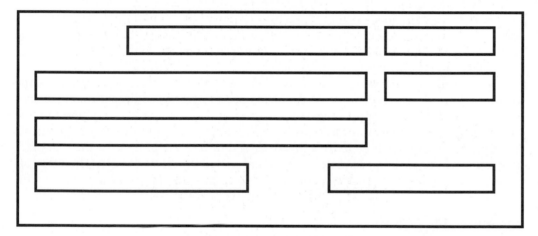

**Fig. 11-4** Check-writing guide.

**Fig. 11-5** Typoscope, a masking device that isolates lines and blocks glare for ease in reading.

for checking these factors, requesting repair information on the equipment, and exchanging information with other specialists.

Some systems are dedicated, which means they were specifically designed for a particular purpose, such as a talking calculator for persons who are visually impaired. Other systems are nondedicated, such as a computer with a screen-reading program and speech synthesizer. Generally, dedicated devices are more durable. For some individuals this factor may be important.

Assistive technology does not have to be complicated to be effective. Because the ultimate goal for all users of assistive technology is self-sufficiency, the assistive technology must be user friendly so that the person does not have to depend on someone else to operate the equipment.

Some manufacturers upgrade the software component of their system at minimum costs. This feature is critical when older assistive technology software does not operate with new programs entering the general market. Without this option, users are at a particular disadvantage in their work environment. If all employees must use a new software program, people with a visual impairment will want to upgrade their systems to accommodate the new software without incurring considerable cost. When major changes occur in the marketplace, however, such as when a new operating system is introduced, adaptive computers may not able to handle the new software programs.

In the selection process for assistive technology, specialists also must consider the manufacturer, warranty, and service support. Many manufacturers start businesses in assistive technology in anticipation of making money, only to be out of business in a short time. Therefore specialists should determine the financial stability of a new manufacturer before a device is purchased; the ability of another business to repair the equipment if necessary also is important. This consideration is not important when the product is a low-cost, low-technology item such as a Braille slate and stylus for writing Braille. However, this factor is critical with high-technology devices.

The length of the warranty of the device is another important factor. If the manufacturer offers only a 30-day warranty, the user may not have enough time to explore all the features of the device and ensure no problems occur. Because equipment is often specialized, the service and support the manufacturer provides is directly related to the cost of the equipment. The reason that assistive technology is so expensive is not because of the components, which are relatively inexpensive, but because of the cost the manufacturer incurs in providing adequate support and service to its customers. Therefore although cost is a factor in assistive technology selection, it should not be the only factor.

## Assistive Technology

Assistive technology for the visually impaired involves low-technology and high-technology devices. *Low technology* refers to any apparatus that is either nonelectronically based or a simple battery-operated item. Examples include magnifiers, rulers with Braille-embossed numbers, battery-operated toys, and tape recorders. High technology involves sophisticated systems that are electronically based such as powered wheelchairs, environmental control systems, closed-circuit televisions, Braille notetakers, optical character recognition systems, screen readers, and speech synthesizers.

## Low Technology

Low-technology devices can enhance educational and vocational opportunities, communication, recreational activities, and independent living (Box 11-6). Some effective devices for persons who are blind are Braille and/or talking watches and clocks, Braille print, and books on tapes. Braille labels affixed to objects help the person who is visually impaired identify the objects. For example, Braille labels attached to food cans result in easy identification in meal preparation. Commonly used objects such as rulers, pill boxes, timers, cooking utensils, popular board games, and playing cards also are available with Braille characters. Individuals who are deaf and blind use these Braille labels as well.

BOX **11-6**

*Low-Technology Devices*

*Educational/Vocational*
Manual Brailler: used to type Braille
Rulers: large numeral or Braille
Calculators: large print
Magnifiers
Books: large print, Braille, or audiocassette tapes
Maps: raised lines and bright colors
Typoscope: cutouts to view isolated lines while reading (see Figure 11-5)
Magnet cards with recorder: cards with adhesive tapes to record messages
Adhesive-backed labels for computer keyboards: large letters, Braille, bright colors/
    contrast
Calendar: large print or Braille
Labeler: large print or Braille to attach to objects
ABC board (child): large letter and Braille
Dictionary/Thesaurus: large print or Braille
Bible: large print or Braille
World Atlas: large print
Adjustable book or paper easel: to improve the angle of viewing
Raised line drawing kit: raises lines drawn on polyester film sheets
Ultraviolet or polarized glasses: changes visual contrast and/or glare
Nonglare filter screens for computers
Acetate yellow overlays: increase reading contrast and reduce glare
Pens with a light: provide additional light when writing
Enhanced visual contrast: large print and sharp contrast between letters and colored back-
    ground (e.g., printing bold black letters on yellow paper)
Telescopic spectacles: prescription spectacles

*Communication*
Raised manual picture communication boards
Writing guides for checks, signatures, letters, and envelopes: provide cutouts where infor-
    mation is written
Braille slates and stylus: used to write Braille

*Recreational/Games*
Dice: raised dot
Monopoly: large print and Braille
Othello: raised ridges, tactile-marked black pieces and smooth white pieces
Scrabble: large print and Braille
Chinese checkers: brightly colored pegs
UNO
    My First UNO (child): large print
    UNO (older child to adult): large numerals and Braille
Dominoes: raised dot
ROOK: large print and Braille
Bingo: large print or Braille
Backgammon: raised divider and tactile pieces
Cribbage: tactile markings
Checkers: round and square pieces
Chess set: raised square
Crossword puzzles: large print
Crossword puzzle dictionary: large print
Connect Four: black pieces with holes
Books
    Children: raised picture and tactile features
    Adult: large print or Braille
Big Bird's Talk to Me Teacher (child): bright colors and Braille
Balls: beeping and musical

*Continued*

## BOX 11-6

*Low-Technology Devices—cont'd*

*Recreational/Games—cont'd*
Basketball: internal bells for ease in locating
Playing cards: large or raised print or different colors for every suit
Poker chips: different colors, shapes, and weight for different amounts
Periodicals (e.g., *Reader's Digest*): large print
Compass: Braille with directional arrow
TV screen enlarger

*Independent Living*
Check register: large print
Address book: large print
Reusable plastic tabs: fit standard hangars that can help sort clothing
Telephones: large numeral
Cooking /food utensils
   Recipe books: large print
   Liquid level indicator: straddles cup and produces tone and vibration as liquid reaches
     1 inch from the top
   Modified sugar dispenser: pores a spoonful of sugar each time it is turned over
   Plate guard: helps to keep food on the plate
   Splatter guard: provides grease from splattering
   Food scale: tactile markings for weighing
   Food timer: large numeral and Braille
   Meat thermometer: tactile
Mirrors: 3X, 4X, 5X, 7X, and 8X magnification
Medical
   Thermometer: large numeral
   Weight scale: large numeral
   Pill dispenser: large letters and Braille
Needle threader
Tactile pen: makes raised pen lines
Canes: folding

Persons with visual impairment can access a variety of low-technology aids, including large numeral watches and clocks, large print books, and large display phone buttons. Writing guides are available for the visually impaired to write letters and checks, write on envelopes, and create signatures (see Figure 11-4). These guides are usually hard plastic cards with open slots. The slots provide a tactile guide to the location where the user can write information such as the date on a check. Writing guides also can help the person with a visual impairment write in a straight line. Leisure activities such as large-print playing cards and a variety of enlarged-print board games can accommodate the user.

Modifications in placement (e.g., use of adjustable paper stands), visual contrast (e.g., printing bold black letters on yellow paper), and size of printed materials (e.g., increasing the standard print size) may enhance the person's ability to see the information. Magnifiers and telescopic spectacles, with various degrees of magnification, also may improve the individual's visual performance. Another option for a person with disabilities is ultraviolet color shields (e.g., gray, green, yellow, orange, or violet) or polarized glasses to change the visual contrast or reduce glare. In addition, a person can use low-technology applications on high-technology devices (e.g., nonglare filters attached to computer screens may improve contrast).

## High Technology

Special high-technology applications for people who are blind may include dollar bill reading machines and talking calculators, VCRs, voltmeters, thermometers, levels, compasses, and oscilloscopes (Boxes 11-7 and 11-8). These devices provide spoken messages

# BOX 11-7

*High-Technology Devices*

*Educational/Vocational*
Devices for persons who are visually impaired
    Closed-circuit television (CCTV): black and white or color
    Text enlargement software/hardware
Devices for persons who are visually impaired and/or blind
    Calculators: talking
    Four track tape recorder
    Talking diary
    Portable notetaker: Braille or QWERTY
    Voltmeters: talking
    Oscilloscopes: talking
    Refreshable Braille display
    Dictionary/Thesaurus: software
    Optical character recognition (OCR): handheld devices or flatbed scanners
    Laptop computer with screen reading program and speech synthesizer: software application that converts computer generated information into artificial speech, which is spoken through the speech synthesizer
    Morse code with speech synthesis and auditory signals

*Communication*
Telephone communication device for the deaf (TDD) with refreshable displays: replaces the standard visual display on a TDD with refreshable Braille
Augmentative communication device with auditory fishing and/or auditory scanning

*Recreational*
Remote control: large and raised numerals
Descriptive video service (DVS)
Compass: talking
VCR: audio programming

*Independent Living*
Cooking Tools
    Recipe books: software
    Microwave oven: tactually marked
    Electric frying pan: Braille control knob
Heating and air conditioning thermostat: large print
Medical
    Thermometer: talking
    Blood glucose monitoring system: large print display or talking
    Weight scale: talking
    Blood pressure monitor: talking
    Tape measurer: talking
Electronic mobility aids
    Audio signage
Electronic mapping software: uses global positioning satellite (GPS)

of information that users would otherwise read on a visual display. For example, a compass may provide the user with digitized speech feedback in English, Spanish, German, or French. A combination of several devices within a single device is available. For example, voice diaries include a talking calculator, clock, appointment calendar, telephone list, and tone dialing output in one small hand-held device.

A person with disabilities can have increased independence in the community through audio signage systems. These systems provide the user with various features from auditory beeps to verbal descriptions or instructions via a pocket-size receiver. One common example is the use of audio beeps at traffic signals, which notify the blind pedestrian when crossing the street is safe. More sophisticated systems can be installed

## BOX 11-8

*Assistive Technology*

*Audio Signage:* A system that gives verbal messages or directions, consisting of transmitters and receivers that transmit information through infrared or radio waves. The transmitters may signal the location of an elevator, door, telephone, etc.

*Braille Embossers:* Produces hard-copy Braille output. Differing features of Braille embossers include the speed of production, the paper size, graphics, and the noise level. In addition, with some embossers, Braille can be produced on both sides of the page.

*Braille Input Computer Devices:* Use of six or eight keys to input computer information through Braille. The keys represent Braille dots.

*Braille Notetaker:* Portable Braille input device for note taking. Additional features for some notetakers include calculators, clocks, calendars, word processing, telephone directories, thermometers, voltmeters, and music compositions.

*Braille TDD:* Provides a refreshable Braille display for each line of text transmitted on the TDD.

*Braille-to-Print Conversion Devices:* Translates Braille characters from traditional Braillers into corresponding traditional orthography.

*Braille Refreshable Displays:* Tactile displays that use retractable pins to form Braille characters. Information on the computer screen is read through tactile Braille feedback.

*Calculator (Talking):* A device that speaks numbers as they are entered and gives the answer to the mathematical problem. Additional features may include a clock and an alarm.

*Closed-Circuit TV (CCTV):* Magnifying system that permits the visually impaired to read and/or write. Provides magnification of any printed text and/or pictures. Magnification ranges from $3\times$ to $60\times$, with monitors ranging from 4 to 20 inches. Positive and negative polarity is available. Selections include black/white and color displays. Some may interface with the computer to provide a split-screen image.

*Descriptive Video Service (DVS):* Offers narrative descriptions of key visual elements in a television program, without altering the audio sounds or dialogue. This includes descriptions of visual elements such as actions, subtitles, scene changes, graphics, and body language. This service also is available for major movies on home video. The viewer must have a stereo TV or stereo VCR, with a second audio program (SAP) channel to receive DVS.

*Enlarged Text:* Hardware and/or software that provides magnification of characters on the computer screen or in the printed output.

*Global Positioning Satellite (GPS):* Used with technology for the blind to guide them to their destination. Satellite receiver continually monitors their current location.

*Large Print Programs:* Hardware and/or software that provides enlarged print on either the computer screen or computer-generated printout.

*Large Print Display:* A computer monitor that enlarges and/or enhances the text that is displayed.

*Liquid Crystal Display (LCD):* A flat computer-type screen.

## BOX **11-8**

*Assistive Technology—cont'd*

*Modem:* A hardware device that permits a computer to communicate with other computers through the telephone lines.

*Optical Character Recognition (OCR):* Scanning of text to a computer or Braille printer for presentation of material in Braille print or synthesized speech. With some models the synthesized speech can be recorded directly on an audiocassette.

*Peripheral:* Hardware that connects to the computer and is controlled through the computer.

*Screen Reading:*
Software and hardware applications that convert computer-generated text to artificial speech, which is spoken through one of many available speech synthesizers. Individual letters, words, paragraphs, or entire documents may be spoken.

*Speech Synthesizer:*
Converts text into artificial or "computer" speech. Options include voices of males, females, or children.

*Spell Checker:*
Words can be typed into this device to determine whether they are spelled correctly. Additional features may include providing the definition, a thesaurus, and the option of speaking the word and definition.

into private offices, public buildings, shopping centers, or parks. With the use of infrared or motion-sensitive features, a person who is blind will receive a verbal message identifying the location of the building, office suite, water fountain, or elevator.

The public can currently receive orientation to the environment through a system that gives verbal directions using a global positioning satellite (GPS) tracking device. A person who is blind, however, cannot access these systems independently because manufacturers designed them for sighted drivers to receive turn-by-turn directions. However, manufacturers have modified GPS units for users who are blind. The adapted GPS system provides directions for users who are blind to get to a specific place via the orientation software, graphic screen reading program, and speech synthesizer.

PBS stations provide descriptive video service (DVS) for various television programs. They give narrative descriptions of key visual elements in a program without altering the audio sounds or dialogue. This includes descriptions of visual elements such as actions, subtitles, scene changes, graphics, and body language. This service also is available for some movies on home video. The viewer must have a stereo TV or stereo VCR with a second audio program (SAP) channel to receive DVS.

People who are blind can read print material by using an optical character reader (OCR). OCRs include hand-held devices or flatbed scanners that convert the printed word to a computer file, synthesize speech, and/or Braille printout. Stand-alone OCRs also are available, and people who are not computer literate may prefer them.

Visually impaired people may use portable notetakers to record notes, word process, and store appointments. Their keyboards may consist of standard typewriter QWERTY boards (see Figure 11-2) or Braille configurations (see Figure 11-3) using six or eight keys and the spacebar. The keys represent Braille dots. The Braille keyboards also are available in ergonomic designs engineered for comfort. The center key on all keyboards serves as the spacebar. Additional features for these devices may include telephone directories, clocks, scientific calculators, alarm clocks, voice calendar reminders, and thermometers. The output modes for these devices consist of speech synthesis and/or refreshable Braille cells (raised Braille characters that display the information the user enters). Some systems also provide dual language capabilities. Therefore users can either listen to the information they entered or read the information through the tactile sense using the refreshable Braille cells.

A person who is blind can use modified computers with various input and output systems. Input systems include standard computer keyboards, Braille keyboards, Morse code with speech synthesis, or auditory signals (e.g., beeps, tones, or key echo). The user can transmit letters, numbers, and punctuation marks to the computer in Morse code, which requires software and/or hardware adaptations using switches. With a single switch, the computer differentiates dots and dashes by the length of time the user presses the switch. In two-switch Morse code, one switch is for dots and one is for dashes. The user also may use a third switch as an entry switch. Individuals who are blind can use this system with auditory feedback, which echoes the letter or command that they entered. Individuals who are blind and physically challenged may select this approach.

Output systems can include screen-reading programs, refreshable Braille displays, Braille printouts, and Braille with traditional orthographic print. A screen reader is a software application that converts computer-generated information into artificial speech, which is spoken through a speech synthesizer. The combination of a screen reader and a speech synthesizer gives the person with a visual impairment access to standard computer programs. Text can appear on the computer screens in two ways: text mode or graphics mode. Screen-reading programs are available that read text and graphic modes. Specially developed Windows screen-reading programs can read Windows programs that use a graphic environment. Different screen-reading versions exist for Macintosh, DOS, and Windows (various versions). Speech synthesizers vary in quality of speech and the way they interface with the computer. They may be either hardware (the individual plugs it into a slot inside the computer or uses one of the computer's serial ports) or software.

Refreshable Braille displays use retractable pins to form Braille characters, which permit users to read information on the computer screen through tactile Braille feedback. The Braille displays may be 80 cells (a full line of computer text), 40 cells (one half the line), or 20 cells (one fourth the line). These devices are particularly beneficial for individuals who are deaf and blind but have good tactile skills.

For individuals who are hearing impaired and blind, a specialist can integrate refreshable Braille displays with telephone communication devices (TDD). Using the fingers, the individual reads the raised Braille characters on the Braille display. This is the same information that appears on the visual display of the TDD. Individuals who are hearing impaired and blind also may use this device to communicate. The person who is hearing impaired reads the visual display as the person who is blind types information via the Braille keyboard, and the person who is blind reads information that the deaf person types via a standard keyboard on the refreshable Braille display.

High-technology applications for the visually impaired include portable and desktop CCTVs to enlarge print material. These are available in a black and white image and/or color. The advantage of a CCTV versus low-technology magnifying lenses is increased magnification, improved contrast, and reversed polarity. An additional feature on one CCTV is an optional keypad, which displays the time, date, and calculator and an address and telephone organizer on the monitor. One alternative in CCTV technology is a hand-held device that attaches to any television set to create enlarged images. Some manufacturers incorporate a computer in the systems to provide a split-screen image of the computer-generated text and material that the CCTV views. This device allows the user to maintain eye contact with one screen rather than shifting between two.

Specialists can modify computer access for visually impaired people by using various input and output systems. Some persons with visual impairment also use many previously described systems that persons who are blind use (e.g., auditory signals: beeps, chirps, or synthesized voice echo of the keys). Other input systems may consist of modified keyboard contrast (e.g., white letters on black backgrounds or vice versa) or large keyboards (with large letters).

Output systems include screen-reading programs with speech synthesizers and text magnification programs. Text magnification programs enlarge the image on the computer screen for the operating systems in DOS, Windows, or Macintosh. These systems also may provide reverse contrast (e.g., white letters on a dark background). The Macintosh computer and Windows offer the accessibility feature of text enlargement within the operating system. Additional accommodations on the computer include enlarged font sizes and large flat screen color display monitors. Flat screen monitors decrease the distortion that may occur with convex screens. By altering the color on the computer screen (e.g., black letters with a yellow background), the user who is visually impaired may be able to view the print more easily. The user also may enhance the mouse control by increasing the size of the mouse pointer or adding a tail to the mouse through the use of special software or accessibility options that some operating systems offer.

All high-technology devices are crucial to enable persons who are blind or visually impaired to function independently. However, many barriers in society still remain. For example, a person who is blind does not know the choices in a standard soft drink machine. Major companies are beginning to respond to these needs. For example, in response to demands by visually impaired consumers, some banks have developed talking ATM machines. Although keys on ATM machines may be labeled in Braille, persons who are blind or visually impaired cannot use the ATM machine independently. Consequently, they have to rely at times on the honesty of strangers to assist them.

## Alternatives to Assistive Technology

Alternatives to assistive technology for persons with visual disabilities include employing people as readers, notetakers, writers, and attendants. The individual's situation dictates the services. The alternatives might be available for persons in an educational setting but are not generally cost effective in the workplace. In California, for example, the law states that school systems must provide readers, notetakers, and writers to persons with visual impairments or dyslexia. They read handouts, chapters, and other printed material in the class. The disadvantage of readers is that they only read the material once; therefore the person with a visual impairment does not have the opportunity to review the material, unlike with assistive technology. If readers record themselves while they read, the person with a visual impairment can at least review the text on tape. This can still be much slower than the visually impaired person using printed material stored on a computer disk because with the appropriate assistive technology, the user may conduct a quick search by key words to locate a specific section for review.

Notetakers record classroom notes that must later be read and recorded on tape or typed on the computer for review with a screen-reading program. Writers record on paper what the person with a visual impairment says aloud. Students frequently use writers when taking tests. In these circumstances, the writer reads the question and then records the answer dictated by the person with a visual impairment. Aides also may provide one-on-one assistance for mobility and/or other ADL, such as meal preparation. Some persons with visual impairment have guide dogs to assist with mobility, provide protection, and/or retrieve objects.

When considering these alternatives, the specialist should ask several questions. Would the purchase of assistive technology be less costly over time than hiring personnel to provide assistance? Does the level of independence that assistive technology provides outweigh any costs? Because readers provide the information only once and notetakers and writers occasionally make mistakes, are these options in the best interest of a person with a visual disability?

## Outcome and Social Validation

Persons with visual disabilities who use low-assistive and high-assistive technology have the potential for increased independence in educational tasks, employment, ADL, recreation, communication, community activities, and socialization. In particular, the Internet has opened many doors for visually impaired people and has enabled them to have the same opportunities as sighted individuals. Through the Internet, they can research information in library catalogues, register for classes, communicate with other people, play interactive games, obtain assistance from manufacturers, and download newspapers, magazines, and books for review without others knowing that they are visually impaired. Several Internet sites focus on issues facing persons who are visually impaired in employment, education, and technology (see Appendix B at the end of the chapter).

Assistive technology also has enabled persons with visual disabilities to increase their productivity level in education and employment. The technology advances for persons with visual impairments has allowed them to independently access, store, and transmit the same information managed by persons with sight.[4] Despite these technology advances, unemployment remains high among people with visual disabilities. Therefore they need to consider other factors that may affect these statistics, including limited funding to obtain the necessary assistive technology, lack of sensitivity of potential employers, and problems with transportation to the work site.

Although one role of the Department of Vocational Rehabilitation is to provide assistive technology, persons with disabilities may have difficulty obtaining funding from some branches of this state agency. This hindrance results in delayed opportunity for the person with a disability to be appropriately trained for employment and increases frustration. Vocational rehabilitation professionals that provide appropriate services not only have to assist visually impaired people to develop the skills they need for the job but also may have to convince employers to recruit, employ, and retain them. With the passage of the American with Disabilities Act and as more people with visual impairments appear in the mainstream work environments, their workplace opportunities may expand.[5]

Even if someone provides an individual with the appropriate technology and offers a job opportunity, an individual may not accept the job because of problems with public transportation in some areas. This is especially true in situations in which some companies have required employees to work at multiple locations in a day. People with visual disabilities may not be able to travel to more than one site during the day using public transportation because of the time involved.

A concern for specialists is whether OCR devices have a negative effect on Braille literacy. Because people enhance much of their language development through reading, no one knows the effect that the absence of Braille will have on grammar, syntax, and vocabulary development of children who are blind. Braille literacy has decreased, however, and these outcomes are developing.

Some technology for the visually impaired is effective for persons with other disabilities and the aging population. Wiener[6] reported that when students with learning disabilities were learning sight words, they absorbed more when the instructor demonstrated written words augmented by speech, such as screen-reading programs, than a visual-only presentation. With the aging of baby boomers, many technologies for persons with visual impairments will be beneficial for adults who are experiencing decreased vision as a result of age or serious eye disorders. Weedman,[7] who lost her sight at age 75 because of macular degeneration, is one example. With the assistance of various low technologies, she was able to continue to lead a productive and independent lifestyle.

As the population ages, persons with visual impairments should have more low-assistive and high-assistive technology options, and the demands should result in a cost decrease. For example, some low-assistive technology for persons with visual disabilities no longer only appears in special catalogues but is available through catalogues distributed by the American Association for Retired Persons (AARP). Although assistive technology, especially most high technology, is not inexpensive, the use of assistive technology can decrease costs for attendant care, readers, notetakers, and writers. The specialist should consider these factors when measuring outcomes.

Public acceptance of persons with disabilities is increasing, in part because of media portrayals of persons with disabilities in television shows, commercials, movies, and documentaries. For example, one celebrity on the television show, *Early Edition,* is blind. In the movie *Scent of a Woman,* the lead character is blind. One television commercial used an individual who is blind and his guide dog in comical situations to advertise cellular phones. In another commercial, Stevie Wonder promoted one manufacturer's reading machine in a nationwide advertisement campaign. Although the primary objective was for the companies to promote awareness and education about the products, these campaigns also helped increase and promote acceptance and knowledge about assistive technology. In addition, in a large metropolitan area the Braille Institute has information commercials about who they serve and the services available. This helps to expand the general knowledge of the various technologies and options available.

## CASE STUDIES

### CASE 1

### *Visually Impaired*

F.G. was a college student majoring in technical writing. She has juvenile macular degeneration (Figure 11-6). The Department of Vocational Rehabilitation requested the assistive technology evaluation.

benefits and other allotments ... impairment are education and training ... Low vision indicates an ... optical correctio ... on. With 20/50 ... ject to see it; wherea ... object a ... tify, interpr ... indiv ... nd train ... sele ... am ... any ... the ... ily livi ... non ... moo ... stylu ... tery opera ... that are ... aille notebool ...

Implem ... of the client's goals, nee ... hrough a comprehensive evalu ... gy can be selected and matched ... owever, only

**Fig. 11-6** Example of macular degeneration.

## GOALS

F.G.'s goals were to increase reading speed, decrease eye strain and pain, and obtain a bachelor's degree. As with most individuals who have some degree of vision, she preferred to use her vision as much as possible.

## FUNCTION AND ABILITY

F.G. had normal cognition and was legally blind. She had no central vision and some peripheral vision. California law stated that she could drive a car within the state if she wore the prescription bioptic lens that attached to standard eyeglass frames. Although she was able to read standard 12-point font print with the assistance of magnification spectacles, she suffered from eye pain and fatigue when reading this size. When the font size was increased to 24-point font print with white on black contrast, her performance improved.

F.G. had difficulty keeping up with the extensive reading assignments that her curriculum required. Although she used readers and requested books on tape, she wanted the technology to give her independence and flexibility.

## CONSIDERATIONS, OPTIONS, AND TECHNOLOGY

F.G. had no high-assistive technology devices. The low technology she used consisted of prescription bioptic and magnification spectacles and a four-track audiocassette tape recorder for recording lectures and listening to textbooks available from *Recording for the Blind*. She used a computer with a text magnification program in the Students with Disabilities University Computer Center but was unable to complete her work during the limited lab hours.

F.G. needed magnification and reverse contrast—from black on white to white on black—to read her textbooks and other printed material and information she typed on the computer. The computer text enlargement program also needed the feature in which a person could enlarge one line of text at a time while still viewing the entire page, which allowed maintenance of orientation to the page. Only one program offered this feature, and a special computer mouse controlled it. Because F.G. did not have a computer, she had to purchase one.

She needed to consider the adaptive technology RAM requirements when selecting the computer. To further expand her access to information, the provider offered a package, including a modem and Internet access. Because F.G. had concerns that her vision might worsen, she also needed a system in which she could add a screen-reading program with a speech synthesizer and an OCR to scan printed text and review it with the screen-reading program.

Because F.G. had problems maintaining her place when reading using a standard CCTV, the provider introduced a unit that also had an automatic viewing table and foot control switch. With this system, she was able to maintain visual contact with the text on the television monitor while advancing the text by line using a foot switch that moved the page forward. She also could move the page backwards and scroll through the text. She was able to interface the two devices so that she could read the information on the computer screen as part of a split-screen image on the CCTV. This feature assisted F.G. in maintaining her place when reading because she was looking at one screen rather than having to shift visual gaze between two. The equipment she selected was durable and available from a well-established manufacturer.

One problem was the funding limitations that the Department of Vocational Rehabilitation imposed. The amount that they were allotting would not adequately meet F.G.'s needs. By appealing through the client assistance program (CAP), she obtained funding. F.G. had the computer set up in her home on a standard computer table after CAP secured the funding.

## OUTCOME AND SOCIAL VALIDATION

F.G. used the system daily to assist her in her educational pursuits, read printed material, and aid in reviewing material that she wrote. F.G. reported that the system was effective because it increased her independence, eliminated readers and writers within the classroom, and assisted in obtaining a bachelor's and master's degrees. Presently, she uses the equipment to help her prepare for class lectures and grade student papers as a university instructor.

## CASE 2

### *Visual, Motor, Cognition, and Speech Impaired*

C.R. was a 5-year-old boy who was cortically blind, nonambulatory quadriplegic, and speech impaired.

### GOAL
The goal was to increase communication by providing more choices.

### FUNCTION AND ABILITY
C.R. was dependent for all ADL. Although C.R. appeared to observe objects and people in his environment, he was unable to interpret what he saw; therefore he could not make choices from visual information alone. He produced different vocal inflections but no speech. He demonstrated the ability to operate a single rocking lever switch when someone positioned it on the right side of his head. C.R. was able to recognize the cause-effect operation of the switch when an aid connected it to a simple battery-operated toy and subsequently to an auditory scanning communication device.

When the teacher presented C.R. with the names of familiar toys and foods through live voice auditory scanning, he became excited, especially when the person presented certain items and simultaneously gave him an opportunity to touch the object with his hands or smell the object at close range. When C.R. demonstrated this behavior, the teacher gave him time to play with the toy or fed him a piece of the food.

### CONSIDERATIONS, OPTIONS, AND TECHNOLOGY
As a result of the cortical blindness, C.R. was not able to use a visual augmentative communication device, and his quadriplegia prevented him from using direct selection. Therefore he needed a switch-activated device that would provide auditory scanning. In addition, the technology had to meet his immediate needs and give him the opportunity to expand its capabilities. The goal was for C.R. to initially have simple choices and then categories from which to choose. At the choice stage, as the teacher presented each object auditorially, C.R. was able to feel the object until he demonstrated a clear understanding of only the verbal name. A teacher later trained him to recognize various categories such as food, drinks, toys, and clothes. Once C.R. selected a category (e.g., drinks), the teacher would present items such as milk, water, and juice in that category. When he selected the particular item, the teacher gave C.R. his choice. In selecting the augmentative communication device, the teacher also had to consider the physical set up in his environment. Because C.R. was in a wheelchair, the teacher addressed mounting considerations so that the device and control switch could easily travel with him. C.R.'s family also initially rented the device with an option to purchase to ensure that he would use it.

During this rental period, specialists trained his parents and school personnel in its use. His parents and school personnel selected the particular device based on their ability to program it to only offer simple choices and then expand it to provide categories and subcategories. Other important factors were C.R.'s ability to operate the equipment, the longevity of the manufacturer, the availability of a rental period, and the durability of the equipment.

### OUTCOME AND SOCIAL VALIDATION
Because C.R. appeared to observe things, his teachers attributed his lack of choice making to limited cognitive functioning and not a severe visual disability. As a result, his family and teachers did not consider a communication system for C.R. until age 5 when his mother insisted that he understood more than he could show, proving that her input was critical and that everyone involved needed to address his visual abilities early.

In this case, once the teacher introduced C.R. with technology, it was successful because it addressed the specific needs of C.R., and he, his parents, and the school system accepted and used it. An electronic scanning communication device is more expensive than live voice scanning of desired items, but the former increased C.R.'s independence, self-esteem, and potential for future development and growth.

## CASE 3

### Visual, Motor, Cognition, and Speech Impaired

L.F. was a 14-year-old girl who was a nonambulatory quadriplegic and severely visually, cognitively, and speech impaired, secondary to anoxia.

### GOALS

The goals of the parent were to integrate L.F. into a regular high school class, increase her participation in classroom activities, develop her ability to communicate "yes" and "no," provide her with a means to make choices, and increase her communication with nonfamiliar listeners. The school staff members, however, felt that because of L.F.'s limited cognitive abilities, she would not be able to achieve much. They agreed to the evaluation because the parent refused to sign the IEP.

### FUNCTION AND ABILITY

L.F. was dependent for all ADL. She was only able to distinguish visually between objects when teachers gave her a two-choice selection. She was able to use her right foot to press a single switch and recognized the cause-effect of switch operation to control a battery-operated toy. She also could make a selection between a visual choice of two objects by using large remote lamps that were next to the objects. L.F. also demonstrated the ability to make a choice when the teacher provided three to four choices auditorially. She could communicate "yes" by clenching her fist and "no" by extending her fingers when the teacher asked simple questions. She also was able to perform some simple gestures for basic communication, such as extending her arms to be picked up.

### CONSIDERATIONS, OPTIONS, AND TECHNOLOGY

One main factor in this case was the adversarial relationship between the mother and the school system. The mother believed that the introduction of technology would resolve all her daughter's problems, and the school objected to the technology because they felt L.F. was not capable of using it. The school system also felt that the mother was more focused on fighting the school than on implementing a particular program.

Although L.F. was severely disabled, neighborhood children who were slightly older took her to the mall when they shopped or drove around at night with her in the car. Her mother was instrumental in developing these relationships.

Because obvious problems existed in the relationship between the school system and L.F.'s mother and because specialists did not know whether she would fully follow any program at home or at school, they initially recommended a low-cost assistive technology solution. Simultaneously, they also demonstrated other assistive technologies that they could introduce in the future once they successfully implemented this first stage.

The proposed assistive technology consisted of a tape recorder that the specialists modified to accommodate a single switch, single rocking lever switch, switch latch timer, loop tapes (outgoing message tapes from an answering machine) of varying lengths, switch mounting at the foot, and a method of attaching the tape recorder to the wheelchair. With this system, the specialists could record someone's voice (they selected another 14-year-old girl) on the tape to read certain poems or stories that L.F. could choose. When the specialists presented the choices to L.F., one recorded voice would speak at a time with a 5-second delay between each one. This provided L.F. with the time needed to press the switch before the next choice would be spoken. Once she pressed the switch, L.F. was given that choice. If L.F. missed the choice on the first presentation, she could hear the choice again because the cassette was a loop tape with a switch latch timer attached.

A switch latch timer is a device that provides an on/off function between the tape recorder and switch. In other words, with this device attached, when the user presses the switch the tape recorder comes on and the tape continues to play until the user presses the switch again to turn the tape recorder off. Specialists made different tapes for different categories: food, drinks, recreational activities, music tapes, etc. They used the poems and story tapes in an English class where the students had to make presentations. With these tapes, L.F. could press the switch to start the poem or story and then press the switch to stop the tape when it was over.

The mounting of the switch to the wheelchair was a concern because someone had to modify the footplate. Because the chair was new, the specialist contacted the wheelchair manufacturer to do the modification, and the wheelchair warranty was not affected. The tape recorder was attached by dual lock to the wheelchair tray. At times, L.F. also carried the tape recorder in a small pouch that was attached to the chair.

The specialist then had to train L.F.'s mother and school personnel in the technology's care and operation. The specialist told everyone that L.F. needed to use the equipment throughout each day to promote success and for L.F. to gain the necessary skills to advance to the next stage of assistive technology.

## OUTCOME AND SOCIAL VALIDATION

The specialist scheduled a follow-up visit months later. The parent reported that she had not spent time working with her daughter on the equipment. Furthermore, the school district staff had not used the equipment with L.F. They stated that they did not understand the way to operate the equipment because they sent the person that they initially trained to another school. This equipment is actually easy to operate, but everyone in L.F.'s environment needed to invest time in the student training. Because no one followed through, the specialist reinstructed the mother and school staff in the equipment's operation and use and again counseled them in the critical need of daily intervention.

This case illustrates that the receipt of technology does not immediately compensate for a person's disability. With assistive technology, everyone involved has the duty to commit the time for training and implementation for it to be successful.

## CASE 4

### *Visual, Motor, and Speech Impaired*

J.V. is a woman who was nonambulatory quadriplegic, blind, and speech impaired, secondary to cardiac arrest after an asthmatic attack during her junior year at college. At the time of the evaluation, J.V. was living in a group home.

## GOALS

The primary initial goal of J.V. and the referring clinician was to increase her independence by providing her with an environmental control unit (ECU). The parents did not share the same goal because a speech-language pathologist who was working with J.V. repeatedly informed them that she had severe memory deficits and was unable to operate any technology. J.V. also was undergoing a series of orthopedic operations to attempt to increase her mobility. As a result, the parents were hesitant about J.V.'s capability of using the technology.

Because of the negative information that one professional gave to the parents and J.V.'s ongoing operations, the family delayed their decision by a year to purchase the system for J.V. Once J.V. gained control of her environment through an ECU, the clinician's next goal was for J.V. to improve written communication so that she could return to the university setting to complete her degree. None of the people involved had a goal of improving J.V.'s speech communication through technology because she could eventually make others understand her.

## FUNCTION AND ABILITY

J.V. was legally blind but could detect lightness and darkness and shapes of people. She was totally dependent for all ADL. She initially demonstrated the ability to operate a single switch using her right foot and could select an item when the ECU auditorially scanned it. Over time and after several operations, J.V. demonstrated the motor skills to use a single switch for Morse code input.

Despite the diagnosis of the speech-language pathologist working with J.V., she demonstrated good auditory memory abilities and was cognitively intact. She learned all Morse codes for letters, numbers, and basic computer commands within 2 weeks. Although J.V.'s speech intelligibility was poor even with familiar listeners, her communication improved when she used appropriate pacing techniques and/or spelled the words verbally she was attempting to communicate.

## CONSIDERATIONS, OPTIONS, AND TECHNOLOGY

The initial and primary goal was to increase J.V.'s independence by providing her with a means to control her environment. Because she could control a device with a single switch and was able to make selections when specialists gave her an array of choices, they considered an auditory scanning ECU. At this early stage, J.V. did not have the motor control to input Morse code. In evaluating which system to recommend, they considered various factors. These included the features of the equipment, reputation of the manufacturer, durability of the equipment, and capability of integrating with other technologies. Because J.V. could depress a single switch at a single input level, specialists selected a dedicated ECU system that provided auditory scanning of choices. The company was well established and the equipment was durable.

Because the system used a combination of infrared and radio transmission technology, specialists had to set up the room to accommodate for the infrared technology. This meant that the ECU box had to be within a direct line of the other infrared devices, which included the television, VCR, cable, and stereo system. To accomplish this, they mounted the system on the wall across the room from the other appliances. Because earthquakes sometimes occur in this geographic area, they also strapped the ECU to the shelf with a bungy cord. J.V. was able to control her environment by pressing the switch when the ECU spoke the desired category, subcategory, and item. For example, the ECU presented the following categories:

- Phone
- Lights
- Appliance
- Television
- VCR
- Cable
- Remote 1 (radio)
- Remote 2 (tape deck)
- Remote 3 (CD)

Once the ECU presented the desired category, J.V. pressed the switch to branch to a subcategory or items within that category. For example, if J.V. selected the phone, the choices would now be the following:

- Answer
- Dial operator
- Hang up
- Mute (places a caller on or off hold)
- Retry (takes the phone off the hook and redials the last number dialed)
- Privacy (disables main speaker so that the telephone conversation can be heard through the headset)
- Dial (enables the user to enter and dial a random number)
- Record (enables the user to program a number for speed dialing)

- Play (enables the user to speed dial a preprogrammed number)
- Volume (enables the user to increase or decrease the listening volume)

From these choices, she could make her next selection. Once J.V. received her system, she was operating it within an hour without difficulty. She also stored 50 phone numbers in the telephone directory over the first month and was able to easily recall each person's phone number she stored using numbers (1 to 50).

After a year with the system, J.V. and her family members were ready to move to the next step, which was computer access. She demonstrated the motor skills at this point to use single switch access to enter Morse code. Because J.V. was visually impaired, she also needed a screen-reading program and speech synthesizer to read back the information she entered into the computer. This required the integration of two technologies. Software-based Morse code entry systems were not compatible with the screen-reading programs. Therefore her family selected a transparent interface hardware-based system. They installed this system into the computer keyboard slot of the computer so that the computer received the same input as if someone were typing keys on the keyboard. The screen-reading program operated in Windows.

Before receiving the computer system, J.V. received Morse code training, which provided two advantages. First, it proved to everyone that she had the cognitive and motor abilities to master Morse code. Second, it meant that once she received her own computer she was ready to start using it. Over a 4-month period, J.V. mastered the commands for the screen reading software. The specialists continuing the training only needed to focus on developing strategies to increase speed of entry. Because J.V. wanted to communicate with others using her computer, they also provided her with a modem and access to the Internet.

J.V. decided that the ECU did not need to be integrated with the computer system because she could control both by alternating between separate single switches. The two separate systems also protected J.V. from losing both systems if one component broke.

## OUTCOME AND SOCIAL VALIDATION

The introduction of the ECU system provided J.V. with independence in being able to control her immediate environment. She no longer had to rely on an attendant to change the channel on her television, to record a television program, or to turn on her fan. She also was able to have private telephone conversations with friends and family and could call people at any hour. Although the ultimate system that the specialists provided was not inexpensive, it did decrease attendant care cost. More importantly, however, it proved to her family that J.V. was cognitively intact and capable of making her own decisions. For J.V., this technology is her lifeline to the outside world.

After J.V. received the computer system, she returned to school and earned her bachelor's degree in music appreciation. She now lives in her own apartment with a live-in attendant but is able to remain alone for hours at a time because of her assistive technology. J.V. is also an avid Internet user.

## References

1. American Foundation for the Blind, *J Vis Impair Blind*, New York, AFB Press.
2. Swenson A: *Beginning with Braille: firsthand experiences with a balanced approach to literacy*, Sewickly, Pennsylvania, 1999, AFB Press.
3. Mueller J: *The workplace workbook: an illustrated guide to job accommodation and assistive technology*, Washington, DC, 1990, The Dole Foundation.
4. Scadden LA: *The changing workplace: view from a disabled technologist*, Proceedings of a National Symposium on the Future of Work for Disabled People: Employment and the New Technology, pp 45–52, New York, 1986, American Foundation for the Blind.

5. Joffee E: *A practical guide to the ADA and visual impairment,* New York, 1999, AFB Press.
6. Wiener R: Computerized speech: a study of its effect on learning, *Technology Horizons in Education* 18:100, Feb 1991.
7. Weedman P: Eighty isn't old, The Braille Monitor 88–90, Feb 1996.
8. American Foundation for the Blind: Product evaluation, *Access World,* New York, AFB Press.

## Appendix A

*Manufacturers of Assistive Technology for the Blind and Visually Impaired*

**Access USA**
242 James Street
PO Drawer 160
Clayton, NY 13624
Telephone: (800) 263-2750
E-mail: info@access-usa.com
**Product description:** Alternative format media supplier, including Braille for all types of documentation and audio description service

**Ai Squared**
PO Box 669
Manchester Center, VT 05255-0669
Telephone: (802) 362-3612
Fax: (802) 362-1670
E-mail: sales@aisquared.com
Website: http://www.aisquared.com
**Product description:** ZoomText XTRA: screen reading and magnification software systems

**ALVA Access Group**
436 14th Street, Suite 700
Oakland, CA 94612
Telephone: (888) 318-2582 or
(510) 451-2582
Fax: (510) 451-0878
Website: http://www.aagi.com
**Product description:** Screen reading and magnifiers for graphic operating systems and text enlargement

**American Thermoform Corp**
1758 Brackett Street
LaVerne, CA 91750
Telephone: (909) 593-6711; (800) 331-3676
Fax: (909) 593-8001
E-mail: atc@atcbrleqp.com
Website: http://www.atcbrleqp.com
**Product description:** Manufactures and distributes Braille embossers, printers, Braille translation software, Thermoform machines, and Graphics machine

**Ann Morris Enterprises, Inc.**
551 Hosner Mountain Rd.
Stormville, NY 12582
Telephone: (800) 454-3175; (845) 227-9659
Fax: (845) 226-2793
E-mail: annmor@webspan.net
Website: http://www.annmorris.agassa.com
**Product description:** Low-tech and high-tech products including talking calculators and clocks, Braille slate and stylus, tactile compass, talking VCR, and note teller

**Arkenstone Products from Freedom Scientific**
11800 31st Court North
St. Petersburg, FL 33716
Telephone: (800) 444-4443
TDD: (800) 444-4443
Fax: (727) 803-8001
E-mail: renee@arkenstone.org
Website: http://www.arkenstone.org
**Product description:** OpenBook scanning and Reading software; vera is a stand-alone OCR that can attach to a TV for text enlargement

**Artic Technologies International**
55 Park Street, Suite 2
Troy, MI 48083-2753
Telephone: (248) 588-7370 (Midwest); (209) 291-3645 (West coast)
Fax: (248) 588-2650
E-mail: info@artictech.com
Website: http://www.artictech.com
**Product description:** Screen access and magnification software, talking notetakers, speech synthesizers, and additional products for blindness and visual impairment

**Beyond Sight, Inc.**
26 East Arapahoe Rd.
Littleton, CO 80122
Telephone: (303) 795-6455
Fax: (303) 795-6425
E-mail: info@senderogroup.com
Website: http://www.senderogroup.com
**Product description:** Atlas, a talking digital map; GPS-talk-accessible GPS system for personal travel for visually impaired and blind

**Blazie, a division of Freedom Scientific**
2850 SE Market Place
Stuart, FL 34997
Telephone: (800) 444-4443; (727) 803-8000
Fax: (727) 803-8001
E-mail: sales@hj.com
Website: http://www.blazie.com/
**Product description:** Braille embossers and translators, notetakers, and refreshable Braille displays

**Brytech**
600 Peter Morand Crescent, Suite 240
Ottawa, Ontario, CANADA K1G5Z3
Telephone: (613) 731-5800
Fax: (613) 731-5812
E-mail: inquires@brytech.com
Website: http://www.brytech.com
**Product description:** Noteteller, identifies money (paper); Universal Bank Noteteller (international currency)

**Columbia Lighthouse for the Blind**
1120 20th Street NW, Suite 750 South
Washington, D.C. 20036
Telephone: (202) 454-6400
Fax: (202) 454-6401
E-mail: info@clb.org
Website: http://www.clb.org
**Product description:** A full-service assistive technology center that includes product sales, assessments, national training, and demonstrations

**Dolphin Computer Access, LLC**
60 East 3rd Avenue, Suite 130
San Mateo, CA 94401
Telephone: (866) 797-5921
Fax: (650) 348-7103
E-mail: info@dolpohinusa.com
Website: http://www.dolphinusa.com
**Product description:** Magnification, speech, and Braille computer-integrated solutions for the visually impaired

**Duxbury Systems, Inc.**
270 Littleton Road, Unit 6
Westford, MA 01886-3523
Telephone: (978) 692-3000
Fax: (978) 692-7912
E-mail: info@duxsys.com
Website: http://www.duxburysystems.com
**Product description:** Braille translation/word processing software including Nemeth (math Braille) and scientific math and foreign language Braille; for use with Windows 98 NT, 2000, Millennium, 10.2 DBT DOS and Macintosh

**Enabling Technologies Company**
1601 N.E. Braille Place
Jensen Beach, FL 34957
Telephone: (561) 225-3687; (800) 777-3687
Fax: (561) 225-3299
E-mail: enabling@brailler.com
Website: http://www.brailler.com
**Product description:** Manufactures Braille embossers, Braille and print devices, and Braille Labeler; Trade-in, demo, and used adaptive equipment

**Enhanced Vision Systems, Inc.**
2130 Main Street, Suite 250
Huntington Beach, CA 92648
Telephone: (800) 440-9476
Fax: (714) 374-1821
Website: http://www.enhancedvision.com
**Product description:** Manufacturer of low-vision products; Max is a portable, hand-held, low-vision magnification product; V-Max is a portable, head-mounted color camera and display system; and Jordy low-vision system enables people with low vision to see objects at a distance up close

**En-Vision America, Inc.**
1013 Porter Lane
Normal, IL 61761
Telephone: (309) 452-3088
Fax: (309) 452-3643
Website: http://www.envisionamerica.com
**Product description:** Manufactures a portable electronic device that uses bar codes to identify home and workplace items for the visually impaired and ScripTalk, a portable handheld electronic device that identifies prescription information

**Eschenbach Optik of America, Inc.**
904 Ethan Allen Highway
Ridgefield, CT 06877
Telephone: (800) 487-5389; (203) 438-7471
Fax: (203) 431-4718
E-mail: catalog@eschenbach.com
Website: http://www.eschenbach.com
**Product description:** Low-vision aids such as magnifiers, telescopes, microscopes, mounted magnification systems, electronic magnifiers, monocular mounting kits, and reading stands; extensive resource for eye care providers and low-vision rehabilitation

**GW Micro, Inc.**
725 Airport North Office Park
Fort Wayne, IN 46825
Telephone: (219) 489-3671
Fax: (219) 489-2608
E-mail: support@gwmicro.com
Website: http://www.gwmicro.com
**Product description:** Screen-reading program with Internet access

**Henter-Joyce, a division of Freedom Scientific**
11800 31st Court North
St. Petersburg, FL 33716-1805
Telephone: (800) 444-4443; (727) 803-8000
Fax: (727) 803-8001
E-mail: info@freedomscientific.com
Website: http://www.hj.com
**Product description:** Screen magnification and Jaws screen-reading software

**HumanWare, Inc. (to be acquired by Pulse Data International)**
6245 King Road
Loomis, CA 95650
Telephone: (800) 722-3393
Fax: (916) 652-7296
E-mail: info@humanware.com
Website: http://www.humanware.com
**Product description:** Screen-reading programs, refreshable Braille terminals, video magnification systems, Braille embossers, and personal notetakers

**IBM Accessibility Center**
11400 Burnet Road
Austin, TX 78758
Telephone: (512) 838-4893
Fax: (512) 838-9367
Website: http://www.ibm.com/able
**Product description:** Computer solutions for persons who are blind and visually impaired, including a talking web browser

**Independent Living Aids**
200 Robbins Lane
Jericho, NY 11753-2341
Telephone: (800) 537-2118
Fax: (516) 752-3135
E-mail: can-do@independentliving.com
Website: http://www.independentliving.com
**Product description:** Low-tech and high-tech products for blind and visually impaired, including color identifier, money identifier, talking VCR, talking caller IDs, and barcode identifier

**InfoCon, Inc.**
2423 West March Lane, Suite 200
Stockton, CA 95207
Telephone: (209) 478-7075; (800) 544-4551
Fax: (209) 478-7074
Website: http://www.infocon-inc.com
**Product description:** Company converts books into large print; the process uses digital technology to generate text and graphics; books are bound with hard cover

**Innoventions, Inc.**
5921 S. Middlefield Road, Suite 102
Littleton, CO 80123-2877
Telephone: (800) 854-6554; (303) 797-6554
Fax: (303) 727-4940
E-mail: magnicam@magnicam.com
Website: http://www.magnicam.com
**Product description:** Magni-Cam, a portable, hand-held electronic magnification system

**Kurzweil Educational Systems, Group**
52 Third Avenue
Burlington, MA 01803
Telephone: (800) 894-KESI (5374);
(781) 203-5000
Fax: ((781) 203-5033
E-mail: info@kurzweiledu.com
Website: http://www.kurzweiledu.com
**Product description:** Kurzweil 1000 scanning and reading tool; magniReader-scans documents for text enlargement on the computer screen

**The Lighthouse International**
111 E. 59th St., 12th Floor
New York, NY 10022-1202
Telephone: (800) 829-0500
Fax: (212) 821-9727
E-mail: info@lighthouse.org
Website: http://www.lighthouse.org
**Product description:** Extensive selection of low-vision aids and high-tech products

**LS & S Group Inc.**
PO Box 673
Northbrook, IL 60065
Telephone: (847) 498-9777;
customer service: (800) 468-4789;
TTY: (800) 317-8533
Fax: (847) 498-1482 (24 hrs)
E-mail: lssgrp@aol.com
Website: http://www.lssgrp.com
**Product description:** High-tech and low-tech vision products including talking watches, large numeral watches, talking thermometers, etc

**MagniSight Inc.**
3360 Adobe Court
Colorado Springs, CO 80907
Telephone: (800) 753-4767
Fax: (719) 578-9887
E-mail: sale@magnisight.com
Website: http://www.magnisight.com
Product description: Manufacturer of CCTVs

**Maxi Aids**
42 Executive Blvd.
Farmingdale, NY 11735
Telephone: (800) 522-6294; (631) 752-0521;
TTY: (631) 752-0738
Website:
http://www.maartdept@hearmore.com
**Product description:** Mail-order catalogue
of low-tech and high-tech products for the
blind, visually impaired, and other disabilities

**Microsoft Accessibility Technology for
Everyone**
Microsoft Corporation
One Microsoft Way
Redmond, WA 98052-6399
Telephone: (425) 703-4929
Fax: (425) 936-7329
Website: http://www.microsoft.com/enable
**Product description:** Manufactures
disability options in operating systems for
the personal computer

**OVAC, Inc.**
67-555 E. Palm Canyon Dr., Unit C103
Cathederal City, CA 92234
Telephone: (800) 325-4488
Fax: (760) 321-9711
E-mail: info@ovac.com
Website: http://www.ovac.com
**Product description:** Vision-aide zoom
lens, low-vision magnification system that
operates off any standard television

**Optelec US, Inc. (acquired by the Tieman
Group)**
6 Lyberty Way
PO Box 729
Westford, MA 01886
Telephone: (800) 828-1056
Fax: (978) 692-6073
E-mail: optelec@optelec.com
Website: http://www.optelec.com
**Product description:** Manufacturer and
distributor of CCTVs

**Pitney Bowes, Inc.**
1 Elmcroft Road
Stanford, CT 06926-0700
Telephone: (800) 672-6937
Fax: (203) 365-6156
**Product description:** Universal access
copier system incorporates speech
recognition, extra large touch screen
interface, with Braille labeling on the
keyboard and control panel

**PulseData International, Inc.**
351 Thornton Road, Suite 119
Lithia Springs, GA 30122-1589
Telephone: (888) 734-8439; (770) 941-7200
Fax: (770) 941-7722
E-mail: PDI_INC@mindspring.com
Website: http://www.pulsedata.com
**Product description:** CCTV's (color and
b/w) stand-alone units or with computer-
interface; "smart keys" and "smart keyboard
organizers" with onscreen displays of time,
day, date, calculator, electronic rolodex,
appointment calendar and memo pad, and
Keynote Gold speech synthesizer

**Repro-Tronics, Inc.**
75 Carver Avenue
Westwood, NJ 07675
Telephone: (201) 722-1880
Fax: (201) 722-1881
E-mail: info@repro-tronics.com
Website: http://www.repro-tronics.com
**Product description:** Hardware and
software for the creation and production of
tactile graphic images; graphic designs can
be produced either as a print or embossed
output

**Sighted Electronics, Inc.**
69 Woodland Avenue
Westwood, NJ 07675
Telephone: (201) 666-2221; (800) 666-4883
Fax: (201) 666-0159
E-mail: sighted@idt.net
Website: http://www.sighted.com
**Product description:** Provides Braille
displays, Braille embossers, Optical Braille
Recognition, and screen-reading programs

**Syntha-Voice Computers Inc.**
304-800 Queenston Road
Stoney Creek, Ontario, CANADA L8G1A7
Telephone: (800) 263-4540; (905) 662-0565
Fax: (905) 662-0568
E-mail: help@synthavoice.com
Website: http://www.synthavoice.com
**Product description:** Screen access
software that supports speech and Braille
for Windows 98, 95, NT, ME, 2000

**Tack-Tiles Braille Systems, LLC**
PO Box 475
Plaistow, NH 03865
Telephone: (603) 382-1904
Fax: (603) 382-1748
E-mail: braille@tack-tiles.com
Website: http://www.tack-tiles.com
**Product description:** Teaching tool for
Nemeth Braille Code (mathematics), Braille
literacy, computer Braille code, and music
notation

**Technologies for the Visually Impaired, Inc.**
9 Nolan Court
Hauppauge, NY 11778
Telephone: (516) 724-4479
Fax: (516) 724-4479
E-mail: tvii@concentric.net
Website: http://www.tvi~web.com
**Product description:** Products for Robotron of Australia and other adaptive devices and hardware for the blind and visually impaired

**Telesensory Corporation**
520 Almanor Avenue
Sunnyvale, CA 94086-3533
Telephone: (408) 616-8700; customer relations: (800) 804-8004
Fax: (408) 616-8720
E-mail: info@telesensory.com
Website: http://www.telesensory.com
**Product description:** Video magnifiers, screen magnification, OCR (scanners), and Reading Edge

**ViewPlus Technologies**
Business Enterprise Center
800 NW Starker Avenue
Corvallis, OR 97330
Telephone: (541) 754-4002
Fax: (541) 738-6505
E-mail: vpt@viewplustech.com
Website: http://www.viewplustech.com
**Product description:** TIGER advantage, a personal computer printer that embosses high-resolution tactile graphics and Braille

**Vision Technology, Inc.**
8501 Delport Drive
St. Louis, MO 63114-5905
Telephone: (800) 560-7226; (314) 890-8300
Fax: (314) 890-8383
E-mail: vti@vti1.com
Website: http://www.freedom-machines.com
**Product description:** Color and black and white CCTVs with auto-focus; hand-held video magnifier and link to IBM compatible computer

## Appendix B

*Organizations*

**AARP (American Association of Retired Persons)**
601 E St. NW
Washington, D.C. 20049
Telephone: (202) 434-2277; (800) 424-3410
E-mail: member@aarp.org
Website: http://www.aarp.org
**Publications:** Product catalogue, through pharmacy services, has low-vision products

**American Council of the Blind**
1155 15th Street NW, Suite 1004
Washington, D.C. 20005
Telephone: (800) 424-8666; (202) 467-5081
Fax: (202) 467-5085
Website: http://www.acb.org
**Publication:** *Braille Forum* is a free monthly newsletter; ACB also sponsors a half-hour monthly radio program

**American Foundation for the Blind**
National Programs and Initiatives
11 Penn Plaza, Suite 300
New York, N.Y. 10001
Telephone: (212) 502-7642; (800) 232-5463
Fax: (212) 502-7773
E-mail: afbinfo@afb.net
Website: http://www.afb.org
**Product description:** Maintains a career and technology information bank (database) of employed blind people willing to discuss their jobs and the technology they use; also conducts evaluations; publications include *Access World,* a monthly technology magazine

**AFB's Braille Literacy Center**
Telephone: (800) AFB-LINE (232-5463)
Website: http://www.aftb.org

**American Printing House for the Blind, Inc.**
1839 Frankfort Avenue
Louisville, KY 40206-0085
Telephone: (502) 895-2405 (voice)
Fax: (502) 895-1509
E-mail: jcarroll@aph.org
Website: http://www.aph.org
On-line newsletter: *APH Technology Update*
**Product description:** Talking software and products for the visually impaired

**Association for Education and Rehabilitation of the Blind and Visually Impaired**
4600 Duke Street, Suite 430
PO Box 22397
Alexandria, VA 22304
Telephone: (703) 823-9690
Fax: (703) 823-9695
Website: http://www.aerbvi.org
**Publications:** *AER Report, AER's Job Exchange* newsletter, Braille instructional materials, *Orientation & Mobility Techniques*

**Florida Instructional Materials Center for the Visually Impaired**
5002 North Lois Avenue
Tampa, FL 33614
Telephone: (813) 872-5281
Fax: (813) 872-5284
Website: http://www.fimcvi.org
**Publications:** Braille instructional materials

**Behavioral Optometry Resource**
Dr. Beth Ballinger, OD
833 Dover Drive, Suite 9
Newport Beach, CA 92660
Telephone: (949) 642-0292
**Description:** Source for listing of behavioral optometrists in the United States

**Blindness Resource Center**
% The New York Institute for Special Education
Office of Development
999 Pelham Parkway
Bronx, New York 10469
Telephone: (718) 519-7000x315 (Mr. Petell)
Fax: (718) 231-9314
Website: http://www.nyise.org
Low-vision website:
http://www.nyise.org/lowvision.htm
Blindness website:
http://www.nyise.org/blindness/htm
**Description:** NYISE provides extensive resources and information on the web

**Braille Institute**
741 No. Vermont
Los Angeles, CA 90029
(Serving Southern and Central California)
Telephone: (800) 272-4553
Website: http://brailleinstitute.org
**Description:** Provides free Braille materials, audio tapes, and catalogues and training for California clients

**The Caption Center at WGBH**
125 Western Avenue
Boston, MA 02134
Telephone: (617) 300-5400
Fax: (617) 300-1026
**Description:** Descriptive video service (DVS)

**Daisy Consortium**
Contact person: Kjell Hansson
Swedish Library of Talking Books
S-122 88 Enskede, SWEDEN
Telephone: (011) 468-399350
Fax: (0111) 468-6599467
E-mail: kjell.hansson@tpb.se
Website: http://www.daisy.org
**Description:** The Daisy Consortium is establishing the international standard for the production, exchange, and use of the next generation of digital talking books and is made up of world-wide organizations serving persons who are blind or print disabled

**Helen Keller National Center**
111 Middle Neck Rd.
Sands Point, NY 11050
Telephone: (516) 944-8900 (voice);
(516) 944-8637 (TTY)
Fax: (516) 944-7302
E-mail: hkncpr@aol.com
Website: http://www.helenkeller.org
**Description:** Provides orientation, mobility, job training, and adaptive technology training for deaf-blind youth and adults

**Lions World Services for the Blind**
2811 Fair Park Blvd.
PO Box 4055
Little Rock, AR 72204
Telephone: (501) 664-7100
Fax: (501) 664-2743
E-mail: training@lwsb.org
Website: http://www.lwsb.org

**The Lighthouse International**
111 East 59th Street, 12th floor
New York, NY 10022-1202
Telephone: (800) 334-5497
Website: http://www.lighthouse.org

**National Association for Visually Handicapped**
22 West 21st Street, 6th Floor
New York, NY 10010
Telephone: (212) 889-3141
Fax: (212) 727-2931
Website: http://www.navh.org

**National Braille Press**
88 Saint Stephen Street
Boston, MA 02115
Telephone: (617) 266-6160
Fax: (617) 437-0456
Website: http://www.nbp.com
**Publication:** National Braille Press Release

**National Federation of the Blind**
1800 Johnson Street
Baltimore, MD 21230
Telephone: (800) 638-7518; (410) 659-9314
Fax: (410) 685-5653
E-mail: nfb@access.digex.net
Website: http://www.nfb.org
**Publication:** *Braille Monitor*

**National Information Center for Children and Youth with Disabilities**
PO Box 1492
Washington, D.C. 20013
Telephone: (800) 695-0285
Fax: (703) 893-1741
Website: http://www.nichcy.org

**National Library Service for the Blind/Physically Handicapped**
The Library of Congress
1291 Taylor Street, NW
Washington, D.C. 20542
Telephone: (202) 707-5100
Website: http://www.loc.gov/nls
**Description:** NLS administers a free library program of Braille and recorded materials circulated to eligible borrowers through a network of cooperating libraries

**National Organization on Disability (NOD)**
910 Sixteenth Street, NW, Suite 600
Washington, D.C. 20006
Telephone: (202) 293-5960 (voice);
(202) 293-5968 (TDD)
Fax: (202) 293-7999
Website: http://www.nod.org

**National Rehabilitation Association**
633 South Washington Street
Alexandria, VA 22314
Telephone: (703) 836-0850 (voice);
(703) 836-0849
Fax: (703) 836-0848
Website: http://www.nationalrehab.org

**National Rehabilitation Information Center (NRIC)**
1010 Wayne Avenue, Suite 800
Silver Spring, MD 20910-3319
Telephone: (800) 346-2742
Website: http://www.nric.com

**Recording for the Blind & Dyslexic (RFB&D)**
20 Roszel Road
Princeton, NJ 08540
Telephone: (800) 221-4792 (for book orders);
(609) 452-0606
Fax: (609) 987-8116
E-mail: info@rfdb.org
Website: http://www.rfdb.org
**Description:** Provides on-loan recorded textbooks at all academic levels; this service is available to members only; a one-time membership fee exists

**RESNA Rehabilitation Engineering and Assistive Technology Society of North America**
1700 North Moore St., Suite 1540
Arlington, VA 22209-1903
Telephone: (703) 524-6686 (voice);
(703) 524-6639 (TTY)
Fax: (703) 524-6630
Website: http://www.resna.org
**Description:** Interdisciplinary organization for persons interested in technology and disability

# Sensory Aids: Hearing Assistive Listening Aids and Signaling Devices for the Hearing Impaired

*Alice E. Holmes*

## Application and Goals

Hearing loss is an invisible disability that affects over 22 million Americans. Estimates on the prevalence of hearing loss vary depending on the population that is part of the study and the criteria that the researchers use to define hearing loss. In the National Health Interview Survey,[1] approximately 1.61% of children under age 18 in the United States reported hearing loss. The prevalence of hearing loss increases as people get older. For people in the age range of 65 to 74 years, approximately 26.6% reported significant hearing loss. This figure increases to 40.3% for those 75 years and older. Many technologic advances have occurred in amplification and assistive technology for those with hearing loss. Hearing aids are the primary rehabilitative tool that researchers use when they identify an individual as having hearing loss.[2] These traditional forms of amplification have improved greatly in the last decade with programmable and digital signal processing and miniaturization. Even with these advances, hearing aids still fall short of restoring normal hearing to those with hearing loss. Unfortunately, background noise and distance from the speaker continue to be challenges.

## Function and Ability

People have designed assistive listening and signaling devices to improve communication of the hearing impaired in instances in which traditional hearing aids are not sufficient. Designers created these devices to help people listen in noise or in the presence of a competing message, improve distance listening, allow independence, and facilitate group conversation when problems exist because of rapidly changing speakers.

With passage of the Americans with Disabilities Act (ADA) in 1990, assistive listening devices (ALDs) are becoming more accessible to people with hearing loss. Employers and public facilities must provide auxiliary aids and services when necessary to ensure effective communication for those who are deaf or hard of hearing.[3] Unfortunately, few individuals with hearing loss are aware that this law applies to them and many are not familiar with the various ALDs available. Audiologists, the trained professionals who can assess, counsel, and fit individuals with various ALDs to aid in their communication, can also educate consumers about the ADA-mandated protection that they are entitled to receive.

## Considerations and Options

### Advantages of Assistive Listening Devices

Any time an individual is in a less-than-ideal listening setting, an ALD may help. If background noise exists, as in a restaurant or noisy work setting, an ALD can reduce the signal-to-noise ratio. With a traditional hearing aid, the speech or desired signal and the noise are both amplified. With an ALD, however, the speech or desired signal has primary amplification, not the competing noise. Additionally, when the individual with hearing loss is not at an optimal listening distance of 3 to 10 feet from the speaker, an ALD can bring the signal directly to that individual via remote microphones. Therefore the user can realize the advantages of ALDs in a number of listening situations such as one-on-one communication in a noisy environment, a lecture in a classroom or meeting, and mass media (theaters, movies, radio, or TV).

### Disadvantages of Assistive Listening Devices

Although ALDs offer many advantages, health care professionals need to be aware that ALDs also have several drawbacks. The physical appearance of ALDs is undesirable to many consumers. Most ALDs are larger and more visible than traditional hearing aids. Franks and Beckman[4] surveyed 100 older adults (50 hearing aid users and 50 nonusers) about their attitudes toward hearing aids. More than 70% of the respondents believed that hearing aids focus attention on the handicap. Some perceive assistive listening devices as focusing even greater attention to the hearing loss than hearing aids and reject them for that reason alone.

Holmes[5] considered the burden factor. Burdens that people have with the everyday use and upkeep of assistive devices can become overwhelming, particularly to older adults. Some burdensome tasks that people can have are changing batteries, removing the hearing aid to use the ALD receiver, and adjusting the volume. Many individuals with hearing loss need extensive training. Some users may also find the cost of some devices to be prohibitive. Professionals who carefully analyze the individual's communication situations and needs can help determine the most effective ALD at the lowest cost with the least burden factor.

### Assessment

Professionals need to first perform a complete audiologic assessment of hearing impaired individuals to determine the most appropriate device. A needs assessment in the form of a questionnaire or case history is invaluable in this process. If the primary concern for individuals is television listening, they could us a device specific to that purpose. If, on the other hand, they have problems with listening to the television and listening in a car, they could use another multipurpose device that would be more appropriate. If possible, professionals should provide individuals with a trial period so that the user can assess the benefit of the ALD in specific listening environments.

### Counseling

Professionals should inform individuals with hearing loss that no device is perfect and that nothing can restore their hearing to normal. These devices are aids not cures. The professional's consultation before, during, and after fitting the individual with an ALD is vital. Self-assessment questionnaires provide individuals with useful and necessary information about the handicap that they perceive. Professionals should talk to individuals with hearing loss and their significant others to help them choose most appropriate ALD. Whenever possible, professionals should include family members and significant others in the counseling process because hearing impairment affects individuals with the loss and their significant others.[6] The significant others should be aware of the benefits and limitations of ALDs. Peoples' attitudes greatly affect society's acceptance of hearing loss and use of rehabilitation devices such as hearing aids and ALDs.

### Technology

Individuals can use assistive listening devices as personal communication aids in one-on-one conversation, in group conversation, with the telephone, radio or television, or in large areas such as in churches and theaters.[7] Simple alerting or signaling devices can inform someone who is hard of hearing of a knock at the door or the cry of a baby. Assistive devices also vary in their internal electronic components from simple hardwired microphone-amplifier units to more sophisticated infrared or FM systems.

## Hardwired Devices

As the name implies, hardwired devices require wires to connect the microphone, amplifier, and receiver/speaker in an earphone or earmold. For personal systems, the amplifier is about the size of a beeper and the hearing impaired person can hold it in the hand or place it in a pocket (Figure 12-1). Listeners can "self-wire" themselves with all parts of the system on their body or can give the microphone to the person that is speaking. By giving the speaker the microphone, communication is enhanced by decreasing the distance from the speaker's mouth to the microphone, hence improving the signal-to-background noise ratio.

Professionals who provide services to individuals with hearing loss (i.e., physician consultations) for personal-use applications (i.e., listening while in the car, at restaurants, etc.) use these personal systems. Personal hardwired devices vary in sound quality and price.[8] People can purchase them at retail audio equipment outlets or through audiologists or hearing aid dispensers.

Individuals with hearing loss can also use hardwired systems in churches or theaters. Typically, the facility wires the microphone from the standard amplifier to personal amplifiers in selected seats. The facility requires the hearing impaired to sit in seats that have the wires and equipment and use a receiver such as a headset or earphone to receive the benefits.

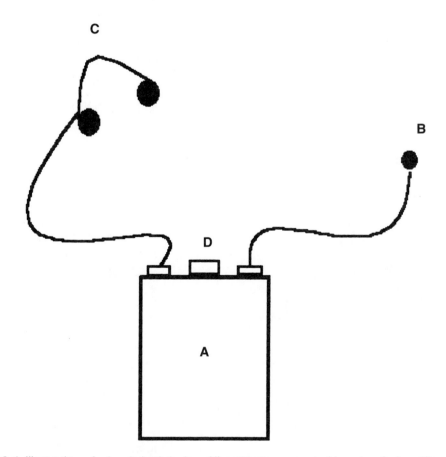

**Fig. 12-1** Illustration of a hardwired device. All parts are connected by wire. **A,** Amplifier. **B,** Microphone. **C,** Receiver headset. **D,** Volume control.

## FM Sound Systems

Free-field, wireless, frequency-modulated (FM) sound systems can improve listening for the hearing impaired in group settings such as meetings, concerts, churches, theaters, museums, and schools. These systems send the auditory message through frequency-modulated radio waves from a transmitter to a small receiver that a listener with a hearing impairment wears (Figure 12-2). Users can then adjust their own volumes and receive a direct signal from the sound source.[9-10]

FM systems can work alone, in conjunction with the sound systems usually found in auditoriums and churches, or with portable PA systems that groups use for meetings and lectures. The wireless transmitters send the signal directly to the listeners' personal wireless receivers. Receivers can be headsets or earphones or users can couple them to hearing aids through direct-input adapters or via teleloop or telecoil induction coupling.

People can use personal FM systems in difficult listening environments such as restaurants, cars, lectures, or meetings. FM systems improve the signal-to-noise ratio and thereby improve the listening environment for an individual with hearing loss. They also vary in cost and quality. FM units tend to be flexible and often have internal settings that people can adjust with changes in hearing loss.

## Infrared Sound Systems

An infrared system transmits the sound to the audience via invisible infrared light waves similar to remote controls on televisions. A transmitter uses light waves to send speech or music to individual wireless headset receivers (Figure 12-3). The receivers are lightweight, and users can wear them anywhere that is in the line of vision with the transmitter and use them with headphones or couple it with some hearing aids. The systems are not subject to electromagnetic interference but they are vulnerable to interference from natural light. Therefore users cannot operate infrared systems in direct sunlight.

Considerable overlap exists in the possible uses of infrared and FM systems. The advantages of infrared include a person's ability to contain the signal within a room, thus increasing privacy of the signal information. Infrared systems can use an unlimited number of receivers and have excellent sound quality. However, unlike FM units, physi-

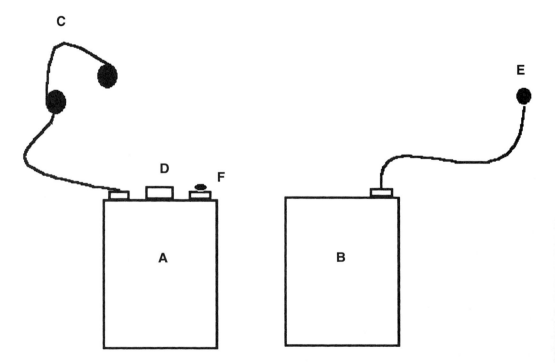

**Fig. 12-2** An FM system. Radio frequency waves are used to send the sound to the receiver/amplifier **(A)** from the transmitter **(B). C,** Receiver headset. **D,** Volume control. **E,** Remote microphone. **F,** Optional environmental microphone.

cal obstruction can block the signal of an infrared system and the system is less portable.[10]

## Audio Loop Systems

An audio loop system transmits sound via a loop of wire that surrounds the seating area. Electric current flows through the loop and creates a magnetic field that the hearing aid equipped with a telecoil (T-coil) switch can receive and then amplify (Figure 12-4). Professionals can permanently install audio loop systems in meeting rooms, theaters, and even automobiles, or they can set up portable loop systems as needed.

The major limiting factor of the audio loop system is the need for the individual to have a hearing aid with a functional T-coil switch. Unfortunately, many hearing aid users do not even know whether their hearing aid has this option and professionals have not instructed them in its proper use.[11] Professional audiology training programs and new-user hearing aid orientation classes need to emphasize the benefits of T-coils for telephone listening and for use with assistive listening devices.

## Telephone Listening Devices

Telephone communication can pose a unique problem for listeners with hearing loss because they have to rely totally on their damaged auditory system rather than being able to benefit from visual cues. Designers have created several ALDs specifically for telephone communication. One of the most common and useful is a telephone amplifier that allows the user to adjust the volume of the telephone receiver. Built-in amplifiers can exist in the telephone or its handset or they can be "in-line" units connected between a standard telephone and the wall jack. Portable snap-on amplifiers are also available. These amplifiers are battery operated and users can attach them to any phone.[12]

Telecommunication devices for the deaf (TDDs) or teletypewriters (TTYs) permit individuals with limited or no useable hearing to type messages through the telephone lines. People at both ends must have a TDD, and each person types a message on a teletype keyboard that is transmitted from a modem through the telephone line to the receiver's keyboard for printout on a screen.[13]

Telecommunication relay systems are available and permit a TDD user to make calls to a standard telephone user and vice versa. A user can call a relay station where a relay operator transmits the message in the proper form.[13]

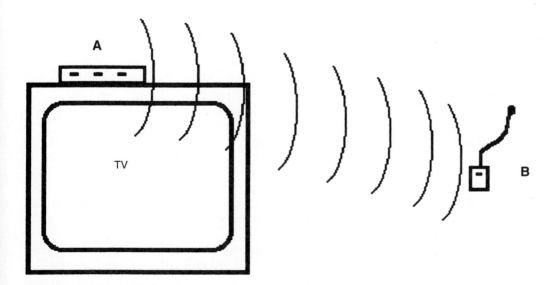

**Fig. 12-3** An infrared system. Infrared light rays send the signal from the transmitter **(A)** to the receiver **(B)**.

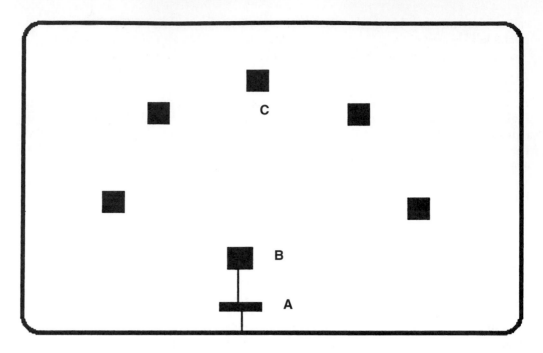

**Fig. 12-4** An audio loop system. Sound is sent to an amplifier **(A)** from the speaker's microphone **(B). C,** An electric current is then sent around the loop to create a magnetic field that can be received and then amplified by a hearing aid equipped with a telecoil (T-coil) switch.

## Television Systems

Alternative listening systems are also available for television. Although FM, infrared, and audio loop systems are hardwired, people can use them in conjunction with television listening. An excellent option for visually impaired people to watch television is closed captioning. By using a television with either a built-in or external caption decoder, viewers can see real-time captions of the auditory portion of a program. Closed captioning is similar to a dubbed movie. As of July 1, 1993, and in accordance with the ADA, all televisions 13 inches or larger that are manufactured or sold in the United States must have closed-captioning capabilities.[14]

## Alerting and Signaling Devices

Alerting devices for the hearing impaired also exist to aid in the detection of convenience and safety/alarm equipment. Users can plug wake-up alarms that use flashing lights or bed vibrators into an alarm clock. Multipurpose light-flashing or vibrating systems are also available for auditory signals such as telephone ringers, doorbells, smoke alarms, and kitchen timers.

## Outcome and Social Validation

Professionals can evaluate the electroacoustic characteristics of the various ALDs. They should complete real ear testing of the gain and output to ensure that the instruments are providing appropriate amplification for the hearing loss. They can also use functional gain measurements.[15]

Beyond these physical measurements, professionals can measure the benefits by functional assessment. Researchers who use various self-assessment measurements to determine hearing aid benefit such as the Hearing Handicap Inventory for the Elderly and its short form can also them to assess ALDs.[16-17] In addition to self-perception scales, researchers can also use traditional speech perception tests to assess the benefit of these devices. They should get ongoing feedback from the person during the fitting process while using various taped background noises. After the initial fitting, researchers should give users the opportunity to try the devices in their unique listening environments.

## Cost and Benefit Analysis

When professionals recommend any ALD for an individual with hearing loss, they must consider the following factors:

1. What are the specific needs of the individual and what specific instruments benefit those needs?
2. What is the burden factor of the device (i.e., how easy is it to operate, how durable is the unit, and how will it be handled)?
3. What is the financial cost of the instrument?
4. Do the benefits outweigh the cost and burden of the system?

The person in need of technology can fulfill each specific need with several systems. The key is for the user to acquire the system that is easiest to operate and offers good quality at a reasonable cost. Each of the devices can range dramatically in price. Users can compromise sound quality, in some cases, if they select the less-expensive units. Additionally, the durability factor can affect cost, but users should not compromise durability when they have a specific need. For example, an adult who occasionally uses an FM system does not need the same durability in a system as a child who wears the system daily in the classroom.

## CASE STUDIES

### CASE 1

K.M. is a 72-year-old widow who lives alone. She has severe bilateral sensorineural hearing loss and wears binaural behind-the-ear hearing aids equipped with T-coils. She reported several concerns. First, her hearing aids whistled or produced feedback when she was on the telephone. Second, she was worried about not hearing the telephone or doorbell ring, particularly when she removed her hearing aids. Finally, she could not understand the TV.

Professionals trained K.M. in the operation of her hearing aid T-coils for telephone use, which solved the feedback problem. They also equipped her telephone with an amplifier handset to increase the signal. They hooked a visual alerting system to her doorbell and telephone ringer so that two lamps would flash (one in her living room and one in her bedroom) at the same time the one or the other was ringing. Finally, she purchased an infrared system for her television so that she could hear a more direct signal at a comfortable loudness. The professionals easily installed these items with the help of her 20-year-old grandson and at a cost K.M. could afford.

### CASE 2

F.S. is a 45-year-old executive who has moderate bilateral sensorineural hearing loss. He wears bilateral in-the-ear hearing aids that professionals equipped with T-coils. He reported having difficulty understanding different speakers at board meetings and at site visits in noisy factories.

Professionals recommended an FM system with several transmitter options for F.S. First, they placed a conference microphone with an FM transmitter on the center of the boardroom's table. He can wear an FM receiver with an audio neckloop that sends the signal to his hearing aid T-coils so that he can now receive direct signals from the conference microphone into his hearing aids from anyone seated at the table.

When he visits noisy environments, F.S. can use the FM system with the standard remote microphone to hear his co-workers without amplifying the competing background noise. He has also found this system helpful when listening to passengers in his car.

## CASE 3

S.Y. is a 10-year-old girl with severe bilateral sensorineural hearing loss who wears behind-the-ear hearing aids that professionals equipped with T-coils in both ears. She uses oral communication and attends school in a regular classroom. S.Y. stated that she was having difficulty hearing the teacher whenever background noise was present in the classroom. She was also having difficulty at home hearing the TV.

Professionals fitted S.Y. with an FM system for the classroom. Her teacher wears a remote microphone and transmitter, and S.Y. wears the receiver directly coupled to her hearing aids. Her hearing aids have a switch that allows the microphones on the hearing aids and the FM system to be active simultaneously. This allows her to hear the direct signal from the teacher's microphone while monitoring her own voice through the hearing aid microphones.

At home, S.Y.'s parents obtained a television with a closed-captioning decoder. This allows her to read any information she misses auditorily. As an added bonus, her parents report that this has also improved her reading skills.

# References

1. Adams PF, Benson V: Current estimates from the National Health Interview Survey, *Vital Health Stat* 10:184, 1991.
2. Bess F, Lichtenstein M, Logan S: Audiologic assessment of the hearing-impaired elderly. In Rintelmann WB, editor: *Hearing assessment,* pp 511-548, Austin, Tex, 1990, Pro-Ed.
3. Strauss KP: The ADA the law, communication assess, and the role of audiologists. In Ross M, editor: *The communication access for persons with hearing loss: compliance with Americans with Disabilities Act,* Baltimore, 1994, York Press.
4. Franks J, Beckman N: Rejection of hearing aids: attitudes of a geriatric sample, *Ear Hear* 6:161-166, 1985.
5. Holmes AE: Hearing aids and the older adult. In Kricos P, Lesner S, editors: *Hearing care for the older adult: a practical approach,* Reading, Pa, 1995, Andover Medical.
6. Hetu R, Getty L: Development of a rehabilitation program for people affected with occupational hearing loss: results from group intervention with 48 workers and their spouses, *Audiology* 30:317-329, 1991.
7. Kaplan H: Assistive devices for the elderly, *J Am Acad Audiol* 7:203-211, 1996.
8. Dempsey JJ: Hardwire personal listening systems. In Ross M, editor: *Communication access for persons with hearing loss: compliance with the Americans with Disabilities Act,* Baltimore, 1994, York Press.
9. Yuzon EV: FM personal listening systems. In Ross M, editor: *Communication access for persons with hearing loss: compliance with the Americans with Disabilities Act,* pp 73-102, Baltimore, 1994, York Press.
10. Ross M: FM large-area listening systems description and comparison with other such systems. In Ross M, editor: *Communication access for persons with hearing loss: compliance with the Americans with Disabilities Act,* Baltimore, 1994, York Press.
11. Centa JM: Telecoils: federally mandated or voluntarily included? *Hear Instrum* 43 (8):43, 1992.
12. Holmes AE: Telecommunications acoustic technology. In Ross M, editor: *Communication access for persons with hearing loss: compliance with the Americans with Disabilities Act,* Baltimore, 1994, York Press.
13. Castle D: Telecommunication visual technology. In Ross M, editor: *Communication access for persons with hearing loss: compliance with the Americans with Disabilities Act,* Baltimore, 1994, York Press.
14. Americans with Disabilities Act of 1990: PL 101-336 Title 42, USC 12101 et seq: US Statutes at Large, 104:327-378, July1990.
15. Comptom CL: Assistive technology for deaf and hard-of-hearing people. In Alpiner JG, McCarthy PA, editors: *Rehabilitative audiology: children and adults,* Baltimore, 1993, Williams & Wilkins.
16. Fino MS et al: Factors differentiating elderly hearing aid wearers vs. non-wearers, *Hear Instrum* 43 (2):6-10, 1992.
17. Newman CW et al: Practical method for quantifying hearing aid benefit in older adults, *J Am Acad Audiol* 2:70-75, 1991.

# PART 3

··········································································

## Technologies for Manipulation

··········································································

*Jack E. Uellendahl*
*Dudley S. Childress*

Manipulation, which feeds the mind and is the main means by which people normally interact with the environment, is at the core of daily existence. Some of the functions that hand and upper limb impairments compromise include a person's ability to perform self-care activities such as eating, dressing, bathing, and grooming, the capacity to communicate through touching, gesturing, writing, drawing, or typing, and the ability to use tools in creating artifacts to alter surroundings.

Hands are wonderfully designed to accomplish a broad range of activities from heavy work to delicate manipulation. With the aid of exquisite sensation, they can exert strong, powerful action or precise, fine movement with elegance and grace. A person's ability to effectively use these matchless tools requires a stable base from which to work and the ability to place the hand accurately in space. Without proximal support and proper placement, a perfectly functional hand may be of little or no practical use.

Part 3 is dedicated to technologies that enable users to physically interact with their environments. Assistive technologies that allow manipulation range from relatively simple adaptive aids such as buttonhooks to complex prosthetic, orthotic, or robotic devices.

As evidenced by the variety of topics and disciplines in this part, for technological interventions to be successful, a qualified team of experts should evaluate each person. Each team member must bring valuable skills and resources to the rehabilitation process. Through close communication, members of the team, the person involved, and family and friends develop interdisciplinary goals and objectives. They should set realistic goals that focus on the objectives and expectations of the user. Because rehabilitation is a temporal process, everyone involved should reevaluate the goals frequently, particularly during the rehabilitation period. Changes in objectives during the process require rehabilitation specialists to be flexible, have a willingness to listen carefully, and alter directions when necessary.

From one point of view, modern technology can offer much to people with impairments. Much advancement has occurred in recent years, from the use of lightweight, strong plastics to the application of computer technology in arm and leg prostheses. Yet, when technologists witness even the most accomplished users operating these sophisticated devices, they realize the tremendous challenges that are ahead when they attempt to mimic the function of the human hand and arm.

# CHAPTER 13

# Seating Intervention and Postural Control

*Jessica Presperin Pedersen*
*Michelle L. Lange*
*Cheryl Griebel*

Optimal sitting is essential when individuals who are nonambulatory and require additional stability, pressure distribution, or body alignment use a wheelchair or another mobility base. Wheelchair positioning is a field of professional intervention that has evolved since the early 1970s. The theoretical approach for intervention and technological strategies has changed throughout the years. Users are now more active in the evaluation and selection processes. Education, focused on wheelchair seating principles and intervention strategies, is readily available for professionals and wheelchair users in many areas of the world.

## Application and Goals

The goals of seating intervention vary greatly depending on the user's needs and expectations. One individual may require significant postural support to perform limited functional tasks using the head to activate a switch, and another person may need a cushion placed on the wheelchair upholstery to provide increased pressure distribution under the buttocks and femurs. A slight increase in spinal extension may change a person's center of gravity when sitting in the wheelchair, allowing for improved wheelchair propulsion. Specific goals of seating may include the following:

- Improved head and/or trunk control
- Improved proximal stability
- Improved gross motor abilities for better self-propulsion
- Improved manipulation skills
- Improved visual motor skills
- Improved oral motor skills (e.g., swallowing, feeding, vocalizing)
- Improved sitting tolerance or comfort
- Improved physiologic function (e.g., respiration, cardiovascular function, digestion, skin integrity)
- Improved endurance (i.e., minimized effects of gravity, increased energy for other tasks)
- Improved psychosocial interaction and/or increased self-esteem
- Reduced influence of abnormal neurologic forces (e.g., asymmetric muscular forces, primitive reflexes, extremes in muscle tone, dynamic posturing)

Technologists note the individual's needs and expectations as goals, which become key factors when they assess outcome measures. Ideally, through appropriate seating, users achieve their desired level of independence in function in a variety of environments such as home, school, work, community, or leisure.[1-9]

## Function and Ability

### *The Team*

As described in earlier chapters, a comprehensive and accurate assessment begins with a multidisciplinary team approach that includes users, their caregivers, and qualified professionals. The service delivery process should be user-centered, making the user and caregivers an essential part of the team. Professionals in the team usually include the referring physician, a licensed therapist (physical and/or occupational), and a rehabilitation technology supplier. In addition, a rehabilitation engineer may be a consistent member of the team. When modifications, custom design, or fabrication are required, the rehabilitation engineer may be a consultant. Other key team members include technical support staff, the third-party payer, and the funding coordinators who compile the necessary paperwork and financial information. The rehabilitation technology suppliers usually employ funding coordinators. The extended team may include the user's primary physical, occupational, or speech therapists, teachers, vocational rehabilitation counselors, employers, other assistive technology practitioners, social workers, nurses, orthopedists, and other physicians.

### Credentialed Professionals

The Rehabilitation Engineering and Assistive Technology Society of North America (RESNA) may credential a practitioner, called an *assistive technology practitioner (ATP)*, specializing in wheelchair seating intervention in the area of assistive technology. RESNA may also credential a supplier as an assistive technology supplier (ATS). A further step in the process of credentialing rehabilitation technology suppliers (suppliers of durable medical rehabilitation equipment) occurs when the individual passes the RESNA certification tests as an ATS and the National Registry of Rehabilitation Technology Suppliers (NRRTS) accepts the individual as a member. This person is called a *certified rehabilitation technology supplier (CRTS)*. When providing wheelchairs and seating systems, the ATP usually partners with a CRTS. For ease in identification, we use the acronyms *ATP* and *CRTS* in the rest of this chapter to refer to these professionals (see Chapter 4).

## Considerations, Options, and Technology

### *The Assessment*

The assessment by technologists is a critical aspect of the seating intervention process. Technologists must have an in-depth knowledge of the current equipment available. However, they should have an understanding of the way to compile information based on an individual's expectations and physical, functional, psychosocial, environmental, and cultural status to formulate the parameters that guide equipment choice. Gaps in this process may lead to technologists making expensive mistakes or equipment abandonment and physical harm to users. Many authors have written books, chapters, and articles describing the evaluation process indepth.[10-13]

Technologists go through a general information gathering process, which may include giving an intake questionnaire (via telephone or mail), having an interview, or engaging in a medical chart review. General information includes the following:

- Diagnosis
- Pertinent medical history
- Pharmacology

- Past and possible future surgeries
- Respiratory status
- Vascular status
- Skin integrity
- Sensation
- Skin management
- Vision
- Hearing

The place the individual uses the equipment is also important. Environmental considerations such as stairs, carpeting, width of doors, accessibility to specific areas in the home, office, or school may determine technologists' recommendations.

Information pertaining to cognition, behavior, or perception may assist technologists in determining an individual's safety in using a powered mobility base, ability to operate a one-armed drive wheelchair, or tolerance of tactile input from the recommended equipment. Orthotic or prosthetic devices that an individual wears when using the seating system influences the technologist's equipment choices.

The technologist should document the individual's ability to participate in activities of daily living (ADL) such as dressing, eating, and going to the bathroom, especially from the chair. Seating equipment that the technologist recommends must not impair a person's functional skills. Ambulation capabilities and transfers of the individual might affect the technologist's choice in seat height or mobility base. The practitioner should record communication status and whether the individual uses any equipment. Answers to the following questions provide the practitioner and supplier with information that helps them determine the required type of wheelchair and seating system:

- In what way will the equipment be transported?
- Where will the equipment be stored?
- Will the person be driving while sitting in the mobility base?

## Current Equipment

The technologist must assess the equipment that the individual currently uses including years of use, manufacturer, model, size, condition, and the reason it does not meet the user's needs. The technologist should thoroughly explain to the third-party payer the reason the user needs equipment modification or replacement. To provide invaluable information to justify third-party intervention, the technologist should include a description and photos of the individual sitting in the current seating system and wheelchair.

## Mat Evaluation

The technologist should always assess individuals when they are outside of the current seating system and wheelchair to obtain accurate information about the body in terms of range, strength, postural control, and purposeful movement. A tablemat works best, although in some facilities and homes, this is not an option and individuals should use the floor and a chair or a bench.

A supine mat evaluation allows the ATP to determine the flexibility of the individuals' trunk, pelvis, and lower extremities. To determine flexibility, the technologist must assess posterior pelvic tilt, anterior pelvic tilt, pelvic rotation, and pelvic obliquity, along with the influence of the hamstrings. The ATP must note whether the pelvis and femur are moving independently or as a unit because of tight hamstrings. This measurement assists technologists in determining the seat-to-back angle and the thigh-to-calf angle (Figure 13-1).[11-12] These angles help technologists determine placement of the seat, back, and lower extremity positioning pieces.

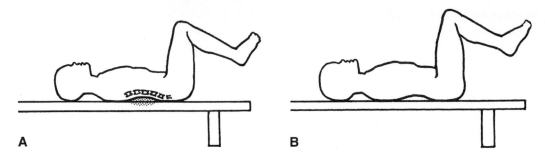

**Fig. 13-1** Seat-to-back angle. (From Bergen AF: Assessment for the seated environment, pp 37-44. In Bain BK, Leger D, editors: *Assistive technology: an interdisciplinary approach,* Edinburgh, 1997, Churchill Livingstone.)

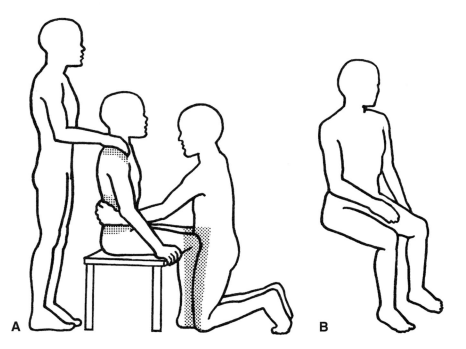

**Fig. 13-2** Preferred position. (From Bergen AF: Assessment for the seated environment, pp 37-44. In Bain BK, Leger D, editors: *Assistive technology: an interdisciplinary approach,* Edinburgh, 1997, Churchill Livingstone.)

When the individual is sitting on the edge of the mat table, the ATP and CRTS can determine how the added component of gravity affects the user's posture. They should ask the person to move into the preferred position.[1,4] Technologists determine whether the individual can sit hands free and use hands for support or is a dependent sitter. The practitioner may palpate the bony landmarks of the pelvis including the ischial tuberosities and anterior superior illiac spine in this position and determine manually whether neutral pelvic alignment is possible. Alignment of the spine may be more clearly identified in this position. They should record scoliosis, kyphosis, or excessive lordosis (Figure 13-2).[11,12,14-16]

ATPs should assess muscle tone, motor control, postural patterns, joint deformity, range of motion, and tolerance of position change in the seated position. They must determine whether the malalignments are flexible and the way external supports influence posture and/or function. Initially, the ATP does this manually by providing support using the hands or body as a contact surface. Placement of the ATP's hands helps other technologists determine placement of the external supports that the seating system needs.

## Simulation

A seating simulation and a trial of recommended equipment may assist technologists in the final equipment decisions. Using a planar simulator, the ATPs and CRTSs can assess the way the person sits with posterior support to the trunk and inferior support to the buttocks. They can try various angles and tilts and test flexibility of the person's body without the dynamic influence of the ATP's body. By adding components such as trunk supports or having the ability to mold along the person's body, the technologist gathers information about the way the person responds to specific intervention.

Once the user is positioned in the seating simulator, the technologist may direct the user to participate in an activity or demonstrate various tasks and functions (e.g., access-powered mobility, a switch-activated toy, or a computer game). The technologist may observe the person's skills of self-feeding, eating, and swallowing in the simulator. This allows the specialist to observe whether the person maintains the best seating position during an activity that might increase stress, excitement, or effort. The technologist should take photos of the individual in the simulator or use any trial products to demonstrate the way these products meet the user's needs.

The technologist may use pressure mapping, which indicates how a person distributes pressure, to determine an appropriate cushion or placement of positioning supports. This is done with the technologist using a sensory array pad connected to a computer. The sensory array can indicate the way the individual's body distributes pressure when sitting still and during activity. After the seating simulation, the ATP should check the user's skin for any signs of redness or pressure, which indicate the need for modification of the components or external support.

## Measurements

If technologists are using a simulator, they should take the individual's measurements during that time (Figure 13-3). If not, they should take the measurements when the ATP supports the individual on the mat. Several books and courses focusing on wheelchair seating intervention provide specific information on they way the ATP and CRTS should perform an assessment, including simulation and taking measurements.[11,17-22]

## Recommendation and Justification

ATPs and CRTSs should conclude the seating assessment by having a summary conference with the user and caregivers. They should provide user-driven versus product-driven or funding-driven recommendations. They should also present the user and the family with the information necessary to allow them to make educated choices in designing the seating system that best suits their environment and lifestyle.

Each component that technologists recommend must meet a specific user need, and thus have a reason for purchase or modification. The evaluation form in this chapter provides the user, family, primary therapists, ATP, CRTS, and third-party payer with a readable document detailing what the technologist assessed and recommended during the evaluation. The form compiles information about the individual, equipment that the user tried, the equipment that the technologist recommended, and the technologist's justification for the recommendations. Used primarily in a check-off and fill-in-the-blank format, the form includes information that the reader and third-party payer can easily find, detailing the process that led the technologist to the equipment recommendations. Photos that the technologist sent along with this document should provide the third-party payer and others with necessary data to determine whether the equipment warrants reimbursement. When the product is delivered, a "final-fit" photo provides the ATP and CRTS with information showing the resulting use of the equipment. Third-party payers appreciate knowing the way others have used the equipment they will be purchasing.

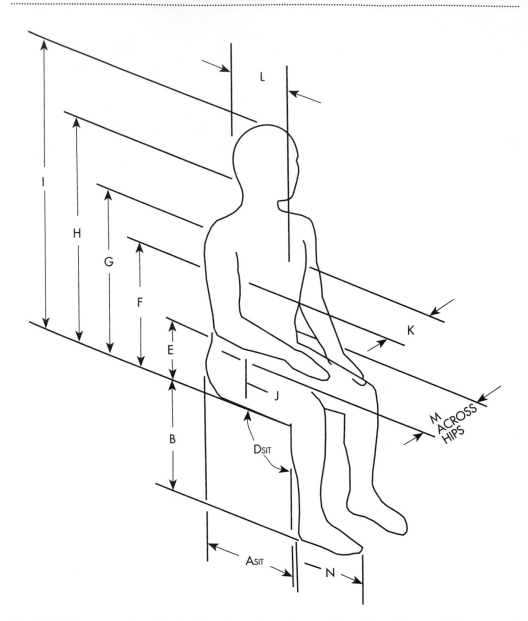

**Fig. 13-3** Measurements added to those taken in supine position. (From Bergen AF, Presperin J, Tallman T: *Positioning for function: wheelchairs and other assistive technologies,* Valhalla, NY, 1990, Valhalla Rehabilitation Publications.)

## Intervention and Technology

Seating intervention options have expanded considerably during the last decade. As with much of assistive technology, the range of product options varies a great deal from the therapist making a seating system out of low-cost triwall cardboard to custom-made seating systems costing thousands of dollars. These options may include commercial purchases, modification of commercial purchases, or custom-designed and fabricated pieces. Combinations of these options may be necessary to meet individual needs. For example, a person may purchase a commercially available cushion to distribute pressure and place it in a seating system that requires custom–fabricated upper–extremity supports. Seating products are introduced each year. Because a chapter written about these products would be antiquated by the time the book was published, we recommend that readers interested in finding out the latest products use the Internet and search for companies and sites that have dedicated pages on seating and positioning.

## Terminology

To ensure consistency when measuring and referring to pieces of equipment, RESNA's Special Interest Group on Seating and Wheeled Mobility developed a uniform terminology guide that professionals involved in the evaluation, recommendation, and delivery of seating intervention can use. The uniform terminology describes body movement, measurements, and seating equipment and its interface with the body. It allows users, therapists, rehabilitation technology suppliers, manufacturers, orthotists, physicians, and third-party payers to share a common language.[23] In 1998, a RESNA/ANSI standards committee was established with the goal of setting standards for wheelchair terminology and seating intervention.

## Seating Angles

Technologists can apply seating supports and components in various planes and also at various angles. The primary angles in seating are seat-to-back rest (hip angle), seat-to-calf rest (knee angle), calf rest-to-foot rest (ankle angle), and overall position in space (recline and/or tilt).

Recline increases the seat to-back rest angle up to 180 degrees. Tilt-in-space retains the seat-to-back rest angle (and other angles described previously) and tilts the seating system back as a unit, usually up to 45 degrees. Some systems combine these features. Occasionally, the technologist can place the entire seating system in a horizontal tilt. This may accommodate asymmetries in the frontal plane such as pelvic obliquities and lateral flexion or convexities of spine, including the neck. For example, if a person has a severe fixed lateral curvature of the spine that is supported by a contoured seating system so that the pelvis is as neutral as possible, the person may actively compensate with lateral flexion of the neck in the opposite direction. By horizontally tilting the system, the head is brought more into midline and is more upright for improved seeing, feeding, and possibly breathing. The person may also access available technology.[24]

## Supports in Reference to the Body

A seating intervention of a person in a wheelchair is generally described in terms of the support provided. Support means "to carry the weight of, especially from below...or to maintain in position so as to keep from falling, sinking, or slipping."[25] The supports in a seating intervention provide contact against the body, which can be used to provide a stable surface, distribute weight, maintain a desired position, reduce extraneous movement, block reflex patterns, or decrease tonal influence on the body.

One of the first things that a technologist should determine in planning intervention is what parts of the body need to be supported and the location the supports should be placed. The therapist's handling and use of the body to support the individual during the evaluation provide a great deal of input. Simulation and trial of these supports also can assist in the decision-making process.

Placement of supports in contact with the body can be posterior, lateral, medial, anterior, inferior or superior. Technologists use posterior supports most commonly and include the seat and back surface and pieces that they place behind the head, arms, and legs. The technologist considers this intervention first because they most often require it and it is the least obtrusive and restrictive. The individual sits on or in front of the supports allowing an observer to see the person first, rather than the equipment.

As the person requires greater support, the surface may come more lateral (to the outside of) to the body and extremities. In some cases such as positioning, the lower extremities the supports may be medial (to the center of/middle). For example, the technologist places the medial knee support between the person's knees to reduce hip adduction. Supports may be anterior (to the front) to the body such as pelvic belts, which technologists commonly use to stabilize the pelvis. Anterior supports may be in front of the chest, forehead, shoulders, or legs, and technologists consider the piece of equipment to be more obtrusive and restrictive as they block more movement because they may view the piece of equipment first rather than the person. Technologists might use anterior supports for short times during the day such as during transportation (for safety) or an activity (to keep the head upright for vision or stability) and they remove them when the user doesn't need them. Persons who require control to maintain the proper seated position may also use them full time.

Technologists place superior supports above the body part as noted with dorsum straps that hold the foot to the foot support. They place inferior supports below the body part such as a chin support that they may use in combination with a head support system.

When naming a piece of equipment, the technologist describes the placement and body part. For instance, a support that the technologist places against the outer side of the upper leg is called a *lateral thigh support*. A support behind the head is called a *posterior head support*. Many seating systems and components provide a combination of supports such as a back support that curves around the trunk. This can be called a *posterior, lateral back,* and *trunk support* (Table 13-1).[2,10,23,26-27]

## Support Systems

After determining the parts of the body that need support and the placement of the supports, the technologist should then determine how much contact the support surfaces should make with the body. The following four main categories describe various support systems, although products may overlap into more than one category[11,15,22,28]:

1. Planar
2. Contoured
3. Aggressively contoured
4. Molded (custom contoured)

Planar systems, sometimes referred to as *linear systems,* are flat surfaces. They are not designed to conform to the user's body and only do so if the foam and covering envelope the body. Flat trunk supports, a plywood and flat foam seat or back, footrests, and a tray are components that use a planar approach. Planar intervention works in situations in which a flat surface provides enough support or is adequate and when the individual wants minimal body contact. In cases in which the user desires more contact against the body, planar surfaces are insufficient. For example, this occurs when an individual sits with a nonflexible posterior pelvic tilt. A planar back only provides the individual with contact against the superior surface of the pelvis, resulting in excessive pressure that may cause skin problems and/or discomfort.

The term *contoured* describes a support that has generically shaped curves. These systems have curves to match the general body shape but are not directly formed to a particular person. The contoured pieces are available in different sizes such as small, medium, and large or fit particular wheelchair sizes in length and seat depth but they have a similarly contoured shape. The contoured approach offers more contact than the planar approach. The seat may provide an individual with a buttock relief area and leg troughs, which serve to center the pelvis and neutralize the placement of the legs and provide more contact and pressure distribution. A contoured back support may provide generic curves that support the lumbar and sacral areas of the spine. Bergen and others[2] described an aggressively contoured system as a generically contoured system with added components to provide more contact around the body. This system is not molded directly to a person's body but usually offers more control and postural support than a generic contoured system. These added pieces may include curved lateral pads, lumbar sacral supports, or lateral hip guides added to the generic support.

During the 1980s, the term *contour* connoted anything that had shape. Therefore the molded cushion product called *Contour-U* (PinDot Products/Invacare) was named based on the strategy of fitting around the individual to get a contoured mold. Since the early 1980s, however, commercially available, generically contoured seats, backs, and components have been developed. When the terms *planar* and *contoured* were used to describe all seating systems, people were confused.

# TABLE 13-1

*Terminology for Postural Supports*

| Body Part | Postural Support |
| --- | --- |
| *Buttocks/Posterior Thigh* | Seat platform/cushion support surface<br>Cushion<br>Posterior buttocks support |
| *Knee* | Anterior knee support/knee blocks |
| *Calf* | Posterior calf support<br>Medial calf support |
| *Shoulder/Humerus* | Posterior shoulder support/scapular protraction blocks<br>Posterior humeral support<br>Anterior shoulder support<br>Superior shoulder support |
| *Pelvis/Hip* | Lateral pelvic/hip support<br>Anterior pelvic support/pelvic stabilizer |
| *Foot* | Inferior foot support<br>Foot plate<br>Foot bucket<br>Foot channels<br>Dorsum foot straps<br>Heel support/guides<br>Ankle straps<br>Toe straps<br>Foot/ankle huggers |
| *Upper Extremity* | Arm support/armrest<br>Arm trough<br>Upper extremity support system (tray) |
| *Thighs* | Medial thigh support<br>Lateral thigh support<br>Superior thigh support |
| *Trunk* | Back support<br>Posterior trunk support<br>Lumbar support<br>Sacral support<br>Lumbar-sacro support<br>Thoroco-lumbar-sacral support<br>Lateral trunk support<br>Anterior trunk support |
| *Head/Neck* | Posterior neck support<br>Posterior head support<br>Posterior/lateral head support<br>Anterior head support<br>Anterior neck support<br>Circumferential head support<br>Inferior chin support |

Toward the end of the 1980s, the term *molded* became common and was used to define supports shaped directly to the person's body. A molded or custom-contoured support surface provides a specific match to an individual's body and provides the most surface area contact. Technologists can mold seats, backs, headrests, armrests, and foot supports depending on the individual's needs. Individuals can use molded systems to "accommodate deformity, promote trunk elongation, distribute pressure more evenly, or can provide specific contact support where desired" (Figures 13-4 and 13-5).[10,17]

Technology has advanced considerably in this area as users, ATPs, RTSs, manufacturers, therapists, medical personnel, and third-party payers become more aware of the benefits of molded surface supports. Several methods are available for technologists to obtain the correct custom shape of an individual's body or extremity and then transfer that information to a finished product. These include technologists hand cutting foam

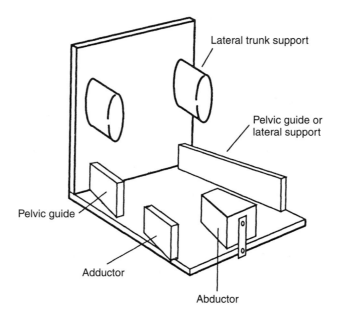

**Fig. 13-4** Planar system. (From Church G, Glennon S: *The handbook of assistive technology,* San Diego, 1992, Singular Publishing Group.)

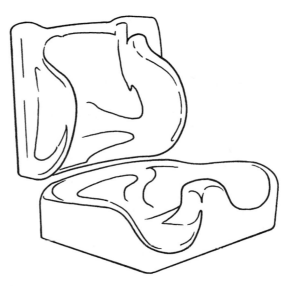

**Fig. 13-5** Custom-molded cushion. (From Bergen AF, Presperin J, Tallman T: *Positioning for function: wheelchairs and other assistive technologies,* Valhalla, NY, 1990, Valhalla Rehabilitation Publications.)

to conform to a person's body, using a chemical combination to fabricate foam that expands around the person (foam-in-place/direct molding), or taking a plaster impression of the person's body or extremity and fabricating the product using a foam-in-the-box method.

Other technologists employ an orthotic approach, using a vacuum consolidation method, simulating using potentiometers that manually or electrically determine the contours of the body, or molding around the person using interlinking materials that they can loosen and tighten to provide and maintain a shape (shapeable matrices). The choice of intervention depends on several factors including time, cost of the equipment used to make and transfer a mold, cost of the final product, skill of the fabricator, skill of the therapist, and product availability. In the orthotic approach, which a certified orthotist usually performs, they use plastics in combination with other materials. Technologists may use this method when the individual wants a combination orthosis and seating system.[9,19,26,28-31]

## Components and Hardware

*Components* refer to the linear or contoured supports that are separate from the seat or back surface. These are usually commercially available, and if necessary the individual can modify them or have them custom-made. They include lateral trunk supports, head rests, lower extremity supports, pelvic belts, anterior chest or shoulder supports, and upper extremity supports. Every component is recommended to provide a specific purpose or goal. When considering the intervention, the user must consider whether the component provides a therapeutic goal such as support, correction, or facilitation/inhibition; accommodation for unchangeable condition, protection/safety; comfort, or function.[15,32] One component may meet many goals. For instance, a lateral trunk support may support the individual decreasing excessive leaning to the left. It may accommodate the individual's fixed convexity while protecting the skin from damage by preventing the rib cage from touching the pelvis and "opening up" the skin folds. The same trunk support may free the person's hands to perform a functional and meaningful task.

*Hardware* refers to the pieces that interface the seating system to the wheelchair or attach specific components to the seating system. Hardware can be fixed or adjustable, removable or nonremovable. It can allow tilt, recline, growth, or other changes. The hardware needs to be compatible with the frame of the wheelchair and the pieces that require attachment.

## Cushions

Technologists should consider cushion intervention separately. Parameters for the cushions can be to relieve pressure, distribute pressure, contain tissue, encourage postural control, increase function, and provide comfort. The cushion materials may disperse tissue, contain tissue, accommodate, or provide support.[27,33]

Sprigle[34] classified cushions by their material and property values. He categorized the materials that cushions are made of into five classifications: foam, viscoelastic foam, solid gel, viscous fluid, and air. Technologists can use these materials in any support system and/or component. Foam (i.e., polyurethane, latex) is the most common material used in cushions. It compresses under weight and is generally light. Light and moisture can damage it and therefore must be protected. Also, foam has good long and short resilience, good dampening, good envelopment, high shear, and poor thermal characteristics. Foam can be planar, contoured, or molded. Each characteristic affects each property.

Solid gel cushions are highly viscous (less movement of molecules). They do not compress under weight and have low shear, poor envelopment, and good thermal characteristics. Sprigle[34] described a viscous fluid cushion as one that has replaced the water cushion. The material in a gel cushion is a creamy fluid that displaces when a person sits on it. Air cushions vary in their appearance, envelopment, and characteristics, depending on the container holding the air and the way users adjust and maintain them. Having an understanding of them and their differences in relation to the material helps them technologists select the most appropriate cushion for a specific individual's needs. The properties of the material include density, stiffness, resilience, damping, and envelopment.[34]

Density is used to describe the weight of a cushion compared with its volume. The density is designated in pounds per cubic foot (between 1.5 and 3 lb per foot). In most instances, a foam cushion that has a greater density also has greater durability and takes longer to fatigue.[28,34]

Stiffness refers to a cushion's hardness and is measured by how far a person sinks into the foam. An indentation load test on the foam measures the force required to indent the foam by one fourth of its thickness. Indentation measures usually range from 30 to 70 lb. Increased pressure may cause foams to be too stiff or too soft.[34] If the cushion is too stiff, the material does not have enough "give" against the person's body. If it gives too much, the foam "bottoms-out," causing the individual to have contact with

## TABLE 13-2

*Cushion Materials Properties Comparison Chart*

| Material | Foam | Viscoelastic Foam | Solid Gel | Viscous Fluid | Air |
|---|---|---|---|---|---|
| Trade example | Polyurethane Latex | Pudgy Sunmate T-Foam | Action | Jay Floam Flo-Fit Avanti | Roho BBD |
| Density | Variable | Variable | Variable | Variable | N/a |
| Stiffness | Variable | Variable | Variable | Variable | N/a |
| Resilience | Good | Fair | Poor | Poor | Good |
| Damping | Good | Poor | Poor | Poor | Good |
| Envelopment | Good | Good | Poor | Variable Depends on container | Variable Depends on design |
| Shear | High | High | Low/ medium | Low | Variable Depends on design |
| Thermal | Poor | Good | Good | Good | Variable Depends on design |
| Other factors | Deteriorates over time Lightweight Damaged by light/moisture | Pudgy can freeze Lightweight Damaged by light/moisture Some are temperature sensitive | Heavy | Heavy Can freeze (except Floam) Can puncture Can change over time Floam is plastic based Others are petroleum based | Pressure varies with altitude Can puncture Lightweight Inflation must be monitored |

**Definitions**

*Density, weight of cushion by volume measured in lb/cubic foot. Seat cushion between 1.5 and 3 lb/ft; Stiffness, relative measurement of how deep a person will sink into the cushion. Indentation load deflection test: force to indent cushion 25%. Cushions typically range between 30 (soft) and 70 (firm) lb; Resilience, ability to recover shape when forces change and ability to maintain properties while in use; Damping, ability of a cushion to soften impacts. Envelopment, ability of the cushion to surround or contain the buttocks and pelvis. Shear, forces that occur when adjacent surfaces slide across one another. Thermal, how well the cushion transfers heat and cold. Adapted from Margolis S: Pressure mapping and alternative materials for wheelchair cushions, 1996, Atlanta, MedTrade (contributions from Stephen Sprigle, PhD). Lange, M, McDonald C: Assitive technology clinics, The Children's Hospital, 1056 E. 19th Avenue, B410, Denver 80218, 303-861-6250, MLange@TCHDEN.org.*

the cushion support surface (flat wood, plastic, or metal). In either case, the pressures against the skin are too great and cause the potential for ischemic problems or skin breakdown.

Resilience describes the "ability to recover shape in response to changing forces...or the ability to maintain force properties after loading."[34] The resilience factor also has a short-term and long-term component. For instance, a cushion has long-term resilience if it recovers its force properties overnight. It has short-term resilience if it continues to recover after the individual bounces in the chair or performs a task requiring movement shifts on the cushion. Sprigle[34] compared the ability of the cushion to dampen with a shock absorber, which is important when technologists consider a cushion for comfort or for response to tissues during movement. Technologists can test the cushion by observing what happens when they drop an object onto it. If the object sinks into the cushion, with the material flowing or compressing around it, dampening occurs. The ATP and RTS need to determine how much dampening they want to occur. Too much dampening means that the cushion may have poor resilience. Envelopment is the ability to contain the tissue. Users may want this to provide better surface area contact around the buttocks and bony prominences (Table 13-2).[34]

## Intervention Strategies

Various intervention strategies exist that technologist may not use "cookbook" style because seating is individual and based on many parameters (Table 13-3). Table 13-3 provides the ATP and CRTS with ideas that they can simulate and try. Often a specific intervention that they try in one area also leads to changes in another. For more information, technologists should refer to books dedicated to seating theory and intervention.[2,12]

The pelvis is the foundation of a seating support system. When individuals have a typical neuromuscular system without any orthopedic involvement, their sitting posture shows the pelvis in a level position with a slight anterior pelvic tilt. Their head should be above the hips, with the spine having its natural curves. The femurs should be in slight abduction with the knees flexed in a functional position and the feet in a neutral position. The specialist may have to accommodate individuals when seating them in a neutral position is not possible because of fixed deformities or the influence of tone on the body. For example, an asymmetric windswept posture of the lower extremities accommodates a fixed pelvic rotation while allowing forward trunk, shoulder, and head orientation. Compromises may occur between the best-looking position and the one that individuals can most tolerate or the one that allows for functional movement.

New materials and components are emerging constantly, requiring the seating specialist to diligently stay informed. However, the most crucial tasks for the specialist are to employ a user-centered approach, involve a team when possible, complete a thorough evaluation, identify the specific seating needs of the user, and recommend strategies to meet those needs using whatever materials and components are available and customizing as needed. Flexibility, creativity, and innovation are the characteristics of a competent seating specialist.

## Outcome and Social Validation

In his keynote address at the International Seating Symposium in 1995, Ferguson-Pell[35] made the following statement:

> Outcomes research is intended to establish in objective terms the effectiveness of a particular methodology (applied to an "intervention group") in achieving specified goals compared to standard methods (applied to an identical "control group") for a defined population of clients.

Ferguson-Pell[35] added that outcome measurements should specify quantitative parameters and an analysis of user satisfaction and use of the seating and mobility intervention.

*Text continued on p. 229*

## TABLE 13-3

*Seating Intervention*

| Problem | Possible Cause | Suggestions for Intervention | Goals |
|---|---|---|---|
| *Posterior Pelvic Tilt*<br>Top of the pelvis is tipped backward. | Low abdominal/trunk tone exists. | Provide support to posterior superior surface of the pelvis to block backward movement.<br>Use an anteriorly sloped seat.<br>Drop the footrests to allow hip extension.<br>Use a biangular back, PSIS pad. | Provide neutral alignment of the pelvis.<br>Support anatomic curvatures of the spine (i.e., prevent kyphosis).<br>Promote weight bearing on ischial tuberosities, reduce pressure risks.<br>Provide best alignment for biomechanical function (e.g., of trunk musculature).<br>Increase proximal stability for function. |
| | Tight hamstrings exist. | Open seat to back angle and/or decrease thigh to calf angle. | |
| | Depth of wheelchair seat cushion or platform is too long. | Provide appropriate seat depth to allow hip and knee flexion. | |
| | Limited range of motion, particularly limited hip flexion exists. | Accommodate fixed limitation in hip flexion by opening seat to back angle greater than 90 degrees.<br>Accommodate asymmetries with contoured or molded seating system. | |
| | Sliding forward on seat occurs. | Provide antithrust or aggressively contoured seat.<br>Stabilize pelvis using appropriately angled pelvic belt or anterior pelvic stabilizer (e.g., subASIS bar). | |
| | Extensor thrust exists. | Stabilize pelvis using appropriately angle pelvic positioning belt or rigid anterior pelvic restraint.<br>Use antithrust seat or aggressively contoured seat.<br>Change position in space if thrust is caused by tonic labyrinthine reflex.<br>Increase hip and knee flexion, hip abduction, and ankle dorsiflexion.<br>Use anterior knee blocks. | Conserve energy.<br>Reduce friction.<br>Maintain alignment with other components. |
| *Pelvic Elevation*<br>Pelvis moves upward off seating surface. | Extensor tone exists. | Use extensor thrust interventions.<br>Use a four-point seatbelt.<br>Remove leverage from under feet.<br>Use hinged footrests.<br>Use dynamic footplates.<br>Remove footplates. | Conserve energy.<br>Reduce shear.<br>Maintain alignment with other components.<br>Provide consistent positioning for access. |

*Courtesy Jessica Presperin Pedersen, OTR/L, MBA, ATP and Michelle L. Lange, OTR, ABDA, ATP.*

TABLE **13-3**

*Seating Intervention—cont'd*

| Problem | Possible Cause | Suggestions for Intervention | Goals |
|---|---|---|---|
| *Pelvic Rotation* One side of the pelvis is forward. | ROM limitation in the hip exists. Abduction exists. Adduction exists. Hip flexion exists. Windswept posture exists. | Align pelvis in neutral and accommodate asymmetric lower extremity posture. | Neutrally align pelvis. Support anatomic curvatures of the spine (i.e., prevent kyphosis). Promote weightbearing on ischial tuberosities, reduce pressure risks. Use best alignment for biomechanical function (e.g., of trunk musculature). |
| | Fixed limitations in spine, pelvis, and/or femoral mobility (i.e., rotational scoliosis) exist. Unequal thigh length exists. Hip dislocation exists. | Pelvis may need to assume asymmetric posture to keep head and shoulders in neutral position. Check measurement from the pelvis to the plane of the popliteal fossa with the pelvis in neutral position, if possible. Create an appropriate seat surface depth for each limb, if fixed. | Increase proximal stability for distal function. Prevent subsequent trunk rotation. Increase pressure distribution over posterior trunk. |
| | Asymmetric surface contract over posterior buttocks and trunk exists. Discomfort exists. | Create contour back surface to "fill-in," if fixed. Identify source and remediate or refer to physician. | |
| | Tone and/or reflex activity occurs. ATNR exists. | Use positioning such as lower extremity abduction with hip, knee flexion, and ankle dorsiflexion. Pull pelvic belt back on forward side of pelvis. Increase thickness of padding of pelvic belt on forward side. Use posterior block on retracted side. Use rigid pelvic positioner. Use anterior knee block on forward side. Use antithrust seat. Use aggressively contoured seat, if fixed. | |
| *Pelvic Obliquity* One side of the pelvis is higher. | Scoliosis exists. ATNR exists. Surgeries have occurred. Discomfort exists. | Change angle of pull of pelvic belt. Use different foam densities (denser under low side). | Use best alignment for biomechanical function (e.g., of trunk musculature). Level the pelvis. |

*Continued*

# TABLE 13-3
## Seating Intervention—cont'd

| Problem | Possible Cause | Suggestions for Intervention | Goals |
|---|---|---|---|
| *Pelvic Obliquity —cont'd* | | Use wedge under low side to correct, under high side to accommodate. | Equalize pressure under the pelvis. Prevent subsequent trunk lateral flexion. Reduce fixing to increase function. |
| *Lateral Trunk Flexion or Scoliosis* Scoliosis may be C curve, S curve, and/or rotational. | Increased tone on one side exists. Musculature imbalance exists, pelvic involvement may exist. Decreased trunk strength or decreased tone exists, causing asymmetric posture. Habitual posturing for functional activity or stability exists. Fixed scoliosis exists. | If flexible: Use generic contoured back Use lateral trunk supports (may need to be asymmetrically placed, one lower at the apex of lateral convexity). Use anterior trunk supports to correct any rotation (see forward trunk flexion interventions). If fixed: Refer to physician to explore medical or surgical procedures/x-rays. Use TLSO. Use aggressively contoured or molded back to allow for fixed curvature of spine and/or rib cage. Use horizontal tilt under seat to right head, if pressure distribution is good. | Neutrally align trunk over pelvis, if flexible. Minimize subsequent deformity in pelvic and lower extremity posture. Level head over trunk for increased vision/social interaction. Increased pressure distribution. |
| *Forward Trunk Flexion or Kyphosis* | Flexion at hips exists. Flexion at thoracic area exists. Flexion at shoulder girdle with gravitational pull downward exists. Problem may occur because of increased or floppy tone, abdominal weakness, poor trunk control, or weak back extensors. Increased tone (i.e., hamstrings) pulling pelvis back into posterior tilt exists. Posterior pelvic tilt exists. | If flexible: Use anterior trunk support. Use belly bands. Use H-straps/butterfly vests. Use Bobath style or backpack straps. Use shoulder retractors. Use tray support with custom wedge or build up supporting anterior trunk or chest. Use chest strap. Use TLSO. May be a rotational component; therefore use posterior trunk support. | Prevent spinal deformity and subsequent pelvic deformity. Neutrally align trunk over pelvis. If flexible, anatomically align. Increase head control. Maintain trunk extension. Maintain pressure distribution. Maintain good visual field. |

*Courtesy Jessica Presperin Pedersen, OTR/L, MBA, ATP and Michelle L. Lange, OTR, ABDA, ATP.*

TABLE **13-3**

*Seating Intervention—cont'd*

| Problem | Possible Cause | Suggestions for Intervention | Goals |
|---|---|---|---|
| *Forward Trunk Flexion or Kyphosis——cont'd* | Habitual seating in an attempt to increase stability occurs.<br>Fixed kyphosis exists. | Correct posterior pelvic tilt.<br>Increase trunk extension with biangular back, PSIS pad, etc.<br>If fixed:<br>Open seat to back angle to match pelvis angle.<br>Use contoured seat.<br>Use tilt seating system to allow upright head. | |
| *Lordosis* | Tight hip flexors or overcorrection of tight hip flexors exists.<br>Increased tone pulling pelvis forward into an anterior tilt exists.<br>Habitual posturing in an attempt to lean forward for functional activities exists.<br>"Fixing" pattern to extend trunk against gravity (e.g., in conjunction with shoulder retraction, etc.) exists. | If flexible:<br>Provide lower back support as needed.<br>Use biangular back.<br>May need to change seat to back angle.<br>Do not over correct limited hip flexion.<br>May require anterior trunk support (see forward trunk flexion strategies).<br>If fixed:<br>Use molded seating system. | Neutrally align trunk over pelvis.<br>Maintain pressure distribution.<br>Reduce subsequent shoulder retraction and fixing to allow function.<br>Reduce subsequent anterior pelvic tilt. |
| *Hip Flexion* | Decreased range of motion of hip flexors exists.<br>Fixing with hip flexors because of lack of hip extension or stability exists.<br>Poor positioning exists.<br>Poor range-of-motion management exists. | If flexible:<br>Use superior thigh pads or strap thighs or feet superiorly.<br>Use padded lap tray (underside).<br>if fixed:<br>Do not overcorrect and cause anterior pelvic tilt. | Prevent anterior pelvic tilt.<br>Prevent lordosis. |
| *Hip Extension* | Decreased range of motion of hip extensors exists.<br>Increased extensor tone exists.<br>Poor positioning exists.<br>Poor range-of-motion management exists. | If flexible:<br>Open seat to back angle.<br>If fixed:<br>Open seat to back angle.<br>Increase knee flexion if hamstrings are tight.<br>Use contoured seating system. | Prevent further loss of range leading to a more reclined and less functional position affecting vision, feeding, and respiratory system.<br>Avoid putting extensors on stretch. |
| *Hip Adduction* | Extensor tone exists.<br>Decreased range of motion of hip adductors exists. | Use medial knee blocks.<br>Use anterior knee blocks.<br>Use leg troughs.<br>Use contoured seat. | Maintain pressure distribution.<br>Anatomically align.<br>Prevent stimulation of stretch reflex or initiation of extensor tone patterns. |

*Continued*

## TABLE 13-3

*Seating Intervention—cont'd*

| Problem | Possible Cause | Suggestions for Intervention | Goals |
|---|---|---|---|
| *Hip Adduction —cont'd* | | | Prevent hip internal rotation. Ease ADLs. |
| *Hip Abduction* | Decreased range of motion of hip abductors exists. Initial low tone exists. Surgeries have occurred. | Use lateral knee blocks. Use lateral pelvic/thigh supports. Use leg troughs. Use contoured seat. | Anatomically alignment. Maintain pressure distribution. |
| *Knee Flexion* | Decreased range of motion of hamstrings exists. Flexor tone exists. Structural knee issues exist. | If flexible: Refer to physician to explore medical or surgical procedures. If fixed: Open seat to back angle. Use anteriorly sloped seat. Decrease thigh-to-calf angle to relieve hamstring pull (e.g., place footrests posterior to front edge of seat and bevel front edge of seat). | Decrease tension in the hamstrings and thus minimize pull into posterior pelvic tilt. Maintain comfort. Clear front castors of wheelchair. Ease transfers. |
| *Knee Extension* | Decreased range in quadriceps exists. Over lengthening of the hamstrings exists. Structural knee changes occur. Extensor tone exists. | If flexible: Refer to physician to explore medical or surgical procedures. Provide alternative positioning to stretch quadriceps. If fixed: Use elevating leg rests. Use custom foot support. | Alleviate pull on pelvis and lower leg. Accommodate in extended position, if fixed. |
| *Lower Extremity Extensor Tone* | Extensor tone exists. Total extensor patterns exist. Reflex activity (i.e., pressure under ball of foot) exists. Spasms occur. Using stable surface at feet to initiate pattern or movement occurs. | Minimize hip extension: See extensor thrust suggestions under Pelvic Posterior Tilt. Minimize knee extension: Use shoeholders with ankle straps. Use anterior lower leg blocks. Remove leverage from under feet: See Pelvic Elevation suggestions. | Prevent initiation of total extensor pattern. Prevent pelvic elevation. Increase endurance. Reduce shear. Reduce wear and tear on equipment. |
| *Lower Extremity Edema* | Feet are consistently lower than knees. | Provide alternative positioning out of the chair to elevate the legs. | Minimize potential for constriction, pressure, or edema. |

*Courtesy Jessica Presperin Pedersen, OTR/L, MBA, ATP and Michelle L. Lange, OTR, ABDA, ATP.*
*ADL, Activities of daily living.*

## TABLE 13-3

*Seating Intervention—cont'd*

| Problem | Possible Cause | Suggestions for Intervention | Goals |
|---|---|---|---|
| **Lower Extremity Edema—cont'd** Fluid retention and/or swelling occurs. | Constriction at knees occurs. Medical issues (i.e., blood pressure, decreased circulatory function) exist. | Open the thigh-to-calf angle if ROM is possible and hamstrings are not put on stretch; must evaluate pull on pelvis. Check that feet are supported. Raise footrests to alleviate pressure on distal thigh or check for pressure areas around proximal lower leg. | Maintain comfort. |
| **Ankle Limitations** | Tonal patterns exist. Lack of weight bearing exists. Surgery has occurred. Discomfort exists. | Use angle adjustable foot plates (sagittal and frontal planes). Use padded foot boxes. Use molded foot support. | Accommodate fixed deformities. Prevent pressure to foot. Protect feet from injury. Maintain comfort. |
| **Shoulder Retraction** Often occurs in conjunction with elbow flexion. | Increased tone in scapular adductors or retractors exists. Weakness of muscles in shoulder girdle with decreased ability to protract shoulder occurs. "Fixing" pattern to extend trunk against gravity, stabilize, or as a righting response exists. Anxiety, startled behavior exists. | Build up posterior back support with wedges or increased foam behind scapular area. Adjust tilt in space. Restrain forearms (trunk must be anteriorly supported). Provide stability elsewhere to break up fixing pattern. | Maintain neutral alignment for function. Reduce risk of injury (arms may get caught in doorways). Break up fixing patterns for function. Reduce neck hyperextension often seen in conjunction with scapular retraction. |
| **Elbow Extension** Often occurs in conjunction with shoulder horizontal abduction. | Muscle imbalance exists. Habitual pattern to laterally stabilize trunk exists. Habitual pattern to extend trunk exists. ATNR exists. Anxiety, startled behavior exists. Effort or stress exists. | Use pad attached to back cushion or tray to block upper extremity laterally and/or posteriorly. Restrain forearms. Use splinting or orthotics. | Neutrally align function. Reduce risk of injury (arms may get caught in doorways). Minimize orthopedic risks to elbow joint. Break up muscle tone patterns for function. |
| **Uncontrolled Movement of Upper Extremities/ Self-Abusive Behavior** | Flailing, uncontrolled movements occur. Increased tone because of effort exists. Athetosis occurs. Self-abuse occurs. Self-stimulation occurs. | Use block or strapping to decrease movement. Use forearm weights. Use dynamic strapping to allow some movement, decreasing extraneous movement. Use distal stabilizer for independent grasp. | Reduce risk of injury to user or others. Allow dependent tasks to proceed such as feeding. Provide stability for independent function. Maintain calm. |

*Continued*

## TABLE 13-3

*Seating Intervention—cont'd*

| Problem | Possible Cause | Suggestions for Intervention | Goals |
|---|---|---|---|
| *Uncontrolled Movement of Upper Extremities/ Self-Abusive Behavior —cont'd* | | Use custom tray, which allows for upper extremities to be placed under tray, movement and function, while promoting safety, stability, and decreasing self-abusive patterns. Use upper extremity orthotics (i.e., to prevent elbow flexion). | |
| *Subluxed Shoulders* Usually occurs in conjunction with upper extremity weakness. | Decreased shoulder or upper extremity strength exists. Decreased muscle control exists. Decreased tone exists. Increased tone exists. | Use UESS tray. Use arm trough. Use desk-style support. Use widened armrests. Use posterior or lateral elbow blocks. Use forearm restraints. Use dual shoulder straps crossing clavicle and acromian process. Use slings. | Prevent subsequent deformity. Maintain comfort. Prevent injury (i.e., arms may fall into wheels). Keep shoulder neutral (not elevated or depressed). |
| *Decreased or No Head Control* | Decreased neck strength exists. Hyperextension of neck in compensation for poor trunk control occurs. Forward tonal pull occurs. Visual impairment, particularly a vertical midline shift, exists. | Use neck rest. Use posterior head support. Assess the weight-bearing aspect of the headrest, noting that a neck rest with pressure at the occiput may actually elicit increased neck extension and may not provide adequate surface area support, particularly in tilt. Change pull of gravity against head by reclining or tilting seating system anterior solutions: Use forehead band or halo. Use chin support/orthosis. Use baseball cap/helmet attached to superior of posterior bar. Use collars. Refer to behavioral optometrist, if appropriate. | Maintain elongation of neck extensors. Maintain capital flexion (e.g., "chin tuck"). Promote visual attention to the environment, peers, etc. Increase function. Improve swallow, feeding, and breathing. Prevent subsequent deformity of neck and shoulder girdle. Prevent overstretching of neck extensors and shortening of neck flexors. |

*Courtesy Jessica Presperin Pedersen, OTR/L, MBA, ATP and Michelle L. Lange, OTR, ABDA, ATP. UESS, upper extremity support system.*

## TABLE 13-3

*Seating Intervention—cont'd*

| Problem | Possible Cause | Suggestions for Intervention | Goals |
|---|---|---|---|
| *Lateral Neck Flexion* | Decreased neck strength exists. Muscle imbalance, tone, and torticolus exist. ATNR exists. Scoliosis exists. Visual impairment, particularly a horizontal midline shift exists. | Use curved headrest with lateral support. Use three-piece headrest with temporal support. Use posterior support with three-point lateral control (either side of head and along jaw line that is deviated laterally). Use custom-molded headrest. Refer to behavioral optometrist, if appropriate. | Prevent subsequent deformity of neck and shoulder girdle. Right head for vision, feeding, and respiratory status. |

Galvin and Wilkerson[36] supported taking appropriate outcome measures noting that "anecdotal stories showing before and after photos are not accompanied by objective evidence of efficacy and cost-effectiveness." Increased justification of effective methodologies would be validated if efficacy and cost-effectiveness were incorporated into the outcome measures. Minkel[13-14] compared two research articles discussing postures of individuals with and without physical impairments with an expert's opinion depicting what a posture should look like. He found that the articles using empirical data demonstrated evidenced-based practice that experts could use to substantiate clinical intervention. On the other hand, expert opinions tended to be viewed as "weak." Scherer and Galvin[37] emphasized the users' roles in outlining specific outcome measures by having them prioritize their own outcomes using measurable changes in perceived quality of life, rather than absence of sickness or the ability to move a body part.

Hammel[38] said the following:

Assistive technology can be applied to address, remediate, or augment an impairment, to maintain or improve functional task performance related to disability (activities of daily living, work, school, play, mobility), and to eliminate or decrease handicaps when performing societal roles as worker, student, parent, or caregiver.

Hammel[38] cautioned against specialists focusing outcome measurements on one level of impact. She also stated that intervention may change over time depending on physical or functional changes of the individual. She suggested using a "portfolio" of measurements to assess the effect on physical and functional status and the cost benefit, user satisfaction, use and maintenance of equipment, and social and cultural environment.

The National Center for Medical Rehabilitation Research (NCMRR) has developed a client-centered model that evolved from the International Classifications of Impairment, Disability, and Handicap (ICIDH) classifications. These are continually evolving and as of 1999, the World Health Organization terminology includes the following[38]:

*Impairment:* Occurs at the organ and organ system level and refers to physiologic, anatomic, mental, or emotional loss.

*Activity limitation* (as opposed to disability): Refers to the inability of an individual to perform an activity in a manner or range considered normal. This would include rolling, sitting, ambulating, reaching, grasping, judging, coping, reading, writing, and performing basic ADLs (dressing, eating, going to the bathroom, hygiene) or instrumental ADLs (shopping, home management, meal preparation, money management, or transportation).

*Participation restriction:* The personal and environmental contextual factors that limit a person's ability to participate in a society or culture.

## Portfolio of Outcome Measures

A portfolio of outcome measurements as they relate to seating intervention can help specialists assess changes affecting an individual's impairment, functional limitation, disability, and societal limitations. When providers groups the outcome measures, using a portfolio unique to the individual and assistive technology they provided, the user and provider have quantitative and qualitative measures to determine the effectiveness of the intervention.

### Impairment

Seating intervention may affect the user at the impairment level. External support to the body may encourage neutral posturing. A cushion may increase surface area support and allow better distribution of pressure. Seating intervention may alleviate pain. It may also enhance physiologic changes such as cardiac output, vital capacity, and swallowing.

Specialists can measure changes in posture using a tape measure or goniometer (for range of motion). They may place lead rules along curvatures of the body and transfer them to paper for angulation measurement. Photographs and video records of the subject with and without the seating intervention may also provide feedback. Axelson and Chesney[39] demonstrated taking posterior spinal measurements for assessing the anterior/posterior curve by manually measuring the horizontal distance between a fixed vertical reference (a flat chair back or wall) and the subject's spine. They used a laser penlight attached to the fixed vertical surface to ensure accuracy. MacKenzie and Devino[40] developed a device to measure lumbar lordosis (the lordosimeter) that specialists can use continuously to evaluate spinal posture during static and active sitting. Specialists have also used MRI, x-ray, EMG, and videotape equipment.[12,28-29]

Specialists frequently measure pressure distribution using static and dynamic methods. Pressure mapping tools provide objective data demonstrating where pressure is greatest at specific times. In an effort to heal a wound, specialists can assess changes in skin condition by looking at photographs and documenting wound stages, time spent out of work, school, or the community, frequency of skin breakdown, and sites of wounds. They can evaluate status of pulmonary and respiratory function by determining forced expiratory volume, forced vital capacity, peak expiratory flow, and pulse oximetry.[12,16,28,29] Inspiration per sentence can also measure respiration.[41] Specialists can determine seating tolerance or pain relief by timing how long the user is seated during one period and how often repositioning needs to occur.

They can measure swallowing and digestion using videoflouroscopy and by documenting consistency and amount of food intake, weight, and number of coughs or gags per meal.[24,42-43] By counting the number of times a person makes a sound or by measuring the volume, they can assess vocalization. Speech pathologists can provide formalized testing to evaluate speech output and clarity.

### Activity Limitation

Seating intervention may have an effect on functional limitations. Specialists providing external support to the trunk may assist in the individual maintaining balance or freeing up the arms for reaching. This may lead to increased ability for the individual to perform fine motor skills such as grasp and release. Proper positioning at the pelvis and trunk may encourage better head control.

By measuring the maximum distance an individual can reach in the forward and lateral directions before losing balance, specialists can assess balance and trunk stability.[39] They can use a stopwatch to time how long the person can maintain a certain posture with varying supports. They can record measurements of how far the individual leans with and without a seating system and can measure reach in different planes for distance, timing, and accuracy. Several standardized tests exist for measuring hand function. Specialists can measure transfers by assessing level of independence, number of caregivers needed, and frequency per day.

Optimal seating intervention may effect a user's ability to complete ADLs and perform tasks related to school, work, or leisure. If functional limitations are decreased, an individual's willingness and capabilities to perform purposeful tasks may also increase.

Fife and others[44] at Sunnyhill Health Centre for Children in Vancouver developed a Clinical Measure of Postural Control for assessing the effects of adapted seating. They measure functional skills using the functional independence measure (FIM). However, Hammel, Galvin, and Wilkerson[36,38] cautioned against using the popular FIM as the only means for an outcome measurement as it gives a lower rating to individuals using assistive technology even if they are independent with the equipment. Smith[45] developed OT Fact, which incorporates the use of assistive technology in its outcome measures. Provan[46] developed a pilot tool with 20 functional subcategories based on the FIM called the *functional outcome measure (FOM)* for wheelchair seating and positioning.

Mobility has several parameters for measurement including speed, distance, incline/decline, indoor/outdoor, level of competency, and level of independence. Specialists can assess community access by determining a person's ability to open a door and measuring the distances traveled on various terrain. They may evaluate communication skills to determine whether the individual can more easily access a communication device, has better eye contact or use of body language, or can talk louder or formulate words better because of seating intervention. By documenting the frequency and type of injuries that the individual or caregiver incurs, specialists can measure safety and judgment using checklists or videotaping.[12,28-29]

## Participation Restriction and Societal Limitations

According to Steinman,[47] subjective information is "directed to values, perceptions, and cultural attitudes of the individual" and effects individuals personally. Research documentation that people specifically write concerning the affects of seating systems and quality of life are scarce. Hammell[48] stated that "quality of life is difficult to define and conceptualize." However, she stated consensus among individuals' perceived quality of life includes engagement in worthwhile productive activity, physical well-being, active leisure pursuits, learning and personal development, interpersonal relationships, community interaction, satisfaction with role functioning, psychologic well being and sense of self-worth, and satisfaction with sexual relationship.[48-49] J. Hammel[50] proposed a client-centered assessment to identify what quality of life means to each individual such as the Canadian Occupational Performance Measure (COPM). Reid and others[51] used the COPM to evaluate occupational performance in children with cerebral palsy using a rigid pelvic stabilizer.

Professionals use the sickness impact profile (SIP) to measure individuals' perceived effect of disability and societal limitations.[47,52] Specialists can implement a user satisfaction survey to determine whether the users met their goals and the way specialists provided services. Scherer and Galvin[37] developed a consumer-responsive outcomes measurement system called the *matching person and technology model (MPT)*, in which individuals prioritize their own outcomes. Specialists use a quality-of-life basis with the theory that function is a means to the achievement of a goal and quality of life.[37] Specialists can also adopt a qualitative approach using focus groups and user satisfaction to provide information based on respondents' views and issues.[50,53] A survey can determine whether individuals are still using the intervention and help the specialist explore reasons for abandonment if it is not. The Cantril Self-Anchoring Striving Scale provides a subjective scale without cultural-specific standards that assesses personal expression of asssistive technology outcomes. People using the equipment defines quality of life based on their own perceptions.[47]

## Assessment of Service Delivery Model

Specialists also need outcome measures to determine whether the model of service delivery is appropriate to the user. They need to assess the cost-effectiveness of the intervention. They can quantify the results compared with the cost of attendant care and the cost of implementation with the number of hours that professionals spend providing the service. Ferrario[54] attempted a cost-outcome analysis on the provision of wheelchairs. He incorporated a number of factors including equipment, services, manpower, and social costs. The analysis also tested the effectiveness and utility of the intervention. The tool used is called *CERTAIN* and incorporates the FIM. CERTAIN includes a data collection structure, processing model, reporting structure, and a database. Countries involved in the development of this study are Italy, Sweden, Norway, and the Netherlands.[54]

Carlson and Ramsey[29] stated the following:

> Much work needs to be done in defining the features and components of postural support systems that reduce impairment, improve function, and increase social access for individuals with severe physical impairments. The societal impact of the use of adaptive seating, as well as of assistive technology clinics and programs, has yet to be studied in detail.

## Conclusion

Specialists should properly assess goal determination and intervention choices by using a user-centered approach to ensure optimal use of the equipment. The user, provider, and payer can gather invaluable information justifying the need for intervention by reviewing societal factors along with objective and subjective data that incorporates the way seating intervention effects the person's physical, functional, and psychologic well being.

Joan Bergman,[55] a physical therapist who was involved in the development of evaluation and intervention techniques for wheelchair seating during the 1970s and 1980s, stated that "positioning in life is everything." She shared this view with users and colleagues throughout the world as she demonstrated that individuals who feel "right" in their position in life use their abilities to the fullest. Positioning intervention is often the precursor to any other assisitve technology intervention. The benefits of optimal positioning, as outlined in the beginning of this chapter, illustrate the way someone's position in life can change with appropriate intervention. The ultimate goal for specialists when they provide seating intervention, therefore, should be to focus on users who have a quest to achieve optimal function, independence, and satisfaction to secure their rightful "position in life."

## References

1. Bazata C, Jones CK: *Developing your seating sense,* New Orleans, Fall 1997, Presentation and Handout.
2. Bergen AF, Presperin J, Tallman T: *Positioning for function for function: wheelchairs and other assistive technologies,* Valhalla, NY, 1990, Valhalla Rehabilitation Publications.
3. Carlson JM, Payette M: *Seating and spine support for boys with Duchenne muscular dystrophy,* Memphis, 1985, Proceedings from RESNA Eighth Annual Conference.
4. Jones CK: *The 10 commandments of seating,* Chicago, 1995, PinDot Training Course.
5. Bock O: *Please be seated,* Minneapolis, 1987, Otto Bock Industries.
6. Presperin JJ: Seating and mobility evaluation during rehabilitation, *Rehab Management* 3 (4):53-57, April/May 1989.
7. Taylor SJ: A clinical framework for evaluation of wheelchair seating, *Occup Ther Prac* 4 (3): 51-58, 1993.
8. Taylor SJ, Monahan L, Abraham J: *A headband system for anterior head support in a seated position,* San Jose, 1987, Proceedings from RESNA Annual Conference.
9. Trefler E: *Seating and mobility for persons with physical disabilities,* Tuscon, 1993, Therapy Skill Builders.
10. Presperin JJ, Pedersen J: Seating and wheeled mobility for OTs. In Hammel J, editor: *Technology and occupational therapy: a link to function,* Bethesda, Md, 1996, American Occupational Therapy Association.

11. Bergen AF, Presperin J, Tallman T: *Positioning for function: wheelchairs and other assistive technologies,* Valhalla, NY, 1990, Valhalla Rehab Pub.

12. Zollars JA, *Special seating: an illustrated guide,* Minneapolis, 1996, Otto Bock Press.

13. Minkel J: *Introduction to evidenced-based practice in seating,* pp 29-30, Orlando, 1999, Fifteenth International Seating Symposium.

14. Minkel J: *Mat evaluation,* pp 39-41, Orlando, 1999, Fifteenth International Seating Symposium.

15. Bergen AF: Chris and his new power chair: a perfect match, *Team Rehab* 9 (5), 26-30, May 1998a.

16. Buck S: *Developing data for justification of assistive technology,* pp 89-90, Orlando, 1999, Fifteenth International Seating Symposium.

17. Presperin JJ, Pedersen J, Lange M: Wheeled mobility and seating: the process of procurement. In Hammel J, editor: *AOTA web based course,* Bethesda, Md, 1999.

18. Bergen AF: *Seating evaluation: demonstration,* pp 59-75, Orlando, 1999, Fifteenth International Seating Symposium.

19. Bergen AF: Just a simple chair and seating system, *Team Rehab* 9 (8), Aug 1998b.

20. Taylor SJ: Evaluating for wheelchair seating. In Angelo J, editor: *Assistive technologies for rehabilitation therapists,* Philadelphia, 1996, FA Davis.

21. Taylor SJ: A clinical framework for evaluation of wheelchair seating, *Occup Ther Practice* 4 (3):51-58, 1993.

22. Zollars JA: *Seating, positioning and mobility: a literature review,* 1991, San Francisco State University.

23. Medhat M, Hobson D: *Standardization of terminology and descriptive methods for specialized seating: a reference manual,* Washington DC, 1992, RESNA.

24. Hardwick K, Handley R: *The use of automated seating and mobility systems for management of dysphagia in individuals with multiple disabilities,* pp 23-24, Toronto, Sept 1993, The Canadian Seating and Mobility Conference.

25. Berube W et al, editors: *Webster's: new college dictionary,* vol II, Boston, 1995, Houghton Mifflin.

26. Presperin J: *Interfacing techniques for posture control,* Vancouver, Feb 1990, Sixth International Seating Symposium.

27. Habasevich J, Presperin J: *Seating and positioning,* Chicago, 1994, Beyond the Basics.

28. Cook A, Hussey S: *Assistive technologies: principles and practice,* St Louis, 1995, Mosby.

29. Carlson S, Ramsey C: Assistive technology. In Campbell S, editor: *Physical therapy for children,* pp 621-661, Philadelphia , 1994, WB Saunders.

30. Post KM: *Evaluation and intervention techniques in seating and mobility, technology review '90: perspectives on occupational therapy practice,* Rockville, Md, 1990, American Occupational Therapy Association.

31. Silverman M: *Commercial options for positioning the client,* Chicago, 1996, PinDot lecture.

32. Ward D: *Prescriptive seating for wheeled mobility,* Kansas City, Mo, 1994, HealthWealth International.

33. Garber S: Wheelchair cushions for persons with SCI: an update, *AJOT* 45 (7): 550-554, 1991.

34. Sprigle S: The match game, *Team Rehab Report* 3 (3):20-21, 1992.

35. Ferguson-Pell MW: *Jay medical lectureship seating and wheeled mobility research: the key to our future,* pp 27-31, Pittsburgh, 1995, Eleventh International Seating Symposium.

36. Galvin J, Wilkerson D: *Do we measure up? Using outcome measures in the quality assurance process: a discussion on the development of a quality assurance process in an assisitve technology program,* pp 123-130, Pittsburgh, 1995, Eleventh International Seating Symposium.

37. Scherer MJ, Galvin JC: Matching people with technology, *Rehab Management* 7 (2): 128-130, Feb/March 1994.

38. Hammel J: What's in an outcome? *Homecare Dealer/Supplier* 4 (5): 87-92, Sept/Oct 1996.

39. Axelson P, Chesney D: *Clinical and research methodologies for measuring functional changes in seating systems,* pp 81-84, Vancouver, 1996, Twelfth International Seating Symposium.

40. MacKenzie T, Devino B: A new device for continuous measurement of the lumbar spine. In Langton, editor: *A proceeding RESNA 95 recreability,* pp 285-287, Vancouver, 1995.

41. Padgitt J, Salm R: *The use of soft anterior pelvic supports to control excessive anterior pelvic tilt,* pp 169-171, Orlando, 1999, Fifteenth International Seating Symposium.

42. Bazata C: Positioning effects on oral motor skills, *Team Rehab* 22-23, Sept 1992; *Positioning for oral motor function,* pp 9-13, Vancouver, 1992, Eighth International Seating Symposium.

43. Chisholm J, Evans J: *The use of pulse oximetry as a positioning tool,* pp 87-90, Vancouver, 1996, Twelfth International Seating Symposium.

44. Fife S et al: Development of a clinical measure of postural control for assessment of adaptive seating in children with neuromotor disabilities, *Phys Ther* 71 (12):981-993, Dec 1991.

45. Smith R: *Outcomes in occupational therapy,* Chicago, 1995, Presentation at AOTA Annual Conference.

46. Provan M: *Measuring functional outcomes for wheelchair seating and positioning,* Shenandoah, Va, 1996, Project for Masters of Science in Occupational Therapy at Shenandoah University.

47. Stienman M: The spheres of self-fulfillment: a multidimensional approach to the assessment of assistive technology outcomes. In Gray D, Quatrano L, Lieberman M, editors: *Designing and using assistive technology* 1998, Baltimore, Brookes.

48. Hammell K: Spinal cord injury; Quality of life; Occupational therapy: is there a connection? *Br J Occup Ther* 58 (4):151-157, April 1995.

49. Abela MB, Dijiker M: Predicting life satisfaction among spinal cord injured patients one to three years post-injury, *JAPS* 17(2):118, 1994 (abstract).

50. Hammel J: *Report of qualitative data analysis of research study on the process of assessment and intervention of the provision of assistive technology,* Orlando, 1997, Annual AOTA Conference.

51. Reid D, Rigby P, Ryan S: *Evaluation of the rigid pelvic stabilizer on occupational performance of children with cerebral palsy,* pp 37-38, Orlando, 1999, Fifteenth International Seating Symposium.

52. Baum C: Achieving effectiveness with a client-centered approach: a person-environment interaction. In Gray D, Quatrano L, Lieberman M, editors: *Designing and using assistive technology,* Baltimore, 1998, Brookes.

53. Pentland W: *Disability over time: the impacts of aging and duration,* Pittsburgh, 1997, Thirteenth International Seating Symposium.

54. Ferrario M: *An attempt of cost-outcome analysis: the provision of wheelchairs,* Pittsburgh, 1997, Thirteenth International Seating Symposium.

55. Bergman J: *Positioning in life is everything,* Memphis, 1987, Third International Seating Symposium.

## Suggested Readings

Brown L: *Achieving client goals in a wheelchair seating clinic,* pp 63-66, Vancouver, 1996, Twelfth International Seating Symposium.

Chesney D, Axelson P: *Measuring functional changes: practical methodologies for use in clinics,* Pittsburgh, 1997, Thirteenth International Seating Symposium.

Curtis K, Kindlin C, Reich K, White D: Functional reach in wheelchair users: the effect of trunk and lower extremity stabilization, *Arch Phys Med Rehab* 76:368-372, 1995.

Engstrom B: *Ergonomics: wheelchairs and positioning, a book of principles based on experience form the field,* Stockholm, Sweden, 1993, Bromma Tryck AB.

Evans J: *Using oximetry to verify positioning strategies,* Pittsburgh, 1995, Eleventh International Seating Symposium.

Ferguson-Pell M, Bain D: *Pressure mapping in the community: detecting sitting behaviors that increase pressure sore risk,* Orlando, Fla, 1999, Fifteenth International Seating Symposium.

Fife S: *Further development of a clinical measure of postural control,* pp 37-40, Vancouver, Feb 1992, Eighth International Seating Symposium.

Fuhrer MJ: *Rehabilitation outcomes: analysis and measurement,* Baltimore, 1987, Paul H Brooks.

Galvin JC, Scherer MJ: *Evaluating, selecting, and using appropriate assistive technology,* Maryland, 1996, Aspen Publications.

Hall K: *Overview of FIM and FAM,* San Jose, Calif, 1995, Santa Clara Valley Medical Center.

Lange M: Low-tech positioning, *OT Practice* 3 (4):49-51, April 1998.

Lange M: Anterior trunk supports, *OT Practice* 3 (12):41-43 December 1998.

Lange M: Positioning the upper extremities, *OT Practice* 4(5):49-50, May 1999.

Miedaner J, Finuf L: Effects of adaptive positioning on psychological test scores for preschool children with cerebral palsy, *Pediatr Phys Ther* 5:177-182, 1992.

Perr A: Elements of seating and wheeled mobility intervention, *OT Practice* 3, Oct 1998.

RESNA/ANSI: *Wheelchair standards—work in progress,* Pittsburgh, 2001, RERC.

Rogers JC, Holm MB: Accepting the challenge of outcome research: examining the effectiveness of occupational therapy practice, *J Occup Ther* 48(10): 871-876, 1997.

Roxborough L: Review of the efficacy and effectiveness of adaptive seating for children with cerebral palsy, *Assistive Technol* 7 (1):17-26, 1995.

Sents B, Marks H: Changes in preschool children's IQ scores as a function of position, *Am J Occup Ther* 43:685-687, 1989.

Scherer MJ: The impact of assistive technology on the lives of people with disabilities. In Gray D, Quatrano L, Lieberman M, editors: *Designing and using assistive technology,* Baltimore, 1998, Brookes.

Sparacio, J: The effects of seating on upper extremity function, *Technology Special Interest Section Quarterly* (9):1-2, June 1999.

Sommerfreund J, Polgar J: *The effects of special seating intervention on the motor function of the high-risk infant,* pp 63-66, Pittsburgh, 1995, Eleventh International Seating Symposium.

Stiens S: Personhood, disablement, and mobility technology. In Gray D, Quatrano L, Lieberman M, editors: *Designing and using assistive technology,* Baltimore, 1998, Brookes.

Wright C: *Seating for hand function in proceedings,* pp 53-63, Vancouver, Feb 1992, Eighth International Seating Symposium.

## Related Web Sites

Abledata Corp: http://www.abledata.com

Adaptive Switch Laboratories: http://www.asl-inc.com

Everest and Jennings Wheelchairs: http://www.coast-resources.com/everestandjennings

Dynamic Controls, Ltd.: http://www.dynamicmobility.co.nz

Invacare Corporation: http://www.invacare.com

Levo manufacturer: http://www.levo.ch

National Pressure Ulcer Advisory Panel: http://www.npuap.org

Bloorview MacMillan Centre (Interfacing Information): http://www.oise.utotoronto.ca/~ortcklt

Permobile manufacturer: http://www.permobile.se

Prentke Romich Company: http://www.prentrom.com

Website focusing on seating and positioning owned by Micheal Silverman, CO, ATP, and Adrienne Bergen, PT, ATP/CRTS, forerunners in the seating and positioning profession: http://www.Rehabcentral.com

RERon Wheeled Mobility: http://www.rerc.upmc,edu

ANSI/RESNA Wheelchair standards: http://www.rerc.upmc.edu.STDsDev/stdsindex.html

Dynavox Systems: http://www.sentient.sys.com

Sunrise Medical Corporation: http://www.sunrisemedical.com

Students in the OT program at the University of Illinois. Provides a case study approach to learning AT. An excellent case study follows concerning seating and mobility. The site is linked with other web sites including manufacturer websites: http://www.uic.edu/~nmintr2/index2html

Information on w/c outcomes: http://www.utoronto.ca/atrc/reference/atoutcomes

Designed by people who use wheelchairs: http://www.wheelchairjunkie.com

Virtual community designed by M.E. Bunning, which provides many links to other sites: http://www.wheelchairnet.org

## Courses and Conferences

International Seating Symposium
Description: Held in even years in Vancouver, odd years in Orlando.
Contact: University of British Columbia
Continuing Education in Health Sciences
Room 105, 2194 Health Sciences Mall
Vancouver, BCCANADA 604-822-2626
or
University of Pittsburgh
School of Health and Rehabilitation Sciences/Technology
5th floor, Forbes Tower
Pittsburgh, PA 15260

RESNA Annual Conference
Description: Held every year in June in rotating cities.
Courses sponsored by SIG 09-Seating and Mobility.
Contact: RESNA
Website: http://www.resna.org

Abilities Expo International
Description: Consumer-centered equipment show held each year in California, Illinois, New Jersey, and Virginia.
Contact: Advastar Communications Inc.
440 Wheelers Farm Rd.
Milford, CT 06460-1847
Telephone: (800) 385-3085
Website: http://www.abilitiesexpo.com

Canadian Seating and Mobility Conference
Description: Held in October in Toronto.
Contact: PO Box 62029
Victoria Terrace PO
North York, Ontario M4A 2WI
Telephone: (416) 759-9046

Medtrade/NHHCE
(National Home Health Care Expo)
Description: Held every November. The location varies from Atlanta, New Orleans, and Orlando. It's the largest home-care trade show in the United States.
Contact: Medtrade Registration
BillComm Expo and Conference Group
Dulles International Airport
PO Box 17413
Washington DC 20041
Telephone: (877) 835-7273
Website: http://www.medtrade.com

NRRTS Continuing Education Programs
Contact: NRRTS
National Registry of Rehabilitation
Technology Suppliers
3223 South Loop 289
Lubbock, TX 79423
Telephone: (806) 797-7299

## Courses Sponsored By Seating and Wheelchair Manufacturers

Contact manufacturers or local suppliers for course information.

# CHAPTER 14

# Upper Limb Orthotics

*Julie Edwards*
*Laura B. Fenwick*

## Application and Goal

As the eyes are an invitation to the soul, the hand is an extension of the mind. Orthoses can never duplicate the infinite functions that the hands and arms perform. In fact, each upper limb orthosis usually serves one simple function. Outcomes are most successful when a well-organized team clearly defines the plans. Team members for upper limb orthotic management include the person who uses the orthosis, the prescribing physician, the occupational therapist, and the orthotist. These team members work together to evaluate, treat, and monitor the progress of treatment during and after a person's rehabilitation.

The primary role orthoses play is to improve function. Functional activities of individuals may improve while they wear an orthosis or because an orthosis prevented deformity. However, no orthosis works well without some user training.

In this section, we delineate functions and indications for upper limb orthotic management and categorize and describe the types of orthoses. Case studies illustrate orthotic recommendations for the specific upper limb disabilities of three individuals. Finally, we identify appropriate resources and references for further study. The National Office of Orthotics and Prosthetics is an excellent resource for information on basic and continuing education programs in this field.

## Function and Ability

Upper limb disability may occur at the shoulder, elbow, wrist, hand, fingers, or any combination of these. Orthoses generally function on the principle of applied forces, specifically three-point pressure systems. Three-point force systems enable orthoses to hold an injured segment, correct a deformity, or assist a weakened muscle (Figure 14-1). Upper limb orthoses use force systems to achieve some specific goals. The following are some of these goals:

- Maintain alignment
- Assist prehension
- Prevent contractures or overstretching
- Protect and stabilize the joints
- Attach functional components
- Increase range of motion
- Correct deformity
- Reduce pain
- Reduce tone
- Immobilize to promote healing

Many orthopedic and neurologic disabilities indicate the use of upper limb orthoses. The same orthosis may function differently for different pathologies.[1]

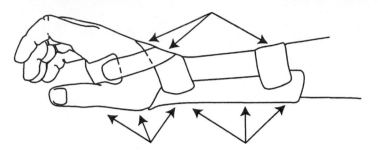

**Fig. 14-1** The orthosis uses three points of pressures to prevent flexion. (From Pedretti LW, Early MB: *Occupational therapy: practice skills for physical dysfunction,* ed 5, St Louis, 2001, Mosby.)

## Fractures

Orthoses function to realign and immobilize fractures. Immobilization can reduce the pain associated with traumatic fractures. Two key principles exist in fracture orthotic management: (1) to create circumferential pressure across the fracture to maintain alignment through total contact and (2) to allow micromotion to stimulate bleeding, which promotes healing.[2]

## Tendon Injuries

Conservative treatment of tendon injuries primarily involves orthotic management. Surgical repair of tendons frequently requires postoperative orthotic management. Orthoses stop motions that overstretch the injured tendon while allowing other motions. This motion control reduces the occurrence of contractures.

## Peripheral Neuropathies

Injuries to the peripheral nerves require orthoses with specific components to function for absent muscle action. Complete recovery is common after traumatic peripheral nerve injury. Maintenance of correct alignment during recovery is a primary goal of treatment. Neuropathy resulting from muscle disease is often progressive. For these neuropathies, improving function is the primary goal.

## Upper Motor Neuron Injury

The primary difficulty in orthotic management of upper motor neuron pathologies is the associated spasticity. Although weakness and deformity require assistance and correction, the upper motor neuron patient's increased tone may prevent orthoses from ideal function and also cause areas of high pressure on the skin. Certain orthoses are specifically designed for spastic limbs and function to facilitate more normal muscle tone or inhibit spasticity.

## Congenital Anomalies

Congenital anomalies often require inventive solutions. In pediatric management of congenital anomalies the technologist should maximize the child's social, cognitive, and emotional development while using minimal orthotic intervention to improve function and reduce deformity.

## Burns

Thermal injury management varies based on the area of involvement and severity (thickness) of the injury. Key principles of management are the prevention of keloid

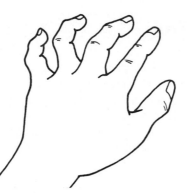

**Fig. 14-2** A claw hand deformity resulting from ulnar nerve paralysis. (From Coppard BM, Lohman H: *Introduction to splinting: a clinical-reasoning and problem solving approach,* ed 2, St Louis, 2001, Mosby.)

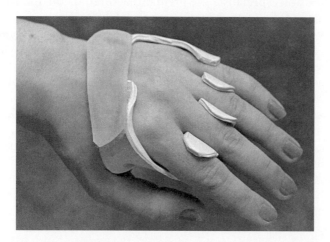
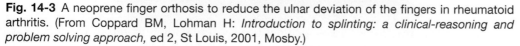

**Fig. 14-3** A neoprene finger orthosis to reduce the ulnar deviation of the fingers in rheumatoid arthritis. (From Coppard BM, Lohman H: *Introduction to splinting: a clinical-reasoning and problem solving approach,* ed 2, St Louis, 2001, Mosby.)

scars and contractures. Garments and orthoses that provide total contact and offer compression help reduce keloid scarring. Neutral (safe) alignment of the upper limb joints reduces contractures and enables increased function.

## Spinal Cord Injury

Upper limb orthotic recommendations for the functional levels in quadriplegia are based on muscular deficit. Specialists frequently use static orthoses to prevent contractures. They use dynamic orthoses to increase function.[3]

## Arthritis

Rheumatoid arthritis works slowly to deform the hand (Figure 14-2). Specialists recommend orthoses for people with rheumatoid arthritis to correct deformities as they are worn (Figure 14-3). Orthoses decreases deformity pain and increases the mechanical advantage of the involved hand. Although orthoses may not reduce the progression of rheumatoid deformities, good evidence exists that the pain reduction and increased strength justifies their use.[4]

## Considerations, Options, and Technology

Specialists must consider many factors before fitting a person with an upper limb orthosis. Most importantly the physician and orthotist must perform a thorough evaluation of the user. The evaluation should include analysis of the person's anatomy including the deformity. They should perform range of motion and manual muscle testing to note any deficits. The treatment team (the person receiving treatment, the physician, the orthotist, and the therapist) should agree on specific orthotic goals before determining the right orthotic recommendation. To increase the user's compliance, they should include the patient in choosing the proper orthosis. Patient involvement improves acceptance of the orthosis. The patient can choose the type of material (metal or plastic), color of plastic, and even the color of straps that the specialists use to fabricate the orthosis.

Specialists often fit upper limb orthoses for temporary use and once they achieve the treatment goals, they discard or alter the orthosis to a less-complex design to achieve a new goal. They often use orthoses made from low-temperature plastics when the user is going to wear the device for a short time. The occupational therapist typically fabricates orthoses. When possible, specialists use premanufactured or off-the-shelf orthoses and modify them to the individual to decrease cost and delivery time.

Specialists may have a difficult time fitting upper limb orthoses because of the anatomy and multiple functions of the upper extremities. The hand has a small amount of soft tissue, and the area that the orthosis encompasses is small; therefore pressures on the skin can cause redness. The specialist should advise the person about proper wearing times and skin evaluation. The person should wear orthoses for short periods at first such as 30 minutes and gradually lengthen the time to increase skin tolerance. If any red marks from the orthosis are still visible 15 to 20 minutes after removal, the user needs to get it adjusted. Because of the diverse motions and functions of the fingers, hands, and arms, specialists usually set multiple orthotic goals. Therefore complexity requires an experienced orthotist to design and fabricate the orthosis. People with low "gadget tolerance" may have difficulty accepting orthoses and thus the specialist should include users in the decision-making process.

### Nomenclature

Proper nomenclature for orthoses includes generic and eponymic terms. Users can easily understand the fit and function of any orthosis when specialists use generic terminology. However, popular manufactured orthoses often come with eponyms that are difficult to avoid.

The most specific, generic terminology are ones that the American Academy of Orthopedic Surgeons (AAOS) accepts. In 1970, a task force of the AAOS created technical analysis forms for the spine, upper, and lower limbs. These forms enabled an orthotist to evaluate and recommend orthoses by following specific evaluation pathways. A system that the task force devised generalized orthotic terminology. It considered two characteristics of orthoses: (1) the area of the body that the orthosis encompasses and (2) the mechanical motion control the orthosis provides. The system was first published in the *Atlas of Orthotics* in 1975. The system can easily name orthoses because they all encompass part of the body and all control motion.

The generic names for upper limb orthoses include the following:

| | |
|---|---|
| SO | Shoulder orthoses |
| SEO | Shoulder and elbow orthoses |
| SEWHO | Shoulder elbow wrist hand orthoses |
| EO | Elbow orthoses |
| WHO | Wrist and hand orthoses |
| WHFO | Wrist, hand, and finger(s) orthoses |
| HO | Hand orthoses |
| FO | Finger(s) orthoses |

The technical analysis form allows the practitioner to define the plane of motion that the orthosis controls and the type of control provided in that plane. Upper limb orthoses are either static or dynamic in one plane. Thus the plane of motion control does not usually describe these orthoses. Of course, the intact upper limb exhibits motion in one to three planes at various joints, and specialists must remember normal motion when the limb is disabled. The goal is to allow as much motion as possible and limit as little motion as necessary for treatment.

The following is a list of types of motion control as originally printed in the *Atlas of Orthotics:*

Free: free motion

Assist: application of an external force for the purpose of increasing the range, velocity, or force of a motion

Resist: application of an external force for the purpose of decreasing the velocity or force of a motion

Stop: inclusion of a static unit to deter an undesired motion in one direction

Hold: elimination of all motion in a prescribed plane

Variable: a unit that can be adjusted without making a structural change

For example, an upper limb orthosis that a specialist uses to replace wrist extensor paralysis is named *WHO, wrist extension assist.* As the orthoses are described, the specialist should consider the plane of motion control and the type of control the orthosis provides.

## Orthotic Options

Although specialists use many different ways to categorize upper limb orthoses, we use the two terms *static* or *dynamic.* Static orthoses hold a segment or segments in a fixed position. Dynamic orthoses allow motion of a joint. Motion that an orthosis allows can be free in a particular plane or designed to stop or limit motion in one direction. Specialists can also fabricate orthoses to assist or resist motion of a joint using springs, rubber bands, and dynamic joints.

### Static

#### Shoulder Orthoses and Shoulder Elbow Orthoses

Specialists commonly refer to static shoulder orthoses as *arm slings* or *hemislings.* Most arm slings have figure-of-eight or figure-of-nine straps and humeral cuffs. Specialists should technically call slings with forearm support straps *shoulder elbow orthoses* (*SEO*) because they hold the elbow in flexion (Figure 14-4). Slings attempt to reduce a

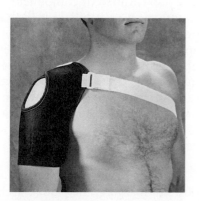

**Fig. 14-4** A SEO sling for positioning in brachial plexus injuries (flail arm) or for painful conditions of the shoulder. (From Coppard BM, Lohman H: *Introduction to splinting: a clinical-reasoning and problem solving approach,* ed 2, St Louis, 2001, Mosby.)

subluxed shoulder, or people wear them to inhibit painful motion at the glenohumeral joint. People also commonly use the SEO for shoulder pain or for flail arm positioning. Shoulder orthoses and shoulder elbow orthoses are premanufactured items, but a person with severe deformity needs a custom design.

### Shoulder Elbow Wrist Hand Orthoses

Specialists typically use the shoulder elbow wrist hand orthoses (SEWHO) to position the shoulder in abduction. They fit this orthosis for a soft-tissue injury or to prevent contracture as in axillary burns. The SEWHO is also known as a *shoulder abduction orthosis* or *airplane splint*. The orthosis consists of troughs or cuffs that supports the volar surface of the hand, forearm, and humerus (Figure 14-5). Weight from the arm is transferred to lateral pads along the chest and iliac crest. The physician suspends and stabilizes the orthosis using straps. The amount of abduction and elbow flexion is adjustable via joints, which the physician should determine for each specific pathology. The SEWHO is an available premanufactured device and has many different design options.[5] For instance, glenohumeral joint selection can be as simple as static or adjustable in all three planes. In difficult cases, a person may require a custom-molded orthosis for example when burns need total contact to prevent keloid scarring.[6]

### Elbow Orthoses

Physicians typically prescribe static elbow orthoses for individuals with contractures. They should custom mold orthoses for contracture management to ensure total contact of the orthosis to prevent pressure points. The orthosis consists of a humeral cuff and a forearm cuff with Velcro straps and an elbow joint (Figure 14-6). When a person needs control of the wrist, the forearm section crosses the wrist (EWHO). The physician gradually increases range of motion using an adjustable flexion/extension joint. Among the joints available, the person's size, vocation, and pathology all influence choice of the appropriate type. The larger or more active individual needs a heavy-duty joint, whereas a smaller or less-active person is more comfortable with a less bulky joint. The severity of the pathology is also important because different joints have different increments of adjustability. The team should decide together what is necessary for each user. Physicians also use elbow orthoses for fracture management. They can readily fit premanufactured fracture orthoses on the appropriate person. In cases of deformity or an unusually sized limb, a certified orthotist should custom mold the orthosis.[7]

### Wrist Hand Orthoses

A wrist hand orthosis functions to stabilize the wrist and maintain the palmar arch of the hand. Wrist hand orthoses are made from plastic or metal (aluminum) and have numerous designs. The orthosis can encompass the volar or dorsal surface of the forearm and hand. Specialists can incorporate different components that are specific to each individual's needs. They use thumb posts to stabilize a flail thumb, opponen bars to place the thumb in opposition, and/or a thumb adduction stop to reduce or prevent web space tightness. They use metacarpal phalangeal (MP) stops to prevent extension contractures of the MP joints. WHOs with utensil channels allow self-feeding, writing, and keyboarding. The user's goals are primary considerations when specialists fabricate the appropriate orthosis and attachments. Specialists should custom mold WHOs or should make specific measurements for each person to ensure proper fit and comfort. In instances in which an individual has low tone and needs an orthosis for simple positioning, orthotic shops can deliver off-the-shelf WHOs to reduce cost and delivery time.

### Hand Orthoses (HO)

Specialists use hand orthoses to maintain the palmar arch, hold the thumb in opposition, and serve as attachment sites for other componentry (e.g., utensil channel, MP stop, or spring assists). They custom mold plastic hand orthoses to a model and fabricate metal orthoses from specific measurements or contour them to fit a positive

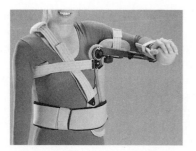

**Fig. 14-5** A SEWHO or "airplane splint" is typically used short term for soft-tissue injuries. (From Coppard BM, Lohman H: *Introduction to splinting: a clinical-reasoning and problem solving approach,* ed 2, St Louis, 2001, Mosby.)

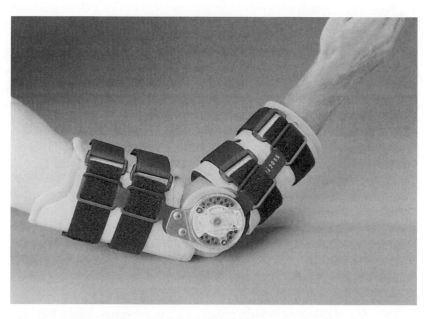

**Fig. 14-6** An elbow orthosis with an adjustable joint and velcro closures. (From Coppard BM, Lohman H: *Introduction to splinting: a clinical-reasoning and problem solving approach,* ed 2, St Louis, 2001, Mosby.)

cast of a user's hand. The therapist and orthotist must work together to determine the appropriate position of the person's hand to most improve function. They fit the individual with the orthosis, and an occupational therapist sees the individual for training sessions with the device. They may need to adjust the componentry many times to perfect the person's ability to function at specific tasks. The team should carefully assess each user's goals before choosing an orthosis and specific components. Premanufactured orthoses are available, and the team should carefully follow the directions. They should fit static hand orthoses to a person with intrinsic muscle loss and good wrist stability. The orthosis holds the hand in a functional position and prevents deformity.

### Finger Orthoses

Specialists can use finger orthoses to stabilize fractured digits and tendon repairs or to correct or prevent a deformity. Common finger deformities include swan neck deformity, boutonniere deformity, and mallet finger.

## Dynamic

### Shoulder Orthoses

Specialists use dynamic shoulder orthoses (SO) to prevent dislocation of the gleno-humeral joint. The SO is typically made from canvas or cloth material and consists of a chest belt and a humeral cuff. The orthosis is available premanufactured, and the orthotist custom fits it to the patient. The orthotist typically fits this orthosis on athletes participating in contact sports.

### Elbow Orthoses

Specialists use elbow orthoses (EO) for fracture management, dislocations, and soft-tissue injuries. The orthosis consists of humeral and forearm cuffs with an elbow joint. Many joint options are available depending on the intended goal of the orthosis. Also, a wide variety of elbow orthoses with adjustable joints are available from manufacturers. A specialist can custom mold them when needed.

### Balanced Forearm Orthoses

The balanced forearm orthosis (BFO) is a prefabricated device also known as a *mobile arm support*. The specialist mounts the orthosis to a wheelchair. It operates on two physics principles: inclined planes and first-class levers. The device consists of a wheelchair assembly bracket, a proximal arm, a distal arm, and forearm trough (Figure 14-7). Other accessories are available depending on the individual's needs. The user needs to have a muscle grade strength of 2+ or better in one or more of the following muscle groups: neck, trunk, shoulder, or elbow.[8]

### Wrist-Hand Orthoses

Although a number of dynamic wrist-hand orthoses (WHOs) are available, we only discuss the following two main categories:

1. The WHO wrist extension assist
2. The tenodesis-style WHOs

Specialists use the WHO wrist extension assist when the patient has absent or weak wrist extensors. They can achieve wrist extension using rubber bands, springs, or premanufactured joints. The forearm and hand components are typically custom made from metal or plastic.

Specialists use tenodesis-style WHOs to achieve three-point prehension. They implement different styles of tenodesis orthoses depending on the musculature available to the user. In this section, we discuss four different types of tenodesis orthoses: (1) the wrist-driven flexor hinge, (2) the Rehabilitation Institute of Chicago-style tenodesis, (3) the ratchet style tenodesis, and (4) the external powered tenodesis.

A person with spinal cord functional level of C6 uses the wrist-driven flexor hinge orthosis. This individual has active wrist extension but no other active motors in the wrist and hand. The first, second, and third digits are held in opposition. Active wrist extension is coupled with passive MP flexion through a parallel linkage in the orthosis. MP flexion against the thumb post achieves three-point prehension. A person must have good shoulder and elbow strength along with wrist extensor strength of at least a 3+ to function with this orthosis.[8] Gravity assists wrist flexion and release of grasp.

The Rehabilitation Institute of Chicago-style tenodesis orthosis consists of a forearm cuff, a separate hand orthosis to oppose the thumb, and a finger orthosis to hold the second and third digits. The physician achieves tenodesis through a linkage between active wrist extension and passive finger flexion. The linkage consists of a cord attached to the volar surfaces of the forearm and finger pieces (Figure 14-8).

Specialists can fit the ratchet-style wrist-driven flexor hinge orthosis on people with poor wrist extensors and no intrinsic musculature. Specialists can achieve prehension by applying force to the proximal end of the ratchet extension. They can maintain pinch by the locking mechanism of the ratchet. A release mechanism and gravity enable individuals to release their grasp on objects.

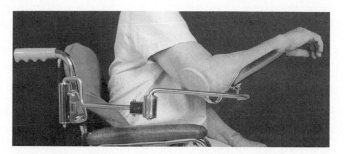

**Fig. 14-7** A balanced forearm orthosis or mobile arm support commonly used to assist a person with upper extremity weakness in feeding. (From Pedretti LW, Early MB: *Occupational therapy: practice skills for physical dysfunction,* ed 5, St Louis, 2001, Mosby.)

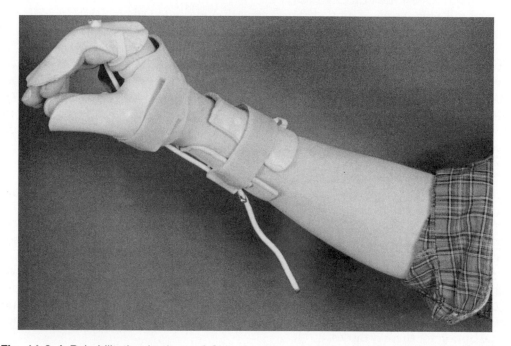
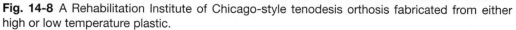

**Fig. 14-8** A Rehabilitation Institute of Chicago-style tenodesis orthosis fabricated from either high or low temperature plastic.

For individuals with absent or weak wrist extensors, specialists can implement external power sources. The most common source for external power is a battery-operated electric motor. Often, because of gadget intolerance, people do not readily accept external power.

## Outcomes and Social Validation

The greatest challenge of orthotic management is cooperation among the user and team members. Cooperation requires clear communication. Practitioners must inform individuals about available options to help them with informed decision making. Users must communicate expectations. All involved must have similar objectives for the management to be successful. If even the most functional orthosis does not meet the goals of individuals for cosmese or comfort, they may discard it.

The ideal orthosis is one that is functional, comfortable, and cosmetic. In reality, an orthosis must be comfortable, should improve function, and may never be as attractive as no orthotic device.

## CASE STUDIES

### CASE 1

#### *Application and Goal*

A 16-year-old teenager came to the clinic after a gun shot wound to the neck. He was in rehabilitation as it was 2 months after the injury. He was seated in a wheelchair and his spine had been surgically stabilized. His goal was to improve upper limb function and performance of activities of daily living.

#### *Function and Ability*

C5 FUNCTIONAL LEVEL ON RIGHT

He had full active range of motion at neck, and shoulder, good elbow flexion, absent extension, trunk stabilized in wheelchair, and poor wrist stability.

C6 FUNCTIONAL LEVEL ON LEFT

He had full active range of motion at neck and shoulder, good elbow flexion and absent extension, trunk stabilized in wheelchair, good wrist extension and pronation, and poor wrist flexion.

#### *Considerations, Options, and Technology*

For the right upper limb, he had many options including materials, style, and functional attachments. A static WHO, Rancho-style with utensil channel for self-feeding and writing, and pointer attachment for keyboarding enabled the young man to function well. A plastic WHO with the same attachments was also a possibility. He would use a ratchet-style tenodesis if the C5 level were his best level of function, however, tenodesis orthoses are too cumbersome for bilateral use.

For the left upper limb, a Rancho-style tenodesis orthosis allowed the patient to achieve palmar prehension, and natural tenodesis developed. He stopped using the orthosis when he achieved natural tenodesis. At that time, a specialist fitted him with a Rancho-style hand orthosis to maintain the thumb in opposition. Polymer is also a material option for these orthoses.

#### *Outcome and Social Validation*

The patient was pleased with the orthoses but developed pressure on the ulnar styloid. The physicians remedied this by selectively cutting away material. The orthotist and occupational therapist worked together to determine the best orientation for the eating utensils, pointer, and penholder. He was especially gratified to discontinue the WHO and replace it with a simple hand orthosis, which demonstrated an improvement in his function. He will continue treatment as an outpatient in the spinal cord injury clinic.

### CASE 2

#### *Application and Goal*

A 21-year-old woman came to clinic after a right midhumeral fracture. The fracture occurred as a result of a horseback riding accident. She also suffered multiple cuts and bruises that were healing well. She was being treated for the fracture, but physicians noted a secondary radial nerve injury. They considered at least two factors in the management of this young woman. The primary consideration was whether the fracture would heal without deformity. Secondly, they needed to manage extrinsic extensor paralysis and prevent contracture. The therapeutic goal was to maintain range and strength and increase strength in the emerging extensors.

## Function and Ability

On examination, her right upper limb shows the following deficiencies: absent wrist extension, absent supination, absent metacarpal phalangeal extension, absent thumb extension, and abduction. The elbow and shoulder had strength and range within normal limits. The triceps were intact.

## Considerations, Options, and Technology

For the humeral fracture, physicians applied a premanufactured humeral fracture orthosis, which the patient used with a sling for 8 weeks. The fracture orthosis maintained sagittal and coronal alignment, and the sling maintained transverse alignment.

For the extrinsic extensor paralysis, physicians used a dynamic wrist-hand orthosis. The orthotist chose a plastic wrist extension assist. Additionally, they also applied removable metacarpal phalangeal extension assist and thumb extension/abduction assist. In therapy, a low temperature, static line orthosis allowed the patient to use the intact finger flexors to grasp and the intact wrist flexors to release. The static line orthosis was too bulky for daily use; therefore she used the wrist extension assist when she was not in therapy.

## Outcome and Social Validation

The injury occurred to the patient's dominant hand, and she was disturbed by the possibility of permanent weakness. Although concern existed that a wrist extension assist might compromise the returning strength of the extensor group, they were unfounded. After a 2-year recovery, she did gain full function without malalignment.

## CASE 3

## Application and Goal

A 68-year-old man came to the clinic with left upper limb weakness after a right cerebrovascular accident (stroke) that had occurred 6 months previously. The physiatrist was concerned about his shoulder alignment and developing contractures in the elbow, wrist, and hand. The goal was to improve the alignment and reduce the developing deformities. He was in outpatient rehabilitation working on gait in physical therapy. In outpatient occupational therapy, he addressed improving range and activities of daily living (ADL) using one hand and arm because he had no active use of his left upper limb.

## Function and Ability

The left upper limb had moderate flexor tone at the elbow, wrist, and hand. At rest, physicians positioned his arm in adduction and internal rotation of the shoulder and flexion at the elbow, wrist, and fingers. Although the patient had full passive range of motion at the shoulder and elbow, he could not extend the fingers when he extended the wrist beyond neutral. Further, a web space contracture existed.

## Considerations/Options/Technology

Physicians fitted the patient with different orthoses for day and night use. At night, he used a resting hand orthosis. They initially positioned it in wrist flexion and modified it weekly to increase wrist extension. In this way, he could maintain his wrist and hand in optimal alignment as he slowly stretched the wrist. For day use, they chose a static WHO with a variable thumb adduction stop. The adduction stop is slowly opened to increase the web space. He will also wear a sling to help reduce the subluxed shoulder.

## Outcome and Social Validation

Approximately 6 months afterward, the shoulder remained subluxed, however, it had not dislocated completely. Passive range had improved in the wrist and hand. He continued to wear the WHO at night but had discontinued the daytime WHO. He remained functionally the same with no improvement in strength or tone.

## References

1. American Academy of Orthopaedic Surgeons: *Atlas of orthotics,* ed 3, St Louis, 1997, Mosby.
2. American Academy of Orthopaedic Surgeons: *Instructional course lectures,* vol XXXVI, 1987, Modern Concepts in Functional Fracture Bracing: The Upper Limb.
3. Malick MH, Meyer CMH: Manual on management of the quadriplegic upper extremity, 1978, Healthcare Harmarville Rehabilitation.
4. Hunter JM et al: *Manual on management of specific hand problems,* Series II, Pittsburgh, 1984, American Rehabilitation Education Network.
5. Hunter J et al: *Rehabilitation of the hand, surgery and therapy,* St Louis, 1990, Mosby.
6. Malick MH, Carr JA: *Manual on management of the burn patient,* Pittsburgh, 1982, Harmarville Rehabilitation Center.
7. Northwestern University Medical School, Prosthetic-Orthotic Center: *Upper limb orthotics manual,* Chicago, 1996.
8. Redford JB et al: *Orthotics clinical practice and rehabilitation technology,* Philadelphia, 1995, Churchill Livingstone.

## Resources

*Professional Organizations*
American Academy of Physical Medicine and Rehabilitation
One IBM Plaza
Chicago, IL 60611-3604
Telephone: (312) 464-9700

American Academy of Orthopaedic Surgeons
6300 North River Road
Rosemont, IL 60018-4262
Telephone: (847) 823-7186

American Physical Therapy Association
1111 North Fairfax Street
Alexandria, VA 22309
Telephone: (703) 684-2782

Orthotics and Prosthetics National Office
1650 King Street, Suite 500
Alexandria, VA 22314-2747
Telephone: (703) 836-7114

*Manufacturers and Distributors*
AliMed, Inc.
297 High Street
Dedham, MA 02026-9135
Telephone: (800) 225-2610
Fax: (617) 329-8392

Becker Orthopedic
635 Executive Drive
Troy, MI 48083
Telephone: (800) 521-2192
Fax: (800) 923-2537

Dynasplint Systems
Telephone: (800) 262-8828

Freeman
900 West Chicago Road
Sturgis, MI 49091-9756
Telephone: (800) 253-2091
Fax: (800) 894-8248

Jaeco
PO Box 75
Hot Springs, AK 71901
Telephone: (501) 623-5944

LMB Hand Rehab Products
PO Box 1181
San Luis Obispo, CA 93406
Telephone: (800) 541-3992
Fax: (805) 541-3996

Maramed Precision Corporation
2480 West 82nd Street
Hialeah, Florida 33016
Telephone: (800) 823-8300
Fax: (305) 823-8304

North Coast Medical
187 Stauffer Boulevard
San Jose, CA 95125
Telephone: (800) 821-9319
Fax: (800) 283-1950

Orthomedics
2950 East Imperial Highway
Brea, California 92622
Telephone: (800) 733-6999
Fax: (800) 733-7005

Ortho-Products
9 Baybrook Lane
Oak Brook, IL 60523
Telephone: (800) 888-6999
Fax: (800) 222-0004

Sammons-Preston
PO Box 5071
Bolingbrook, IL 60440

Silver Rings Splint Company
PO Box 2856
Charlottesville, VA 22902-2856
Telephone: (804) 971-4052
Fax: (804) 971-8828

Smith and Nephew Rolyan, Inc.
One Quality Drive
PO Box 1005
Germantown, WI 53022-8205
Telephone: (800) 558-8633
Fax: (800) 545-7758

Truform Orthotics and Prosthetics
3960 Rosslyn Drive
Cinncinnati, OH 45209
Telephone: (800) 888-0458
Fax: (800) 309-9055

Ultraflex Systems
362 Technology Drive
Malvern, PA 19355
Telephone: (800) 220-6670
Fax: (610) 647-7015

CHAPTER 15

# Adaptive Aids for Accessing Technology

*Christine R. Jasch*

## Application and Goal

Assistive technology requires input from a user to make it function. The user must use some method to control the device. Cook and Hussey[1] refer to this method as "the human/technology interface," which they define as "the boundary between the human and the assistive technology across which information is exchanged." All forms of assistive technology, both low tech and high tech, require a defined method to exchange information. For the standard computer keyboard, the method a person uses is touching a key. For a power wheelchair, the person may use a joystick and for a communication device, the person may use a switch. In this chapter, this method or human/technology interface is called the *access method,* which a person uses to interact with the device.

The access method must be identified for optimal integration between the user and the device. An access method should allow the client to use the technology in the fastest, most efficient, and functional manners.

### Considerations for Optimal Access

Technologists must ask the following questions to ensure that the user has optimal access:

- Can the user perform the motion(s) required to complete the task within a functional time?
- Can the user cognitively understand the access method?
- Can the user use visual, auditory, or tactile outputs? Does the access method provide the feedback?
- Can the user stabilize the device to access it?
- Can the user access the device in all desired locations?

## Function and Ability

### Definitions

Access can be broken into two selection methods: direct selection and indirect selection. Two categories within indirect selection are scanning and encoding. Scanning types include row/column, linear, and step scanning. Morse code is one example within encoding.

*Direct selection* refers to a client being able to directly interface with a device. The user places a hand on an augmentative communication device, touches the letter K, and the device produces a K. This requires that the user have muscle strength to lift the arm to the device, coordinated movements to isolate one finger or to control a tool such as a typing stick, and control to push just one button. The user needs sensation to feel the depression of the key and intellect to know which key to press. The user can achieve direct selection through means other than the hand manipulating a device. Examples of alternative direct selection methods are an alternative pointer such as a typing stick or even an alternative mouse device such as the HeadMouse.

If an individual does not have the strength or control to direct select, an indirect selection method may be an appropriate alternative. *Indirect method* refers to any method such as scanning and encoding that does not include the direct manipulation of the device.

Automatic scanning allows a person to have access to the device via a single or dual switch. The person activates the switch, which causes the devices to present an item in a preselected order. The user makes a second activation when the device presents targeted item or items. The preselected order determines how many switch hits the device needs to arrive at the targeted item. The user must activate the switch three times to reach the desired letter K. Client need and device characteristics determine the order of selection and the grouping of the selected items. Examples of various scanning orders include linear, rotary, or group scan.

Step scanning requires the person to switch hit to advance the scan by item. The user can do this with a single switch or dual switches. This type of scanning should be easier for a cognitively impaired user, however, it is physically more demanding. Inverse scanning begins the scan when the person activates the switch and continues to scan as long as the person activates the switch. To make a selection, the user releases the switch. This method is useful for the user who has difficulty activating the switch but can maintain the switch activation and release it in a timely manner.[2] Directed scanning allows the user to define the path of the scan using a multiple switch such as a joystick.

Scanning requires that the user have focused attention, concentration, and switch skills. *Switch skills* refer to the person's ability to hit and release a switch in a timely manner. This requires motor control and endurance to perform a motion repetitively. Typically the user must be able to visually track the scanning array. If this is not possible, some devices provide auditory feedback.

Scanning can be adapted to meet individual needs. The timing of the scan can often be adjusted. The switch acceptance rate (how long the user needs to hold down the switch) can usually be adjusted.

*Encoding* refers to a person using a code to produce a desired result. Each series of codes represents a different result or action. Morse code is an example of encoding. A series of dots and dashes each represent a different letter or result. In two-switch Morse code a person activates one switch and the machine produces a dot while the other switch produces a dash. When a person activates these switches in a specific sequence the device produces a letter. For example, a dash-dot-dash sequence produces the letter K (Figure 15-1).

Direct selection is usually the fastest method of input unless the movements that the machine requires are fatiguing to the user or cause too many inaccuracies. Encoding can be considered the next fastest input method, however, it requires that the user have a high level of cognitive skills. Scanning is considered the least efficient method because of the waiting time necessary for the cursor to reach the selection that the user desires before the person can activate the switch.[3]

## Access Method Determination

The access method to a piece of technology should be the easiest, most direct path available.[4] The user should be thinking about what the technology can offer, not the way to access it. In other words, if students are spending too much time and effort attempting to hit the correct key of a keyboard and not on thinking about spelling homework, they should explore an alternative method to allow the focus to be on the end product, not the access method.

The technologist should know the capacity of motor skills along with the cognitive, perceptual, and visual abilities of the user to determine the most appropriate access method. Because optimal movement of the user is maximized with a stable base, the technologist should begin the assessment by determining the appropriateness of the seating system and the various positions the user will be in when operating the device. An appropriate seating system and proper trunk support should allow the user to have optimal use and control of the extremities. Other areas the technologist should consider

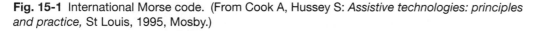

**Fig. 15-1** International Morse code. (From Cook A, Hussey S: *Assistive technologies: principles and practice,* St Louis, 1995, Mosby.)

are vision (including visual perception, accuracy, double vision, and color blindness), sensory abilities (including proprioception and light touch and auditory function), and motor skills (including tone and coordination of movements). To determine motor skills, the technologist must evaluate each position in which the user will operate devices such as from a wheelchair, the floor, a bed, and a stander.

The technologist should consider direct selection first. If motor control is limited, the user has alternative choices to increase success. These include the user changing the acceptance rate and/or repeat rate of a key, adding a keyguard, using an alternative means of direct access or changing the position of the device. The *acceptance rate* refers to the time a user needs before activating a selection. For example, for individuals with decreased coordination, they may randomly hit many keys before the target key. The technologist can lengthen the acceptance rate so that the device ignores the random hits and only accept the target hit if the user depresses the key for a set length of time. The repeat rate is the amount of time the user activates the key before it repeats itself. If the user has difficult time releasing keys, the technologist increasing the repeat rate decreases the likelihood of the user getting multiple activations.

Keyguards, which are typically constructed of plastic and lay over the device providing a square or circle around each selection option, can reduce the number of misstrikes the user makes because of decreased coordination. They are available for augmentative communication devices, environmental control devices, and the computer keyboard. An alternative means of direct access could be a pointer such as a T-bar fabricated out of low-temperature plastic or a wrist support with a projection (Figure 15-2). Other alternatives for the user, which could assist in the absence of a functional finger point, include the following:

- An optical indicator for selections with an augmentative communication device
- A mouse-input device for use with an augmentative communication device or an on-screen keyboard on a computer
- The voice for computer and/or environmental control access

The technologist should consider the positioning of the device and the layout of the targets for successful access. If clients are unable to optimally reach for a device, they can-

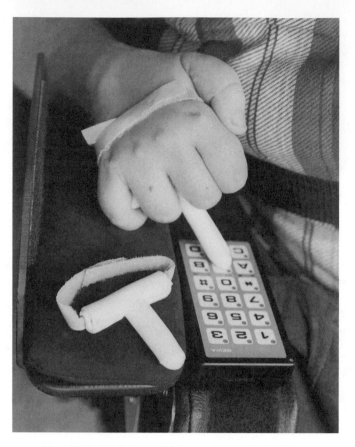

**Fig. 15-2** A fabricated T-bar or an optical pointer.

not achieve optimal access. If the client is ambulatory, several options are available for the client for optimal mounting of devices to wheelchairs and beds (Figure 15-3). If a client has difficulty reaching an area of a device, for example the upper left corner, this corner could be left empty, with all the targets within reachable range.

For a direct selection method to be successful, a client must have sufficient control and endurance to repeat the motion through task completion. For a low-level augmentative communication device user, this may be hitting a single message device two times. For a high-level computer user, this may be typing a full page of text using a typing stick.

The user's environment may play a role in the access methods. An augmentative communication user may need access from the wheelchair and the bed. This may require a primary and secondary access method.

If direct selection is not ideal, the technologist considers an indirect access method. To use an indirect access method, the technologist should identify a switch site and decide on the indirect access method (Box 15-1).

When the client uses an indirect access method, as opposed to a direct access method, the task becomes inherently more difficult. Therefore, the effort that device requires the user to use with the indirect access method should be easy, and the user should focus on what will occur when reaching the target.

The indirect access method may also play a role in the technologist's placement of the switch site. The *indirect access method* refers to the type of scanning or encoding that the client will use. The technologist can ask the following questions:

- Does the client have the cognitive abilities to perform an automatic scan or will a step scanning method be required? (Step scanning is cognitively less challenging but requires more motor control.)
- Will the technologist need to identify one switch site or two switch sites? (A dual switch may make step scanning easier for the user.)

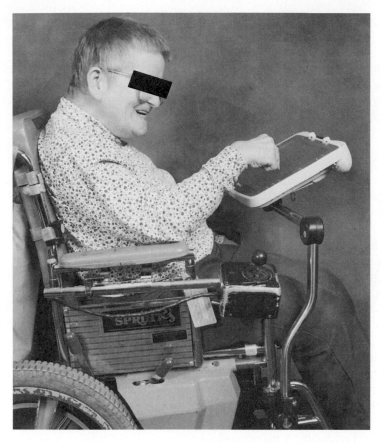

**Fig. 15-3** A device properly mounted on a wheelchair with the user directly accessing it.

BOX **15-1**

*Questions the Technologist Should Ask When Deciding on a Switch Site*

*For All Potential Switch Sites*
Does the user have sufficient endurance to repeat the motion consecutively?
Do reflexes exist that will interfere with the motion the user needs to hit a target?
Is tone present that will interfere or enhance the user getting to a target?
What is the available range at each site and which is less restricting?
Are the available movements the user controls able to hit a target and release in a timely
    manner?
How can the technologist position the switch for optimal activation?

*Specific Body Parts*
Body parts are listed in order of preference for switch site
*Hand function*
What kind of isolated or gross finger movement is available for a fine motor switch?
Can the user activate a switch if it is in the hand secured with a strap or splint?
Can the user control a pointing device?
*Arm placement*
What kind of arm placement is available for a gross motor switch site?
*Head and neck*
Does the user still have visual contact with the device with switch activation?
*Lower extremities*
Does adequate sensation exist if visual input is not available?

• Can the person perform a directed scanning array? (This would require the user's ability to manipulate multiple switches or a multiple input switch.)

The technologist should not independently decide which indirect access method is ideal and where to place the switch. The technologist's determination of the indirect access method may be a direct result of the way the client is able to handle activating the switch consistently.

### Switch Site Determination

Two important parts to the switch assessment process include the technologist identifying the most efficient body movement and placement of the switch and identifying whether the user has functional switch skills.

The technologist should begin the assessment of an appropriate switch site without the presence of technology. This approach reduces the complexity of the task so that the technologist's initial focus is on the effort that the user needs to access the switch. The technologist should first observe available user motions through either a functional activity such as turning on a radio or switch-toy or working with a cognitively intact adult through interview and discussion. Through these observations, the technologist should identify the most consistent quality movement available. In order of preference, the ideal motions of the client would be in the hand or arm, head or neck, leg, foot, or toe. Based on the motions available, technologists can try switches at each location they identified. The user and the clinician should remain flexible regarding access options and reassess regularly (Figure 15-4).

The user must have functional switch skills to accurately reach a scanning target or to input an encoding signal in a timely manner. The user should be able to do the following:

• Activate the switch only when desired
• Wait while the desired item is scanned
• Activate the switch in a timely manner

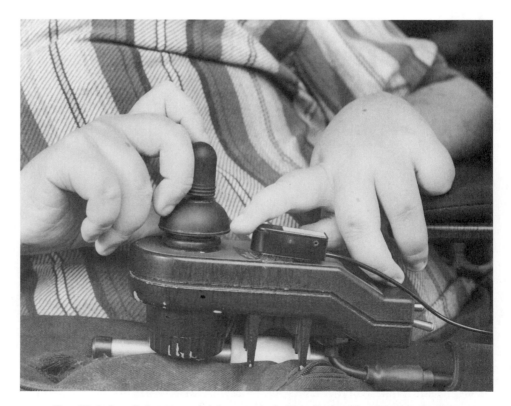

**Fig. 15-4** A switch appropriately mounted either for hand or head activation.

- Release the switch in a timely manner
- Ability to sometimes hold the switch for a set time

The user must also have switch skills for encoding, which include the following:

- Activate two switches quickly in succession
- Operate one switch at variable lengths of time

## Considerations, Options, and Technology

### *Switches*

A switch can be broken into three parts: (1) the connector plug (typically a ⅛-inch mono plug or stereo plug for dual switches), (2) the cord, and (3) the switch mechanism. Most switch mechanisms consist of two wires that must connect in some manner for the user to close or activate the switch. The types of switch mechanisms vary considerably thus the user has a wide variety of switch type options. User knowledge of the variety of switch characteristics should assist in the determination of the appropriate switch (Box 15-2).

### Size and Shape

The type of movement (fine motor or gross motor movement) that the user needs to activate the switch indicates the size of the switch. The smaller the user's movement, the smaller the switch size is. The larger the user's movement, the larger the switch size is. The switch location may determine the shape.

### Force Needed for Activation

Some switches require no force to be activated, others can tolerate a great amount of force without breaking.

### Range Needed for Activation

Range needed for activation refers to how far the user needs to move the before activation. For an individual with limited range of motion or strength, 0.3 inches may be too far to push a lever for activation. Other individuals may need a longer range to decrease unwanted switch hits.

### Feedback Provided

Auditory, visual, and/or proprioceptive cues can assist some switch users to be more accurate. Other individuals may find these cues distracting.

### Type of Force Needed for Activation

The user activates most switches through contact with a body part, for example, from the pressure of a hand or a finger. The user controls pneumatic switches through air pressure either through a sip or a puff of air from the mouth or squeezing air through a tube from a handgrip. Specialized switches allow for the user to generate force by a single muscle twitch or eye blink.

### Number of Controls Needed

Most switches are single switches allowing the user control of one input. Dual switches provide the user with two input controls. These may be useful if the individual uses an

## BOX 15-2

*Examples of Switches*

**Push Switch**
AbleNet's Jellybean, Big Red, Spec, and String switches
Tash's Buddy buttons
Micro Light, Leaf, Pillow, Soft, and Cup/mini-cup switches
Don Johnston's LT and Elipse switch
Zygo's Plate, Lever, and Lolly switches
Prentke Romich's Rocking levers

**Push Pull**
Prentke Romich Wobble
Enabling Devices Ultimate, Wobble and Pull switches
Zygo's Leaf switch
Tash's Flex switch

**Touch Activated**
Tash's Plate switch
Adaptavation's Taction and Pal pads.

**Pneumatic**
Zygo's CM 3 Pneumatic single, CM 3-3 Pneumatic dual, and rubber ball switches
Tash's Pneumatic and Grasp switches
ATP's Air cushion switch
Prentke Romich's Pneumatic

**Light Touch (0.0-0.4 oz)**
Tash's Micro Light, Tip Switch
Enabling Devices Ultimate and Twitch switches (check on twitch)

**Heavy duty (10 oz +)**
Tash's Tread, Soft, Treadle, and Pillow switch
Zygo's Thumb switch

**Gravity Dependent**
Tash's Tip switch
Enabling Devices' Tilt switch

**Specialty Switches**
Prentke Romich P-switch
Words Plus IST switch
Proximity switches from various vendors
Enabling Devices Whisper and Movement sensor switches
ASL Fiber optic switches

encoding method or step scanning. The user can pair two or more separate switches with an interface to provide access to one device (i.e., mouse emulation). If the user needs five switches for control, a multiple switch can provide multiple switch inputs housed into one switch, which may be useful for directed scanning or mouse control. Examples include joysticks, a waver switch, or a penta switch (Figures 15-5 and 15-6).

Equally important is where and how the user will position the switch. A switch mount should allow the user consistent access to the switch, a stable surface for the switch, and easy removal or repositioning of the switch to ease transfers or position changes. The switch mount should also be as unobtrusive as possible.

The user can hold smaller switches in the hand or position them with a splint or elastic strap into the palm of the hand. They can be fixed to a number of surfaces using Velcro, including a wheelchair armrest, laptray, or the side of the joystick. A number of

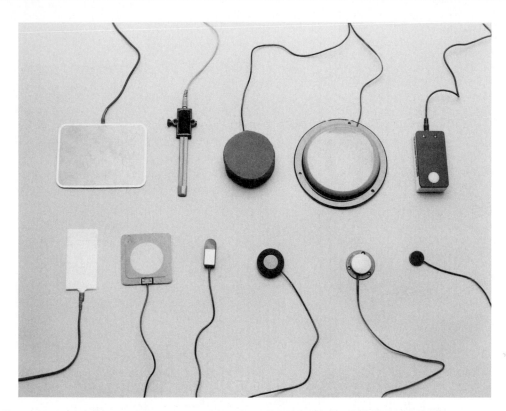

**Fig. 15-5** A variety of switches are available. Some examples are above beginning in the top row from left: pal pad, ribbon, soft switch, big red, and L.T. switch. On the bottom row from left the switches include: taction pad, plate switch, microlight, capswitch, spec, and minicap.

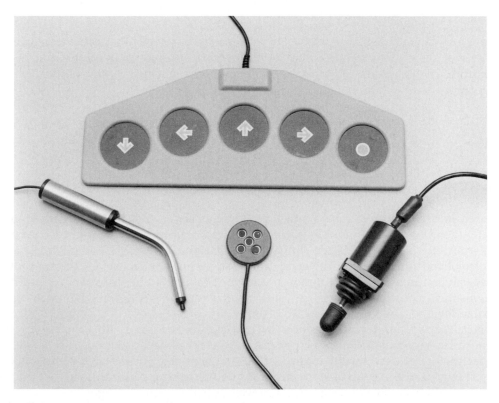

**Fig. 15-6** Dual and multiple switches are available; for example the wafer board is on the top row, and on the bottom row beginning from left are the pnuematic, penta switch, and joystick.

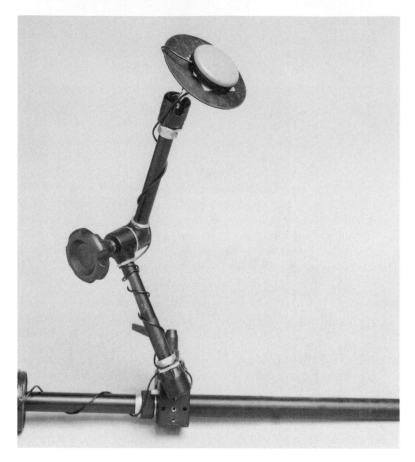

**Fig. 15-7** A magic arm with a switch.

commercial universal switch mounts are available that provide quick setup and release. These can attach to the frame of a wheelchair, a tabletop, or a bed frame. Specific hardware for switch mounting is available from most manufacturers who produce them (Figure 15-7).

## CASE STUDIES

### CASE 1

J.H. is a 38-year-old man who had a cardiovascular accident and had been classified as "locked in." He appeared to have intact cognition as he made facial expressions appropriate to conversations around him. He was able to recall switch use from each session and was aware of errors he made with a communication device. J.H. had no arm placement or hand function with the exception of some minimal active left thumb movement. He had minimal head rotation towards the left, no ability to verbalize, and had been using eye blinks to answer "yes" and "no." He was referred for augmentative communication and computer access.

Initially, the technologist introduced partner-assisted scanning with a letter board for an immediate communication method. Because of J.H.'s decreased motor capabilities, the technologist determined that direct selection would not be possible for him and explored switch sites. J.H. was able to activate a spec switch strapped around his left thumb by hitting it against his index finger. However, because of quick fatigue and decreased stability of the switch, the technologist needed to come up with alternatives. J.H. was able to activate a buddy button secured by Velcro to a Magic arm switch mount attached to his wheelchair and positioned at his left temple. He caused frequent misactivations

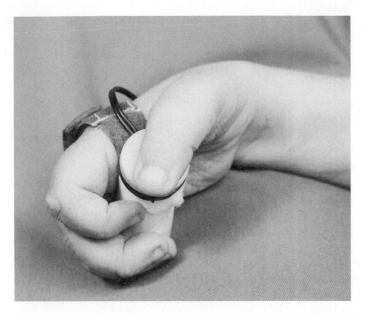

**Fig. 15-8** A fabricated switch mount with the spec switch on it.

when he coughed or breathed heavily. He also demonstrated decreased endurance for this motion. The technologist explored sip/puff, however, J.H. did not like having any devices in front of his face. The technologist decided to further explore the switch site at his thumb and attempted a Micro Light switch because of its reduced pressure requirements. However, the technologist had difficulty mounting it into position. The technologist mounted a flex switch via a Tash switch clamp, however, this required J.H. too much travel (0.5 inches) and force to activate. A grasp switch was too inconsistent for him and a string switch was too difficult for easy setup. The technologist fabricated a cone shape out of low temperature plastics and attached a Velcro strap to go around his palm (similar to a universal cuff) (Figure 15-8). The technologist mounted the spec switch to the end of the cone, and J.H. was able to activate this consistently when the technologist positioned his arm correctly on his armrest.

With more practice, his endurance and accuracy grew. Over time, his hand strength increased to allow him to position the switch in the palm of his hand with a Velcro/elastic strap activated with his thumb.

J.H. was initially successful with a row/column array on a communication device. During his exploration of various devices, he tried single-switch Morse code and single-switch scanning with EZ-Keys, a program that allows augmentative communication, computer access, and environmental control via the same device. In the end, he used a laptop computer with EZ-keys accessed via a single switch held in his left hand. He used single switch scanning with a half-scan array for entering text and used HeadMouse with Dragger for all mouse control. He used the program for augmentative communication and computer access. The technologist mounted the laptop on his chair using a rigid wheelchair mount and plugged the HeadMouse and laptop into his power wheelchair battery.

## CASE 2

D.G. is a 26-year-old woman who a physician diagnosed with cerebral palsy and developmental delays. She was nonverbal, used a manual wheelchair, and was dependent for mobility and all her activities of daily living (ADL). She came to the clinic with large fluctuating tone and the presence of reflexes that influenced her movements, specifically a pronounced asymmetric tonic neck reflex (ATNR), which resulted in her turning her head with the extension of an arm. She had a fluctuating grasp and was able to open her hand when relaxed, however, she was unable to open or release on command. Using active, intentional movements, her tone increased thus making her movements uncoordinated, inaccurate, and difficult to control. Through observations and interviews with the family members, the technologist noted that she had some increased movement and control with her left arm. According to her mother, D.G. was able to use a letterboard with partner-assisted scanning for selection, which she could not demonstrate.

D.G. came to the clinic with a Macaw augmentative communication device mounted to her wheelchair positioned at midline. She had no functional means of accessing it. The family had purchased the device, however, D.G. had not yet been able to use it. She was unsuccessful with traditional direct selection because of uncoordinated movements and the loss of visual contact on extension of her arm. The addition of a keyguard and a technologist increasing the acceptance rate only slightly improved her accuracy.

The technologist attempted auditory linear scanning and presented a mounted Jelly-bean switch on a Magic arm switch mount. The technologist attempted various positions, including her left fist, left hand, and her head. D.G.'s limitations included decreased ability to activate the switch in a functional amount of time and the inability to release the switch on command.

Initially, the scanning array consisted of eight items. After several attempts, the technologist noted that D.G. did not have the cognitive ability to functionally scan despite her mother's report of intact cognition. She seemed to hit the targets without discrimination for the message.

The technologist then decided to further pursue direct selection. To provide increased stability to the wrist complex with the intention of increasing a functional finger point, the technologist attempted several wrist supports. These were variably successful based on D.G.'s tone. A T-bar fabricated out of low-temperature plastic was not successful either. She pointed the pointing end of the T-bar in various positions depending on the way the tone influenced her pronation and supination. The technologist tried a plastic three-point knob, which massage therapists often use. She was able to grasp the knob at the center and have three available points at any given time depending on what position her wrist was in when it made contact with the device. This became her alternative direct selection access method. The technologist changed the position of the device to the left side of her chair (close to her body). This allowed her to maintain visual contact with the device and access it with her elbow flexed. D.G. became successful with direct selection from a field of six choices. The technologist developed three different overlays.

## ADDITIONAL CASE STUDIES

### Other Unique Access Options

R.R. is a 62-year-old man who had a brain stem cardiovascular accident. He was confined to bed in an extended care facility. No movement, except for eye gaze and minimal right thumb movement with wrist stability, was available. The technologist fabricated a left resting hand splint, punched a hole out of the thumb piece, and fixed a minicup switch into position. R.R. was able to access a scanning augmentative communication device with this setup.

B.D. is a 3-year-old girl who a physician diagnosed with spinal muscular atrophy. She had minimal movements throughout her body including the lack of head control. She came to the clinic with weak active finger movements but no arm placement. She had a functional seating system including a laptray. She required access to single messages with the development of multiple messages with a simple scanning setup. B.D. was able to activate a Micro Light switch, however, she needed precise positioning each time. Because her arms were in slightly different positions each time, the technologist could not fix the switch to a permanent spot on her laptray. The alternative was for the technologist to use a medium-strength theraputty to hold the switch in place for her use. When she not in her chair, the therapist could store the theraputty, which proved to be a functional mounting setup for this client.

O.H. is a 46-year-old man with spinal stenosis resulting in limited proprioception and light touch with his hands. He is also legally blind. He had functional ROM and strength in both hands and generalized weakness in his legs. He ambulated household distances at home and used a manual wheelchair for community mobility. His goals included computer access. Conventional keyboarding was not an option because of his limited sensory abilities. He tried an alternative keyboard (the BAT) with fabricated key guides made of low temperature plastic; however, the proprioception limitations greatly reduced success. Using his voice for access was not consistently successful because of a strong fluctuating accent and technical difficulties with a screen reader. The technologist attempted Morse code as an alternative input method, and the client demonstrated a good ability to learn and use this encoding access system. He used a sip/puff switch to accommodate for the decreased sensation. After trials of several types of technology, Morse code with auditory feedback using a sip/puff switch proved the most functional access for him. The client was able to successfully input data using this setup.

## References

1. Cook A, Hussey S: *Assistive technologies: principles and practice,* p 313, St Louis, 1995, Mosby.
2. Beukelman D, Mirenda P: *Augmentative and alternative communication: management of severe communication disorders in children and adults,* p 65, Baltimore, 1995, Brookes.
3. Hedman G: *Rehabilitation technology,* p 101, Binghamton, NY, 1990, Haworth.
4. Galvin J, Scherer M: *Evaluating, selecting, and using appropriate assistive technology,* Gaithersburg, Md, 1996, Aspen.

## Resources

Adaptivation, Inc.
2225 W. 50th Street
Sioux Falls, SD 57105
Telephone: (800) 723-4445

AlelNet, Inc.
1081 10th Ave S.E.
Minneapolis, MN 55414
Telephone: (800) 322-0956

APT Technolgy, Inc.
236 A North Main Street
Shreve, OH 44676
Telephone: (303) 567-2001

Don Johnston Development Equipment, Inc.
26799 West Commerce Drive
Volo, IL 60073
Telephone: (800) 999-4660

Enabling Devices
385 Warburton Ave.
Hastings-on-Hudson, NY 10706
Telephone: (800) 832-8697

Prentke Romich Company
1022 Heyl Rd.
Wooster, OH 44691
Telephone: (800) 262-1984

Tash, Inc.
Unit 1, 91 Station Street
Ajax, Ontario CANADA L1S 3H2
Telephone: (800) 463-5685

Words +
1220 West Avenue J
Lancaster, CA 93534
Telephone: (800) 869-8521

# CHAPTER 16

## Upper-Limb Prosthetics

*Craig W. Heckathorne*

### Application and Goal

The daily environment is designed to be handled. People are surrounded by objects that they must grasp, push, pull, rotate, put together, take apart, pick up, or put down in order for the objects to be useful. People must wash, groom, use the toilet, eat, and dress. Most people do these actions with their hands and arms. They use their hands to act on the objects and perceive their physical attributes. They use the joints of the arms to position the hands in space and orient them to most effectively engage the object "at hand."

Traumatic amputation of the hand or arm or the absence of some portion of the hand or arm at birth results in a person's loss or impairment of manipulative ability. Therefore one of the primary goals for an upper limb prosthetist is the restoration of or augmentation of a person's manipulative function. This is achieved by the prosthetist matching a set of integrated prosthetic components to the individual's abilities and intentions and training the person in the efficient and effective operation of the prosthesis.

The way a prosthetist achieves this goal is generally not straightforward. Complete restoration of the function, appearance, and feel of the lost or absent hand and arm is technically not possible. Consequently, the design of any upper-limb prosthesis represents a limited set of functions or characteristics that the prosthetist chooses from the multitude of functions and characteristics associated with the physiologic hand and arm. Achievable goals for the individual receiving prosthesis include the following:

- Restoring the ability to perform many routine daily activities
- Participating in vocational and avocational activities that require manipulation
- Augmenting existing function to improve performance in some specific activity
- Having an acceptable appearance, although not always physiologically cosmetic

### Function and Ability

The primary cause of upper-limb amputation is trauma. Industrial and farming accidents are the leading sources. Motor vehicle accidents, civilian gunshot injuries, and military action (injury from gunshot, shrapnel, or land mines) also account for a significant number of amputations. A smaller number of persons have hand and arm amputations resulting from disease processes such as cancer and vascular insufficiency, which are the leading causes of amputations in this category.

Most traumatic amputations occur when people are within the ages of the late teens to the early 40s. Most persons who experience these amputations are men and most are unilaterally involved. Persons with bilateral amputations are estimated to be less than 5% of all those with arm amputations.

The most common level of amputation is distal to the elbow, with amputations through the forearm (transradial) and at the wrist (wrist disarticulation) accounting for 50% to 60% of arm amputations. The second most common level of amputation is through the upper arm (transhumeral), which accounts for 20% to 30% of arm amputations. Approximately 5% of people have amputations through the shoulder (shoulder disarticulation). Amputations through the elbow (elbow disarticulation) and total arm amputations including the scapula and clavicle (interscapulothoracic) also occur but with less incidence.

The absence of part or the entire upper limb at birth (congenital limb deficiency) is estimated at about 5% of all persons with upper-limb amputation or deficiency. Deficiencies at the forearm level are most common (about 60%).

Statistically, the person with an upper-limb amputation has commonly experienced a traumatic amputation, is an adult man in the latter stages of education or is employed at the time of amputation, has only one arm affected, and is twice as likely to have an amputation distal to the elbow than proximal. A person who can benefit from a hand or arm prosthesis has the following characteristics:

- Has lost a limb or limbs resulting from trauma and is seeking to reacquire some level of manipulative function and restored appearance
- Has congenital absence of an upper-limb segment or severe malformation of a segment and sees an opportunity to augment existing skills and abilities

## Cosmetic

People with unilateral amputations generally use cosmetic prostheses principally to restore appearances of physiologic limbs. The contralateral limb manually positions joint components, and the prosthetic hand has no active grip function. These prostheses are usually lighter than any other type of prosthesis, often have a soft foam cover enclosing skeletal-like components (endoskeletal construction), and have an external plastic finish approximating the appearance of skin.

## Body Powered

Body-powered prostheses use mechanical components positioned through cable and harness systems that transfer physiologic movement and forces to prosthetic components (Figure 16-1). The harness, which is made from fabric straps, fits over the upper torso and provides an anchor point for the cable. The cable then crosses a physiologic joint, most often the shoulder on the amputated side, as it is routed to the component. Forward flexion of the residual limb at the shoulder or scapular abduction (shoulder protraction) causes the cable to be pulled from the anchor point, thus actuating the component. A single cable can actuate several components sequentially if the prosthetist uses locks to constrain the movement of the unintended components.

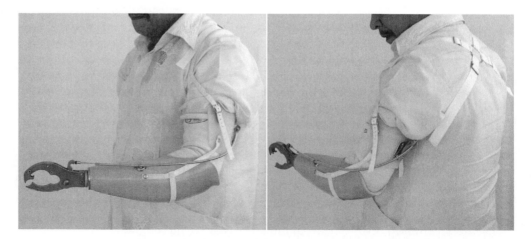

**Fig. 16-1** A body-powered transradial prosthesis. The control cable is anchored at one end to a body harness made of straps and to a mechanical prehension device at the other end. Forward flexion of the arm at the shoulder pulls on the cable and actuates the prehension device.

## Electric Powered

Electric-powered prostheses use motorized components powered by batteries. The only commercial electric-powered components currently available are prehension devices, wrist rotators, and elbows. No electric-powered components are commercially available for individual fingers, wrist flexion, humeral rotation (the inward and outward rotation of the forearm about the axis of the upper arm), or shoulder movement. A person can control electric-powered components through electronics using myoelectricity, the electrical signals that a person's muscle contractions produce (Figure 16-2). Typically, myoelectric control uses the muscles in the limb segment through which the amputation was done. A prosthetist also uses force transducers, linear potentiometers, switches, and other force and movement transducers to control electric-powered devices.

## Hybrid

Hybrid prostheses combine body-powered and electric-powered components within a single prosthesis. A common example is the hybrid transhumeral prosthesis (Figure 16-3). This system incorporates a mechanical, body-powered elbow and an electric prehension device. A cable and harness system actuates the elbow using flexion of the arm or scapular abduction. The prehensor is actuated using myoelectric signals from the

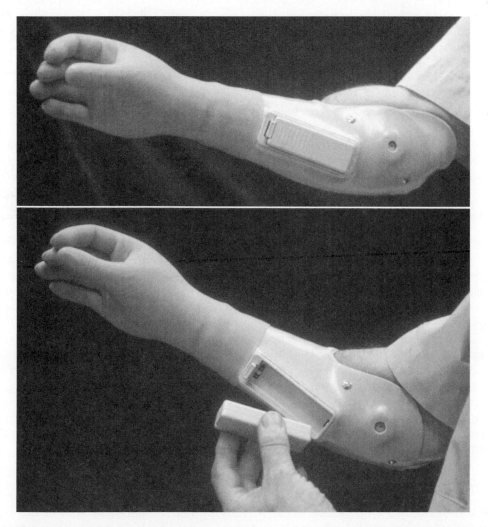

**Fig. 16-2** A transradial prosthesis with an electric-powered hand controlled by myoelectric signals. The signals are produced by the contraction of muscles in the residual limb and are detected at the skin surface with electrodes built into the prosthesis. A removable battery powers the electronics and the motor of the hand.

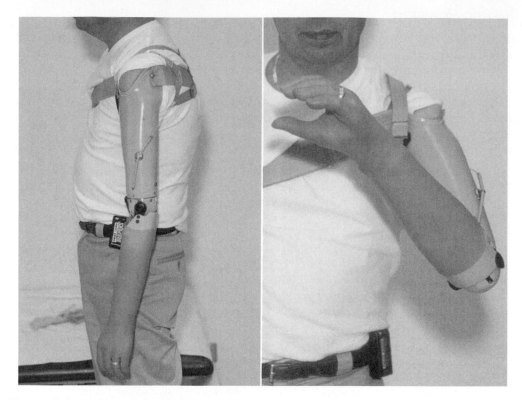

**Fig. 16-3** A hybrid transhumeral prosthesis. The mechanical elbow is linked to the body by a control cable and harness and is positioned by forward flexion of the arm at the shoulder. The electric-powered hand is controlled by myoelectric signals produced by contracting remaining portions of the biceps and triceps muscles in the residual limb.

residual biceps and triceps muscles. A person is often able to produce coordinated movement of the components of a hybrid prosthesis because the control sources are independent of one another.

## Special Function

Prosthetists construct special-function prostheses for a particular activity, commonly a sport. These prostheses tend to be constructed for the activity and are rarely physiologic in appearance, functioning more like tools. Examples include prostheses with swimming paddles or special attachments for people to handle bows or rifles. Some people also use special-function prostheses to drive cars and motorcycles or to pilot airplanes. These prostheses typically serve as extensions of the residual limb for people to use the controls in vehicles.

All prostheses use a socket and suspension system to secure the prosthetic components to the body. The socket, generally made of plastic or composite materials, encloses the distal limb segment, stabilizing the prosthesis on the limb. The socket also allows for the transfer and distribution of forces over the limb surface while pushing, pulling, or holding something with the prosthesis. Depending on the level of the amputation and type of components the prosthetist uses, the socket may be suspended by the bony structures of the joint proximal to the amputation site, by atmospheric suspension using airtight elastomer sleeves, or by straps securing the prosthesis to the upper torso.

## Functional Limitations

Because most arm amputations occur in early or middle adulthood and result from trauma rather than disease, a person is likely to be in good health at the time of the amputation. This contrasts with persons who have lower limb amputations. These are generally people more than age 50 at the time of amputation who have had the amputation because of the effects of a prolonged systemic disease. A person with an arm amputation may also be ambulatory, with an intact arm and hand. Consequently, this person is able to move about and perform many one-handed activities. Such a person has retained many abilities and is not hampered in the rehabilitation process by the debilitating effects of disease.

However, the specialists involved should not assume that a person is in good health after the amputation and therefore retains the functional capabilities typical of a person of similar age and physical build. In addition to the status of a person's general health before and after the amputation, the traumatic event that resulted in the amputation may have caused other injuries to the body, possibly involving the joints proximal to the amputation level, the contralateral limb, the lower limbs, and/or the spine. Associated injuries are likely in motor vehicle accidents and encounters with powerful equipment such as farm machinery. The presence of coincident musculoskeletal injuries compound and sometimes overshadow functional limitations resulting from the amputation. Sensory deficits before or resulting from the trauma, especially those involving vision, touch, or kinesthesia, also affect the level at which a person can function and the options for prosthetic restoration.

Persons with bilateral arm amputations, especially proximal to the elbow or with upper and lower limb amputations, have lost a significant amount of body surface area. These people generally cannot give off heat as readily as people without amputations. Therefore they may be susceptible to overheating and have limited tolerance for sustained activity, particularly in warm environments.

## Prerequisite Skills and Abilities

Among the types of upper-limb prostheses, most combine active and passive components to provide a prehension device and the joints for positioning and orienting the device.

*Passive components* refer to devices that a person can grasp and position directly with the contralateral hand if the amputation occurs on only one side. Consequently, the condition of the contralateral limb is crucial to the quick and efficient positioning of these components. Alternatively, a person may push or pull these components against a part of the body or some stable object in the environment. This, however, is generally more cumbersome and intrudes more on the task that a person performs.

*Active components* refer to the body-powered or electric-powered devices that some action associated with the same side of the body as the amputation site, usually the residual limb, positions or controls. The controlling action might be movement of the residual limb segment, force that the limb segment produces with minimal movement, or myoelectric signals that muscles produce either in the limb segment through which the amputation has been made or by muscles in the torso if the amputation is through the shoulder. A sufficient number of control sources (or actions) must exist for the intended active components. The control sources should be reliable and under consistent voluntary control and preferably independent of one another. The sources should also not interfere with the use or function of other intact limbs.

A user operating a prosthetic component must have the cognitive ability to correlate the action of a physiologic control source with the operation of that component. A prosthesis with multiple active components also requires a user to be able to coordinate multiple control sources or sequence the use of a single control source.

Persistent pain is sometimes also a consequence of the traumatic injury that resulted in the amputation. A person experiencing severe pain cannot be expected to use a prosthesis well or consistently. The physician should effectively manage a person's pain first but without significantly impairing cognitive ability.

## Considerations, Options, and Technology

As in the application of any assistive technology, the specialists involved must determine the goals and objectives of the intended user and weigh the technical options according to the likelihood of a person meeting those objectives. The decisions, however, should not be left entirely to a user. A person with a recently acquired amputation is going to have difficulty visualizing the way life will be and the way various prosthetic choices might affect life. Fears of incapacity and concerns with body image and reactions of family and friends will be prominent feelings for a person. Education and support are essential for a person to put those concerns into perspective and are the foundation for realistic decision making.

The rehabilitation team, which includes the physician, the prosthetist, the occupational therapist, the social worker, the vocational counselor, and others, are responsible for providing their patients information, materials, and opportunities to educate them about choices and possibilities. Brochures illustrating componentry and photographs of persons with prostheses are useful and can be helpful for the team as visual references for discussion. However, opportunities to meet people who have similar amputations and life circumstances can have a far greater influence on patients achieving perspective. If the team does not know appropriate persons who can serve as peer counselors, they can sometimes find people through support groups representing or serving persons with amputations. Of course, the team is more likely to find a peer counselor in a highly populated area. Instructional videos of and by persons with amputations are available from a number of sources, and people can use them when peers are not an option or as an additional resource.

The team must also learn about the patient. They should make a detailed physical assessment of the person's health. They should functionally assess the strength and range of motion of all remaining joints of the affected and unaffected limbs. They should also make a psychologic assessment, especially in the case of a person with a recently acquired amputation. Successful prosthetic restoration depends on a person's willingness to actively participate in the decision making and evaluation of prosthetic options. A person's unresolved fears and anger or a passive attitude only impedes or negates any possibility of success. The team must also become informed about the person's social environment, home situation, and education or vocational setting to make appropriate recommendations.

## Technical and Clinical Expertise

A certified prosthetist (CP) that the American Board for Certification in Orthotics and Prosthetics (ABC) accredits should develop and fit the prosthesis. CPs are trained through an accredited university program followed by a 12-month residency. At the completion of training, a comprehensive three-part examination that the ABC administers tests their competency. Only those who pass are permitted to identify themselves as certified prosthetists and use the initials CP.

Individual CPs may not have the opportunity to work with many persons with arm amputations because the number of such persons is considerably smaller than those with leg and foot amputations. A person with an arm amputation should seek out a CP who has become skilled in upper-limb prosthetic fittings and is familiar with a broad range of componentry and control options.

A certified and licensed occupational therapist should carry out the training and use of a prosthesis. The therapist should be familiar with persons with upper-limb amputations or work under the supervision of a therapist with this experience. The therapist should also be knowledgeable about the components and control methods that the CP implemented for the individual user and know the capabilities and limitations of the prosthetic system.

The therapy protocol is generally designed to improve a person's control of the prosthesis, help a person achieve competency in common daily activities, and address a user's functional goals. In addition to training in the use of the prosthesis, the therapist also trains a user to accomplish common tasks without the prosthesis and advises in the use of adapted equipment to augment function with or without the prosthesis.

The relatively low incidence of persons with bilateral amputations suggests that most CPs and therapists do not have experience with these individuals. These persons, especially those with bilateral amputations proximal to the elbow, can often receive superior service at one of several centers specializing in bilateral fittings.

## General Considerations

When providing services to children, the therapist should consider their age and developmental readiness for different prosthetic options. Although many more components are currently available for children than 10 years ago, it is still true that within any category of components, such as prehension devices, wrist units, and elbow mechanisms, fewer types are available for children than for adults. Of those available, the force and range of motion requirements to operate some components may be greater than the norm for younger children or even for a particular older child. Complex control procedures or sequences for multiple components may be inappropriate for the normal cognitive level of young children.

Any movement impairment of the child's or adult's proximal joints of the residual limb or in the ability to exert forces with the residual limb affects the control options and types of components that the prosthetist can consider for the prosthesis. A person's inability to contract the muscles of the residual limb—to produce myoelectric signals—or reliably and consistently control the contraction of those muscles also influences control and component choices.

The prosthetist has more difficulty providing prosthetic restoration for more proximal or higher levels of limb loss or absence. In these situations, the prosthetist has to replace more physiologic joints with analogous prosthetic joints but have enough control sources to operate all the components. Also, greater tactile and kinesthetic sensory loss exists, which typically increases the mental effort that a person needs to manipulate and handle objects effectively. For similar reasons, a person has more difficulty if both arms are involved (bilateral arm amputations) or if one arm has an amputation and the other is neurologically or orthopedically impaired.

Persons with amputations resulting from thermal or electrical burns may have difficulty wearing prostheses comfortably because of injuries to the skin surfaces touching the sockets or suspension systems of the prostheses. Wearing a prosthesis may not be possible for some people because of discomfort or fragility of skin. The prosthetist takes special care during the initial phases of fitting the prosthesis to assess a person's tolerance and the integrity of the skin. For this reason, the CP often constructs diagnostic prostheses of clear socket materials so that the therapist can monitor the condition of the skin during use. Improvements in skin grafting, skin expansion and coverage, and new socket interface materials have enabled more persons with burn injuries to use prostheses.

Although prostheses may move like physiologic limbs, they lack the kinesthetic and tactile sensory systems of limbs. The prosthesis user perceives forces through the socket interface and control harnessing and uses those perceptions during activities. Vision, however, remains a critical factor in a person's ability to use the prosthesis effectively. Consequently, a person with blindness or poor vision finds that arm and hand prostheses do not help much.

A person with cognitive impairment may not be able to understand the relationship between a required control action and a desired action of a prosthetic component. The difficulty is compounded by the absent or reduced sensory feedback from the prosthetic limb. This can be true of a person with a developmental impairment or someone who sustained a head injury during the trauma that resulted in the amputation such as a motor vehicle accident. Cognitive impairment associated with stroke or disease affecting the brain could also render a previously successful and consistent prosthesis user unable to use the device effectively. Drugs (medical or otherwise) may also temporarily interfere with the cognitive ability a person needs to use a prosthesis.

## Technical Considerations

The prosthesis should assist a user and not be an additional impairment. A person needs to have training in the functional use of a prosthesis. For a person with a newly acquired amputation, the prosthesis is an unfamiliar tool, even if a person participated in its selection and implementation. A person's ability to actuate or operate the prosthetic components does not necessarily translate into functional use. A person needs supervised guidance and assistance in problem solving to provide the basic skills that lead to proficiency.

In choosing components, the prosthetist should consider compatibility with a user's environment. For example, myoelectric control systems are susceptible to electromagnetic interference from electrical equipment and transmission sources. The degree of susceptibility depends on the type of system used, the type of interference source, the proximity to the interference, and the implementation of the control system within the prosthesis. Therefore the prosthetist may have a difficult time knowing in advance if interference will be a problem in a suspect environment but the prosthetist can use a diagnostic prosthesis to evaluate the susceptibility. As another example, because most prosthetic components are not sealed against moisture, a user should not expose them to water, especially salt water. This is particularly true for motorized components and electronic controllers. CPs make some special-function prostheses that persons use for swimming or sail boarding that are designed for the water environment. The prosthetist should also consider the documented performance of components under consideration. Newer components with limited clinical application are best used for persons who will be tolerant of possible problems.

All used prostheses require service or adjustment occasionally. A user should be aware of the typical service turnaround times for different systems and the availability of loaner components or backup prostheses. A user, family members, or friends might be able to make simple repairs such as replacement of mechanical control cables or lubrication of parts. More complex repairs or adjustments in the socket or suspension likely require a person to travel to the CP. If users have to travel long distances or make difficult travel arrangements, they may desire systems that presumably require fewer adjustments.

A prosthesis is not just a function of manipulation. It is a tool that is worn by a person, which the CP intimately couples to the body. As such, the prosthesis reflects the qualities and attitude of a user. Therefore the prosthesis also serves the function of appearance, presenting a user in certain ways.

Different people weigh the two functions of manipulation and appearance differently when choosing the characteristics of their prostheses and never completely disregard one for the other. Almost all users have had to accept trading aspects of one function to achieve some preferred level in the other. For many persons, the tradeoff in either manipulative function or the function of appearance becomes unacceptable in a single prosthesis. These people are most successful with two or more prostheses intended for different purposes. Each prosthesis embodies different characteristics that emphasize either the manipulative or appearance functions.

## *Technology*

### No Tech

At the no-tech level, a person forgoes the use of a prosthesis or any equipment the therapist might suggest to adapt for use. This person relies on remaining physiologic function and the nonadapted tools, utensils, and appliances available to the general populace. Adults with unilateral congenital limb deficiencies below the level of the elbow often are functional without any specialized assistive devices, prostheses or otherwise. A person with acquired amputations who takes this approach, particularly with higher-level and bilateral amputations, generally requires help from family members and caregivers to implement certain activities (sometimes routine).

### Low Tech

Persons who opt for the low-tech approach use special tools that extend the range of the residual limb, allow them to hold objects in proximity to the limb (such as a utensil cuff), or provide an opposition surface against which they grasp an object with the residual limb. Relatively simple modifications to the environment such as adapted kitchen utensils or extensions on appliance controls to facilitate their operation also qualify as low tech.

## High Tech

High tech involves componentry that requires a person to use specialized tools or material treatments to construct and replace and requires a skilled and experienced practitioner to implement them effectively. It is a misunderstanding of technology to equate high tech with whether a device is newly designed or decades old, is more or less expensive, or is mechanically operated by body movement or by a motor and battery. Prosthetic components of all kinds are highly technical devices, and prostheses are highly technical systems. They require specialized training to design, implement, and maintain.

## Prehension Devices

Prosthetic components that provide a user with prehension, or the function of grasp, have many categories. One of the more obvious divisions is between devices that appear similar to the physiologic hand and devices that do not.

Hand-like devices can be passive, mechanically actuated, or electric powered. Passive prosthetic hands, sometimes called *cosmetic hands,* have no mechanism for active grasp and primarily create the appearance of a physiologic hand. Although an object cannot be grasped directly, a person can push lightweight objects between the opposing thumb and fingers, and the compliance of the prosthetic digits can retain it. Some passive hands also incorporate an armature of wire or metal linkages. This allows a user to shape the position of the fingers of the prosthetic hand using the contralateral intact hand. A passive hand can be made to look remarkably similar to the physiologic hand through appropriate shaping, coloring, and using artificial hair and nails. In general, the more closely the hand matches the physiologic hand, the more expensive it is because of the skill and time to achieve the lifelike effect.

Mechanically actuated prosthetic hands and electric-powered hands generally use similar arrangements of thumb and finger mechanisms to produce three-point grasp patterns with the distal palmar surfaces of the thumbs opposing the distal palmar surfaces of the index and middle fingers. Studies have shown that this prehension pattern, referred to as *palmar prehension,* is the most common pattern that a person uses for the dominant and nondominant physiologic hands.

A person cannot move the thumb alone or move individual fingers with commercially available prosthetic hands. Typically, the thumb and fingers are linked to move simultaneously when a person opens and closes the hand. Some mechanical hands use a stationary thumb, with only the fingers moving as a unit to open or close.

As with all body-powered components, a cable linkage to a control harness that a user wears over the upper body actuates mechanical hands with arm or shoulder motion on the amputated side. Hands can either be voluntary opening or voluntary closing. Voluntary-opening hands are operated by pulling on the control cable and closed with springs when the control cable is relaxed. The force of the spring determines the maximal prehension force. Voluntary-opening prosthetic hands can hold an object without effort because the spring provides the closing force.

Persons close voluntary-closing hands by pulling on the control cable and open them with a low-force spring when they relax the cable. The prehension force is determined by how hard a user is pulling on the control cable. Voluntary-closing hands require that a user maintain tension on the cable to hold an object within the hand. Although effort is required to hold objects, voluntary-closing hands provide a user with a perception of the grip force because that force is proportional to the force with which a user is pulling on the control cable.

Mechanical hands have a relatively low efficiency or mechanical advantage compared with non–hand-like mechanical prehension devices. Because of the hand-like shape, the lever arrangement of the mechanism is constrained, resulting in operating forces that are much greater than the prehension force. Consequently, few people elect to use mechanical hands.

Electric-powered hands use motors that batteries power to actuate the thumb/finger mechanism and generate the prehension force. Some motorized hands can achieve grip force for palmar prehension comparable with that of the physiologic hand of the average adult male, about 111 N (25 lb-force). A variety of control options are available for a person to operate the hands. A person most commonly uses myoelectric control or switch control. With myoelectric control, a person is able to have proportional control of the speed of movement of the fingers and the rate at which prehension force increases once grasping an object. Stronger contractions of the controlling muscles produce faster movement and a quick buildup of force; weaker contractions produce slower movement and a slow buildup of force. Neither switch control nor myoelectric control gives a user any direct perception of contact with an object and the grip force a person exerts. Users watch the response of their hands and the objects they grasp and gauge their controlling actions based on what they see and on previous experience with similar objects.

Plastic-molded gloves that give the appearance of the hand's skin surface cover mechanical hands and electric-powered hands. Gloves are made of either polyvinyl chloride (PVC) or silicone and are available in a variety of colors approximating various skin tones. Although PVC gloves are durable, common substances such as ink, dyes, and grease can stain them. Silicone gloves are less durable but do not easily stain. Gloves can be color customized, but the process is expensive and must be redone each time a user replaces them.

The other category of prehension devices, called *nonhand prehensors,* are those that do not resemble the physiologic hand. These devices offer different prehension patterns from prosthetic hands and have more durable surfaces and construction. People prefer them in environments that might damage the cosmetic covering of a hand-like device. As with prosthetic hands, nonhand prehensors are available as either mechanical devices that body-power actuates or as electric-powered devices. The mechanical nonhand prehensors can be either voluntary opening or voluntary closing. These devices are more efficient than mechanical hands and have a higher ratio of prehension force to operating force. They can also be lighter than electric-powered hands and obstruct less of the work area visually because of their streamlined utilitarian shapes.

The cable-actuated split hook is the most common nonhand prehensor with the voluntary-opening version more common than all other prosthetic prehension devices (hand-like devices and nonhand devices) in North America. Rubber bands or springs provide the closing force, and the number of bands or springs determines the maximal grip force. Although the number of bands a person uses varies, most persons use four to six bands that give a prehension force of about 27 to 40 N (6 to 9 lb-force). Split-hook prehension devices are available in a variety of sizes and styles with different finger shapes, rubber-lined gripping surfaces, and modifications to facilitate a person holding hand tools. They are typically made of aluminum or steel (aluminum is lighter, but steel is more durable).

Nonhand devices that voluntarily close are also available in a variety of forms, including a version with hook-like fingers. The grip force depends on the force with which a person is pulling the control cable. Strong individuals can readily achieve grip forces at the finger tips in excess of 222 N (50 lb-force). As with voluntary-closing mechanical hands, nonhand devices that voluntarily close provide a user with a perception of the force being applied to the object.

People use nonhand devices that are electric powered either when they need compatibility with electric-powered hands or when hand-like devices are inappropriate but they need higher grip forces or different control arrangements than can be achieved with voluntary-opening split-hook devices. In the former case, a user interchanges the prosthetic hand and nonhand device according to the type of task (Figure 16-4). In the latter case, the shape and prehension patterns of an electric hand may not meet the user's needs. This is often the situation with persons who need bilateral upper-limb amputa-

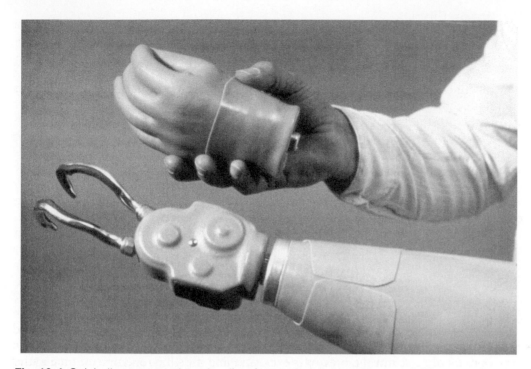

**Fig. 16-4** Quick disconnect wrist units allow for one-handed interchange of different prehension devices. The units incorporate mechanical and electrical couplings.

tions. Several models of nonhand, electric-powered devices are available, and each model has its own unique characteristic.

Another category of devices that a person uses as a substitute for functions of the physiologic hand but which are not prehension devices because they do not have a grasp mechanism are tools or adapters designed for specific purposes and are commonly referred to as *terminal devices*. A person may use them for example to attach a camera to the end of a prosthetic forearm or use them to interconnect modified hand tools with the wrist unit of the forearm. A variety of devices of this kind are made for a number of specialized applications, including sports and recreation.

## Wrist Units

Prosthetic wrist units are designed to provide a user with a mechanism for attaching the prehension or terminal device to the prosthetic forearm. They also incorporate a rotation joint and for some units a flexion joint for orienting the prehensor.

Wrist rotation units are available that a user can position manually, by cable actuation with body movement or by electric power. A person selects the particular type of unit for use based on compatibility with the prehension device, the length of the residual limb if the amputation level is transradial (through the forearm), and the availability of a control source to operate the wrist if it is not manually positioned.

Wrist flexion units are only available as mechanical devices that a person manually positions or by body-powered cable actuation. The most common units offer several positions of flexion in which a person can lock the unit. Flexion devices are generally more useful to a person with bilateral amputations than to a person with a unilateral amputation. They are especially helpful in the performance of body-centered tasks such as dressing, engaging in oral and facial hygiene, toileting, and shaving.

Ball and socket wrist units provide the greatest variation for a person orienting the prehension device. These friction-type joints generally do not hold their position securely enough for adult use, although they are adequate in a cosmetic limb. They are most useful for children who need to rotate, flex, and deviate their prehension devices to engage bicycle handlebars and other play equipment.

## Prosthetic Elbows

Several categories of prosthetic elbows are available, including manually positioned elbows, mechanical body-powered elbows, and electric-powered elbows. Manually positioned elbows incorporate locking mechanisms so that a person can maintain the position of the elbow at a desired angle of flexion. The contralateral hand is intended to operate the lock mechanism. Typically, a person uses a manually positioned elbow with a cosmetic prosthesis. Therefore the most common design is a modular (or endoskeletal) elbow with a shaped foam cover. The lock is activated with a lever placed along the medial side of the forearm tube (or pylon). With one motion, a user can grasp the forearm to unlock the elbow, reposition the forearm, and relock the elbow. Manually positioned elbows with shell-like forearms (exoskeletal design) are also available. A person who wants the convenience of a manually positioned elbow but needs a more durable external covering typically uses these.

A person positions body-powered elbows with a control cable that the CP attaches to the prosthetic forearm (near the elbow axis) at one end, routes across the shoulder joint, and attaches to a body harness at the other end. Flexion of the arm at the shoulder or scapular abduction moves the elbow. A locking mechanism maintains the position of the elbow. In a transhumeral fitting, a separate control cable that a CP routes along the anterior surface of the upper arm and anchors to the same body harness that is used to suspend the prosthesis actuates the lock. A complex motion involving depression of the shoulder and abduction and extension of the arm cycles the lock mechanism. This arrangement of two control cables, one for positioning the elbow and one for cycling the elbow lock, is called the *dual control system*. In a shoulder disarticulation fitting, a CP routes the elbow lock control cable to a control lever, called a *nudge control*, that is mounted on the socket and actuates with the chin.

A CP that uses the control cable to position a body-powered elbow can also route the cable more distally and attach it to the control attachment of a cable-operated prehension device that voluntarily opens (Figure 16-5). When the elbow is unlocked, a user's control motions position the elbow. When the elbow is locked, the same control motions open the prehensor.

The harness and control system of a body-powered elbow provides a user with direct feedback of the action of the elbow. During flexion, the movement of the prosthetic elbow is directly coupled to the movement of a user's controlling arm or shoulder joint. Therefore the position and speed of a user's physiologic joint determine the position and

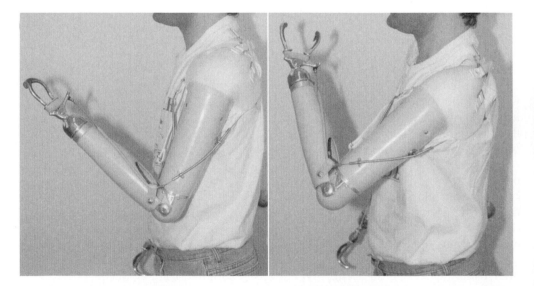

**Fig. 16-5** A body-powered transhumeral prosthesis. Forward flexion of the arm at the shoulder pulls on the control cable anchored to the body harness. When the elbow is unlocked, this motion causes the elbow to flex. With the elbow locked, flexion of the arm at the shoulder causes the split hook to open.

speed of the elbow. The user immediately feels forces exerted on the prosthetic forearm and elbow through the connecting control cable. This proprioceptive feedback of position, speed, and force is one of the chief advantages of a person using body-powered devices that cables actuate.

The lever arrangement of the prosthetic forearm, body-powered elbow, and control cable constrains the amount of weight a user can lift with elbow flexion. A typical setup requires forces on the control cable 8 to 10 times greater than the force equivalent to the weight of the object that a person lifts. Most users are therefore limited to objects weighing less than ½ kg (about 1 lb). People can only lift heavier objects using leg and trunk movements while they keep the elbows locked.

People can use electric-powered elbows to achieve greater lifting capacity. They are also advantageous to persons who do not have the force and shoulder range of motion they need to operate body-powered elbows.

A person can operate electric elbows with a variety of electronic controllers, but myoelectric control and switch control are the most common. At the transhumeral amputation level, a person could possibly use remnants of the biceps and triceps muscles for myoelectric control. At the shoulder disarticulation level, a person could possibly use the pectoralis major and infraspinatus muscles or a remnant of the deltoid muscle, if the surgeon preserved it. A person could actuate a switch controller by flexion of the arm at the shoulder or by scapular abduction. Although these are the same movements that a person uses to operate a body-powered elbow, a person's range of motion and actuating force to operate a switch is considerably less.

Some electric elbows incorporate controllers that integrate operation of the elbow with operation of an electric prehension device and/or electric wrist rotator. In these systems, a person is able to use the same control source or action to operate each device, but sequentially. Although a person's coordinated motion of more than one component is not possible, this arrangement can be useful when control sources are few.

Two primary disadvantages exist for electric elbows, first of which is their weight. The elbow mechanism, controller, and battery pack alone can weigh approximately 0.7 to 0.9 kg (1½ to 2 lb). The second disadvantage is the limited feedback to a user. Controllers that a person commonly uses with electric elbows do not provide the position, speed, and force feedback that is available to a user of a cable-actuated mechanical elbow. Electric elbows, as is the case with any motorized component, are more expensive to purchase and maintain than mechanical components.

## Humeral Rotation Mechanisms

A humeral rotation joint for inward and outward rotation of the forearm about the axis of the upper arm is generally provided in the design of prosthetic elbows. The joint is typically an adjustable friction joint incorporated where the elbow is secured to the upper arm segment. A person with a unilateral amputation pushes or pulls the forearm to change its position. Persons with bilateral amputations use objects in the environment or their trunk or legs to push or pull against.

Locking humeral rotation units are also available but they are not as well known and people use them less commonly. Mechanisms that lock are most advantageous to persons with bilateral amputations. When locked, the device contributes to the prosthesis becoming an extension of users' bodies through which they can exert high forces. If CPs were to adjust friction components to resist high external forces, users would have difficulty changing their position when needed.

## Mechanical Shoulders

All commercial shoulder joints are mechanical and manually positioned. Most shoulders use friction joints that are either arranged as compound joints with flexion/extension and abduction/adduction or as ball and socket joints. One type of shoulder joint provides locked positions in flexion/extension (abduction/adduction is friction) and is most appropriate for persons with bilateral amputations or persons with unilateral shoulder disarticulations who want the advantage of easy positioning but high resistance against external forces.

## Outcomes and Social Validation

### Measuring Success

A specialist can use many approaches to measure successful implementation of upper-limb prosthetics from counting the number of hours a person wears a prosthesis to quantifying performance on standardized manipulation tasks to asking the person if the quality of life has improved. These approaches are useful because each one offers a specialist a part of an answer about the value and importance of prostheses as assistive tools. But, a specialist can often measure success of an individual user's device by getting answers to the following three questions:

1. Does it have an acceptable appearance?
2. Is it comfortable to use?
3. Can anything be done better with it than without it?

A person's successful restoration of manipulative function can only be possible if the CP considers comfort and appearance in the design and fitting of the prosthesis. If the user is physically uncomfortable wearing or using the prosthesis or if it causes pain, the user is likely to underuse or reject it. If the control of the prosthesis places an undue burden on the user's attention, which is a distraction from performing needed actions, the user is not likely to incorporate the prosthesis into activities. Finally, and to many users most importantly, if the prosthesis' appearance is not acceptable, the user will not use it. For some users, an acceptable appearance is having the prosthesis closely match the look of physiologic limbs, as much as possible. Other users prefer a more technical or nonphysiologic appearance.

If people like their appearance with the prosthesis and find them comfortable to use, they are likely to wear them even if they do not use them much as a manipulative assist. However, if the prosthesis' appearance is not acceptable for the user and wearing it is uncomfortable, the person will rarely use it regardless of how much it improves manipulative abilities.

When a CP successfully fits a person with a prothesis, the success is likely temporary. This is especially true for a person who has recently experienced traumatic limb amputation and who may have considerable difficulty setting priorities and realizing the implications of certain prosthesis choices. Over time, changes in a user's perspective, physical abilities, or circumstances and in available componentry and implementation encourage the user to reassess the factors that culminated in the selection of the prosthesis, which the person is using or has given up using. When a CP must refabricate a prosthesis (generally every 3 to 5 years for an adult) because of cumulative wear and tear or because of a child's growth, the user should reconsider the choices. No definitive prosthesis exists. Prosthetic restoration or augmentation is a dynamic process that occurs over a person's lifetime. It should be periodically punctuated by reassessment and fabrication of a new prosthesis.

### Social and Demographic Trends

Trauma is the leading cause of upper-limb amputations. Therefore the reduction in trauma incidences will likely reduce the number of persons who have upper-limb amputations. Better safety requirements and greater attention to existing requirements in certain occupations can reduce injuries. Occupations of particular concern are farm work, high-voltage electrical work, machine operation in manufacturing plants, and construction work. Improvements in highway safety and gun control will also likely reduce the number tf persons with arm amputations. Avoiding or reducing the number of major military conflicts will also decrease the incidence of amputations. Specialists often do not know the cause or causes of congenital limb deficiencies. As long as they do not understand the underlying mechanism, the incidence of limb deficiencies is likely to persist.

## CASE STUDIES

### CASE 1

D.J. was a business executive and sailing enthusiast who was injured in a power-boating accident, resulting in a unilateral amputation of the nondominant limb at the transradial level. He was concerned about his appearance in his business dealings and expected to continue sailing.

The business and sailing environments presented different demands on prosthetic restoration that a single prosthesis could not curb. Appearance was paramount in the business environment, and manipulative ability and exposure to water were critical factors in the sailing environment.

The "business prosthesis" served as D.J.'s general-use prosthesis. A specialist team recommended an electric-powered hand to achieve prehension function and hand-like appearance. Because the amputation was in the middle or proximal third of the forearm, the CP was able to incorporate an electric wrist rotator, otherwise the CP would have to install a manually positioned wrist. A proportional myoelectric controller controlled the hand and the rotator sequentially from two muscle sites. The socket was self-suspending using a supracondylar design. The CP finished the prosthesis with a custom-colored glove to match the appearance of the contralateral hand.

D.J. needed active prehension in the "sailing prosthesis," but electric components do not hold up in the water environment. The specialist team recommended a body-powered prehension device that voluntarily closes to provide the possibility of high-grip forces and perception of the applied force. D.J. used a nonhand prehensor for greater mechanical efficiency. To prepare for the possibility of a different prehensor or specialized terminal devices, the CP incorporated a quick disconnect wrist. Suspension was atmospheric using a silicone sleeve that locked into the prosthetic forearm. The only harness proximal to the elbow was a figure-9 harness that anchored the prehensor control cable to the contralateral shoulder.

The loss of the nondominant limb was significant because D.J. did not have to transfer the dexterous skills of the dominant hand, especially writing and artistic manipulation, to the remaining physiologic limb. His touch-typing skills and ability to play a musical instrument, which are bimanual dexterous activities, were affected; therefore he had to consider alternative techniques.

### CASE 2

L.O., a farmer, had an accident with a piece of equipment that resulted in a unilateral amputation of the dominant arm at the transhumeral level. His primary concern was to continue farming.

A specialist team recommended a complete body-powered prosthesis with a split-hook prehensor that voluntarily opened and a heavy-duty mechanical elbow. The heavy-duty elbow had fewer locked positions than the standard mechanical elbow but was more rugged and could withstand heavier loading. A quick disconnect wrist allowed for interchange of adapted tools and other voluntary-opening prehension devices. The CP suspended the prosthesis with a chest strap harness and shoulder saddle. The shoulder saddle secured the prosthesis against downward displacement under heavy loading and distributed lifting forces over a wider area of the body.

Because L.O.'s amputation was through the distal third of the upper arm, he had sufficient leverage to use a farmer's split hook. This device had adaptations to accommodate hand tools but was heavier, was made of stainless steel, and was rugged. The quick disconnect wrist unit also offered the possibility of L.O. using a cosmetic hand for certain situations. The CP installed an anchor on the forearm to secure the control cable when L.O. used the hand.

Alternatively, a second prosthesis of hybrid design might have been useful. This prosthesis would have had an electric-powered hand that L.O. controlled myoelectrically using the biceps and triceps muscles. The elbow would have been mechanical and cable actuated. A counterbalancing unit in the forearm would have reduced the force needed to lift the forearm and hand and increase the weight of objects that L.O. could have lifted.

## CASE 3
An electrical worker, S.F., had traumatic loss of both limbs at the transhumeral level. No impairment of shoulder motion existed.

The specialist team suggested likely success with bilateral body-powered prostheses that incorporated cable-actuated mechanical elbows, locking wrist rotation units, locking wrist flexion units, and split-hook prehensors that voluntarily opened because of experience with bilateral fittings at this level. S.F. needed the flexion units to facilitate body-centered activities because he was bilaterally involved.

The locking wrist and elbow components allowed the CP to use a single control cable to position all four components using the same control motion. S.F. actuated the lock for the elbow through the control and suspension harness using the complex shoulder motion. S.F. actuated the lock for the wrist rotator by a lock reciprocator mounted in the forearm by pressing a lever, extending from the side of the forearm against the torso. The lock release for the wrist flexion unit extended from the base of the unit, and S.F. operated it by pushing it against the side of the body or leg.

If the elbow and wrist units were locked, S.F. pulling on the control cable using flexion of the arm or biscapular abduction opened the split hook. If the elbow was unlocked, S.F. pulling on the cable flexed the elbow and relaxing the cable allowed the elbow to extend with gravity. If the wrist rotator was unlocked, S.F. pulling on the control cable supinated the wrist. His relaxation of the cable allowed a spring within the forearm to pronate the wrist. When he unlocked the wrist flexion unit, S.F. pulling on the control cable pulled the unit into flexion and relaxing the cable allowed a rubber band to pull it back into extension. Both prostheses were set up the same way, and the CP connected them with a figure-8 harness for suspension and control.

## Suggested Reading

Atkins DJ, Heard DCY, Donovan WH: Epidemiologic overview of individuals with upper-limb loss and their reported research priorities, *J Prosthet Orthot* 8:2-11, 1996.

Atkins DJ, Meier RH: *Comprehensive management of the upper-limb amputee*, New York, 1989, Springer-Verlag.

Bowker JH, Michael JW: *Atlas of limb prosthetics: surgical, prosthetic, and rehabilitation principles*, St Louis, 1992, Mosby.

Mooney RL: *The handbook: information for new upper extremity amputees, their families, and friends*, Lomita, Calif, 1995, Mutual Aid Amputee Foundation.

# CHAPTER 17

# Robotics and Manipulators

*Richard F. ff. Weir*

Although numerous researchers have taken initiatives to develop robotic aids for persons with significant disabilities, few of these initiatives have resulted in commercially available devices. However, research and development must occur for products in the field of medical manipulators and rehabilitation robotics to be available. The main barrier to the success of these devices and the dominant area of research has been the control interface. For example, how does a person with high-level quadriplegia who can barely move the head control a mechanical arm that may have shoulder rotation, humeral rotation, elbow flexion or extension, wrist supination or pronation, wrist rotation, and a hand or terminal device that opens and closes? The level of available technology and the degree of the user's physical impairment determine the control interface. Other factors affecting this interface are the proposed tasks, projected cost, aesthetics, and operator safety.

Medical manipulators or rehabilitation robots are considered a special class of artificial limb replacement, and many of the same issues apply to these devices as artificial limbs. Rehabilitation manipulators are generally mechanical arms that attempt to allow persons with high-level quadriplegia to interact with their environment. Because the primary benefactors of this technology have severe disabilities, the current generation of devices cannot replace caregivers. Rather, these robotic aids augment personal care and possibly provide some independence by enabling persons to perform limited numbers of activities of daily living (ADL). Psychologic makeup of the individual often determines the benefit of these devices. For some people, the extra time and effort involved in using these devices is vital to their sense of self and psychologic well being. But for another individual, the independence these devices might afford may not be important.

Computer-controlled wheelchairs with obstacle avoidance and automatic navigation capabilities are another class of rehabilitation robots. The main beneficiaries of these "intelligent" wheelchairs are persons with severe mobility disabilities, such as serious spasticity (cerebral palsy), excessively weak residual physical capacities (tetrapelgia), or some cognitive impairments (head trauma). Conventional wheelchairs sometimes cannot aid these conditions. Researchers also are exploring robot-assisted surgery (e.g., total joint replacement)[1] and the use of robots in the treatment of people undergoing range-of-motion physical therapy.[2,3] Rehabilitation robotics range from robotic manipulators and intelligent wheelchairs to dedicated interfaces for household and vocational devices. This chapter is limited primarily to information about medical manipulators and intelligent wheelchairs.

## Application and Goal

The primary objective of rehabilitation robotics is the full or part restoration of a disabled user's manipulative function through the use of a robot arm or manipulator. Unlike traditional industrial robots, which run under program control, the user operates the manipulator from within the manipulator's own workspace. This enables the user to directly interact with the environment.

Persons with disabilities may use these devices to help them eat, wash, and perform other ADL either with or without the aid of a personal attendant. For safety reasons, manipulators used in rehabilitation are smaller and have less power and thus less physical capabilities than their industrial counterparts. In addition, more stringent sensory and computational requirements are needed to ensure operator safety. Safety is always a primary concern when a person has to coexist within the workspace of a robot because a robot is only as good as its controlling program and is a rigid object. If the program crashes and the robot goes out of control, a person could be seriously injured if the requisite fail-safe mechanisms such as physical range of motion "stops" and supervisory program control are not present.

In theory, the ideal outcome of manipulator application is for a person to have complete restoration of manipulative function. In practice, the device is deemed successful if it can help the user to perform limited daily routines such as grooming and eating or if use of a dedicated workstation enables a user to return to work. The ultimate test of whether a device is successful is if it benefits users and consequently they use it regularly. Disabilities based on partial or total loss of upper-limb function are particularly serious because of the consequent reduction or loss of manipulative function. This kind of disability is the most significant impediment to people accomplishing common, everyday activities such as personal hygiene, work, and hobbies. When a person also has reduction of or loss of lower limb function, the physical and psychologic loss of control is profound, and the disabled user becomes dependent on others in virtually every respect. Rehabilitation robotics tries to alleviate this situation by using manipulators to restore manipulative function and intelligent wheelchairs to provide mobility.

## Function and Ability

To use this technology, the user must have sufficient means to control each joint or degree of freedom (DOF) of any given device. Possible control sources include voice control, air pressure in the mouth (sip and puff), and head, body, or trunk movement. Other possibilities include the following:

- Myoelectric control: Isolated and controllable electric signals generated as a byproduct of normal muscle contraction
- Ocular tracking: Monitoring of the position of the eyeballs
- EEGs: The electric signals detected on the surfaces of the skull emitted as a byproduct of the brain's natural functioning

All these schemes assume potential users have sufficient cognitive abilities to correlate physiologic control sources with the operation of robotic components. They also assume potential users have the ability to coordinate multiple-control sources or the sequential use of one control source if they are to control multiple components.

Persons with either developmental cognitive impairment or cognitive impairment associated with trauma that resulted in quadriplegia may not be able to understand the relationship between a required control action and a desired action of a manipulator component. In general, persons with blindness or poor vision cannot use these devices. Visual feedback is an important factor in persons controlling many of these devices successfully. The complex control procedures required of some multiple-joint manipulator systems may render them inappropriate for elderly people and young children. A medical manipulator is still a robotic arm and a young child being within its workspace may be unsafe. The assistive technology specialist should consider the following additional factors:

- The user's degree of disability: These systems must be flexible enough to be adapted to each user's capabilities
- Modularity: The method used to control the system must be easy to add or remove according to each user's needs

- Reliability: The system must be dependable
- Cost: The system must be affordable

## Consideration, Options, and Technology

The first and most important step in assistive technology specialists ensuring the success of any rehabilitative aid is to determine the goals and objectives of users and the involved caregivers. Next, they should determine the realism of these goals given the limitations of the technology and the consistency of the goals of all parties. Once realistic goals have been set, the specialist can obtain a better idea of the systems to provide. A detailed physical assessment including range of motion of remaining joints is important in specialists ascertaining the realism of the goals. The physical assessment is an important factor in specialists determining the way users will control manipulators. Psychologic assessments of the users also are important in specialists determining the validity of the goals. Successful outcomes depend on users' willingness to participate in decision making and evaluating solutions. Active participation from users is vital to successful outcomes.

### *Types of Manipulators*

Rehabilitation manipulators comprise four categories: powered orthoses, desktop systems, wheelchair-based systems, and mobile roving units. The first category consists of powered orthoses, in which a user wears a manipulator and it physically moves an arm. Specialists recommend this device only in cases in which the user retains a sense of touch. Potential dangers to the user exist and problems may occur that are associated with controlling the orthosis because of the additional weight of the arm. These risks typically do not warrant this type of device. In instances in which the user has some sensation, the level of function possible with a powered orthosis may supersede anything possible with a regular robotic manipulator, justifying the potential risks.

### Powered Orthoses

Researchers of rehabilitation manipulators initially focused on developing powered orthoses. These were essentially externally powered exoskeletons that moved the arm of a person who was paralyzed to perform a desired manipulation.[4,5] Reswick and Mergler[4] pioneered this work. The Rancho Los Amigos Manipulator or Golden Arm built on these early efforts and achieved some success fitting a number of persons with polio enabling them to accomplish activities of daily living (Figure 17-1, *A* and *B*).[6,7] A gentleman who had been using his Golden Arm for many years recently told the author that it enabled him to paint and he now needed spare parts because the arm was beginning to fail (Figure 17-2). The limited success of these early powered orthoses can be attributed to fittings on people who had intact sensation. However, the primary target group for this type of assistive technology is persons with high-level quadriplegia, and they do not retain a sense of touch. As a result, a greater risk of injury exists with this type of device. The orthosis could drive the user's arm beyond its physiologic ranges without the user's awareness. In addition, because the mechanism moves the paralyzed arm, the stability of the mechanical arm could be in jeopardy. The additional dead weight of the arm can make the system prone to oscillations. Maintenance for these early systems was also a problem as they were not robust. Any technology should aid the user; therefore the user should not be subservient to the aid. Currently, no commercially available powered orthotic arms exist beyond powered hand orthoses, although researchers are revisiting the idea for persons who retain a sense of touch but do not have the ability to move their arm by themselves.[8]

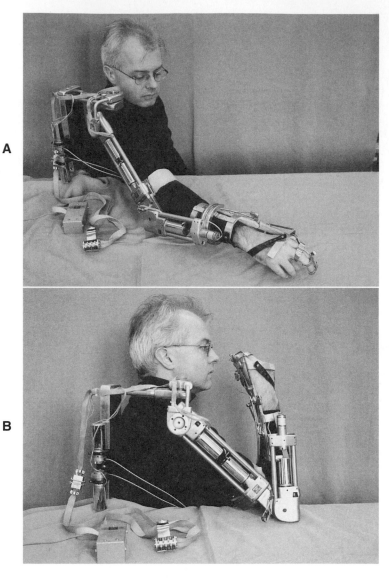

**Fig. 17-1** The Rancho Los Amigos Manipulator or Golden Arm was an externally powered orthoses worn by the user. It had seven joint rotations, each with the kinematic range limitations of the corresponding human arm joint. Control was through an array of seven bidirectional tongue switches. One switch controlled each joint rotation independently. Many persons with polio successfully used these arms for ADL. (Courtesy Northwestern University Rehabilitation Engineering Research Center, Chicago, Ill.)

## Desktop Systems

The second category of assistive manipulator is the desktop system that operates in a dedicated or highly structured environment. In this system, a person uses a robot arm mounted on a desktop to retrieve objects such as books from predefined positions and to deposit them at another predefined position, such as a book rest, which enables the user to read the book. Predefined locations for objects and the resulting predefined paths that the robot takes to grasp and move these objects greatly reduces the computational overhead required to control the robot. It also serves to limit the usefulness of the robot for anything other than predefined tasks. A person placing the wrong object in the wrong place causes problems because the computer/robot cannot recognize these different objects. A person uses a computer with a sequential menu system and a sip-and-puff, point-click device to control the robot, resulting in even the simplest task taking a long time.

The Cambridge University Robot Language (CURL)[9] and Lees' and Leifer's investigation[10] of a "story board" graphic interface are attempts at making developing tasks for

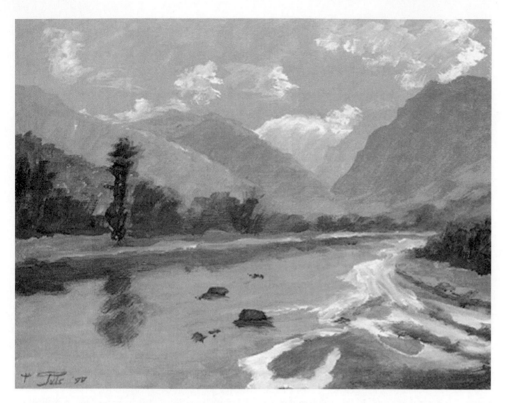

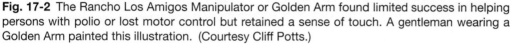

**Fig. 17-2** The Rancho Los Amigos Manipulator or Golden Arm found limited success in helping persons with polio or lost motor control but retained a sense of touch. A gentleman wearing a Golden Arm painted this illustration. (Courtesy Cliff Potts.)

the robot easier for nontechnical persons. CURL is a task-level programming environment designed specifically for rehabilitation applications. It is interactive and employs a natural language. The "story board" graphic interface consists of a series of pictograms displayed on the screen, each causing the robot to move in a predetermined manner, which the user can be combine to execute more complex tasks.

Desktop systems represent the high end of the price spectrum for rehabilitation manipulators. An individual may justify the cost by amortizing the expected benefit over a number of years.[11] A need exists for these systems in such areas as vocational assessment and placement. However, although a dedicated desktop system might be suitable in a work environment, such a system could dominate a user's home.

Research began on manipulators that were physically isolated from users as a result of experience gained with powered orthoses and a movement away from the idea of physical arm replacements. Many systems of this type exist. The most significant include the following:

- In Germany, the University of Heidelberg was the first to use an industrial manipulator for rehabilitation purposes[12]
- In the United States, the Applied Physics Laboratory Rehabilitation manipulator at John Hopkins University (APL/JHU), evolved from a shoulder-level arm prosthesis[13]
- In France, the Spartacus and MASTER projects set up in the Advanced Robotics Engineering Unit (UGRA) of CEA, the French Atomic Energy Commission were important projects that sought to examine the role that manipulators could play in assisting the severely disabled[14]

The Palo Alto Rehabilitation Research and Development division of the Department of Veterans Affairs Medical Center and Stanford University have the most developed desktop or workstation systems. Their DeVAR system, formerly known as *the Stanford Ro-*

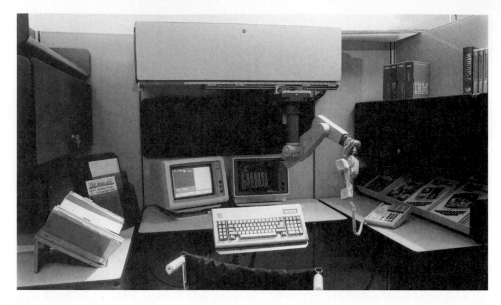

**Fig. 17-3** The DeVAR desktop system is the most advanced system of this kind. The current system consists of a Unimation PUMA-260 arm mounted to the center of a wheelchair-accessible table. Control was through an early form of voice control in addition to mixed hierarchical control software running five independent microcomputers. Manipulandum, sensors on the arm, and a smart sensate hand provided additional control inputs. The smart sensate hand supported reflex control of grasp, object localization, and object avoidance. The system could mix voice-initiated motion with joystick (head control unit) inputs during real-time manipulation. (Courtesy HFM Van der Loos, Rehabilitation Research and Development Center, Palo Alto, Calif.)

*botic Aid,* has undergone a number of iterations throughout its evolution (Figures 17-3 and 17-4).[15] Currently, teaching and vocational assessment are the primary roles for the DeVAR system and although DeVAR is not generally commercially available, a few have been sold to sites for these purposes or to research institutes for extended evaluation.[16]

In Europe, the robot for assisting the integration of disabled people system (RAID) is the current incarnation of the Spartacus and MASTER desktop projects. It is a dedicated workstation manipulator for use within office environments.[17] As with the other systems in this category, it is a system for use in a highly structured environment. Trials of the prototype system revealed that a smaller workstation and the application of the RAID concept in more common vocational activities were needed.[18]

These systems are technologically intensive and tend to be expensive rehabilitation manipulators. They have had limited success as educational and vocational training systems and as tools for further research. The exception to this trend is the Handy Series of Rehabilitation Robots from Rehab Robotics Ltd., Staffordshire, England (Figures 17-5 and 17-6). These systems are comparable in price to a high-end wheelchair or a midrange manipulator system and can be loosely defined as *desktop-type medical manipulators.* They consist of a robot arm and a food tray mounted on a wheeled base unit. The arm executes preprogrammed movements to scoop or pick up items at specific locations on the tray. Users choose these movements using a single scanning switch mechanism with a number of lights that illuminate in sequence. In this sense, the system operates in a structured mode. The means of interfacing between the person and the robot is the only part of the system that is different for each individual. This enables almost any part of the body to operate the Handy system. The Handy system presents food to the user at mouth level, then lets the user use gross trunk movements to take the food from the machine. This devices success can be attributed to this idea of presenting objects rather than trying to be a mechanical arm replacement. The Handy has been shown to improve the eating skills of regular users over time because of the consistency with which it presents food.[19,20] Over 60 units have been placed with individuals of varying ages and disabilities for evaluation.[18] More recently, the aid has been considered for

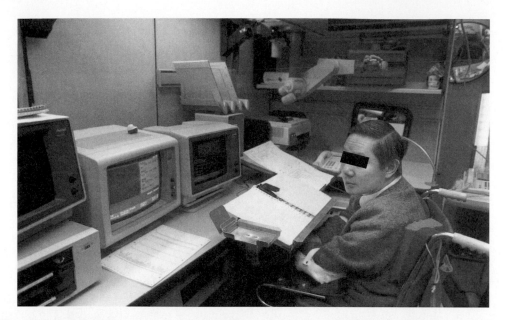

**Fig. 17-4** The DeVAR system in operation. Initial evaluation results showed that sensor-driven reflex control loops were needed to decrease the mental burden on the operator. Intelligent motion planning was also needed to reduce the dependence on a structured environment and to reduce the mental burden on the operator. Evaluations of the system concluded that the system was indeed useful to persons in gaining independence in the performance of ADL, but that further research was necessary to evaluate the system for individuals with other severe physical disabilities. (Courtesy HFM Van der Loos, Rehabilitation Research and Development Center, Palo Alto, Calif.)

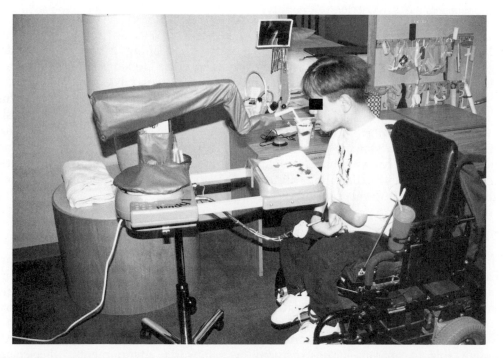

**Fig. 17-5** The Handy 1 Rehabilitation Robot from Rehab Robotics Ltd., Staffordshire, England, is the first commercially available robotic aid capable of assisting the severely disabled with everyday tasks such as eating, drinking, and shaving. Developed at Keele University, this device is successful because of the simple nature of the interface between the user and the device. A single switch is the sole mode of control and is the only part of the system that may be different for each individual person. Because of this, almost any part of the body can operate the Handy 1. (Courtesy Rehab Robotics Ltd., Staffordshire, England.)

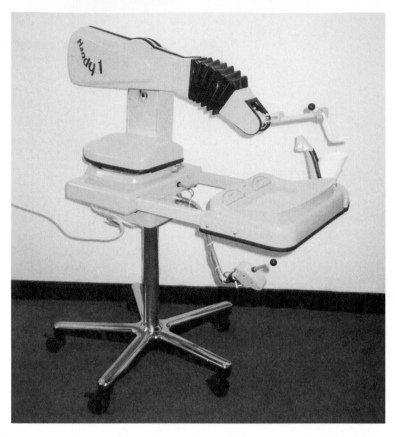

**Fig. 17-6** The Handy 1 Rehabilitation Robot. This device does not try to feed the user but instead presents the user with food. (Courtesy Rehab Robotics Ltd., Staffordshire, England.)

other activities including drinking, shaving, and teeth cleaning. It was originally designed for persons with cerebral palsy but has now been used to aid persons with motor neuron disease, stroke accident, multiple sclerosis, and muscular dystrophy.[21]

User experiences with the Handy fell in three categories[20]: (1) people who never had the ability to eat for themselves used the device to achieve something that they had previously been unable to do; (2) people who lost the ability to do things for themselves in the short term used the device to achieve a measure of independence while in a therapy program; and (3) people who had the ability to do things for themselves but have lost it permanently viewed the device with expectations that were too high. To date, this is one of the few rehabilitation manipulators that is commercially available for persons with disabilities.

## Wheelchair-Mounted Manipulators

The third category of rehabilitation manipulators is wheelchair-mounted manipulators that operate in the highly unstructured world of daily activities. One of the most significant conclusions of the previously mentioned Spartacus project was that when a specialist mounted it on a wheelchair, the effectiveness of a rehabilitation manipulator would increase. The combination of electric wheelchair and manipulator offers functional compensation for the impairment of mobility and upper limb functions. Although able to operate in unstructured or real world environments, wheelchair-mounted devices have tended to suffer from technical problems associated with accuracy and a lack of a user-friendly arm controller. The development of the Veterans Administration Prosthetic Center (VAPC) wheelchair-mounted manipulator did not use an anthropomorphic shape for its manipulator.[22] Instead, they used a prismatic, or telescoping, shoulder joint to enable it to reach objects on the floor and above the user's head. While the idea was novel, Corker and others[23] evaluated the device and found that

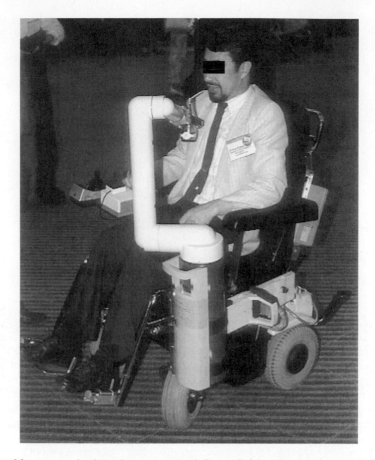

**Fig. 17-7** The Manus manipulator is a commercially available wheelchair mountable rehabilitation manipulator. The combination of electric wheelchair and manipulator offers functional compensation for the impairment of mobility and upper-limb functions. It was designed to work on a wheelchair or a table to reach shelves somewhat above eye level and to reach the floor over a small area next to the wheelchair. The fully stretched arm can lift objects with a weight of 1.5 kg. Exerted torques are limited by slip couplings on the shoulder, elbow, and wrist joint drives to protect the user and system against excessive forces. (Courtesy CW Heckathorne, Northwestern University Rehabilitation Engineering Research Center, Chicago, Ill.)

it was not sufficiently reliable for clinical tests. This device succeeded somewhat as a research test bed in the study of alternative approaches to the man-machine interface.

Currently, the only wheelchair-mounted system that is commercially available is the Manus manipulator, developed in The Netherlands and available from Exact Dynamics bv., The Netherlands (Figures 17-7 and 17-8). The impetus for the Manus system arose from the conclusions of the Spartacus Project.[24] Manus was designed to work on either a wheelchair lapboard or a table to reach shelves above eye level and on the floor next to the wheelchair.[25] The control system is modular, to make it adaptable to people with severe disabilities of all four limbs. Manus has been extensively evaluated within rehabilitation centers for several years. Although commercially available, Manus has not been widely used partly because of its high cost. Some of the problems encountered with early systems included the following:

- Suspension of the manipulator on a wheelchair made the chair too wide to pass through doors.
- The arm when unfolded prevented the chair from moving under a regular table.
- Mounting of the device on one side of the chair added asymmetric weight, influencing driving on inclined surfaces.
- With spring-suspended wheelchairs, the movements of the user made the base move and hence, also the arm and the gripper.[24]

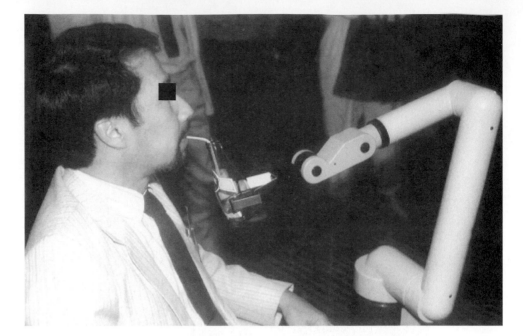

**Fig. 17-8** The Manus in operation. The control system is modular to make it adaptable to people with severe disabilities of all four limbs. Individually selectable controls and reconfigurable microcomputer assisted procedures are used to control gripper and wheelchair movements in a unified way. Initial tests revealed the suspension of the manipulator on the side of a wheelchair made the chair too wide to pass through doors and also made the weight asymmetric, influencing driving on inclined surfaces. In addition, the unfolded arm prevented the chair from moving under a regular table. Another problem encountered with spring-suspended wheelchairs was that the user's movements jostled the arm and gripper. All of these issues have been or are in the process of being solved. (Courtesy CW Heckathorne, Northwestern University Rehabilitation Engineering Research Center, Chicago, Ill.)

## Robotic Assistants

The fourth and last category of rehabilitation manipulators pertains to free-roaming robotic assistants or computer-controlled autonomous roving units. For some persons with severe disabilities, assistive manipulators may not be practical. Free-roaming robotic aids seek to remedy this situation but are still in the early stages and have not evolved beyond the laboratory. One of the conclusions of the initial evaluation of the DeVAR workstation manipulator was the need for a mobile robot to extend the robotic work aid sphere of operation beyond the tabletop workspace.[26] To this end, researchers explored the idea of a mobile component known as *MOVAR*, but this device never evolved beyond the laboratory (Figure 17-9).

Another research initiative in this area is the mobility and activity assistance systems for the disabled project (MOVAID), which is an example of a mobile robotic assistant for severely disabled bedridden users. The system is designed to interact with task-specific workstations or to be able to interact with a range of user interfaces for appliances. It features a mobile base equipped with a robot arm and sensory systems for navigation and obstacle avoidance.[18] Presently, no commercially available mobile robotic attendants exist.

The telematics for improving the quality of life of disabled and elderly people (TIDE) initiative in the European Union has funded much of the research in this area. This initiative was aimed at improving the quality of life for disabled and elderly persons. The MOVAID project was funded under this initiative as was the office wheelchair with high maneuverability and navigational intelligence for people with severe handicap (OMNI) project. The OMNI project is an example of an intelligent wheelchair. The system uses

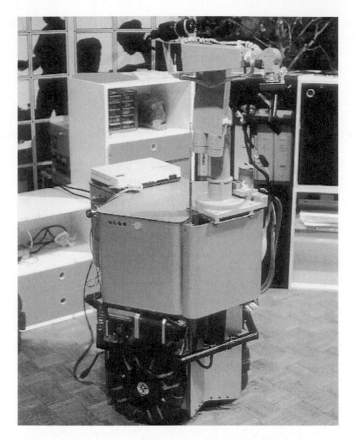

**Fig. 17-9** The MOVAR mobile robotic aid. Evaluation of the DeVAR desktop mounted system indicated the need for a vehicle to extend the robotic work aid's sphere of operation beyond the tabletop workspace. MOVAR was the result of the effort to meet this observation. However, this device has not evolved beyond the laboratory (Courtesy CW Heckathorne, Northwestern University Rehabilitation Engineering Research Center, Chicago, Ill.)

ultrasonic and infrared sensors for environment analysis and obstacle avoidance. This project is still in its infancy.

## Outcomes and Social Validation

Few commercially available rehabilitation robots exist. Essentially only the Handy System from Rehab Robotics, Staffordshire, England and the Manus Manipulator from Exact Dynamics, The Netherlands, are commercially available. Numerous devices and systems have been tried and are undergoing development. Seeing where these systems came from and examining what may be available in the future are important for researchers.

On a more practical level, specialists should remember that these devices are mechanical and as with any mechanical device, are prone to failure. Hence, an important factor in the choice of device is access to maintenance facilities for servicing and repair. Another consideration is the ability of the user or a family member to do occasional repairs. A manipulator is a complex electromechanical device. Therefore a person needs knowledge of robotics, electronics, computers, and mechanics to service and maintain it properly.

Those who are possible benefactors of robotic technology do not have many options. The alternative to this technology is a full-time caregiver to perform ADL. Simple alternatives that enable limited interaction with the environment include mouthsticks and specially modified utensils to aid in grasping. Often the user uses a mouthstick or headstick to interact with the electronic and computer interfaces to control powered manipulators. The single biggest measure of success of a device in this field is how often the user uses it. Often times these devices require more effort than the user can provide. What seemed like a good system at the initial fitting slowly fades into disuse as the user discovers the benefit-to-effort ratio.

Presently, commercially available robotic systems cannot replace an attendant. They can provide a measure of independence that may be an immeasurable psychologic benefit to a user by enabling self-sufficiency. This depends on the psychologic makeup of the individual, and the specialist must evaluate each person. The hindrance for the majority of rehabilitation robots is the transition from the laboratory into clinical usage or commercialization. These systems have been commercially unsuccessful because of a lack of reliability and utility, high cost, poor user interface, or any combination of these.

Harwin, Rahman, and Foulds[11] noted that many devices are programmed so that contact with the environment is minimized to protect the device. But the purpose of a manipulator is to enable the severely disabled user to interact and have contact with the real world. According to consumers, the effectiveness of the robot is a primary criterion for success. This relates directly to the human-machine interface and the ease with which a person can control a manipulator. A person will not use an interface that is difficult to learn and control. The user should not have to focus on the way to control the robot but should be able to focus on the current task.

# References

1. Dario P et al: Robotics for medical applications, *IEEE Robotics and Automation Magazine* 3 (3):44–56, Sept 1996.
2. Erlandson RF: Applications of robotic/mechatronic systems in special education, rehabilitation, therapy, and vocational training: a paradigm shift, *IEEE Trans Rehabil Eng* 3 (1): 22–34, March 1995.
3. Hogan N: Guest editor, special issue on rehabilitation applications of robotic technology, *J Rehab Res Dev* 37 (6):ix-vi, Nov/Dec 2000.
4. Reswick JB, Mergler K: *Medical engineering progress report on case research arm aid*, Rep No EDC 4-64-3, Cleveland, 1962, Case Institute of Technology.
5. Corell RW, Wijnschenk MJ: *Design and development of the case research arm-aid*, Rep No EDC 4-64-4, April, 1969, Engineering Design Center, Case Western Reserve University.
6. Allen JR, Karchak A, Jr, Nickel VL: *Orthotic manipulators: advances in external control of human extremities*, Belgrade, 1970, Yugoslav Committee for Electronics and Automation.
7. Karchak A, Allen J, Nickel VL: The *application of external power and control to orthotic systems: advances in external control of human extremities*, Belgrade, 1970, Yugoslav Committee for Electronics and Automation.
8. Romilly DP et al: *Analysis and development of a powered upper-limb orthosis*, pp 87–92, Wilmington, Del, 1994, Fourth International Conference on Rehabilitation Robotics, Applied Science and Engineering Laboratory.
9. Gosine RG, Harwin WS, Jackson RD: *Development of a task-level robot control language*, pp 97–118, Wilmington, Del, 1990, International Conference on Rehabilitation Robotics, AI DuPont Institute.
10. Lees DS, Leifer LJ: *Experimental evaluation of a graphical programming environment for service robots*, pp 19–23, Wilmington, Del, 1994, Fourth International Conference on Rehabilitation Robotics, Applied Science and Engineering Laboratory.
11. Harwin WS, Rahman T, Foulds RA: A review of design issues in rehabilitation robotics to north American research, *IEEE Trans Rehabil Eng* 3 (1):3–13, March 1995.
12. Roesler H et al: *The medical manipulator and its adapted environment: a system for the rehabilitation of the severely handicapped*, pp 63–77, Rocquencourt, France, Sept 4–6, 1978, Colloques IRIA, Proceedings First International Conference on Telemanipulators for the Physically Handicapped.
13. Schneider W, Schmeisser G, Seamone W: A computer-aided robotic arm/worktable system for the high level quadriplegic, *IEEE Computer* 14 (1):41–47, Jan 1981.
14. Detriche JM, Lesigne B: *The integral system MASTER,* pp 161–175, Wilmington, Del, 1990, International Conference on Rehabilitation Robotics, AI DuPont Institute.

15. Leifer L et al: Robotic *aids for the severely disabled needs assessment,* pp 19–34, Rocquencourt, France, Sept 4–6, 1978, Proceedings First International Conference on Telemanipulators for the Physically Handicapped.

16. Van der Loos HFM, Hammel J, Leifer LJ: *DeVAR transfer from R&D to vocational and educational settings,* pp 151–155, Wilmington, Del, 1994, Fourth International Conference on Rehabilitation Robotics (ICORR94), Applied Science and Engineering Laboratory.

17. Dallaway JL, Jackson RD: *RAID,* (ICORR '92), Keele, 1992, A Vocational Robotic Workstation, Proc of the third International Conference on Rehabilitation Robotics.

18. Dallaway JL, Jackson RD, Timmers PHA: Rehabilitation robotics in Europe, *IEEE Trans Rehabil Eng* 3 (1):35–45, March 1995.

19. Topping MJ: Early experience in the use of the "Handy 1" robotic aid to eating, *Robotica* 11 (6):525–527, 1993.

20. Topping MJ: *The development of Handy 1: a robotic aid to independence for the severely disabled,* pp 2/1–2/6, Digest No 1995/107, Dundee, Scotland, May 17 1995, Proceedings of the IEE Colloquium "Mechatronics Aids for the Disabled" University of Dundee.

21. Makin J, Smith J, Topping MJ: *A study to compare the food scooping performance of the "Handy 1" robotic aid to eating, using two different dish designs,* Lille, France, July 9–12 1996, Proceedings of the IMACS International Conference on Computational Engineering in Systems Applications CESA 96.

22. Mason CP, Peizer E: Medical manipulator for quadriplegics, pp 309–312, Colloques IRIA, Rocquencourt, France, Sept 4–6, 1978, Proc First International Conference on Telemanipulators for the Physically Handicapped.

23. Corker K, Lyman JH, Sheredos S: A preliminary evaluation of remote medical manipulators, *BPR* 10 (32):107–134, Fall 1979.

24. Kwee HH: *Rehabilitation robotics: softening the hardware,* pp 69–79, Wilmington, Delaware, 1990, International Conference on Rehabilitation Robotics, AI DuPont Institute.

25. Kwee HH: SPARTACUS and MANUS: telethesis developments in France and the Netherlands. In Foulds R, editor: *Interactive robotic aids - one option for independent living: an international perspective,* pp. 7–17, Monograph 37, New York, 1986, World Rehabilitation Fund.

26. Van der Loos HFM, Michalowski SJ, Leifer LJ: Design of an omnidirectional mobile robot as a manipulation aid for the severely disabled. In Foulds R, editor: *Interactive robotic aids - one option for independent living: an international perspective,* pp 61–63, New York, 1986, Monograph 37, World Rehabilitation Fund.

# PART 4

Technologies for Mobility and Locomotion

*Carol A. Sargent*

Movement is fundamental to an infant's development of self-awareness, investigation of the environment, and basic health. As movement and later mobility are experienced, the child learns control and mastery of self and develops skills to access environments such as home, school, and the playground.

*Locomotion*, a word derived from the Latin *loco* (from a place) plus *motion*, is the ability of a person to move from place to place. Ambulation, the use of a manual wheelchair, a powered mobility device, and personal transportation, are all methods of locomotion. Assistive technologies that enable an individual with disabilities to have improved or independent mobility are crucial for that individual's self-awareness, self-esteem, and ability to access various environments (including school, work, and the community). These technologies are often necessary for the individual to live independently.

Before the provision of any assistive technology, a specialist needs to thoroughly evaluate the individual user's skills, needs, environments in which the individual functions, and tasks the individual wants to accomplish. Central to the effective use of these technologies is the specialist matching the identified personal and environmental needs of an individual with the features and functions of a device, or combination of devices, to address the desired tasks. The assistive technologies that enable mobility and locomotion for persons with disabilities are numerous with ever-increasing technologic advances, which provide improved features and functions. Therefore as product lines evolve and technologies change, the rehabilitation professional must focus on the advances in features and functions relevant to the user's needs.

The chapters in this part provide practical information about the problem-solving processes applied to a specialist matching user needs to features and functions of assistive technologies. The needs addressed by assistive technology in these chapters include posture and positioning, personal mobility, way finding for persons with visual impairments, and personal transportation. Sensitive to the value of device features, the contributing authors have provided examples for the reader to match a feature or group of features to a particular need with the rationale supporting the match. The case study examples also may assist the reader in deriving a problem-solving approach to assistive technology service delivery and practice.

Access to mobility via improved positioning, assisted ambulation, wheelchair mobility, way finding, and transportation remains essential for a person's personal development, achievement, and well being. Assistive technology features, when successfully matched to the functional mobility needs of persons with disabilities, can diminish barriers and enable independence.

# CHAPTER 18

## Lower Limb Prosthetics

*Mark L. Edwards*

## Application and Goal

The primary objective of a prosthesis is to provide persons with lower limb amputations the ability to return to functional lifestyles. Prosthetics technology varies from simple prostheses such as passive and cosmetic devices to more sophisticated and dynamic technology. These sophisticated prostheses allow individuals with lower limb amputations to walk, run, and participate in many different activities. The individual who sustains an amputation relies on this technology to perform activities that were once second nature. For optimal use, the prosthesis must become an extension of the person's body. This occurs with a comfortable prosthesis that the person can wear for sufficient periods. A prosthesis that is comfortable and distributes forces in an even pattern assists an amputee to ambulate with a more natural gait. Amputation level, residual limb geometry, muscle and skin padding, and components and materials that are incorporated into the design of the prosthesis often dictate comfort.

Another goal for a person using a prosthesis is attainment of normal function. Symmetry, speed, efficiency, and balance have an effect on function. The function of the prosthesis should not be considered independent from comfort. A comfortable prosthesis allows the person to achieve function more easily. Furthermore, a well-functioning prosthesis feels more natural and comfortable to the amputee. These two objectives have a secondary effect of making the appearance of the prosthesis more natural and anatomic. A successful lower-limb prosthesis is one that combines comfort, function, and appearance. Many factors have an effect on an amputee's ability to realize these goals and objectives.

## Function and Ability

The prevalence of lower limb amputation has remained relatively consistent over the past 20 years. Amputations at the transtibial level (below the knee, between the ankle joint and the knee joint) represent over 50% of the amputee population.[1] Although amputations can occur at any age, most amputations occur between the ages of 51 and 80.[2] Some statistics estimate the total number of amputees in the United States ranges from 300,000 to 1.8 million.[3] Amputation can result from disease, trauma, or congenital deficiencies. The leading cause of lower limb amputations is vascular disease, specifically diabetes and arteriosclerosis.

Transfemoral (above the knee, between the knee joint and the hip joint) amputations make up approximately 30% of the amputee population.[1] In general, traumatic lower limb amputations occur in younger people, usually between the ages of 21 and 50.[2] Congenital, lower-limb deficient patients represent less than 5% of the total amputee population.[1] The most common congenital lower limb abnormality is partial or complete loss of the fibula.[2] Lower-limb amputations include partial foot, ankle disarticulation, transtibial, knee disarticulation transfemoral, hip disarticulation, and hemipelvectomy.

Specialists should evaluate the presence of sufficient strength, balance, and cognitive ability to fully assess an amputee's level of ambulation potential. They use common

## TABLE 18-1

*Function Levels of Rehabilitation*

| Classification | Description | Example |
| --- | --- | --- |
| Level 0 | Has little or no potential for ambulation or transfer, safely with or without assistance | Nonprosthetic user |
| Level 1 | Has the ability or potential to use a prosthesis for transfers or ambulation on level surfaces at fixed cadences | Limited household ambulator |
| Level 2 | Has the ability or potential for ambulation with the ability to traverse low level environmental barriers (curbs, stairs, etc.) | Limited community ambulator |
| Level 3 | Has the ability or potential for ambulation at variable cadence in the community | Unlimited community ambulator |
| Level 4 | Has the ability or potential for prosthetic ambualtion that exceeds basic ambulation skills, exhibiting high impact, stress, or energy levels | Typical of the prosthetic demands of a child, active adult, or athlete |

functional levels of activity and ambulation to help assess this potential (Table 18-1). Because many amputees are between the ages of 51 and 80, their general medical condition, amputation level, and number of amputations are critical variables in the ability to successfully wear prostheses. Generally, the more proximal the amputation, the more effort or exertion the user needs to use a prosthesis. Amputation at the most proximal levels such as ankle/knee (AK) and hip disarticulations may cause some individuals to never reach a functional level of ambulation. People who have sustained multiple amputations (bilaterals) often have difficulty with balance and have decreased energy. Surgeons must have an understanding of forces, lever arms, and gait mechanics to make the appropriate decision regarding the optimal level of amputation. This expertise enables them to produce a residual limb that is suitable for prosthetic fitting.

## Considerations, Options, and Technology

Gait studies have demonstrated the efficacy of preserving the anatomic knee joint in amputations.[3] Energy costs increase when surgeons perform amputations above the knee. It has also been documented that transtibial amputees are the most successful users of prosthetic technology. Therefore amputation level is critical in optimizing the patient's ability to return to a normal lifestyle. In addition to the level of amputation, limb shape, soft-tissue padding, muscle strength, and balance help assess the future rehabilitation potential of a particular patient. To begin the process of achieving a functional gait pattern, a certified prosthetist (CP) performs the necessary measurements and evaluations on a patient. The CP has received training through an accredited university program and completed a 12-month residency program. The CP has also passed a rigorous 3-part examination to be certified by the American Board for Certification in Orthotics and Prosthetics (ABC).

A properly fitted prosthesis is necessary for maximum comfort and function. The most critical component of any prosthesis is the interface between the residual limb and the prosthesis. This is often referred to as *the socket*. A socket that does not fit properly can result in many different problems, including residual limb edema, pain, skin breakdown, and gait deviations.[3] The prosthetic socket acts to transfer loads from the pros-

TABLE **18-2**

*Prosthetic Feet Catagories*

| Classification | Indications | Advantages | Disadvantages | Examples |
|---|---|---|---|---|
| Solid ankle cushioned heel | Majority of lower limb amputees Pediatric Limited ambulators | Low cost Durable Many sizes and styles | Less flexible Nonresponsive Does not conform to terrain | |
| Single axis articualtion | For individuals who require increased knee stability | Enhances knee stability | Heavier Higher maintenance | |
| MultiAxis articulation | For traversing uneven terrain For special recreational activities | Conforms to terrain Provides torque absorption | Heavier Higher maintenance | |
| Flexible/elastic heel | For community ambulators | Provides smooth rollover Durable | Increased cost Limited responsiveness | |
| Dynamic responses | For high activity levels For more than one speed of walking | Increased level of responsiveness | Increased cost Limited sizes and styles | |

thesis to the amputated limb. Pressure distribution is adjusted by the prosthetist to load pressure-tolerant areas of the limb while unloading pressure sensitive areas. Many patients have diminished sensation and cannot tell if pressures are too high. The need for objective evaluation of the limb is necessary. Prosthetists identify the antalgic, sensitive, or insensate areas and through the manipulation of the forces on the limb, they can eliminate or keep them low.

Strong, lightweight materials have been developed that have expanded the choices of materials that the prosthetist can use. These technologic advances have contributed to reduced prosthetic weight and have greatly benefited patients. A prosethtist can make the interface (socket) that incorporates a soft-padded material to further increase comfort. This is often referred to as *a liner*. Among some of these options are, foam, silicone, or urethane elastomers. By using one of these padded materials in the socket, the prosthetist helps to spread the pressures on the limb over a larger area thereby increasing overall comfort. CPs routinely uses liners in many prostheses today.

Most prosthetic componentry options are categorized under general headings (i.e., feet, knees, suspension, socket design interface materials.) The options available to the lower-limb amputee range from low-cost, low-function designs to high-cost, high-function designs. Many prostheses are available for every level of amputation. The CP prescribes the type of prosthesis based on the individual patient's vocational and avocational needs.

## Feet for Lower Limb Prostheses

The objectives of prosthetic feet are to provide shock absorption at heel contact, support the body through stance phase, allow a smooth transition to toe off, produce a dynamic push off, and if possible provide triplanar motion at the ankle (Table 18-2). Some feet have one or two functions and others try to incorporate all of them. The foot is important because it has a mitigating effect on the forces that are generated at the socket-limb interface.[3] The foot should be lightweight, durable, and relatively simple in its design to decrease repairs and the need for replacement. The CP should consider other features including comfort, appearance, and cost. In general, with more proximal amputations, the

CP should incorporate a foot that has a softer heel into the design of the prosthesis because of the relationship between heel stiffness and knee stability (i.e., a soft heel tends to improve stability). Feet that allow inversion and eversion are good for uneven terrain and feet that offer transverse motion are good for sports and recreation. Other factors for the CP to consider when selecting a prosthetic foot are amputation level, patient weight, foot size, activity level, and cost.

## Knees for Lower Limb Prostheses

Prosthetic knee mechanisms should restore gait to as close to normal as possible. The patient's limb length and muscle strength are key factors in the CP determining the type of knee component to use. A variety of options for knee mechanisms exist (Table 18-3). The main objectives for knee components are stance phase stability, swing phase control, and toe clearance. These goals are accomplished through the CP's design of the knee mechanism and the alignment of the knee within the prosthesis. The CP prescribes knee components by evaluating the patient's ability to control a mechanical knee and the inherent stability that the CP designs into any one particular knee. Some knees are simple in their design and offer little or no inherent stability, and other designs are sophisticated and offer varying degrees of stability. The stability of the knee derives from the alignment of the prosthesis and the patient's use of the hip extensors in stance phase to stabilize the knee. Transfemoral amputees that have extremely short residual limbs and weak or atrophied musculature require knees that have a high degree of built in stability. This guideline ensures that a patient with limited volitional control and/or shortened lever arm can still ambulate with confidence.

The CP should fit amputees who have gait patterns that require fast walking or running with fluid control mechanisms. These knees offer either hydraulic or pneumatic re-

## TABLE 18-3

*Prosthetic Knee Catagories*

| Classification | Indications | Advantages | Disadvantages | Examples |
|---|---|---|---|---|
| Single axis | Single-speed ambulators<br>Pediatric<br>Good voluntary control | Low cost<br>Durable | No inherent stability<br>Fixed cadence | |
| Weight-activated stance control | For individuals who require increased knee stability<br>Less voluntary control | Enhances knee stability | Difficult to unweight on stairs<br>Increased maintenance | |
| Polycentric (4-bar) | Same as stance control<br>Very short or very long amputations | Excellent inherent stability<br>Provides good toe clearance | Increased weight<br>Increased maintenance | |
| Manual locking | General debility<br>Poor balance and voluntary control | Maximum knee stability | Unnatural gait | |
| Fluid control | For high activity levels<br>For more than one speed of walking | Variable cadence<br>Smoothness of swing | Increased cost<br>Increased weight<br>Increased maintenance | |

sistance to control swing-phase gait mechanics. They are classified as cadence respon-sive, meaning that the resistance increases or decreases as the walking speed varies. The most intricate and sophisticated designs incorporate multilinkage designs with stance phase stability and hydraulic swing phase control. This technology allows above-the-knee amputees to function at high activity levels and participate in many recreational ac-tivities. Many knee components are available with low technologic designs. CPs use sim-ple single-axis mechanisms with manual locking features to provide maximum stability when locked. The patient is able to release the lock for sitting. Unfortunately, this type of knee produces an uncosmetic, unnatural gait pattern. CPs use this for extremely debili-tated amputees for balance and transfer activities. They can incorporated this manual locking design into most knee mechanism categories and eventually remove them as the person's rehabilitation progresses.

## Construction of Lower Limb Prostheses

Construction designs generally are classified as either endoskeletal or exoskeletal. A hard plastic outer shell identifies exoskeletal prostheses. This shell functions as the supporting structure of the prosthesis. Exoskeletal prostheses are usually heavier, more difficult to make adjustments or changes to, and are used for heavy-duty work environments.[4] An inner tube or pylon that makes up the support structure identifies endoskeletal prosthe-ses. A cosmetic foam cover shaped to represent the anatomic features of the contralateral leg covers the inner tube. Endoskeletal designs are usually lighter weight, more natural looking, have adjustable capabilities, and are considered less durable because of the foam covering. CPs can make the inner tube and the adjustable components from stainless steel, aluminum, titanium, or carbon composites. The materials CPs use to fabricate and design exoskeletal and endoskeletal prostheses range from simple polyester resins to complex carbon and kevlar composites (Figures 18-1 and 18-2).

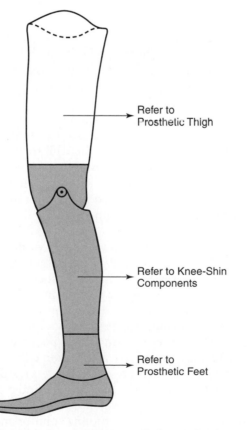

Refer to Prosthetic Thigh

Refer to Knee-Shin Components

Refer to Prosthetic Feet

**Fig. 18-1** Exoskeletal lower limb prosthesis.

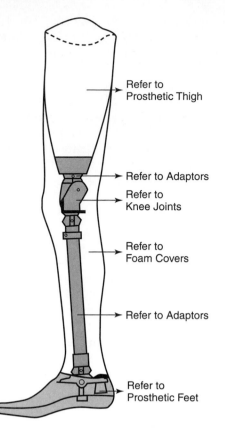

Refer to
Prosthetic Thigh

Refer to Adaptors

Refer to
Knee Joints

Refer to
Foam Covers

Refer to Adaptors

Refer to
Prosthetic Feet

**Fig. 18-2** Endoskeletal lower limb prosthesis.

## Socket Designs for the Lower Limb Prostheses

### Transtibial Socket Designs

The geometry of the interface as it contacts and encapsulates the amputated limb is important for the distributions of forces while the user is walking. The CP taking a wrapped cast or impression of the patient's limb determines this geometry. The cast is prestressed or contoured to allow the CP to identify bony structures and compress soft tissue areas. Using highly specific measurement and modification procedures, the prosthetist plans the shape of the socket. The patella tendon bearing (PTB) socket is the standard socket used for the transtibial limb. Its use has been well documented and has been used successfully since 1959. The objectives of the PTB socket include loading the pressure tolerant areas of the limb relieving the pressure-sensitive areas, placing the limb in a flexed position for increased anterior weight bearing, and maintaining total contact with the limb. Maintaining total contact is required in all lower limb sockets. Failure to support the distal soft tissue results in fluid pooling that may lead to more complicated skin problems.

CPs often use PTB sockets in conjunction with soft or padded liners that they place between the sockets and the limbs. Soft liners add cushioning to bony, atrophied limbs. CPs fabricate soft liners from a variety of materials, such as closed cell foams, silicone, and urethane. Because the majority of lower limb amputations result from vascular diseases, soft, flexible liners can decrease pressure and improve comfort. In general, the PTB prosthesis attempts to achieve a comfortable fitting socket through basic biomechanical principles. Forces are spread over as wide an area as possible. This design seems simple enough to apply. However, the area of force application can vary greatly with each individual. Individuals with firm musculature can tolerate pressure better compared with individuals who have atrophied limbs. The socket shape and contours are important factors that allow individuals to tolerate this pressure distribution.

Today, transtibial socket designs that incorporate contour and shape and that are considered "hydrostatic" or fluid loading are popular. This principle is good when the CP

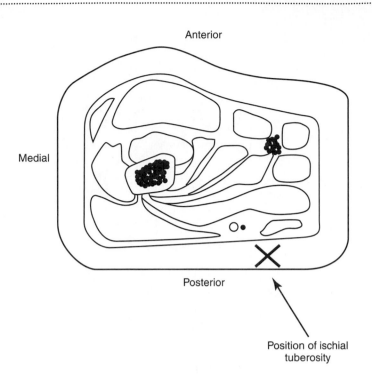

Anterior

Medial

Posterior

Position of ischial
tuberosity

**Fig. 18-3** Quadrilateral socket design.

needs to stabilize the bony anatomy within the soft tissue. The CP uses a pressurized casting procedure to elongate the soft tissue and stress the fluid to a uniform volume. This technique is often referred to as *total surface bearing,* which suggests that the entire limb is being used for pressure distribution. The CP routinely uses these two techniques for transtibial prostheses.

### Transfemoral Socket Designs

Two basic socket shapes are available for the transfemoral amputee: the quadrilateral design and the ischial containment design. The CP can achieve basic biomechanical principles that apply to transfemoral amputations by using either socket design. These principles are comfortable containment of the amputated limb in a receptacle (socket), support or transfer of body weight when walking, control of the prosthesis during all phases of walking, and contact maintenance with the entire limb.[6] The prosthetics research group at the University of California at Berkeley developed the quadrilateral socket design in the early 1950s. Its rectangular shape characterizes this quadrilateral socket design. Each of the walls or sides of this rectangle has specific functions and objectives. A combination of ischial weight bearing, gluteal weight bearing, and hydrostatic loading accomplishes the transfer of vertical loads. To keep the ischial tuberosity in its proper location on the posterior shelf, the anterior wall must apply a posteriorly directed force against the soft tissue of the anterior thigh. This compression causes the quadrilateral shape to be somewhat narrow from anterior to posterior and thus the medial to lateral dimension is usually wider (Figure 18-3).

Ivan Long, CP, first created the ischial containment socket shape, and John Sabolich, CP, further developed it in the 1980s. This design is characterized by having the ischial tuberosity lie inside the socket for increased M-L stability. Compared with the quadrilateral shape, in which the ischial tuberosity is supported on a shelf, the ischial containment socket encapsulates the tuberosity on the posterior and medial aspects (Figure 18-4). This is theorized to improve lateral displacement of the femur and decrease pelvic list at midstance. When patients have M-L stability difficulties, they compensate by moving their center of mass over the prosthesis. This is often referred to as *lateral trunk bending.* Most transfemoral amputees exhibit varying degrees of this deviation from normal walking.

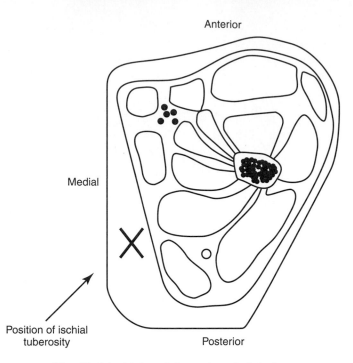

**Fig. 18-4** Ischial containment socket design.

These two transfemoral socket designs are appropriate for all levels of above-the-knee amputations. However, short transfemoral amputations would seem to benefit more from the increased stability and residual control while using an ischial containment design. A CP using ischial containment sockets on the bilateral above-the-knee amputee has proven to be better for increased comfort and freedom in the perineum because of the shape and dimension of the socket proximally. The quadrilateral design is somewhat wider in this M-L dimension and may cause discomfort when the bilateral patient is walking (see Figure 18-3).

## Suspension Techniques for Lower Limb Prostheses

### Transtibial Suspension Techniques

The methods and techniques of suspension are applicable to all the socket designs previously discussed. The ability to hold the prosthesis on the limb is one of the most critical functions of the prosthesis. A prosthesis that has good suspension feels much lighter and allows the amputee to ambulate with more confidence. The basic means of transtibial prostheses suspension is through the use of straps (Table 18-4). The CP uses the supracondylar cuff suspension for many preparatory or temporary prostheses. It is adjustable and the CP achieves suspension by positioning the cuff above the patella. The cuff is allowed to swivel through the swing phase of gait and hold the prosthesis on to the limb. The CP can design this strap in a variety of styles. For the cuff to be successful, the patella must be relatively prominent. If the thigh is large and the patella is not easily palpated, the CP may add an additional waist belt to assist the cuff in holding the prosthesis on.

The CP also uses elastic external sleeves for suspension and makes these suspension sleeves from materials that provide high friction against slipping from the person's thigh and the outside surface of the prosthesis. The transtibial amputee uses sleeves to conceal the proximal trimlines, eliminate straps, and minimize pistoning. Common sleeve materials are latex rubber, neoprene rubber, elastic, and silicone. The CP commonly uses this method for more active amputees. The main disadvantages for the user are allergic skin reactions to the material and heat and perspiration retention.

The next category of suspension techniques uses the bony structure of the knee for suspension. The PTB supracondylar (SC) and supracondylar-suprapatellar (SC/SP) designs are in this category. The nomenclature describes the area of the knee that the

## TABLE 18-4

*Transtibial Suspension Systems*

| Classification | Indications | Advantages | Disadvantages | Examples |
|---|---|---|---|---|
| Supracondylar cuff | Long limb length Good muscular control | Adjustable | Additional straps Some inherent pistoning May need auxiliary belts | |
| External sleeve | Long limb length Good muscular control | No straps or buckles Hides trimlines under clothes | Skin reactions to material Difficult to don | |
| Anatomic | Medium-short limb Slight degree of laxity | Provides more support Increases overall contact | Limites knee ROM May be difficult to don | |
| Silicone suction | Most transtibial levels Stable volume | Very good suspension Silicone material provides shear control | Difficult to don Some skin reactions to materials | |
| Joints and corset | Short or damaged residual limb High degree of laxilty | Maximum knee support Maximum axial support | Heavy Bulky Inherent pistoning | |

socket encompasses. Medial and lateral walls that cup above the femoral condyles, specifically the contour of the medial femoral condyle, characterize the supracondylar suspension. The CP usually achieves this suspension by using a wedge that is added to the soft liner of the socket. The PTB SC design provides good suspension and also increases knee stability and the overall weight-bearing surface of the amputated limb. The PTB SC/SP design encapsulates the entire knee above the condyles and the patella. The SC/SP design is indicated for short residual limb lengths. This design has the added benefits of providing suspension, M-L stability, and an increased area for loading over the patella. Patients find this valuable in late stance-phase loading as it prevents the tendency for recurvatum to occur. However, it can limit the range of motion of knee extension for individuals with long stride lengths.

The next suspension technique uses silicone liners with pin attachments to secure the prosthesis on the limb. This method is often referred to as *silicone suction suspension*. Silicone sleeve liners are manufactured in a variety of sizes to fit most amputated limbs of the transtibial level. The sleeve has an attachment pin that engages a spring-loaded locking mechanism in the bottom of the socket when the CP positions it into the socket. The user can release the pin by pressing a button on the side of the prosthesis, which is a secure means of suspension. The patient experiences little pistoning during walking because the liner is made of silicone. Torque and shear dissipate between the outside of the silicone liner and the socket instead of interfacing with the patient's skin. This is important for the patient with poor sensation or adherent scar tissue. The silicone suction liner and suspension system works well with the pressurized casting procedure in which hydrostatic fluid loading is the principle means of weight distribution.

The last suspension category uses outside joints and a thigh lacer attached to the prosthesis. This method is not a good suspension option. The thigh corset cannot grip the thigh sufficiently to resist pistoning. The CP is often required to add a belt and fork strap for this thigh corset and side joints design. Other disadvantages are the added weight and bulk and constriction of the thigh. The main indication for a CP using a joints and corset design is to increase the weight-bearing surface by taking up vertical loads through the corset. The side joints also add to knee stability on the amputated side (see Table 18-4).

### Transfemoral Suspension Techniques

The socket designs of either a quadrilateral or ischial containment accept all the following suspension methods and techniques, and the above-the-knee prosthesis may be suspended by the following (Table 18-5):

1. Suction/silicone suction
2. Suction/partial suction with auxiliary suspension
3. Belts, straps, and sleeves

## TABLE 18-5

*Transfemoral Suspension Systems*

| Classification | Indications | Advantages | Disadvantages | Examples |
|---|---|---|---|---|
| Suction | Long limb length<br>Stable limb volume | Provides best suspension and ROM | Requires stable limb volume<br>Difficult to don | |
| Silicone suction | Long limb length<br>Stable limb volume | Material reduces shear | Skin reactions to material<br>Difficult to don | |
| Straps | Used as auxiliary suspension<br>When suction alone is not available | Adjustable<br>Provides added security<br>Provides rotational control | Added straps and buckles<br>Inherent pistoning | |
| Hip joint and pelvic band | Short limbs<br>Weak hip abductors | Maximum ML support<br>Provides rotational control | Heavy<br>Bulky<br>Inherent pistoning | |
| Suspenders | Previous wearers<br>Abdominal scarring | Eliminates abdominal pressure | Uncomfortable<br>Inherent pistoning | |

Once again, suction appears to be the best method of suspension for the majority of transfemoral prostheses. It is indicated for patients with long residual limb lengths that are well shaped and stable in volume. The inherent positive quality of suction or silicone suction is that it allows the patient better control of the prosthesis. The CP achieves suction suspension in the transfemoral prosthesis with an airtight seal at the proximal brim by compressing the tissue of the upper thigh and creating a seal. The patient pulls the tissue beyond the seal by means of a pull sock. The CP positions a one-way valve at the distal end, which creates the distal seal. The patient can expel air through the valve by pushing a button and must have good balance and upper limb strength to perform the proper donning procedure. The CP can also use a silicone sleeve with a distal pin, as in the transtibial design. This method eliminates the difficult donning procedure, and the patient can still adjust the fit with additional prosthetic socks.

The CP commonly uses auxiliary belts and straps with suction designs. The belts often give additional security and can control rotation of the prosthesis on the soft tissue. By adding a belt to the lateral wall of a transfemoral prosthesis, the CP can give better M-L stability for patients with shorter limbs. The CP can use a mechanical hip joint and pelvic belt for auxiliary or primary means of suspension, which offers M-L stability. The amputee with weak hip musculature, short residual limb, or poor balance can benefit from this component. In rare instances, the CP uses none of the suspension techniques if the patient is excessively obese, pregnant, or has scar tissue, skin disorders, or abdominal pathologies. In these circumstances, the CP may use a shoulder harness to attach to the prosthesis and suspend it over the shoulder.

## Outcomes and Social Validation

The ability of amputees to ambulate comfortably and perform their daily activities while using their prostheses demonstrates the efficacy of this technology. The amputee population remains constant largely because of the proliferation of vascular diseases in the United States. The rehabilitation team must evaluate, prescribe, and continually monitor the efficacy of its recommendations. The team must not view the individual who has sustained an amputation as a failure in terms of medical care. They should give the patient the opportunity to develop and become an independent member of society. The team uses prosthetics technology from standing and balance activities to participating in athletic and recreational endeavors to assist in this rehabilitation process.

Functional outcomes and validation differ for various levels of amputations. In general, a reasonable goal for many amputees today is the ability to ambulate in and around the community in a comfortable and efficient manner. The functional outcome of this process has a tremendous effect on a person's quality of life. When appropriate and well-designed prosthetic technologies are used, an amputee who is initially debilitated and dependent on others is transformed into a more independent, functioning, and productive member of society.

## CASE STUDIES

### CASE 1

#### *Application and Goal*

M.T. is an 18-year-old unilateral transfemoral amputee. His amputation occurred as a result of a motorcycle accident. His residual limb is of medium length (midthigh) level with good tissue coverage and padding over the end of the femur. The uninvolved leg and upper extremities are intact and functioning normally. He has no other medical complications and is motivated and eager to begin walking again.

Management of the individual who experienced a traumatic limb loss and is otherwise young and healthy allows the team to incorporate innovative and functionally appropriate prosthetics technology. The treatment plan and objectives allow M.T. to perform most tasks and activities at levels that he accepts. These objectives go beyond basic ambulation and include ambulating in the community, walking on uneven terrain, changing cadences, and independent caring of residual limb and prosthesis. This young, active individual with traumatic amputation above the knee is expected to become a successful rehabilitation candidate with few obstacles to overcome.

## Function and Ability

M.T. should progress to a high level of function because of his age, health, and residual limb status. The prognosis for a return to independence is good. He should become a community ambulator without assistance at the minimum and if desired should be able to participate in sports and recreational activities. Specialists should place few functional limitations on him. Amputations that occur above the anatomic knee joint present limitations to normal walking and running. The knee joint is critical to energy conservation, balance, and volitional control of the prosthesis. Literature suggests that energy costs rise as much as 30% to 80% above able-bodied people when a surgeon performs amputation above the knee. This rise in energy cost causes most transfemoral patients to slow their speed of walking to decrease the total energy cost. This is often referred to as a *self-selected walking speed (SSWS)*.

## Considerations and Options

M.T. should begin early preprosthetic care including ROM, muscle strengthening, and balance activities. Early prosthetic intervention promotes healing, shapes the residual limb, and increases pressure tolerance. The team of specialists should take care to prevent a hip flexion contracture from developing. With the proper preprosthetic care and training this individual will be ready for early prosthetic fitting. The technologic options for this particular prosthesis are numerous. Factors that the team should consider are the person's vocational and avocational needs. Often a prosthesis that is good for a particular work environment is not good for recreational activities. If he needs a prosthesis for work and play, the technology must adapt for this dual function. The construction of the prosthesis is another factor to consider. The endoskeletal design looks more natural but may not be durable enough for high-level activities. The specific material that the CP uses must be able to withstand the demands of a teenager in activities of daily living (ADL). Componentry options should match the functional requirements that the CP places on the prosthesis. This particular candidate pushes the technology to keep up with his activity. Failure to use components and designs that are not durable, functional, and dynamic may result in rejection of the prosthesis.

## Technology

The CP indicates an ischial containment socket design for M.T. to increase the stability and comfort that he needs for functioning at high activity levels. Today, a CP uses many socket designs that have the needed biomechanical principles to stabilize the pelvis and femur during ambulation with a prosthesis. The CP suspends the prosthesis by suction for improved proprioception and control. The prosthetic knee component that the CP uses is a polycentric knee mechanism with fluid friction for stability and cadence responsiveness. The prosthetic foot that the CP uses is a carbon fiber dynamic response design for increased cadence and weight savings. The construction materials of the prosthesis that the CP uses are high tech, lightweight, and high strength. The CP uses an endoskeletal construction for its cosmetic features.

## Outcomes and Social Validation

M.T. is functionally independent in all phases of ambulation. He can increase his walking velocity up to running for short distances. He participates in recreational activities with his prosthesis. Private insurance covers the prosthesis, which needs routine maintenance and repairs. M.T. is satisfied with the outcome. The cosmetic appearance of the prosthesis is satisfactory, but the foam covering and cosmetic stockings continue to need frequent replacement.

## CASE 2

## Application and Goal

G.H. has sustained bilateral transtibial amputations secondary to diabetes and vascular disease. Diabetes and vascular diseases account for a large percentage of lower limb amputations. G.H. is 68 years old, has a history of high blood pressure, peripheral vascular disease, and mild osteoarthritis. He needs to ambulate for short distances in his home independently.

## Function and Ability

G.H. has poor circulation and sensation in both remaining extremities. His upper limb strength is fair, limb length is average, and muscular strength of the thigh is good. He will be unable to ambulate during the early part of the rehabilitation process. The rehabilitation team should use an amputee wheelchair for increased mobility during the time G.H. is unable to walk.

## Considerations and Options

G.H. begins preprosthetic care, limb shaping, desensitizing, and upper limb strengthening. After this process, a CP will fit him with preparatory prostheses for early weight bearing and balance training. Because of sensation difficulties, G.H. may require materials that allow for increased interface cushioning and shear force control. The CP often uses a urethane-based interface for more even distribution of forces over the residual limbs in the prostheses. A bilateral amputee needs to be concerned with total body height while wearing the prosthesis. The center of body mass rises as the surgeon amputates the leg segments; thus the CP must lower the person's overall height to compensate. G.H. will need to use an assistive device to ambulate independently. He also will need physical therapy for gait training and to ensure that no contractures develop.

## Technology

The CP should fit G.H. with bilateral PTB prostheses incorporating silicone liners for added cushioning. The CP will achieve suspension by sleeve suspension for simplicity and security. Construction will be endoskeletal for adjustability and appearance. The CP will incorporate SACH feet for stability and durability because the CP expects that G.H. will be a single-speed ambulator.

## Outcomes and Social Validation

G.H. ambulates for short distances with two canes. He is independent and continues to perform simple daily activities. He uses the wheelchair for long-distance mobility and to unload his residual limbs. Medicare paid for 80% of the prostheses cost, and the patient paid the remainder. G.H. was extremely satisfied with the outcome. He can continue to live in his current home and not be forced into an extended care facility.

## References

1. Winchell E: *Coping with limb loss,* Garden City, NJ, 1995, Avery Publishing Group.
2. Wilson AB: *Limb prosthetics,* ed 6, New York, 1989, Demos Publications.
3. Bowker J, Michael J: *Atlas of limb prosthetics, surgical, prosthetic, and rehabilitation principles,* ed 2, St Louis, 1992, Mosby.
4. Sanders G: *Lower limb amputations: a guide to rehabilitation,* Philadelphia, 1986, FA Davis.
5. Moore W, Malone J: *Lower extremity amputation,* Philadelphia, 1989, WB Saunders.
6. New York University Medical Center: *Lower limb prosthetics,* New York, 1990, New York University.

## Resources

American Academy of Orthotists and Prosthetists
American Board for Certification in Prosthetics and Orthotics
American Orthotic and Prosthetic Association
International Society of Orthtotists and Prosthetists: http://www.oandp.com

# CHAPTER 19

## Wheelchair Mobility

*David Kreutz*
*Susan Johnson Taylor*

## Application and Goal

Mobility is a necessity. Many children never have the opportunity to walk because of a variety of neuromuscular diseases or conditions. Adults may lose the functional use of their legs because of traumatic injuries or a variety of disabling diseases. Mobility restrictions can occur in many forms and to various degrees. Therefore specialists should consider each individual based on functional limitations rather than on specific diagnoses.[1] When ambulation is no longer functional, people require assistive devices such as ambulatory aides or wheeled mobility. According to the National Center for Health Statistics, 1,363,026 noninstitutionalized Americans with mobility impairment rely on manual wheelchairs and another 160,103 rely on either powered wheelchairs or power-operated vehicles (scooters) for mobility.[2] This chapter focuses on wheeled mobility options to improve a person's ability to access the home and community.

The primary goal of wheeled mobility is to provide safe, functional, and energy-efficient mobility in the household and community. This goal allows the person to achieve secondary goals such as increased independence, health maintenance, enhanced self-esteem, the attainment of an education and vocation, and a better quality of life.

For many, the need to be mobile ranks second only to the need to communicate. Unfortunately, the goal of independent mobility is not possible for everyone. The two basic categories of wheelchair mobility are independent and dependent wheelchair mobility. Independent wheelchair mobility is possible through a vast array of technology options including manual wheelchairs, powered wheelchairs, and scooters. The majority of dependent mobility is through manual wheelchairs, strollers, and travel chairs. A far less common form of dependent mobility is a powered wheelchair with an attendant control. Attendant-controlled powered wheelchairs are exceptions but can prove extremely beneficial for individuals who experience severe fatigue or are not safe given a particular situation or environment. A person may select dependent mobility despite the demonstration of independence in powered wheelchair mobility. For example, factors such as the availability of accessible transportation, technology tolerance, funding, and personal preference may override the goal of independent mobility.

### Specific Goals for Independent and Dependent Forms of Mobility

Specific goals for independent and dependent wheelchair mobility vary among individuals. "Medical necessity may set the limits on which wheelchairs are appropriate, but individual personalities, attitudes, living situations, and personal preferences will ultimately determine when and how the equipment will be used."[3] A determining factor in individuals establishing specific goals is the type of mobility they select, which can be manual or power.

Goals and outcomes leading to independent use of equipment vary depending on the person's physical ability, personal motivation and desires, and the type of manual or powered wheelchair selected. The following list of goals addresses mobility and other

BOX **19-1**

*Outcome Evaluation Factors for Wheelchair Mobility*

Has the mobility goal been achieved relative to performance, covering travel distances in an appropriate amount of time, and accessibility to desired environments (e.g., to home, school, and work)?

Is the person comfortable in the seating and mobility system? Is sitting tolerance appropriate for daily living activities, including weight shifts?

Is the user/caregiver able to manage environmental obstacles?

Is the user/caregiver able to transport the wheelchair? Have they achieved independence with loading and unloading the wheelchair in the vehicle?

Is the user/caregiver satisfied with the evaluation process, including personal level of participation in setting goals and participation in equipment selection and trial?

Has the user/caregiver obtained funding? Was the user made aware of personal expenses and the processes surrounding billing?

Is the user/caregiver able to identify the supplier of the equipment? Do they understand the responsibilities of the supplier versus the clinician? Do they know who to contact in the event of a problem, either functional or equipment related?

Is the user/caregiver able to state and/or demonstrate maintenance procedures to keep the mobility device safe and operational?

functions directly related to a manual or powered mobility base, each requiring an objective measure to quantify the level of independence:

- Level of independence in propulsion indoor and outdoor on level surfaces and side slopes (sidewalks and streets)
- Level of independence ascending and descending a 1 : 12 ramp
- Level of independence in management of environmental barriers such as ascending and descending curb cuts, ramps, curbs (specific heights), stairs, and various types of surfaces
- Level of independence loading and unloading the wheelchair from a vehicle
- Level of independence in transfers to and from the wheelchair to various surfaces
- Ability to operate component parts of the wheelchair as related to functional activities
- Ability to manage or communicate knowledge needed to maintain equipment
- Ability to identify a supplier (for repairs) and funding sources

To determine how well the mobility system meets the needs of the individual, clinicians perform an outcome assessment (Box 19-1). The outcome assessment should look beyond individual satisfaction with the equipment and solicit information on the entire delivery process. Positive outcomes depend on the thoroughness of the assessment, discussion of goals and personal preferences, success with training, skill development, and the person's knowledge acquisition.

## Function and Ability

People who have physical impairments that result in nonfunctional ambulation or functional ambulation that is limited by poor endurance could benefit from manual or powered mobility. Individuals with complete paralysis differ from those whose functional ambulation is limited by endurance, balance disorders, pain, and/or safety-related problems. Nonfunctional ambulation as a result of lower-extremity paralysis or severe weakness is obvious to the clinician. The clinician can easily justify alternative mobility being medically necessary when physical impairment has resulted in nonfunctional ambulation. Functional ambulation limited by endurance, pain, or safety requires more careful observation from the clinician and alternative mobility may be more difficult to justify. For example, individuals with postpolio syndrome or multiple sclerosis may walk into a clinic without an ambulatory aid or any apparent difficulty. Subjectively, they may report episodes when they have been stranded and unable to walk because of fatigue or a sudden relapse in their condition. A wide range of assistive technology exists to enhance mobility needs. The selection of specific technology depends on the individual's physical abilities and lifestyle.

......................................................... C A S E   S T U D Y .........................................................

## CASE 1

A neurologist referred a 30-year-old man with a diagnosis of multiple sclerosis for a manual wheelchair and training. He had the ability to transfer independently and ambulate household distances by cruising furniture. However, he demonstrated an ataxic gait pattern and poor endurance. He also complained of occasional falls. His primary goal was to maintain a nondisabled appearance. Safety, conservation of energy, and household and community wheelchair mobility were not issues of primary concern to him. He denied his disability and refused to use any assistive technology. More importantly, he perceived the use of crutches, a rolling walker, or a wheelchair to contribute to a "handicapped" appearance. Provision of a wheelchair would not have guaranteed that he would use it. The wheelchair would have probably ended up in a closet with the previously purchased crutches and walker. Approximately 3 months after the initial visit, this man realized the way the fatigue and lower extremity weakness limited his mobility and he ultimately obtained a manual wheelchair. He continues to use the wheelchair 2 years later and is convinced it has improved his quality of life.

Clinicians must carefully assess and recognize the physical ability of individuals to use the equipment and their willingness to accept and handle mobility technology including canes, crutches, walkers, rolling walkers, manual wheelchairs, scooters, and powered wheelchairs. Proper application of this technology requires that clinicians listen carefully to people's needs and thoroughly understand the basic application principles of manual and powered mobility.

## Principles of Manual and Powered Mobility

Manual and powered wheelchair performance depends on the design of the wheelchair and the way it is set up for the specific user. The clinician must understand a few basic principles about wheelchair performance before making recommendations. The first and most important principle is for the clinician to try the device before allowing the client to use it. Significant harm and loss of trust can result quickly if a wheelchair is unstable, too fast, fails to work, or is difficult to operate. Furthermore, by using the device, the clinician is able to understand and anticipate the way the wheelchair will respond to user input. The next most important principle is for the clinician to observe and assess the client's positioning needs and the skills required to operate the device. Understanding the way a power or manual wheelchair will respond (to user input and on different terrain) will allow the clinician to appropriately match the technology to the person's needs.

Regarding wheelchair performance, the clinician should answer the following key questions:

1. How can the wheelchair be made stable for the user to ensure safety?
2. How can the wheelchair be made more efficient to maximize the user's ability during propulsion?

## Stability

Stability and mobility are inversely proportional in manual wheelchairs. As stability is increased, mobility efficiency is decreased. In wheelchair stability, the more centered and lowered the person's mass is between the front and rear wheels, the more stable the wheelchair becomes. When the clinician displaces the rear axle well behind the center of mass, rearward stability increases. The greater the perpendicular distance between the rear axle ($Z$) and the vertical line drawn through the center of gravity ($Y$), the more stable the wheelchair becomes (Figure 19-1). Conversely, when the clinician moves the rear axle forward (or the person back) the stability of the wheelchair decreases. Terrain can also affect stability. As the person ascends a ramp or incline, the center of gravity is displaced rearward causing the wheelchair to be less stable. The person must lean forward to compensate for this instability.

This same principle applies to traction in powered wheelchairs. Simply, the more weight over the drive wheels, the better the wheelchair traction especially outdoors on steep uphill and downhill grades and on wet or icy surfaces. For example, a rear-wheel

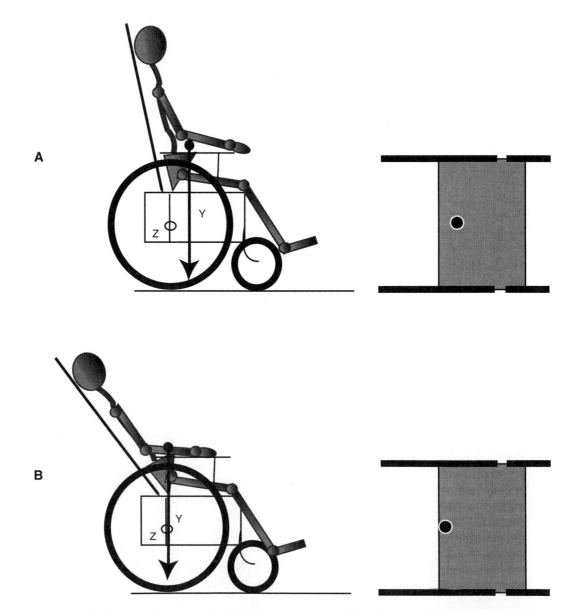

**Fig. 19-1 A,** Side view of a semirecliner and top view of the base of support and projected center of gravity when the chair back is upright. **B,** Same two views when the chair back is fully reclined. (Greene DP, Roberts SL: *Kinesiology: movement in the context of activity,* St Louis, 1999, Mosby.)

drive powered chair is able to climb fairly steep grades provided it does not tip backwards because of the increased traction caused by the rearward shift in center of gravity. Conversely, the same wheelchair descending steep grades or ramps with a low friction coefficient may lose traction and begin sliding because the center of gravity is shifted off the drive wheels and onto the casters. A front-wheel drive mobility system would demonstrate just the opposite response. One way to compensate for changes in stability in manual and powered wheelchairs because of terrain is for the user to lean forward when ascending inclines and lean backward when descending inclines. A midwheel drive powered wheelchair places the drive wheels more directly under the person and provides antitip devices at the front of the wheelchair. Although midwheel drive wheelchairs are stable in a rearward direction, they tend to tip forward more easily than a front-wheel drive or rear-wheel drive wheelchair.

The clinician may also adjust lateral stability on certain manual wheelchairs. Stability to prevent the wheelchair from tipping to the side depends on the height of the center of mass and rear wheel camber (Figure 19-2). The lower the mass and the wider the base of support, the more stable the wheelchair. Wheel camber describes the vertical orientation of the rear wheel. The clinician adjusts typical wheel camber so that the top of the rear wheels is angled in toward the user while the bottom of the rear wheels slopes away. This brings the wheels closer to the user's hands for better accessibility to the wheels and a more efficient propulsion stroke. Generally, people use large degrees of camber (usually 6 to 8 degrees or more) in sports such as wheelchair tennis, basketball, and road racing to improve lateral stability and access to the handrims. The disadvantage of camber on everyday-use wheelchairs is that it increases the overall width of a wheelchair causing accessibility problems. The overall width of the wheelchair increases by about 1 to ½ inches for every 3 degrees of camber.

## Mobility

A clinician shifting the axle forward (relative to the person) or the person rearward (relative to the rear axle) can improve efficiency of mobility. When this is done, propulsion efficiency, maneuverability, and a decrease in the downhill turning tendency improve.[4] The primary reason for this improved performance is the reduction in weight and resistance on the front casters. A decrease in downhill turning tendency means that tracking

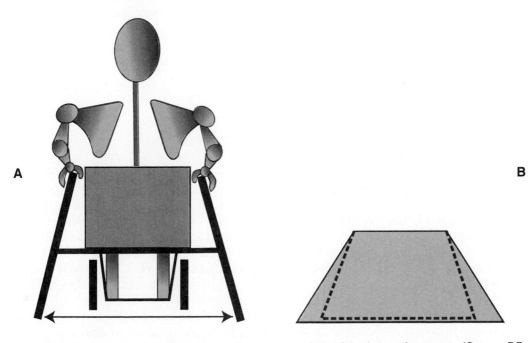

**Fig. 19-2 A,** Rear-wheel camber. **B,** Its effect on the width of the base of support. (Greene DP, Roberts SL: *Kinesiology: movement in the context of activity,* St Louis, 1999, Mosby.)

a straight course on sidewalks and other surfaces will be easier for the user when traversing a slope.

Wheel alignment, surface composition, tire pressure, and tire material affect propulsion efficiency.[4] The wheels must be parallel on a wheelchair if the chair is to roll efficiently. Rear-wheel alignment must be parallel to reduce drag. Rear wheels that toe in or toe out can result in a wheelchair that is much more difficult to propel. Toe in occurs when the wheels are closer together at the front than in the rear. The distance between the rear wheels at the height of the axle (at the front and rear of the wheel) should be of equal dimensions if the clinician properly aligned the wheels. Causative factors for toe in or toe out include a bent frame or poor folding frame design, improper axle and/or axle plate alignment, and modifying the rear wheel camber. Whenever the camber is changed on a manual wheelchair, the clinician must make a measurement for toe in and toe out. Manufacturers use different methods to correct toe in and toe out.

Propulsion efficiency is also affected by tire pressure, tire material, and surface composition. Tire pressure affects the rolling resistance by reducing the amount of friction. Generally, the greater the tire pressure, the lower the rolling resistance. As tire pressure decreases, the person must use more effort to propel the wheelchair. The surfaces that a person rolls over also greatly affects the amount of effort needed to propel the wheelchair. Firmer surfaces are easier to push over than soft surfaces because less friction exists. Sandy or boggy soil increases the amount of friction. The user must consider tire size, tire pressure, and method of propulsion when using a wheelchair on surfaces where the wheel tends to sink rather than roll across the surface.

With the exception of camber, the principles outlined previously also apply to powered mobility. However, powered mobility forces the clinician and wheelchair user to consider additional performance characteristics such as maximum forward speed, turn speeds, acceleration, deceleration, "cruise control" (driving in latched mode), and tremor dampening (Table 19-1). Basically, all powered wheelchairs have a controller that communicates with the motors (Figure 19-3). The clinician programs the controller to various extents, depending on the manufacturer and style of the wheelchair, to adjust the performance to the user's physical and cognitive skills. Most powered chairs offer a choice of two separate programs that allow the supplier/clinician to provide the user with two distinct performance parameters.

Clinicians need to understand the relevance of these controller functions and be able to apply them appropriately. Significant differences exist in controller functions with each manufacturer and model of wheelchair. Identifying the input device and necessary performance characteristics are two of the most important steps the clinician makes in selection of a powered wheelchair. The clinician must determine which of these features are important for the wheelchair user to efficiently manage and safely operate the wheelchair.

## Considerations, Options, and Technology

Many factors influence the selection of a mobility system for an individual. Some factors that can influence the decision are diagnosis, prognosis, medical complications, function, cognitive status, transportation, environment, funding, service, personal goals, lifestyle, and ability to care for and maintain the chair. One of the first branches in this decision tree is for the user to decide between powered and manual mobility. Today, the determination of manual versus powered mobility looks beyond the typical dividing line of whether or not the person has impaired upper extremity function. The "use it or lose it" mentality of previous years has, in some cases, resulted in higher levels of dependence (increasing disability) because of years of overuse. Clinicians and the person with a disability should discuss the desired form of mobility and the possible physical long-term effects. Secondary complications such as carpal tunnel syndrome, bursitis, tendonitis, chronic pain, and arthritis have been attributed to manual wheelchair propulsion.[6]

## TABLE 19-1

*Wheelchair Performance Characteristics and Functional Implications*

| Performance Characteristic | Definition | Functional Implications |
|---|---|---|
| Speed | Speed is how fast the chair moves. In some wheelchairs, the clinician/supplier can separately set maximum forward, reverse, and turn speeds to improve operation and safety. | Maximum top speed may be important to some. Young, old, and new users of specialty switches may be more concerned with how slow they can set the top speed for safe operation. Speed adjustment may be crucial for management of thick carpet or other barriers. Someone attending college may need increased speed to arrive to class on time. |
| Acceleration | Acceleration describes the amount of time it takes to reach top speed from a standstill. The user programs this separately for forward, reverse, and turning. | A short acceleration time results in a responsive chair. The person must have good control and be able to respond quickly. A short acceleration also provides the user immediate feedback. A user can combine a short acceleration time and slow speeds for learning new input commands. A long acceleration time provides better control of the wheelchair for someone who has difficulty adjusting to abrupt changes in speed. |
| Deceleration | Deceleration is the amount of time it takes the chair to stop once the user has ceased input to the chair. The user programs this separately for forward, reverse, and turning. | A short deceleration time results in abrupt stops, and a long deceleration time slows the wheelchair gradually to a stop. People with good control and balance prefer short deceleration so that they can stop suddenly and do not overshoot their target, particularly in areas that have tight accessibility. People with poor head and trunk control may require a long deceleration time to prevent them from losing balance. |
| Cruise control or momentary versus latched | Cruise control defines the user's need to maintain contact on the input devices to operate the wheelchair. Momentary control operates only when the user maintains contact. Latched control allows the user to select and maintain a set forward and/or reverse speed by activating the switch once. The user stopping and making directional changes require additional input. | A person uses latched control most frequently with specialty digital switches such as pneumatic and various forms of single switches. Functional gains in control of the wheelchair, improved efficiency of operation, and conservation of muscle strength are some of the reasons for a person to use a module that has switch latching ability. Turns are never latched. They remain momentary while forward and/or reverse are latched. A person must always use a safety switch and place it in location, which immediately cuts power to the wheelchair. The client can access it 100% of the time because this is the only input that allows the client to stop the chair immediately in an emergency. |
| Tremor dampening or switch sensitivity | Tremor dampening permits the controller or module to average erratic signals from the input device, which results in smoother driving. This only works with proportional systems.[5] | Tremor dampening allows a person with upper extremity tremors and spasms to use a proportional joystick. The user can engage the tremor-dampening feature to remove extraneous right and left signals to maintain a relatively straight course. |

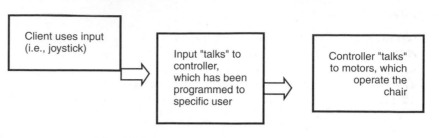

**Fig. 19-3** Power wheelchair control process.

TABLE **19-2**

*Manual Mobility Versus Powered Mobility Considerations*

| Consideration | Manual Mobility Questions | Powered Mobility Questions |
|---|---|---|
| Function | Is the person able to propel a manual w/c using upper and/or lower extremities at household and community distances? Has the person been given an opportunity to use technology that would maximize potential to propel a manual w/c (e.g., an adjustable w/c that has been set up appropriately for the person)? | Is the person's strength or endurance such that manual w/c propulsion is not possible? Does the typical daily routine require propulsion beyond the limits of the individual's endurance or place the person at high risk of orthopedic problems? Will use of a manual w/c result in secondary complications (i.e., pelvic obliquity or scoliosis)? |
| Transportation | What kind of transportation is available for a manual w/c? Will the person load the w/c independently? What w/c frame and components will improve independence? | Does the person have access to transportation (personal or public) for powered mobility? Are tie downs and a lift device available and appropriate for powered mobility? Is obtaining powered and manual mobility feasible for the person? |
| Environment | Will the person primarily use the w/c inside the home? Is the user able to self-propel in the community or rely on assistance? What is the terrain like in the community (e.g., hilly, flat, rocky, etc.)? | Is powered mobility necessary for independence because of the distances traveled or difficult terrain? |
| Cognition | Is the person able to safely propel a manual w/c? Because of poor judgment or safety concerns, does the clinician need to restrict accessibility? | Does the person understand cause and effect? Does the person exhibit cognitive impairments in memory, problem solving, or impulse control that may prohibit the use of a power w/c? Is the intended user only safe in familiar environments? |
| Vocational | Can the person manage daily routines including work and school activities using a manual w/c? | Is powered mobility necessary for the person to efficiently manage work and school activities without being exhausted? |
| Medical complications | What medical complications are present that would inhibit the person's ability to use a manual w/c? | Does the person have cardiopulmonary problems? Is the person unable to sustain functional cardiac output to push a manual w/c household distances? |

*W/c,* wheelchair.

Another consideration is the person's endurance, or how much effort it takes to propel a manual wheelchair over distances. School-age children and adults may be expending too much of their energy resources just moving from one place to another, resulting in a decreased ability to concentrate or complete other tasks such as activities of daily living (ADL) or school work. Some individuals with diagnoses of multiple sclerosis or postpolio syndrome risk permanent damage if they push beyond their limits over time. Clinicians who treat children must remember that the children have many years of mobility in the future. Clinicians and users need to give ample consideration to the decision of manual versus powered mobility (Table 19-2).

The user must consider the following general factors before selecting a specific-powered or manual-mobility wheelchair model to improve function and lifetime of the equipment:

- Will the user need to modify the wheelchair? This is particularly important if the intended user is a child or a person who has lost significant weight after a traumatic injury. Children are not the only ones who may need modification ability. Rehabilitation stays are currently short; therefore some people can gain or lose significant amounts of weight and/or function after being discharged and receiving their wheelchairs. In addition to knowing whether the wheelchair can be modified for growth, the user also needs to know the way to achieve this and how much the cost will be to accomplish it.

What other equipment will the mobility base need to be compatible with to maximize function, accessibility, and transportation? First and foremost is for the user to be compatible with the seating system. For example, if a person has a hip contracture allowing only 45 degrees of hip flexion, the seat-to-back angle accommodating this limitation is essential. Possible solutions include the person using a reclining wheelchair or integrating the seating/mobility system to achieve 45 degrees of recline. Other compatibility issues might include consideration of van lifts and tie-down systems that are required for transportation. In addition, the person may need support trays for a communication system, computer, oxygen concentrator, ventilator, and ventilator battery. Other factors include integration of an environmental control unit, communication system, and/or powered seating systems that allow the person to use the input device to perform multiple functions.

Will the mobility base be able to adapt to address changes in functional status over time? Prognoses can vary greatly from one person to the next despite similar diagnoses. Trends with certain disease processes have helped clinicians forecast changes and build in adaptability to mobility bases. The user anticipating these changes can enhance the lifetime of the mobility base.

## CASE STUDY

### CASE 2

A 30-year-old man with a diagnosis of Guillain-Barré syndrome showed slow yet steady improvement during his rehabilitation stay. At discharge, he could ambulate 20 feet in parallel bars with the assistance of one but relied on a power wheelchair for household and community mobility. His limited upper-extremity strength and endurance prohibited manual wheelchair propulsion. However, transportation was available for a manual wheelchair only. To maximize his independence, he used a manual wheelchair with a power add-on unit. As his condition improved, he could lower the manual wheelchair base to allow lower-extremity propulsion. He can also use the power component, which is necessary for long distances. In this way the wheelchair remained functional longer and served as an adjunct to therapy.

## *Manual Mobility Systems*

### Dependent Mobility

Persons with disabilities should use dependent mobility as an alternative to independent mobility only after they have tried all forms of independent manual and powered mobility or when they are not capable of independent mobility. The inability of the user to operate a powered wheelchair or propel a manual wheelchair is not the only reason for selecting a dependent mobility system. Other reasons might include a user's inability to transport a powered wheelchair, the ease of transporting a manual wheelchair or stroller, the personal preference of the user, a lack of home accessibility, environmental considerations, or a lack of funding to obtain powered mobility.

A powered wheelchair with a powered tilting or reclining system can weigh up to 250 lb or more. Dimensions for a similar chair may start at approximately 25 inches in overall width and 46 inches in overall length. These weights and dimensions have serious implications for a person's transportation and accessibility. Lack of transportation, a living situation that requires ascending and descending stairs, inadequate floor support, or a small living space are reasons people have declined a power wheelchair. Dependent mobility options include pediatric and adult strollers, travel chairs, manual wheelchairs, manual reclining wheelchairs, positioning chairs, and tilt-in-space wheelchairs.

### Strollers

Strollers come in many varieties. Some include their own seating components, and others accept various manufacturers' seating inserts. One feature of strollers that specifically relates to dependent mobility is the adjustable stroller handles that allow the person pushing the stroller the ability to adjust the height for comfort. The main advantage of strollers is that they tend to be lighter and more portable than wheelchairs. In addition, parents of young children with disabilities may find the stroller a more socially acceptable solution to a child's positioning and mobility needs. The disadvantage is that strollers promote dependence if the child is capable of propelling a manual wheelchair. Options for removable seating systems that interface with positioning frames, floor sitting frames, and high chairs broaden their application potential and cost effectiveness.

### Travel or Transport Chairs

Travel chairs are similar to strollers in that they have four small wheels. Like strollers, travel chairs are considerably lighter than wheelchairs, weighing approximately 15 lb. The weight and folding characteristics, similar to that of lawn chairs, make these chairs easy to transport. Persons use transport chairs primarily when they require assistance ambulating long distances or fatigues easily. They should use these chairs on solid, level surfaces because managing obstacles such as loose terrain and stairs can be difficult.

### Manual Wheelchairs

Manual wheelchairs function well as dependent mobility systems. They are built for the caregiver to propel and for stability to protect the user. The large rear wheels can make curbs and other obstacles easier to manage. Most of the low-cost standard manual wheelchairs have a fixed, rear axle position. This vertical orientation of the seat requires the user to maintain sitting balance. Some of the moderately priced wheelchairs have semiadjustable rear axles allowing for vertical movement. The operator can use this vertical adjustment to change the orientation of the wheelchair seat in space and allow gravity to assist in positioning and balance, giving the person increased stability. This option can allow individuals with poor sitting balance a more compact and more transportable alternative to the bulky manual reclining and tilt-in-space mobility systems.

### Reclining and Tilt-in-Space Wheelchairs

Reclining and tilt-in-space wheelchairs are designed to serve as dependent mobility systems and positioning systems. These wheelchairs are intended for individuals who cannot sit in a vertical position for extended periods. They may need to change positions for the following reasons:

- Pressure redistribution to prevent decubiti
- Compensation for episodes of orthostatic hypotension
- Compensation for dependent sitting balance
- Accommodation of orthopedic deformities at the hips and spine

Because of the reclining and/or tilting feature, the overall length of the wheelchair base must be longer for stability. Placement of the rear wheels far behind the user's center of gravity ensures stability, however, it does impede efficient propulsion. This same principle of offsetting the center of mass in front of the rear wheels also impedes the caregiver's management of the wheelchair, especially when descending ramps and ascending curbs. Some tilt-in-space manual wheelchairs are designed to allow the user to shift the weight (thereby shifting the center of gravity) forward on the base as it tilts. This assists in reducing the overall length of the wheelchair by 4 to 6 inches. The user may have difficulty transporting these wheelchairs because of their weight and size. Most tilt-in-space systems do not fold like conventional cross-frame wheelchairs and therefore take up significant cargo space. Some reclining and tilt-in-space wheelchairs offer a relatively lightweight frame with removable rear wheels that allow storage in a large trunk space or in a van without a lift.

## Independent Mobility

Independent wheelchair propulsion is possible when a person uses the upper extremities, an upper extremity, and the lower extremities, one upper and lower extremity, and even one lower extremity. Each of these methods requires the user to set up different equipment to optimize efficiency and function. Although propulsion may be possible under institutional or indoor conditions, some of these methods do not necessarily guarantee a functional outcome. For example, propelling a manual wheelchair with an asymmetrical approach can result in a person having secondary complications such as scoliosis, pressure sores, or dysfunction of a limb, and therefore should not be considered as independent or functional. Hundreds of manual wheelchair options exist. Commercial literature, selection guides, and wheelchair standards all exist to aid the intended user and clinician in selecting appropriate equipment.

### Conventional Wheelchairs

Conventional frame wheelchairs weigh 35 lb or more and have a cross brace to allow a person to fold the wheelchair. This type of wheelchair is best suited for temporary use, such as after a hip fracture or other lower extremity impairment. Conventional wheelchairs have a fixed, rear axle position set behind the center of mass of the user for maximum stability and safety. However, this axle position does allow independent propulsion.

### Semiadjustable Wheelchairs

Semiadjustable wheelchairs have a folding frame construction and typically weigh between 28 and 35 lb. The term *semiadjustable* refers to the limited vertical/horizontal adjustment of the rear axle. A person adjusting the rear axle higher up on the frame results in an increased degree of fixed seat tilt. This vertical adjustment is applicable for persons who lack functional sitting balance. Horizontal adjustment brings the wheel slightly closer to the user and can shorten the overall wheelbase by about an inch. Propulsion efficiency in this wheelchair may be slightly better than the conventional frame because of the person's improved balance and the reduced wheelchair weight.

### Fully Adjustable Wheelchairs

Fully adjustable wheelchairs allow for rear axle adjustment in a horizontal and vertical plane (usually about 4 inches in both directions). This affects stability of the wheelchair, access to the wheel for propulsion, and the overall length of the wheelbase for horizontal adjustment. Most designs also allow for toe-in/toe-out and camber adjustment of the rear wheel. These four adjustments combine to impact propulsion efficiency, static and dynamic stability, and maneuverability of the wheelchair. The frames of these wheelchairs can be either folding or rigid with a weight of between 18 to 30 lb. Application is not restricted to "the active wheelchair user" as is so often assumed. These wheelchairs are often called *sports chairs,* a great disservice to the function this chair can provide. Persons with C-5/6 quadriplegia or generalized weakness from aging could show significant gains in mobility if they use fully adjustable wheelchairs that are properly adjusted to meet physical and functional needs. If properly adjusted, a person who could not function in a conventional frame wheelchair might be able to propel a fully adjustable wheelchair at household levels because of improved efficiency and access to the rear wheels. Additionally, long-term orthopedic problems such as shoulder pain may be reduced.

### Hemi and One-Arm Drive Wheelchairs

*Hemi* and *one-arm drive wheelchairs* refer more to the seat height and the method of propulsion and do not truly warrant a separate wheelchair category. For example, the term *hemi* refers to a particular seat-to-floor height of 17 inches. The clinician can achieve this seat-to-floor height using wheelchairs from each of the three previous categories and should determine the optimal seat-to-floor height for lower extremity propulsion (Box 19-2). The individual should be able to sit on a cushion in the wheelchair with a foot or feet flat on the floor and cushion fully supporting the thighs. A seat that is too high results in the person having to slide down on the cushion to reach the floor to propel. Many semiadjustable and fully adjustable wheelchairs can provide a wide range of seat-to-floor heights.

Similarly, *one-arm drive* also refers to the method of propulsion. With this type of propulsion, the user propels and steers the wheelchair using only one arm. The most common form of a one-arm drive system is an optional component that a clinician can add to some of the wheelchairs in the three previous categories. However, one model of a one-arm drive is unique and the user can only use it as a one-arm drive mobility system. This wheelchair uses a lever drive/steering column combination to operate. It is also one of the few manual wheelchairs that is equipped with a true braking system. Both types of one-arm drive systems require full function in an upper extremity to operate the wheelchair. The clinician should remember that this is not an easy method of propulsion, as the person is propelling body weight plus the chair weight with one arm. Therefore persons must have ample opportunity to evaluate this method of propulsion within their expected environments.

### Manual Wheelchair Components and Characteristics

Manual wheelchairs are available in either folding or rigid frame designs. Folding-frame wheelchairs have basically the same design as previous years with a cross brace that allows a person to fold the wheelchair and load it into a vehicle. Wheelchairs load into a car with less width than a rigid frame, although it takes up more length in the cargo space. Another advantage of the cross-frame design is the capability to change seat width over time. The cross-frame design also allows the frame to flex so that all four wheels remain in contact with the ground on uneven surfaces. This flexibility does, however, result in less efficient propulsion because much of the energy the user puts into propelling is lost in the flexing of the frame.

Rigid frame wheelchairs are usually welded into a box frame and have little flex in the frame. The clinician may alter the seat plane angle in rigid wheelchairs for balance, stability, and seating through coupled or uncoupled adjustment. Coupled adjustment means that the clinician must alter the wheel position while changing the seat angle. Conversely, the clinician accomplishes uncoupled adjustment through a hinge mechanism in the seat rail and requires no corresponding adjustments to correct wheel and

## BOX 19-2

*Wheelchair Height Considerations*

Appropriate seat height for foot propulsion equals length of user's lower leg minus the cushion height measured at the front of the cushion. For example, if a person has a 17-inch lower leg length and a 3-inch cushion height, the seat height (floor to top of seat rail) would need to be 14 inches.

caster stem alignment. The combination of frame design, quick-release wheels, and a fold-down back can make loading and unloading a rigid wheelchair into a car possible for the user with good upper extremity strength. Components and safety features vary significantly depending on the manufacturer. Options include wheel types and sizes, caster sizes, wheel locks, front and rear antitip devices, armrests, push handles, footrests and legrests. Component parts are essential in postural support, mobility, and transfers. The user should base selection of components on the ease of operation and management.

## Powered Mobility

Powered mobility technology has advanced tremendously in the past few decades. Improvements in frame design, computer technology, energy storage systems, circuitry, and switches are a few of the reasons that this area of technology is growing. The clinician selects a specific power wheelchair for a person based on physical ability and planned use of the equipment. The clinician should consider a number of factors when selecting a powered mobility system. Besides seating, the most important components are the input device and the controller (control module is the part of the wheelchair that tells the motor how to respond to the user's input). The clinician must answer the following questions when selecting an input device:

- What functional ability does the user have for operating the input devices to drive the powered wheelchair?
- Which is the most consistent site for operation? Do multiple sites exist where the client can operate the chair using individual single switches?
- Where does the clinician need to place the input device to allow the best control? How will the clinician position the input device?
- Does the user need commercially available or customized hardware?
- What parameters (speed, acceleration, etc.) does the user need that provide function, safety, and efficiency in operating the powered wheelchair?

## Input Devices

The user should determine the type of input device (i.e., control interface, joystick, switch) before selecting the mobility base. Certain basic power wheelchairs do not accept specialty input devices. Input devices are either proportional or digital. A proportional input device is similar to a dimmer switch allowing the user to vary the amount of light or, in the case of a wheelchair, speed. Much like the accelerator pedal on a car, the further the user deflects the input device, the faster the chair will move. Digital input devices are on/off switches similar to a standard light switch. The person has only one speed with a digital input device. Adjustment of performance parameters such as acceleration, deceleration, and speed is important on digital systems, as the user is not able to grade the parameters. The chair will immediately respond to the controller as programmed. Proportional input devices include most joysticks and a variety of head control systems. Digital systems include pneumatic switches (sip and puff), individual single switches, and microswitch joysticks.

### Proportional Input Devices

The input device for proportional control of a powered wheelchair that a person most commonly uses is a joystick. A joystick serves three functions: (1) variable speed control, (2) multidirectional steering, and (3) stopping the chair. A joystick is typically placed for optimal hand control, provided the person has the upper-extremity strength and range of motion to use a joystick. Functional prerequisites for the user include being able to place the hand on and off the joystick, moving the joystick throughout its 360 degree range with some degree of fine motor control, and understanding the way to stop the wheelchair by removing the hand from the joystick. The location, resistance to deflection, and the range of deflection are factors that the user can change to address the previously described prerequisites. Short throw occurs when the user decreases range of deflection. A short-throw joystick decreases the deflection necessary for full range and function in either forward/reverse and/or left/right, depending on the user's patterns of movement and strength. For example, a child with a diagnosis of spinal muscular atrophy and severe weakness may require a short-throw joystick with little resistance to movement. The clinician should place the short-throw joystick in a position where the child exhibits the greatest strength and least postural deformities to compensate for weakness.

The clinician can place joysticks by the user's hand, head, chin, elbow, knee, and foot for control. Site selection requires the clinician and supplier to research the availability of different joystick sizes, positioning hardware to mount the joystick, and the programming capability of the module before selecting a powered wheelchair. The most common placement of the joystick for hand control is on the outside of the armrest. If range or strength of the user necessitates a more midline position, use of a standard joystick may be prohibited because of its size. A clinician can place a remote joystick (a smaller joystick with multiple mounting orientations) inside the armrest on a removable support tray or swing-away hardware.

A person who has good head control and range of motion but no upper-extremity and lower-extremity function has several options for proportional input. The simplest and least expensive is the chin control interface. The clinician mounts the remote joystick to a swing-away support or on a bib worn around the person's neck. Disadvantages for the user include strain on the cervical musculature, difficulty achieving consistent positioning for optimal access, and interference with other functional activities. If foot control is the most functional movement, the clinician also may place a modified, heavy-duty joystick at the foot. However, the foot joystick needs to be heavy duty because a standard joystick is not able to withstand the forces that the lower extremity applies. Because of the thickness of most foot-controlled systems, the clinician must take care to ensure adequate footrest clearance.

Proportional head-operated systems can be low tech, such as a standard joystick with a headrest or occipital control interface. They can also be high tech, such as the Peachtree Head Control. This input device is a headrest that tracks a person's head position and detects movement of the head in a 180-degree transverse plane. The user selects emergency stop, two forward-drive programs (high and low), reverse drive, and other integrated components by tapping the head against the headrest. The user then achieves direction and speed control by head movement and not by contact with the headrest. The head movement required is primarily neck flexion/extension and lateral neck flexion. The head movement the user needs to operate these input devices varies. Joystick head systems require head rotation, and the Peachtree Head Control requires lateral head flexion. With all head control drives, the user must have good proximal stability. All head-operated input devices allow the user to drive in only three directions at one time. The same head movement generally controls forward and reverse directions. The standard joystick requires head retraction or cervical extension against the input device to make the chair move forward or backward. This resistance provides some sensory feedback to the person. The Peachtree Head Control requires head flexion away from the headrest to make the chair move forward or backward. Both of these input devices require special module electronics to allow the user to select between forward and reverse directions.

### Digital Input Devices

A digital input device that the user activates provides operation in one direction at a preset, constant speed. Some joysticks, single switches, switch arrays, and pneumatic systems are examples of single-switch controllers. Digital input devices work best when the individual lacks fine motor control or one consistent location where the person has the physical ability to operate a proportional system. The single-switch systems offer the user less control to gradually change speed for moving through tight spaces. Two methods for the user to improve efficiency in digital-switch systems include activating two switches at the same time to achieve a turn while moving forward or using latching forward and/or reverse. Both methods require the user to have fairly fast response time. Use of latched mode in any of these digital systems requires that a clinician position a safety switch to stop the chair if the user should lose access to the controller.

Single switches offer a lot of diversity. Besides abundant shapes and sizes, these switches may vary in method of activation and transmission, sensory feedback, and location. A person may activate single switches through pressure, detection of movement toward the switch, eye movement, eye blink, and muscle contraction. Direct wiring typically permits transmission of the input signal to the module. However, some switches transmit to a receiver, which transmits the signal to the module, such as in the New Abilities Tongue Touch Keypad. Probably the biggest advantage of single switches is the ability to place them almost anywhere that the user has function. Depending on the method of activation, a clinician can mount these switches basically anywhere the user has functional movement: to upper-extremity support trays, headrests, inside the user's mouth, overlying a specific muscle, and about the user's eye. The more complex the technology is to drive the chair, the more parts, pieces, and repairs will likely be necessary. Clinicians should ensure that their clients understand the levels of complexity they are recommending.

Air pressure from the user's mouth typically controls a pneumatic switch, commonly called *the sip and puff,* rather than the muscles of respiration. Good, consistent oral motor control is a necessity. A person who has absent-to-severely limited extremity and head control usually chooses a pneumatic controller. The user may be ventilator dependent and still operate a pneumatic input device by sipping and puffing commands through a straw. A hard puff causes the wheelchair to move forward; a hard sip stops forward movement; another hard sip activates reverse; and soft puff and soft sip results in right and left turns, respectively. Pneumatic systems are easiest to operate when the user latches them in forward and/or reverse while right and left turns remain momentary. The user must have a great deal of energy (and breath-holding ability) to operate a pneumatic system set entirely in momentary operation. Learning to use pneumatic systems may be somewhat difficult for some people because they may have difficulty differentiating between hard and soft commands or committing the commands to memory. Some powered wheelchairs offer biofeedback and programming capability to preset hard and soft commands for each user to improve success with a pneumatic system.

## Types of Powered Mobility

Powered mobility options include power add-on units, scooters, standard conventional wheelchairs, and power-base wheelchairs. These powered mobility systems are presented in ascending levels of complexity.

### Power Add-On Units

A clinician can mount power add-on units on certain manual wheelchair bases to convert them to powered wheelchairs. The intent is to provide manual and power mobility that the user can transport without a van. By removing the power add-on unit and batteries, the person can achieve efficient manual wheelchair propulsion. The most common form of add-on units relies on friction between the rear wheels and motors. Because of this, powered mobility may be less than optimal under certain environmental conditions, such as rain or snow, or when tire pressure is low because the friction required to move the rear wheels tends to result in less-than-optimal tire pressure. Likewise, power-base wheelchairs that convert to manual wheelchairs provide less-than-optimal manual wheelchair mobility.

Of the two basic designs, the first has a mounted unit off the back of the wheelchair with the motors resting on the rear wheels. This design uses tension straps to apply friction between the drive motor and the rear wheel to propel the wheelchair. The second design has the motors built into the hubs of the rear wheels and is direct drive. A person controls both systems by using a two-battery powered standard joystick that the user can remove for folding the wheelchair for transport. The clinician should verify the warranty of the wheelchair with the wheelchair manufacturer before mounting one of these systems on a specific manual wheelchair. Because most manual wheelchairs were not designed to endure the added stresses that the frame must withstand at the higher speeds of powered mobility, an add-on power pack often voids the warranty of the manual wheelchair on which the pack rests. The friction drive systems also add significant wear to rear tires and wheels.

### Scooters

Scooters (or power-operated vehicles) are different from powered wheelchairs. The majority of scooters have three wheels that support a long and narrow platform with a swivel seat at the rear and a tiller or steering column in the front. The combination of three wheels and narrow overall width make scooters inherently unstable but mobile for tight, indoor environments. The user combining high speed and moderate-to-sharp turns can cause the scooter to ride on two wheels or roll onto its side. Four-wheel versions are available and are much more stable but tend to be longer and require more space for the user to maneuver it.

Scooters are available in front-wheel drive and rear-wheel drive. The front-wheel drive systems are usually the smallest options. They do, however, offer considerably less power and traction and therefore are intended primarily for indoor use. The advantage of the front-wheel version is its relatively small turning radius. The rear-wheel drive scooters have greater traction because the user's mass is just in front of the drive wheels. The traction actually improves when the user is ascending ramps because the center of gravity passes almost directly through the drive wheel. Another reason that rear-wheel drive scooters offer more power and range is that they generally contain two 12-volt batteries compared with a single 12-volt battery on front-wheel drive scooters.

Steering and speed are separate functions on most scooters. The user accomplishes steering with a tiller and controls acceleration and speed using thumb levers or finger triggers. For many people, this combination is easier to understand than the joystick on most powered wheelchairs. This method of operation requires the user to have good sitting balance, proximal stability, shoulder mobility to steer, and fine motor control to operate the accelerator. Speed control on scooters can be either proportional or single switch (fixed speed). Switch options to allow alternative methods of control are not available.

Because the foot platform is not adjustable, the user should be able to adjust the height of the scooter to ensure proper thigh and foot support. The manufacturer mounts scooter seats to a single post, actually a tube within a tube, to allow quick although somewhat awkward disassembly for transport. The user also can adjust the height of most of these seat posts. Powered seat lifts are optional on some scooters. The powered seat lift can aid in transfers and accessibility but may restrict the user in lowering the seat to accommodate short lower extremities. In addition to being height adjustable, the scooter seat also swivels and locks in place for transfers and access. One of the major recent advances in scooter technology has been improved seating. Wheelchair-like seat frames and customized seating options are now available.

### Transportable-Powered Wheelchairs

Transportable-powered wheelchairs refers to the lightweight power wheelchairs that are designed for disassembly and transport. They weigh approximately 100 lb with batteries. Although the concept is wonderful, the outcome may not be. Almost all of these chairs, when broken down for transport still have a frame and motor unit that weighs around 60 lb, almost twice the heaviest component of a typical scooter. A clinician should show the users and caregivers the process of folding the wheelchair. Caregivers need to learn this task to have a clear understanding of what is involved to assemble and disassemble the wheelchair.

Transportable-powered wheelchairs have been more effective in addressing cost containment issues than in providing a more portable wheelchair. Transportable wheelchairs provide the fewest options of all the powered wheelchairs, as they are designed to meet the lowest funding criteria. They provide excellent household and limited community mobility. Programmable electronics are available but may be limited to only certain adjustments. Switch options may be available, depending on the manufacturer. Standard joystick operation is the typical input device. Unique features such as 12-inch rear wheels and the possibility of flip-back armrests can make a difference in level of transfer dependency.

### Conventional-Powered Wheelchairs

Manufacturers originally made conventional-powered wheelchairs by adapting motors and reinforcing the frames of conventional-style manual wheelchairs. Each large-drive wheel has a large pulley attached to it and is belt driven by a motor attached to the side frame of the wheelchair. These rear-drive wheels actually steer the chair while the front caster wheels freely rotate. The standard input device is a proportional joystick. The electronics vary considerably, from little or no adjustment to a wide range of driving parameter adjustments. The major differences between conventional wheelchairs and the previously described wheelchairs is the possibility for the user to change electronic adjustments to alter driving response, use alternative specialty switches, and integrate specialty seating systems such as manual, powered, and recline seating systems. The potential to integrate these optional switches and seating systems varies considerably and is directly proportional to the cost of the wheelchair. Some of the conventional frame-power wheelchairs are designed for weight capacities exceeding the limits of all the other categories of power wheelchairs.

### Power-Base Wheelchairs

The main concept of power-base wheelchairs is not new. These wheelchairs offer a modular design, or a power mobility base and separate seating system. The advantage is that the user can change the seating system over time to address different functional needs without having to change the power base. Furthermore, the overall width of the mobility base remains the same despite the width of the seating system. A few manufacturers of power base wheelchairs also offer seat elevation and power-standing options that have therapeutic and accessibility benefits. The clinician should check for potential compatibility before selecting a power base, especially if changes in the client's condition over time are anticipated. A short frame length or specific frame design may prevent the clinician from integrating a particular seating system.

Power-base wheelchairs have direct-drive motors. Unlike conventional belt-driven wheelchairs, the motors on direct-drive wheelchairs are connected directly to the wheels. Therefore the direct-drive wheelchairs provide more power. Because the power to the wheelchair does not have to be translated from the motor to the wheels through a belt, they also run more efficiently. Manufacturers of power-base wheelchairs have always extolled the superiority of power-base systems for outdoor mobility. Most power-base wheelchairs use a smaller diameter but wider tire to achieve a larger overall footprint for better traction. Power-base wheelchairs are designed with either the drive wheels located in the front, middle, or back of the wheelchair. Front-wheel drive systems tend to offer better maneuverability in tight spaces. The disadvantage with front and midwheel-drive wheelchairs is that they tend to fish tail unless the user has a steady hand and has programmed the wheelchair to reduce the sensitivity of the joystick.

Midwheel-drive systems were created to shorten the turning radius for accessibility and to improve maneuverability. The drive wheels are directly under the user. A set of rear-mounted casters allows the chair to turn. A set of front casters (antitip wheels) also prevents the wheelchair from tipping forward. The disadvantage of a midwheel system is that the wheelchair rocks forward when the user stops it abruptly on flat surfaces or on downhill slopes. Midwheel-drive wheelchairs are also difficult for the user to maneuver over a curb. Rear-wheel drive systems outperform front and midwheel systems in maximum speed and ability to climb steeper grades. Some rear-wheel drive systems have adjustable rear-wheel positions to alter the weight distribution relative to the rear axle. A person can use this adjustment to alter the wheelchair's performance and accessibility. Compatibility with seating systems (particularly powered tilt, recline, seat elevation, and standing), input devices, types of specialty electronics available, and compatible tie-down systems vary among manufacturers. The clinician should address the need for these items when the user is selecting the wheelchair. The clinician can convert some power-base wheelchairs to manual wheelchairs for dependent or limited independent mobility when the power system fails or if transportation of the power base is not possible.

## Outcomes and Social Validation

Several functional scales such as the Functional Independence Measure (FIM)[7] exist to provide the clinician with tools to classify a person's level of performance specifically related to mobility. Unfortunately, when the clinician evaluates wheelchair mobility, these scales are insufficient. Although this scale provides a gross representation of the patient's mobility, it does a poor job of accurately depicting the person's ability to propel a manual or powered wheelchair within a home or community setting. Specific functional skills that the user has are not components of this scale, such as propelling up the 1:12 maximum slope requirement for ramps,[8] maneuvering over a 1-inch door threshold, descending ramps and curb cuts, and propelling a specified distance per unit of time. A more specific grading scale could be beneficial in helping the clinician identify levels of performance given specific functional disabilities. This information would in turn help the clinician to justify the need for a particular assistive mobility device to the client. A tremendous need exists for more studies in this area; clinicians have performed the only efficacy studies for mobility with children, focusing on justification for powered mobility at an early age.[9]

Clinicians must take an active role in determining the cost effectiveness of this technology, which has been funded primarily on the basis of medical necessity in the past. Third-party payers, specifically some insurance carriers, are now excluding or putting caps on durable medical equipment coverage, specifically wheelchairs. This is occurring more with managed care and cost containment.

### CASE STUDY

### CASE 3

A 19-year-old man with a diagnosis of C-4/5 tetraplegia had an insurance policy that would only pay for 50% of the powered wheelchair. This person's family was financially unable to afford the remaining 50%. Despite combined efforts of the therapist, case manager, supplier, and manufacturer to reduce the total cost of the wheelchair by more than 50%, the insurance company representative refused to authorize the purchase of the powered wheelchair. Furthermore, the justification was that the family now qualified for Medicaid and could obtain full funding for the equipment through the state. The result was that the person suffered and society incurred the cost. Unfortunately, without public awareness of these deficits in health care, the clinical team and supplier have difficulty being the advocates for the intended user's needs.

Clinicians have to prove to able-bodied people first and payers second the benefit of this technology. Additionally, they must be able to clearly justify functional and medical necessities of chairs and components. If clinicians cannot answer the question, "Why is this needed?" to each component on a prescription, they must evaluate why it is listed. If clinicians cannot explain why their clients need certain devices, justifying the need to third-party payers is dubious. The following cost-effective outcomes can occur for patients when clinicians use technology:

- Improve function thereby reducing the need for nursing/attendant care
- Reduce or decrease the occurrence of medical complications such as decubiti or lung ailments such as pneumonia

- Provide an ability to perform activities in the wheelchair that could not be performed without the wheelchair, which improves quality of life such as allowing a person to return to work or care for family
- Provide access to public transportation versus expensive medical transportation
- Reduce length of stay in a rehabilitation center or a faster transfer to home-based therapy
- Provide equipment that is modular in the frame and electronics so that a person with a progressive disease or condition does not require a whole new wheelchair when conditions change

Another trend that can have a detrimental affect on quality provision of mobility technology is *preferred providers*. In some cases, these contracts result in failure to provide a person with proper equipment and adequate service, primarily because the provider is unqualified to provide high-end rehabilitation equipment. To address this concern, suppliers of rehabilitation equipment have formed a registry called the *National Registry of Rehabilitation Technology Suppliers (NRRTS)*. In addition, certification testing of suppliers and clinicians is available through RESNA to promote a higher standard of care in the service and delivery of rehabilitation technology. The demand for this technology continues to rise as the population ages and medical advances increase life spans. Social acceptance also increases as more individuals experience the freedom and independence that mobility technology can promote.

## References

1. Warren CG: Powered mobility and its implications, *J Rehab Res Dev Suppl* 2:74–85, 1990.
2. Jones ML, Sanford JA: People with mobility impairments in the United States today and in 2010, *Assistive Technol* 8 (1):43–45, 1996.
3. Krause SJ: Changes in wheelchair technology: a consumer commentary, *Topics Spinal Cord Inj Rehab* 1 (1):66–70, 1995.
4. Thacker J, Sprigle S, Morris B: *Understanding the technology when prescribing wheelchairs,* Washington, DC, 1994, Resna Press.
5. Taylor SJ: Powered mobility evaluation and technology, *Topics Spinal Cord Inj Rehab* 1 (1):23–36, 1995.
6. Pentland W: The weight bearing arm, *New Mobility* 41, 1992.
7. Functional Independence Measures (FIM): *Uniform data systems for medical rehabilitation,* Buffalo, NY, 2001.
8. Americans with Disabilities Act: Accessibility guidelines, part 36, *Nondiscrimination on the basis of disability by public accommodations in commercial facilities,* sect 4.8, Washington, DC, 1990.
9. Butler C: *Augmentative mobility: Why do it?* Vancouver, 1994, University of British Columbia, Proc of the 10th International Seating Symposium.

## Internet Resources

http://www.rehabcentral.com
http://www.wheelchairnet.org
http://www.wheelchairjunkie.com
http://www.RESNA.org
http://www.nrrts.org
http://www.udsmr.org

# CHAPTER 20

# Spatial Orientation and Individuals with Visual Impairments

*Richard G. Long*

## Application and Goal

The ability to travel places safely and efficiently is important to a person's vocational, social, and personal success. Visual impairments including low vision and blindness result in a variety of travel-related challenges. In this chapter, I discuss these challenges and describe strategies and technologies that aid visually impaired people in achieving travel-related goals. I also discuss new orientation-related technologies currently in development. The term *visual impairment,* which I use in this chapter, refers collectively to individuals without vision and to individuals with legal blindness who are able to use their impaired vision to obtain information useful in guiding their travel. The term *low vision* refers to individuals with legal blindness who use their impaired vision to obtain information useful in guiding their travel. The term *blind* refers to individuals who rely on nonvisual perceptual input during travel.

## Function and Ability

### The Visually Impaired

Visual impairment affects a significant proportion of middle-aged and older Americans. A total of 1 in 6 adults, or about 13 million Americans, report some form of vision impairment.[1] About half of them report that they are severely visually impaired, that is, they cannot recognize a friend at arm's length or read a newspaper even with corrective lenses. A total of 15% of them report that they are totally blind.

The leading causes of visual impairment in the United States are macular degeneration, diabetic retinopathy, cataracts, and glaucoma. These eye diseases occur most often in older individuals. The aging of the population in the United States, particularly the projected growth of the number of individuals living to age 80 and longer, has significant implications for vision rehabilitation services in the twenty-first century. Many service programs have only recently begun to meet the growing need for services to visually impaired elders, and elders often are severely underserved because of lack of trained personnel.

Although most new cases of visual impairment occur in older individuals, some children are born with visual impairments resulting from retinopathy of prematurity, a condition associated with premature birth. Other children experience vision loss because of congenital glaucoma or congenital cataracts, and some experience vision loss of unknown etiology. Vision loss in childhood can also result from trauma or infection. Approximately half of all children with visual impairment have multiple impairments, including limitations in cognition, motor abilities, and other domains.

### Services for Visually Impaired Individuals

Many individuals with visual impairments benefit from services designed to reduce the disability resulting from their impairment, including disability in orientation and mobility (O&M). *Orientation* refers to travelers' knowledge of their location in space, the locations of destinations they wish to travel to, and the routes that take them efficiently to each place. *Mobility* refers to accomplishment of travelers' tasks such as detecting and negotiating obstacles and changes in elevation such as stairs. Determining appropriate times to cross streets is also a mobility task for persons, although they must also have good orientation skills for safe and efficient street crossing.[2]

Most school-age students who are visually impaired and do not have additional disabilities attend regular classes. Teachers of the visually impaired work with students and their classroom teachers to ensure that teachers meet educational goals. For example, teachers of visually impaired children may produce material in Braille or large print and may assist with other educational modifications as needed. Teachers also teach specialized skills such as Braille reading and writing. O&M specialists also usually work with visually impaired students. Along with parents, these specialists have specific training in and are responsible for helping students learn to move about safely and efficiently in their homes, schools, and communities. For example, O&M specialists assist students in understanding the spatial and object concepts that are important in traveling efficiently with impaired vision or in the absence of vision. Students should have good concept development, which contributes to safe and efficient travel. For example, specialists should consider the concept of "behind" and answer the following questions:

- What does it mean for an object to be behind another object?
- How would a blind child develop a generalized concept of behind?

O&M specialists, with support from teachers and parents, help students learn spatial concepts.

O&M specialists also help students learn environmental concepts. They help students understand what an intersection is, what a traffic light is, and where parking lots are typically located in relation to businesses at a strip mall. O&M specialists are skilled in guiding students to acquire the concepts and skills necessary to travel by themselves in familiar and unfamiliar areas of their communities by using their senses of hearing, touch, and proprioception and to a lesser degree, smell. O&M specialists also often introduce students to the long cane and teach the strategies for using it. They usually initially train young children indoors in familiar areas such as the home and school building, although children benefit from exposure to travel in a variety of environments.

O&M specialists teach students with low vision to use their vision along with their other senses efficiently during travel. For example, they may teach students to visually "follow" a curb or other environmental features such as an intersection some distance away. Many students with blindness and low vision learn to use a long cane to detect and safely negotiate obstacles and changes in elevation such as stairs and curbs. Older blind students learn to monitor movements of traffic and to cross streets safely, primarily by using their hearing. Warren[3] has researched the development of spatial abilities, and readers interested in a detailed overview of research about visually impaired and blind children should read his work. Scholl[4] and Blasch, Wiener, and Welsh[5] include a more extensive overview of general issues in the education and rehabilitation of visually impaired individuals in their work.

Visually impaired adults receive a variety of rehabilitation services that enable them to meet the complex physical, psychologic, and social demands of home, work, and school environments. In addition to O&M instruction, visually impaired adults often receive counseling services such as vocational guidance and psychologic adjustment to the onset of a disability and rehabilitation teaching services such as training in communication, leisure time, and home and personal management skills. Visually impaired adults learn in a variety of settings. For example, private, not-for-profit agencies provide day services in many metropolitan areas in the United States. The U.S. Department of Veterans Affairs provides residential centers and itinerant-based services for vision rehabilitation, and many states also have center-based and itinerant service programs that federal and state rehabilitation funds support. Through comprehensive vocational rehabilitation programs, many adults with visual impairments acquire the skills they need to achieve success in their vocational and personal goals.

Optometrists, ophthalmologists, and individuals trained in low vision provide adults with low-vision care, which is another important vision rehabilitation service that can aid in successful orientation and mobility. For example, adults who use telescopic low-vision aids can often dramatically improve their skills in reading signs or locating landmarks while traveling such as fixed objects or environmental features. Their improvement in these areas can have a significant effect on travel confidence and safety. With the exception of some low-vision care that optometrists and ophthalmologists provide, most third-party sources do not reimburse visually impaired adults who receive rehabilitation services, although third-party reimbursement is growing as the benefits of these services become more evident. Most of the not-for-profit vision rehabilitation programs rely on various sources of support, including the United Way, personal and corporate contributions, and client fees. As is common in many areas of allied health, the programs often underserve people in rural areas.

## Orientation and Mobility

*Orientation* refers to a person's knowledge of location or position in space relative to locations or places in the environment such as a destination a pedestrian is walking toward. O&M specialists sometimes use the term to refer to a person's skill of moving efficiently by relatively direct routes from each place. Psychologists often refer to a person's purposeful movement from each place as *wayfinding.* The term *mobility,* in the context of O&M, refers primarily to a person's ability to move about safely. For example, the ability of a blind pedestrian to detect and safely negotiate a newspaper box on a sidewalk is primarily a mobility-related problem. Long and Hill[2] provide an extensive review of issues related to O&M and visually impaired individuals, and Blasch and others[5] provide information about other aspects of travel for individuals with impaired vision.

The overall goal of O&M services for visually impaired individuals is to enable them to travel independently and safely in their homes, communities, and the other environments in which they want or need to travel. This includes travel in familiar and unfamiliar environments. The Association for Education and Rehabilitation of the Blind and Visually Impaired (AER) certifies people in O&M, who then usually provide orientation and mobility services. Certified O&M specialists have completed a course of study in O&M at one of the 17 colleges and universities in the United States that the AER accredits. Most of these individuals earn a master's degree, although some programs offer post-baccalaureate courses of study. Some programs in the United States prepare O&M specialists at the baccalaureate level. Distance education programs are becoming increasingly popular.

The demands of travel are complex and multifaceted for people with impaired vision and without vision. Individuals who teach O&M require specialized training. Consequently, a certified O&M professional should only teach most O&M skills. The theoretic and practical training that university-based O&M programs provide to students enables them to give effective instruction. For example, students in university-based O&M programs spend many hours traveling while blindfolded and while wearing low-vision simulators to learn first-hand the skills they will be teaching. Typically sighted and visually impaired individuals enroll in university-based O&M training and work as O&M specialists. Although most O&M specialists are sighted, the number of AER-certified instructors who are visually impaired is gradually increasing. Individuals can find additional information on O&M instruction in Blasch and others[5], Pogrund and others[6], LaGrow and Weessies[7], and Jacobson.[8]

O&M specialists teach a variety of orientation and mobility-related skills and tailor their instruction to the particular needs and goals of their students. They usually provide O&M assessment and instruction "one-to-one," although small group lessons may be useful for some travelers. An O&M specialist may introduce the concept of an intersection to a blind student in a relatively safe indoor setting where two hallways intersect (e.g., four corners, 90-degree turns usually required to change the direction of travel). Once students have mastered basic skills in indoor travel, O&M specialists guide students in practicing skills in environments that are spatially more complex. These environments may include complex unfamiliar buildings such as office buildings or malls and may occur outdoors in residential and small business areas. Training in safe street crossing is an integral part of outdoor travel for most students. O&M instructors rely heavily on directed questioning and student-initiated problem solving as they support students' efforts toward greater independence in travel.

One important variable that often affects the development of O&M skills is an individual's age at the onset of visual impairment. Individuals without visual experience in childhood often experience difficulty in developing generalized concepts about space such as concepts of shape, size, and spatial relationships among objects. For example, children who do not understand the concept that they can arrange objects in a line will probably have difficulty forming an accurate mental image of the arrangement of stores along a block. In addition, the presence of other disabilities can have a negative effect on a person's orientation. Impairment of cognitive functioning, for example, may limit a person's skill in acquiring and generalizing various spatial concepts and in effectively using O&M strategies and technologies.

Another important factor affecting O&M instruction is a person's type and degree of visual impairment. Some eye conditions such as macular degeneration result in impairment primarily in a person's central visual field. The central visual field aids in the resolution of visual detail and color. As a result, individuals with central visual field losses may experience particular difficulty with tasks such as reading, watching television, or looking at photographs. Impairment of the peripheral visual field is associated with eye conditions such as glaucoma and retinitis pigmentosa. Individuals with impaired peripheral visual fields but relatively intact central fields may experience difficulty in O&M. This is because the peripheral field is important in a person detecting moving objects and objects to the side, below, and above. For example, a student with impairment of the lower visual field may have difficulty detecting a curb or a step. The peripheral visual field also plays a key role in vision at night or in other conditions of low illumination. Experts have conducted a substantial body of research on the relationship of the degree and location of visual loss and O&M. They have also done research about the psychologic and environmental factors affecting the travel of individuals with visual impairments.[9–10] O&M specialists are skilled in evaluating the functional effect of low vision and other personal and environmental factors that may influence a traveler's need for O&M training and the skills they have to teach.

Visual impairment among older individuals may result in limitations in quality of life in several areas, including the ability to move independently about in the home and community.[10] The O&M goal for some older adults who experience the onset of visual impairment later in life may simply be to learn to move about in their house comfortably or to get their mail independently. Older adults with visual impairments may lose the capability to accomplish these simple tasks, and a brief period of O&M training can often provide the skills and confidence they need to accomplish them. Many adults including some older adults may want and need a comprehensive program of O&M to enable them to travel independently, safely, and efficiently. They may want to travel independently to work or school and to various social and recreational activities. In addition, they may want to learn the O&M skills necessary to travel on a bus or a train to an unfamiliar store, make a purchase, and return home. To accomplish relatively complex travel tasks like these, adults may need to learn and practice skills such as obtaining and following directions that others provide, using cardinal directions, and locating and negotiating stairs, curbs, escalators, and other potential hazards. They may also need to learn how to cross streets safely at a variety of types of intersections, to locate subway stations or bus stops, and to board the correct bus or train.

Many individuals with low vision and almost all individuals who are blind use a primary mobility device such as a long cane or a dog guide. Some legally blind individuals with relatively mild impairment rely only on visual and other sensory information when traveling. Individuals who are functionally blind and some with low vision primarily use the long cane mobility device. Long canes are usually slightly taller than midchest when the teacher holds it vertically in front of the student. They are generally made of aluminum, fiberglass, or carbon fiber. White reflective tape usually covers them except near the bottom where red reflective tape covers them. Canes are tipped with replaceable metal or fiberglass tips of various shapes. People can fold or collapse some canes for ease of storage. Some individuals with visual impairments may choose to use a support cane and a long cane.

The long cane serves to extend the perceptual "reach," or preview, of blind pedestrians and provides them with a means to safely probe the environment. The cane is useful for locating landmarks that provide individuals with information about location and orientation (Figure 20-1). It also aids in individuals safely negotiating obstacles in the travel path and changes in elevation such as curbs and stairs. *The primary O&M technology that visually impaired individuals use is the long cane, combined with the various techniques for probing the environment with the cane.* Individuals can use a variety of cane techniques, depending on the demands of a particular travel situation. For example, blind individuals who are attempting to locate a landmark adjacent to the travel path move the cane differently than when they are walking across an open area in a mall. The techniques involved in long-cane use are important for individuals accomplishing travel goals. O&M specialists are skilled at assisting learners in using the cane as an effective tool for information gathering and protection.

Relatively small percentages of visually impaired individuals use dog guides, another primary mobility aid. Although professionals usually train dogs to locate a few environmental features on command such as a door or stairs and to distinguish the commands for "left" and "right," a blind individual must give a dog guide commands to turn at specific points or to move toward specific features in the environment. People with dog guides must have good O&M skills to effectively use their dogs and to avoid becoming disoriented. Dog guides are available through specialized not-for-profit agencies located throughout the United States.

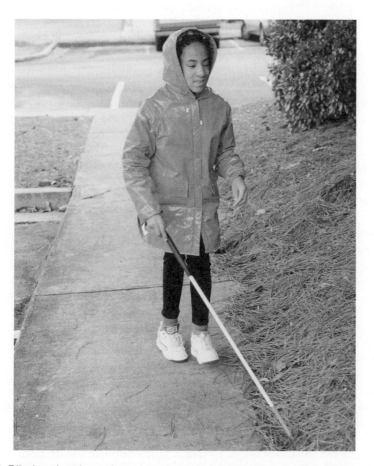

**Fig. 20-1** Blind pedestrian using a long cane to locate edge of sidewalk for orientation.

Finally, all blind people occasionally use human guides. Although the long cane and the dog guide permit independence in travel, human guides are often the most convenient mobility aid, particularly in unfamiliar areas.

## Orientation and Wayfinding: Issues, Options, and Technologies

This next section provides answers to the following questions:

- What kinds of orientation problems must visually impaired pedestrians solve?
- How do impaired vision and other personal characteristics that interact with the characteristics of environments where people travel affect orientation?
- What resources including technologies can visually impaired pedestrians bring to bear to solve orientation-related problems, and how are users "matched" to appropriate technologies?
- How is the effectiveness of orientation technologies measured?

### Using Landmarks

All travelers, whether visually impaired or not, use landmarks to confirm their location and the direction they are facing. Using landmarks is a key strategy for individuals maintaining orientation. Landmarks are fixed reference points in space such as buildings, objects, or changes in surface texture. They are perceptually distinguishable from their surroundings and they convey spatial information. In other words, for persons to "know" a landmark means they recognize it and recall its location (e.g., "I feel the carpet under my feet; therefore know I have reached the elevator lobby." "I hear the elevator door open and know that I am facing it."). Pedestrians often locate and remember landmarks at points along a route where they must turn. They relocate these landmarks on subsequent trips to ensure that they are enroute to their destination. The ability of visually impaired travelers to recognize landmarks and to estimate the approximate distance they have traveled along a route are important orientation strategies.

### Recovering from Disorientation

To use landmarks effectively for orientation, visually impaired travelers must rely on their sensory/perceptual skills and their cognitive skills. Travelers recognize that they are disoriented when what they perceive no longer fits with their expectations of what they should perceive as they travel a route. This is usually based on their previous experience in traveling the route. When disoriented, travelers must engage in problem solving to reorient themselves. This usually means relocating the travel path and determining which way to walk to continue toward their destination. Recovery from disorientation is akin to hypothesis testing. Travelers make educated guesses about what they must do or which way they must move to acquire information about where they are and where they want to go.

For example, they may simply stop and listen for a moment, using auditory cues for reorientation. They may reverse direction or search systematically until they locate a landmark, ask others in the area for help in locating a landmark or in identifying their location, and read signs or use a tactile or auditory map to determine their location, facing direction, and desired direction of travel. They may also use orientation devices such as talking compasses or satellite-based navigation systems to assist in recovering from disorientation. The strategies and technologies they use for reorientation depend on their skills in using perceptual information that their senses obtain and the orientation information that devices provide.

### Traveling a Familiar Route

To travel familiar routes efficiently, pedestrians simply recall the distances and directions they must walk to reach a destination. They recognize landmarks along the way that confirm their location and their direction of travel (e.g., "The bakery is on my left so I am heading toward my destination. I make a right-hand turn onto Sunrise Drive at the next intersection."). As they walk, pedestrians mentally note the location of traffic. Because they know the side of the street they are on, they can confirm the direction they are walking (e.g., "I am on the east side, or bakery side, of the street. I know I am walking toward my destination because traffic is on my right."). Traveling familiar routes is often relatively automatic and requires little mental effort for travelers. They can demonstrate their knowledge of familiar routes by traveling them efficiently, by describing them to others, or by drawing maps that accurately depict them. By identifying and using landmarks, travelers remain oriented as they move along familiar routes.

### Spatial Updating and Cognitive Maps

Travelers also use the strategy of mentally retaining their location and facing direction relative to landmarks in the surrounding areas. Psychologists who study spatial orientation and O&M specialists refer to the individuals' skill of keeping track of changes in location that movement causes as *spatial updating*. Specialists can help travelers by having them envision a scenario in their heads (Figure 20-2):

Imagine that you are standing on the street in front of your house and facing it. You know that your sister's house, which is out of view, is also in front of you. It is two blocks away on a street running parallel to the street your house is on and slightly to your right. When asked to point to it, you point to your right a few degrees. If you move several hundred yards to the left down the street, face the same direction as before, and point to your sister's house, you then point much farther to the right. Your knowledge of the changing straight-line self-to-object spatial relationships is evidence of your spatial updating skill. In other words, your knowledge of the location of your sister's house in relation to your new position shows your ability to keep track of changes in spatial relationships that occur with self-movement.

Another important concept that helps individuals understand O&M issues is a *cognitive map*. Psychologists often refer to individuals' knowledge of straight-line or "as the crow flies" distances and directions from each place as a *cognitive map*. The term cognitive map does not imply that individuals envision a map-like structure in their heads, but in-

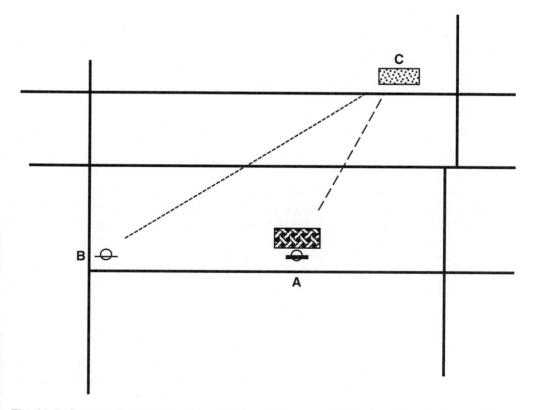

**Fig. 20-2** Graphic depicting spatial updating. *A*, The viewer's initial position. *B*, The position after moving to the left. *C*, The destination (the sister's house).

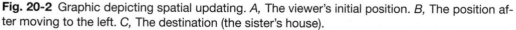

stead it is a metaphor for people's knowledge of object-to-object spatial relationships. Specialists can help travelers with the concept of cognitive map in the following scenario:

> Imagine standing with your back to your refrigerator and pointing to your stove. Your ability to do this accurately, even though you are not actually standing with your back to your refrigerator, is evidence that you have a relatively accurate cognitive map of the spatial arrangement of objects in this familiar space.

Individuals having spatial updating skills and the ability to form accurate cognitive maps of places too large for them to perceive from a single vantagepoint are essential elements in establishing and maintaining orientation. For example, travelers should consider the way an accurate cognitive map can aid in determining an efficient route between several landmarks.

## CASE STUDY

### CASE 1

## *A Person with Visual Impairment*

Specialists can help visually impaired travelers understand this concept by giving them the following case study to ponder.

Suppose a visually impaired traveler wanted to travel from the bank to the grocery store several blocks away. Assume this traveler knows the route from the bank to the post office and from the post office to the grocery store but she has not walked from the bank to the grocery store. Her cognitive map of the area aids in determining a direct route from the bank to the grocery store and in traveling it.

In short, the skill of individuals traveling efficiently along a novel route between familiar locations depends in part on their knowledge of the layout of the locations and the related ability to determine an efficient route.

### Traveling in Unfamiliar Environments

In unfamiliar places or complex travel environments where few landmarks are known or few exist, travelers may use a variety of strategies to establish and maintain orientation. They may also use one of the O&M technologies that appear later in this chapter. For example, travelers sometimes call stores or other businesses they have never visited to get directions. Sometimes their destinations are in cities where they have never been. Several issues are relevant for travelers when they are requesting and following directions that others give. One issue of course is the accuracy of the directions. Sometimes people give inaccurate directions to travelers when they solicit aid; therefore travelers must seek additional information to reach their destination.

Additionally, people can use different reference systems when giving and receiving directions. These reference systems are important in a discussion of various technological aids for O&M. To better help their students, specialists should consider the way people give directions. Perhaps the most common means of providing directional information is for people to use the terms "right" and "left." Although these terms are familiar to most travelers, they can cause confusion because they are "egocentric," or relative to the direction a person is facing (e.g., an object or location on the specialists' left is on the students' right when specialists are facing students). People also can use various prepositions to describe distances and directions to locations in a large space such as *beside, behind, next to,* and *further than.* Similar to right and left, spatial relationships that people describe with prepositions can be ambiguous because they do not depend on a fixed reference system. For example, people do not always have an easy time determining which entrance is the front entrance to a large building with multiple entrances.

Cardinal directions (north, south, east, west) are different in that a permanent reference system (i.e., magnetic north) fixes them; therefore they are independent of the observer's frame of reference. However, some travelers (visually impaired and typically sighted) and some people giving directions have difficulty using cardinal directions.

Distances can also pose difficulties when people are giving and receiving directions. For example, a clerk may tell a caller how many miles it is from the caller's location to the store, but the clerk is more likely to tell the caller how many blocks the store is from the caller's current location. The clerk is also likely to give landmarks instead of or in combination with distance and direction information when giving the traveler directions. One difficulty visually impaired travelers encounter is that individuals giving directions are often accustomed to providing visual landmarks. Visually impaired individuals learn (from O&M specialists and from their own experience) the way to ask questions that yield the kind of information that is most useful to them. A blind individual may ask whether a business is in the middle of a block or on the corner and may ask whether an awning, carpet, or distinctive texture on or near the entryway exists that could serve as a nonvisual landmark. Locating landmarks in unfamiliar places is sometimes difficult for travelers because they are not familiar with the distances and directions from each landmark. Travelers are also not familiar with the environmental clues that could aid them in locating landmarks efficiently. For example, they may not know on an initial walk in a new place that parking meters exist in a particular area along the walk. Once they know that parking meters are present in a particular location, travelers can use them during subsequent trips to determine what block they are on.

### Veering from the Travel Path

Blind travelers sometimes encounter another type of orientation problem not usually experienced by sighted travelers. Sometimes they veer off the sidewalk or travel path and they can veer while crossing streets. They can usually remain on the travel path easily when the path is a sidewalk with grass that borders each side or another surface that is different tactually from the walking surface and one that the traveler can easily detect underfoot or with the long cane. However, sometimes the sidewalk or path is indistinguishable from the surface around it. In these circumstances, a blind pedestrian may veer into a parking lot or driveway that blends with the sidewalk. Pedestrians may detect that they are no longer on the sidewalk when their cane contacts a parked car or when they perceive that cars on the street they are walking along seem to sound farther away than they should if they were on the sidewalk. O&M specialists teach their students to apply various strategies to recover from these kinds of disorientation. Individuals with low vision can often see the edges of the sidewalk or curb and can "follow along" the available environmental guidelines.

## *Goals of Assistive Technology for Orientation and Wayfinding*

## Technologies That Can Help Visually Impaired Travelers Meet Those Goals

The overall goal of assistive technology for O&M is to enable visually impaired persons to travel efficiently from each place. The ideal outcome would be travel that is always quick and efficient. That is, technology would permit travelers to travel efficiently by helping them plan efficient routes and recognize and correct their route when they veer from the travel path.

Orientation and wayfinding can be broken down into the following two primary components:

1. Travelers determining location in space and the route they need to walk to reach a desired destination. Usually they are not able to walk in a straight line from one destination to another because of intervening walls or buildings.
2. Travelers relocating the travel path after veering from it.

Technologies that visually impaired pedestrians use for orientation are generally low tech. Most pedestrians rely on the long cane or a dog guide, in combination with their perceptual and cognitive skills, to establish and maintain orientation. One reason for this is that visually impaired pedestrians like other pedestrians often travel familiar routes with known landmarks. They do not commonly become disoriented along these routes.

Several new technologic solutions have been introduced in the past few years that may prove to be useful to travelers. They include tactile maps and signs such as those that the Americans with Disabilities Act and its implementing regulations require, detectable tactile warning systems, audible signage, audible street crossing signals, light guides, audible and tactile compasses, and satellite-based O&M technologies.[11–13]

## Tactile Maps

Tactile maps are raised line maps that are usually labeled with Braille. People can make tactile maps in many ways. Some maps are homemade from string or other material that people can attach to a surface with glue, and people can make other maps from kits specifically designed for this purpose. Some maps are designed to be accessible to individuals with blindness and those with low vision and thus incorporate tactile and visual information. O&M specialists typically provide their students with at least an introduction to the use of tactile or raised-line maps, and some instructors assist students in developing tactile maps of areas where they are likely to travel. The legibility of tactile maps depends on a variety of factors, including the traveler's experience with them and the characteristics of the map such as the amount of information that the map conveys. Travelers' experiences with map use, their preferences for the way they learn orientation-related information, and their travel experiences presumably affect their ability and interest in using tactile maps. Issues such as information density, the legibility of tactile and visual labels, and the strategies individuals use to explore maps affect the usefulness of maps as wayfinding aids. Bentzen[12] provides individuals with a comprehensive description of the steps for making and using tactile maps.

## Tactile Signs

Tactile signs can provide information to blind and low-vision pedestrians such as room numbers, restroom labels, and special rooms, such as auditoriums. According to Bentzen,[13] ADAAG 4.30.4 standard requires signs with standard-size Grade 2 Braille in addition to high-contrast raised characters (an experienced Braille reader can read Braille much faster than raised print). Locating tactile signage sometimes can be problematic for visually impaired individuals. In an attempt to standardize the location of tactile signs, AADAG 4.30.6 requires that signs be placed 60 inches from the floors and on the latch side of doors (to avoid obscuring the sign when the door is open). Bentzen[13] noted that tactile signage can be useful to individuals who are deaf and blind. She also suggested that tactile signs are not effective for providing those individuals with directional information, largely because of problems in standardization of placement of these signs.

## Detectable Tactile Warnings

Detectable tactile warnings provide tactile information to cane users and dog-guide users about the presence of specific travel hazards. People can find standards for the design and installation of these warnings and locations in Section 4.29.2 of the ADA Accessibility Guidelines (AADAG). Detectable tactile warnings are typically raised, truncated domes made of a rubberized material installed on the walking surface (Figure 20-3). To meet the requirements of AADAG, detectable tactile warning surfaces must contrast visually with the surroundings and must differ from the surrounding surface in resiliency and in sound-making properties it makes when a person taps it with a long

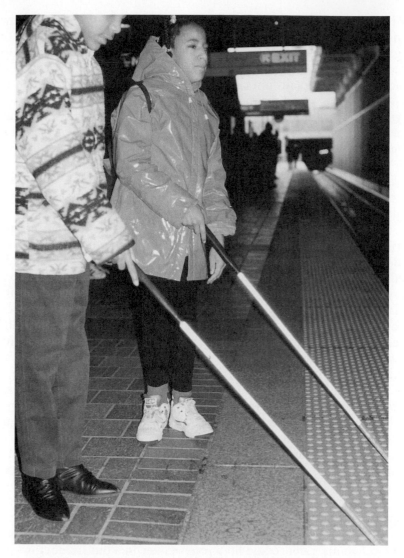

**Fig. 20-3** Detectable tactile warning strip on an Atlanta subway platform.

cane. Detectable tactile warnings must be installed at platform edges of new transit stations or stations undergoing significant renovation. The warnings also are sometimes installed at boundaries between walkways and adjoining driveways or streets, especially where other detectable features that alert blind pedestrians to the presence of a hazard are not present.

Detectable tactile warnings are likely to be beneficial to visually impaired pedestrians and to other pedestrians. However, a controversy among professionals and visually impaired consumers currently exists regarding where and to what extent detectable tactile warnings should be installed. Bentzen and Barlow[14] provide an overview of the detectability of curb ramps for visually impaired pedestrians. Some curb ramps may be difficult to detect underfoot or with the long cane, and consequently some visually impaired individuals may be unaware that they have walked from the sidewalk into the street. This is an important issue when the installation of detectable tactile warnings is considered.

## Audible or "Talking" Signs

Another relatively recent environmental support for visually impaired pedestrians is audible signage.[15] Audible sign systems provide a way for visually impaired individuals to access information on signs from considerable distances away, rather than only on direct contact as in the case of Braille signage.

Although relatively few installations of audible signs have occurred in the United States to date, a commercially available system exists that has been shown to be effective as a wayfinding tool for visually impaired individuals. Engineers and blind individuals at the Smith-Kettlewell Eye Research Institute in San Francisco designed this system, called *Talking Signs*. Talking Signs, Inc. markets Talking Signs. The system includes an infrared transmitter that conveys information (i.e., a brief audible message such as "information desk" or "telephone") to a handheld receiver that a blind person carries. The receiver receives and "speaks" the message when a person points it toward a transmitter. Transmitters are located near doors, information desks, restrooms, and other important features in a building. By sweeping the receiver in front of the body or by turning around, the user of Talking Signs can scan an environment and locate transmitters.

Because it is an infrared-based system, Talking Signs operates on line of sight, and the signal does not penetrate obstacles that may be between the user and the transmitter. The Talking Signs system has many positive features, including that it is audible when needed and silent when unnecessary and audible only to the user. In addition, it is lightweight, easy to use, and free to the user. Perhaps the greatest benefit of Talking Signs is that it is directional. Unlike radio frequency-based systems that are omnidirectional, the infrared-based Talking Signs system permits users to "hone in" on a transmitter as they walk toward it. Users pick up a message and then walk while moving the receiver slightly to the left or right to maintain a clear signal. This enables them to walk in a relatively straight line to the transmitter.

Blind individuals often ask bus drivers for the bus name or number when it arrives at the stop, but technologic solutions to identifying bus stops, bus names, and route numbers have also been developed. For example, travelers use Talking Signs transmitters and receivers for information about the names and locations of bus stops. Simple annunciators that travelers place near the door can automatically identify a bus each time the bus driver opens the door. Alternatively, speakers that announce bus information can be mounted on the top of a bus. A radio signal from the stop can activate the speakers automatically as the bus approaches each stop. Conversely, a radio signal from a bus that activates speakers could be placed at bus stops. Finally, satellite-based locator systems can provide travelers with information about where particular buses are located along a route. In these systems, riders could lift a receiver, key in a bus number or route name, and learn the location of the bus along the route. This is possible because a satellite can continuously track a bus using technology widely used today to track over-the-road tractor-trailers. Schedule information can also be presented audibly at bus stops. These technologies will likely receive wider use as the costs of technologies drops, as their benefit to all travelers is demonstrated, and as disabled consumers advocate them.

## Accessible Pedestrian Signals

Accessible pedestrian signals provide information to visually impaired pedestrians about the status of a traffic signal when relying on the "traditional" cue for initiating a street crossing is not possible (i.e., the surge of traffic moving beside pedestrians and in the direction they want to travel). For example, some traffic signals are actuated. This means that they change in response to the presence of vehicles, rather than a timer controlling them on a fixed cycle. If only one or two vehicles are waiting when a signal turns green, the signal may turn back to red quickly thus leaving a pedestrian "stranded" in the middle of the street with oncoming traffic having a green light. To avoid this problem, traffic engineers install pedestrian signals and call buttons that activate them. One of the functions of this pedestrian signal system (i.e., the "WALK/DON'T WALK" signal) is to extend the cycle when pedestrians push the button so that they have time to cross regardless of vehicular volume. Traffic engineers typically assume that pedestrians need one second of "signal time" to move 4 feet; thus a 28-foot street would have a minimal pedestrian phase of 7 seconds.

Blind individuals and those with severe low vision can benefit from accessible signals that make sounds when they activate the walk cycle for the street they want to cross. Evidence exists that the redundant information that accessible pedestrian signals provide may benefit all pedestrians.[16] Some signals produce a "cuckoo" sound in one direction and a "chirp" in another direction, to avoid confusion regarding which street has the green signal. Other signals emit tones, and systems such as Talking Signs and Relume (a Troy, Michigan-based manufacturer of accessible pedestrian signals) convey signal information via a hand-held receiver. Locating the pushbutton can be problematic for pedestrians in some circumstances, and some accessible pedestrian signals incorporate a locator tone into the pushbutton as an aid to blind pedestrians. Vibrating audible pushbuttons are available and can be useful to individuals who are deaf-blind. Finally, in addition to providing information about signal status, accessible pedestrian signals also can provide information to blind pedestrians about their line of travel as they cross the street. If the sound of the signal is highly localizable, pedestrians can use the sound as a homing beacon. This may reduce the likelihood of them veering during the crossing (a common problem, particularly at wide streets, streets with little flow of traffic in the direction they are walking, or at intersections where the streets do not intersect at right angles).

People in Europe and Australia have used accessible pedestrian signals extensively, and they are becoming more common in the United States. As Bentzen[17] notes, federal code accessibility standards in the United States do not yet include scoping or technical requirements for these signals. Active collaborative efforts from consumers, blindness professionals, and transportation planners and engineers are currently underway to develop standards for these signals. Accessible pedestrian signals may prove to be useful for pedestrians at intersections located near facilities for people who are blind and near transit stops. The planners should also consider them when individuals request them at particular intersections or when pedestrian accident rates are high for a certain intersection.

Some visually impaired travelers oppose the installation of audible traffic signals because they believe that they may mask the traffic sounds they rely on to initiate crossings and to maintain a straight line of travel during a street crossing. Travelers also argue that the signals foster a belief among the general public that visually impaired individuals require special aids to be able to travel safely, a belief they reject. Readers interested in additional information on accessible pedestrian signals should consult the state-of-the-art monograph recently published by Bentzen.[17]

## Light Guides

Light guides are thin, fiberoptic lights that when installed along the baseboard of a wall or along a building line or imbedded in a street provide a brightly illuminated path that aids individuals with low vision (and presumably typically sighted individuals). These lights are intended to reduce the likelihood that a traveler with low vision will veer off the travel path. To date, no installations of light guides have occurred in the United States other than for research and demonstration purposes. However, they have been installed in a few locations in Japan.

## Electronic Talking Compasses and Braille Compasses

Compasses that provide information, which travelers can access readily via touch or hearing can be useful in establishing or confirming their facing direction. Compasses may be particularly useful in unfamiliar places or when disorientation occurs.

## Satellite Locator Systems and Computer-Based Route Planners

One of the most exciting developments in technology for visually impaired travelers is the linkage of digital map databases and satellite-based locator systems. These systems are currently under development in the United States and Europe. In principle, they offer visually impaired travelers the ability to determine their location at any time or continuously track their location using a small handheld device. The systems enable travelers to determine directions to a location in an unfamiliar area by entering an address or destination on keyboard. One such system called *Strider* was beta-tested in the United States in 1996 and is undergoing continued development (Figure 20-4). Little information is available about the actual effect of systems such as Strider on orientation-related needs of visually impaired and blind individuals and other pedestrians as well. However, these systems are unlike any existing O&M technology and they have the potential to revolutionize the way that visually impaired and other travelers travel, particularly in unfamiliar places.

The satellite-based systems involve integration of two types of relatively new technologies. One technology is the collection of digital map databases that the U.S. Bureau of the Census initially developed. These databases became available approximately a decade ago to private-sector companies seeking to develop various computer-based mapping products. They contain the latitude and longitude coordinates of virtually every known street and street address in the United States. Persons can store the databases on CD-ROM disks or, for smaller geographic areas, on floppy disks. With the aid of sophisticated, computer-based route-planning algorithms, persons can determine the route from any address or other landmark in the database to any other address. They can print directions in text or in graphic (i.e., map) format. Systems such as Strider and its European counterpart called *MOBIC* provide computer-generated verbal direction for blind users to access spoken directions. For example, when people query these devices to provide directions from their hotel to a nearby restaurant might say, "Walk 1.3 miles

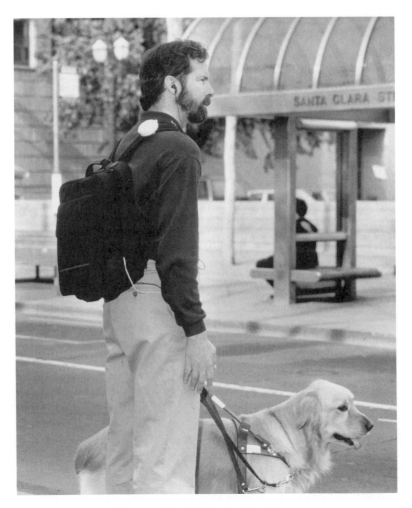

**Fig. 20-4** The Strider system in use.

north on Peachtree Street. Turn left on Dorsey Drive and walk 0.6 miles. Turn right on Northshore Drive and walk 0.1 miles to the restaurant, located on the east side of the street." Users also can add personal points of interest to the database.

The other technology "packaged" with systems such as Strider and MOBIC is the satellite locator system, usually referred to as *the global positioning system,* or *GPS.* It is designed to provide the digital map database with a "starting point" for routing when users do not know their current location. GPS was developed initially for military applications. The system now has wide application for truckers, surveyors, and farmers. It also aids boaters in determining their location and provides wayfinding information in wilderness areas. In recent years, applications of this technology in the surveying, mining, and construction industries have become commonplace.

GPS is based on a network of satellites located in fixed, precise orbits around the earth. With a handheld receiver, the individual can send a signal to three or more satellites. The satellites then determine the transceiver's position by calculating differences in the time of arrival of the signal transmitted from earth. The accuracy of positioning ranges from about 50 to 100 m, although with supplemental earth-based signals, the accuracy can be improved to within a few meters.

Strider and MOBIC use essentially the same GPS-based satellite locator system and the digital map systems now available in some luxury automobiles that people use to track the locations of over-the-road trucks. The developers of Strider refer to it as *a talking personal map.* By using the GPS transceiver and map database integrated into Strider, visually impaired pedestrians can determine their location (e.g., distance and direction to the nearest address) and if they move a few steps, they can determine their direction of travel. The system can then guide users to their destinations by giving prompts. For example, the system can prompt users when they reach a particular intersection where they must make a turn and it prompts them regarding the direction of the turn. It will also prompt users when they reach their destination (within the range of error inherent in the system).

These devices may be most useful when people are traveling in unfamiliar areas. They also may aid travelers who have cognitive difficulties that limit their problem-solving abilities and their abilities to recall and follow route directions. It is conceivable that portable map databases may also eventually include information about physical accessibility and thus may prove beneficial to individuals with physical disabilities. The technologies are in the process of being developed and commercialized, and much growth will likely take place in the next few years. In addition to the development of the technologies themselves, a need exists for training tools, development of plans for implementing training, and development of evaluation research to assess the effectiveness of high-tech orientation devices.

## Outcomes and Social Validation

This chapter illustrates the importance of orientation for independent travel of persons with visual impairments. Despite its importance, relatively little research has been conducted on the orientation-related challenges experienced by visually impaired pedestrians or the technologies available to solve them. As a result, little is known about the outcomes or the effectiveness of various low-tech and high-tech solutions to orientation problems. Research and product development should proceed in several areas. First, the effect of environmental features such as lighting, color, and contrast should be considered. The concept of universal design, in which all architectural elements are accessible or adaptable to all persons including those with disabilities, should be an integral part of the design and installation of buildings, pedestrian areas, and transit facilities.[12] For example, the availability of sidewalks and other defined walking paths, the design of curbs and transitions between walking and vehicular surfaces, and construction of travel environments to include nonvisual landmarks are important considerations for blind and visually impaired travelers.[9]

Second, visually impaired individuals have traveled safely and efficiently for many years using the long cane or dog guide. Clearly, they can establish and maintain orientation without the aid of high-tech devices. They cannot accomplish this, however, without the skills and knowledge necessary to use the long cane or dog guide effectively. One of the most important strategies for ensuring that visually impaired individuals have the skills and knowledge they need for orientation is to ensure that all individuals have access to certified O&M instruction that specialists provide. This is particularly important for children. Children with visual impairments must acquire a complex set of concepts about spatial orientation and mobility to travel independently. Some O&M specialists specialize in services to young children and others are experienced in providing instruction to school-age students. These instructors, the parents of visually impaired students, and the students themselves can be valuable resources for allied health professionals who work with individuals with visual impairments.

Third, as previously described, several promising technological developments may dramatically change the nature of orientation-related challenges experienced by persons with visual impairments. The way travelers will use these devices and the way changes in technology will affect the devices is not evident. One factor that affects opportunities for social validation of these technologies is the lack of measurement tools to evaluate orientation in a reliable and valid way. In addition to developing technologies, scientists must also work to improve measurement technology.

## CASE STUDY

### CASE 2

### *Illustrating the Goals and Technologies for Orientation*

L.M., a visually impaired woman, wants to travel to a store she has never visited before. It is in an unfamiliar part of town. She calls the store, asks for the street address, and then calls the bus company to determine which bus she needs to take. L.M. then calls the store again to obtain directions from the intersection at which she will get off the bus to go to the store. She must determine where the bus stop is relative to the intersection and must know which way to walk as she gets off the bus. As she walks toward the store, she veers gradually off the sidewalk and into a parking lot. She relocates the sidewalk, comes to an intersection, and must cross the street. She veers slightly into the intersection rather than crossing directly to the opposite corner. She corrects the veering problem and continues on toward the store. Although the store gave L.M. a landmark to locate the store (an awning that shades the sidewalk), she has difficulty using this particular environmental feature to locate the store because of the cloudy day. She asks a passing pedestrian for information, and the pedestrian tells her that her destination is the second door in the building to her left. She stands so that the building is to her left and then follows the building with her long cane and locates the second door. With the assistance of store personnel, she makes her purchase. She then reverses the route and returns home.

A blind traveler is unlikely to experience all the problems or situations cited here on a single trip. However, the vignette illustrates the variety of challenges that can occur. L.M.'s objective was to locate a store in an unfamiliar area of town. To do so, she may call the store for directions before leaving home or she may consult the routing programs on her home computer. She may obtain bus schedule information not only by phone but also from a voice-activated, interactive information system located at the bus kiosk. The "talking" bus "announces" its arrival by name and number as it approaches the stop. When the bus is near the destination, the traveler disembarks and turns to walk toward it. She knows that the bus was traveling south on the west side of the street, so she uses this information to establish her facing direction as she gets off the bus (a cognitive "strategy" for wayfinding). If uncertain about her facing direction or the location of the store, she may ask the driver or another passenger where the bus stops in relation to the intersection or she may use Strider or an electronic talking compass to establish her direction.

As L.M. walks toward the store, she veers slightly into an intersection rather than crossing directly to the other corner. She corrects the veering problem with the aid of an audible traffic signal and continues toward the store. Other street crossings are aided by detectable tactile warnings, which alert her that she is at the street in places where other information to alert her (e.g., curbs, movement of traffic, slope of the curb cut) is unavailable or difficult to interpret. Although she knows a landmark to locate the store (the awning), she has difficulty detecting it because of the cloudy day. By recalling that the store was the fourth business from the corner, she is able to locate the door. She enters the store and makes a purchase with the assistance of store personnel.

## Conclusion

Although sometimes challenging, visually impaired travelers establishing and maintaining orientation and moving about efficiently will probably become easier with the aid of the strategies, training, and technologies I described in this chapter. However, to establish and maintain orientation, visually impaired travelers will always have to rely on their cognitive and perceptual skills such as their ability to gather environmental information using their primary mobility device (i.e., the long cane or dog guide). They will also rely on the strategies that aid them in problem solving when disorientation occurs, as it inevitably does for all travelers on occasion. With the advent of new technologies, the comfort, safety, and efficiency of travel should continue to improve for all, including individuals with visual impairments.

## Acknowledgment

I gratefully acknowledge Dr. David Guth of Western Michigan University and Dr. Duane Geruschat of the Maryland School for the Blind for their helpful comments on this chapter.

## References

1. The Lighthouse: *The lighthouse national survey on vision loss,* New York, 1995.
2. Long RG, Hill EW: Establishing and maintaining orientation for mobility. In Blasch BB, Wiener WR, Welsh, RL, editors: *Foundations of orientation and mobility,* ed 2, New York, 1997, American Foundation for the Blind.
3. Warren D: *Blindness and children: an individual differences approach,* New York, 1994, Cambridge University Press.
4. Scholl GT: *Foundations of education for blind and visually handicapped children and youth: theory and practice,* New York, 1986, American Foundation for the Blind.
5. Blasch BB, Wiener WR, Welsh RL: *Foundations of orientation and mobility,* New York, 1997, American Foundation for the Blind.
6. Pogrund R, Healy G, Jones K et al: *Teaching age-appropriate purposeful skills: an orientation and mobility curriculum for students with visual impairments,* Austin, 1993, Texas School for the Blind.
7. LaGrow SJ, Weessies M: *Orientation and mobility: techniques for independence,* Palmerston North, New Zealand, 1994, Dunmore Press Limited.
8. Jacobson WH: *The art and science of teaching orientation and mobility to persons with visual impairments,* New York, 1993, American Foundation for the Blind.
9. Long RG: Housing design and persons with visual impairment: report of focus-group discussions, *J Vis Impair Blind* 89:59–69, 1995.

10. Long RG, Boyette LW, Griffin-Shirley N: Older persons and community travel: the effect of visual impairment, *J Vis Impair Blind* 90:314–324, 1996.
11. Farmer LW, Smith DL: Adaptive technology. In Blasch BB, Wiener WR, Welsh, RL, editors: *Foundations of orientation and mobility,* New York, 1997, American Foundation for the Blind.
12. Bentzen BL: Orientation aids. In Blasch BB, Wiener WR, Welsh RL, editors: *Foundations of orientation and mobility,* New York, 1997, American Foundation for the Blind.
13. Bentzen BL: Environmental accessibility. In Blasch BB, Wiener WR, Welsh RL, editors: *Foundations of orientation and mobility,* New York, 1997, American Foundation for the Blind.
14. Bentzen BL, Barlow JM: Impact of curb ramps on the safety of persons who are blind, *J Vis Impair Blind* 89:319–328, 1994.
15. Bentzen BL, Mitchell PA: audible signage as a wayfinding aid: verbal landmark versus talking signs, *J Vis Impair Blind* 89:494–505, 1995.
16. Van Houten R, Malenfant J, Retting R: *Using auditory pedestrian signals to reduce pedestrian and vehicle conflicts,* Washington, DC, 1997, Transportation Research Board Publication Number 1578.
17. Bentzen BL: *Accessible pedestrian signals,* 1998, US Access Board Publication No. A-37.

## Further Readings

Blasch BB, Welsh R, Davidson T: Auditory maps: an orientation aid for visually handicapped persons, *New Outlook Blind* 67:145–158, 1973.

Connell BR et al: Home modifications and performance of routine household activities by individuals with varying levels of mobility impairments, *Technol Disabil* 2:9–22, 1993.

Cratty BJ, Sams TA: *The body-image of blind children,* New York, 1968, American Foundation for the Blind.

Edman PK: *Tactile graphics,* New York, 1992, American Foundation for the Blind.

Guth DA, Hill EW, Rieser JJ: Tests of blind pedestrian's use of traffic sounds for street-crossing alignment, *J Vis Impair Blind* 83:461–468, 1989.

Hill EW: Orientation and mobility. In Scholl GT, editor: *Foundations of education for blind and visually handicapped children and youth: theory and practice,* New York, 1986, American Foundation for the Blind.

Hill EW, Ponder P: *Orientation and mobility techniques: a guide for the practitioner,* New York, 1976, American Foundation for the Blind.

Hill EW et al: How persons with visual impairments explore novel spaces: strategies for good and poor performers, *J Vis Impair Blind* 93:295–301, 1993.

Hunter-Zaworski K: Accessing public transportation: new technologies aid persons with sensory or cognitive disabilities, *TR News* 175, Nov–Dec 1994.

Jansson G: The control of locomotion when vision is reduced or missing. In Patla AE, editor: *Adaptability of human gait,* Amsterdam, 1991, Elsevier.

Klatzky RL et al: Acquisition of route and survey knowledge in the absence of vision, *J Motor Behav* 22:19–43, 1990.

Long RG: Orientation and mobility research: what is known and what needs to be known, *Peabody J Educ* 67:89–109, 1992.

Rieser JJ: Development of perceptual-motor control while walking without vision: the calibration of perception and action. In Bloch H, Berenthal B, editors: *Sensory motor organization and development in infancy and early childhood,* Amsterdam, 1991, Kluwer.

Rieser JJ, Garing AE: Spatial orientation. In *Encyclopedia of human behavior,* vol 4, New York, 1994, Academic Press.

Rieser JJ, Guth DA, Hill EW: Sensitivity to perspective structure while walking without vision, *Perception* 15:73–188, 1986.

Schone H: *Spatial orientation: the spatial control of behavior in animals and man,* Princeton, NJ, 1984, Princeton University Press.

Special issue on orientation and mobility, *J Vis Impair Blind* 83 (9), 1989.

Strelow ER: What is needed for a theory of mobility: direct perception and cognitive maps: lessons from the blind, *Psychol Rev* 92:226–248, 1985.

Tellevik JM: Influence of spatial exploration patterns on cognitive mapping by blindfolded sighted persons, *J Vis Impair Blind* 92:221–224, 1992.

Uslan MM et al: *Access to mass transit for blind and visually impaired travelers,* New York, 1990, American Foundation for the Blind.

Zimmerman GJ: Effects of microcomputer and tactile aid simulations on the spatial ability of blind individuals, *J Vis Impair Blind* 84:541–546, 1990.

## Web Sites of Interest

The Access Board: http://www.access-board.gov/
American Council of the Blind: http://www.acb.org/
American Foundation for the Blind: http://www.afb.org/
The American Printing House for the Blind: http://www.aph.org
Association for Education and Rehabilitation of the Blind and
   Visually Impaired: http://www.aerbvi.org/
National Federation of the Blind http://www.nfb.org/
Smith-Kettlewell Eye Research Institute (Talking Signs): http://www.skeri.org
Talking Signs, Inc. (includes information regarding locations where these systems have
   been installed): http://www.talkingsigns.com

## Other Resources

AER
4600 Duke Street Suite 430
PO Box 22397
Alexandria, VA 2230
Telephone: (703) 548-1884
E-mail: aer@laser.net

A link to hundreds of web sites regarding all aspects of visual impairments:
http://www.seidata.com/~marriage/rblind.html

A state-of-the-art monograph recently published by Bentzen[17] in conjunction with the
U.S. Access Board: http://www.access-board.gov/

Additional information on adaptive aids and materials for visually impaired individuals, including tactile map kits: http://www.lgu.ac.uk/psychology/ungar/intact/

The AADAG guidelines can be viewed in their entirety at the web site of the US Access
Board: http://www.access-board.gov

For information on purchasing an electronic talking compass, contact:
IAT USA
250 H Street
Blaine, WA 98230
Telephone: (800) 688-9538

# CHAPTER 21

# Driver Evaluation and Vehicle Modification

*Jürgen Babirad*

## Application and Goal

Personal mobility and access to private vehicles is a rite of passage that most people take for granted. This modern privilege can influence and shape who people are and what they do. For some people, personal transportation is a means to an end, supplying them with a reliable means of getting from one place to another. Other people go further and develop a close bond with their vehicles, which become an extension of their personalities. The rest of the people lie somewhere in between. Most people would find their lives negatively affected if driving privileges were suddenly interrupted or restricted. For thousands of motorists, this happens everyday. Age, trauma, and disease may instantly change lives or slowly evolve, changing the way they do things. Other people are born with congenital disabilities and face restrictions of mobility all their lives. These disabilities require that physical modifications be made to already manufactured vehicles so that they can safely operate them.

Figures vary, but the American Automobile Association (AAA) estimates that 500,000 licensed drivers with significant physical impairments exist in North America. Another 1.5 million drivers, many above the age of 55, have lesser disabilities.[1] No fewer than 15 manufacturers of hand controls exist that allow individuals to use their hands instead of their feet to drive.[2,3] Modifications to the steering gearbox and brake boosters are commonly applied to vehicles using relatively simple methods.[4,5,6] Designers, developers, and rehabilitation technicians have provided innovative solutions to compensate for even the most severe impairment. Unistick vehicle control has filtered down from NASA's Technology Utilization Program[7] and has encouraged several commercial manufacturers to design and develop their own "joystick" control interfaces.[8]

Adaptive driving technology not only has assisted people with physical limb impairments but also has extended into the area of optic prosthetics or bioptic lenses for individuals with low vision. Approximately 10 million Americans have significant visual impairments.[9] The majority of them have distance visual acuity in the 20/50 to 20/200 range. Most states require corrected visual acuity of 20/40 or better to be eligible for a driver's license.[10] The introduction and use of bioptic telescopic spectacles (BTS) has facilitated access to private transportation for individuals who have been carefully evaluated and taught to use these devices. As of June 1994, 29 states permitted driving with the use of BTS.[11]

Even larger numbers of individuals have multiple impairments. Individuals with cerebral palsy or spina bifida often have physical disabilities that are relatively easy for clinicians to identify and recommend use of adaptive driving devices. More often than not this group also requires careful neurologic assessment because they also may have less-obvious perceptual and cognitive involvement. Many people are unable to compensate for the perceptual skills associated with changes of speed and direction that are imperative for safe motor vehicle operation. The same difficulties may occur in individuals who have suffered strokes or traumatic brain injuries. Evidence exists that many people who have sustained high-level spinal cord injuries also may experience the deficits of brain injuries.

Evaluation, driver rehabilitation, driver education, vehicle modification prescription, and independent driving are steps that organizations need to apply uniformly and in proper sequence to maximize road safety for individuals with disabilities and the general public.[12] The first operator's license ever issued was in 1896 in the state of Indiana. The first automobile fatality in this country occurred in New York City in 1899. As early as 1906, the *Journal of the American Medical Association* urged the following[13]:

> The numerous accidents from motor cars call for special legal requirements as to those who handle them. Special senses and general physical condition should be required to be in as good a state as those of the locomotive engineer. If an automobilist is out of health, nervously weak, defective in sight and hearing, or under the influence of drugs or stimulants, he is not a safe man to run an automobile . . .

In 1923, the AMA created the Committee on Physical Standards for Drivers of Motor Vehicles, which reported the following at the June 1924 meeting[14]:

> We as a profession, should insist on the passage of laws in each state, with a view of restricting the granting of licenses to operate motor vehicles to such persons as may submit themselves to physical tests at the hands of properly qualified medical and surgical practitioners and have demonstrated their physical fitness. As the opinions of practitioners regarding such physical ability may vary, it is necessary that a standard be adopted of a minimum amount of efficiency below which it would, in the majority of instances, be unsafe for applicants to operate such vehicles.

Definitions and interpretations of these basic principles have changed as technology and education has evolved. However, the basic premise of the AMA's 1906 position has not changed. In October 1992 the New York State Education Department, Vocational Educational Services for Individuals with Disabilities (VESID), appointed a committee to recommend evaluation and training procedures for individuals that they serve. With input from other rehabilitation organizations such as the Association for Driver Educator's for the Disabled (ADED), they developed several definitions that will be used throughout this chapter.[15]

## Driver Evaluation

An interdisciplinary assessment of an individual's abilities and/or potential to become a safe, independent driver, the driver evaluation is the preparatory phase for all other services within the field of driver rehabilitation. A clinician's request for a driver evaluation implies that a concern exists regarding increased risk when an individual is independently operating a motor vehicle. The clinician uses the driver evaluation to assess an individual's current level of risk and, if appropriate, to predict the effectiveness of future treatment (driver rehabilitation) or education (adapted driving instruction). The driver evaluation includes medical review, clinical screening of physical functioning, visual perception, and, where applicable, an assessment of cognition or wheelchair seating. Successful performance on the clinical driver evaluation includes an on-the-road assessment of the individual's skills and abilities in an actual driving environment using equipment similar to that which a clinician will prescribe.[16]

## Driver Rehabilitation

After the successful completion of a driver evaluation, a driver rehabilitation program must use a vehicle that is matched to the driver's individual needs. It must assist the individual in developing behind-the-wheel competency in a variety of actual traffic situations. A trained clinician should provide or supervise driver rehabilitation. The person responsible for services must be knowledgeable in understanding clinical diagnosis and prognosis and is considered accountable for the outcome of the program.[17] Driver rehabilitation is applied to individuals who have been previously or are currently licensed and have suffered a traumatic accident that does not allow them to drive as they previously had.

## Adaptive Driving Instruction, or Driver Education

A clinician provides adaptive driving instruction, or driver education after successful completion of a driver evaluation, including a determination of license eligibility. The program must use a vehicle that is matched to the driver's individual needs. It must encompass behind-the-wheel competency in a full range of roadway environments and institute classroom learning governed by NYS Department of Education and the NYS Department of Motor Vehicles. A certified NYS driving instructor with educational or experimental background in the driver rehabilitation field should provide the program. The driving instructor should be accountable for the results of the program.[18] Adaptive driving instruction is applied to individuals who have congenital disabilities and have never driven before.

This chapter identifies various types of driver rehabilitation programs and describes specific evaluation considerations and basic methods for clinician assessment and screening. A description of compensatory techniques to improve performance through rehabilitation, education, or a combination is included. The discussion is general with some known specifics given on driver rehabilitation and education methods. The way for a clinician to apply appropriate levels of assistive technology is discussed at the many levels that disability and subsequent impairment present themselves. Driver rehabilitation can occur in a number of settings and they often define the type of programs that evolve.

## Models of Service Delivery

Most driver rehabilitation programs begin with some type of formal referral and procedure. Seven models exist through which a clinician delivers assistive technology.[19] Driver rehabilitation programs typically occur in four of these settings, but certain elements may exist within a private driver education program. The procedures vary based on the type of model under which the program operates.

## The Department within a Comprehensive Rehabilitation Program

Many programs are a component of a comprehensive rehabilitation program. They may be based at the host hospital, but most are multidisciplinary. A common referral model is the medical model, evaluation and treatment under a physician's order. This ensures that a medical professional is part of the decision-making process related to an individual's care and treatment. Programs operating in these settings typically serve a wide geographic area and work with a variety of diagnoses. Most programs tend to specialize in driver rehabilitation and do not serve drivers who do not have a diagnosis. The most common diagnoses within these programs include (1) stroke, (2) head injury, (3) spinal cord injury, and a variety of amputees and people with cerebral palsy, multiple sclerosis, and muscular dystrophy. Most programs operate under specific hospital policies, and outside accreditation agencies such as the Commission on Accreditation of Rehabilitation Facilities (CARF)[20] or the Joint Commission on Accreditation of Healthcare Organizations (JCAHO) may be audit them.

## State Agency-Based Programs

Driver rehabilitation services are often a concern of state government executives because they purchase assistive driving technology through their Vocational Rehabilitation (VR) departments. Most states support driver rehabilitation programs in the private sector through contracts, fee-for-service agreements, or in some cases establishment grants to develop evaluation and training facilities that assist in the selection and training of appropriate driver rehabilitation services. A few states offer driver evaluation and training services directly through their state VR agencies.

## Programs within a University

A few driver rehabilitation programs are based within a university system. These programs typically have a large research component and the service delivery programs found in the medically based programs. Federal or state money fund most of these centers that were or are rehabilitation engineering centers (RECs). Previous RECs for driving included the University of Michigan in Ann Arbor, Louisiana Tech University in Ruston, and most recently the University of Virginia in Charlottesville. No REC is currently assigned for driving. Louisiana Tech continues to operate a model service delivery program in a university setting with funding from a variety of third-party sources.

## Local Affiliates of a National Nonprofit Disability Organization

Programs also operate out of national nonprofit organizations such as the Association for Retarded Citizens, United Cerebral Palsy and other community-supported rehabilitation organizations. Programs based in these organizations have a primary purpose and mission founded on helping individuals with disabilities. Most of these organizations tend to serve the populations they were originally formed to serve, however, some of them have developed diversification plans to serve individuals who are not disabled.

## Private Commercial Driving Schools

Commercial driving schools traditionally provide services for individuals without disabilities. As a means to fill a need or to diversify their services, some of these programs install hand controls, left accelerator pedals, and spinner knobs into their vehicles and provide driver training to individuals who contact them directly for services. Most of these programs do not have a formal evaluation component and rely on standardized teaching methods to develop skills in motor vehicle operation. The programs usually are packaged to offer a fixed number of lessons, and the student either passes or fails the program based on performance in those lessons. Programs differ in the way their staff delivers services, but services typically involve an interview, in-clinic tests, and behind-the-wheel components.

## Function and Ability

### *Interview*

Before the first appointment and interview, most programs require minimum documentation. Typical documentation includes a physician's order for the assessment (if an OTR, PT, or other licensed allied health professional is involved in the service) and medical and specialists' reports describing the diagnosis and prognosis. Prerequisites include the individual being seizure-free for a minimum of 1 year.

Many driver rehabilitation programs restrict their services to previously licensed drivers and have additional requirements such as age limitations and requirements that the driver have a valid driver's license or history of having a driver's license. The program format and intent are designed to provide rehabilitation through the use of customized rehabilitation modalities and adaptive technology training and do not emphasize the driver education requirements that new drivers need.

Once the clinician receives a proper referral, the individual has an interview. The scheduled interview may begin with information the clinician obtained through a questionnaire. The goals of the interview often include the interviewer obtaining the following:

- Additional pertinent information about the individual's residual abilities, tolerance to testing, and expectations for adaptive driving[21,22]
- Self-perceptions of the individual's ability to operate a motor vehicle and family support
- Self-reported medical considerations such as medication contraindications, occurrence of seizures and spasms, and use of other mobility equipment
- Reported driving history and license information

The clinician collects this information in a casual narrative format, allowing the individual to relax and feel at ease. The individual must feel comfortable with the interviewer. The purpose of evaluation is for the interviewer to identify and isolate contributing factors of potential driver risk. Once the interviewer identifies these issues, a team can form to lessen or resolve them through rehabilitation or the introduction of assistive technology. In most cases, the individuals are unclear about the intention of the assessment and often feel that the interviewer will use results against them or that they will revoke their driving privileges because of their responses and performance in the evaluation. The evaluator should establish a careful balance by developing a sense of trust with the individual so that the assessment will have meaning to both parties and serve the interests of public safety.

If the individual's impairment is too severe and direct rehabilitation or the application of assistive technology cannot compensate this, the interviewer should share the results with the referring physician and in extreme cases the department of motor vehicles. Interviewers should never make decisions such as these on the sole basis of interviews, however, they should discuss with individuals the possibility of releasing information within the context of initial discussions.

In many programs, the individual signs a release that allows program staff to direct results and recommendations to state motor vehicle departments.[23] If the evaluation reveals compelling, valid evidence that the driver has a high probability of posing a public risk, the evaluator must report the individual. In cases in which the evidence against the person independently driving is strong and documented, the case law suggests that courts regard the protection of the public as superior to confidentiality when the two are in conflict.[24]

## Inclinic Tests

### Vision and Vision Testing

Vision and vision screening are essential to establish the most basic element of developing a person's driving skills. A person must be able to see to successfully drive a motor vehicle. Driving involves dynamic vision necessary for a person to control a moving vehicle in relationship to its environment, which includes other moving and stationary objects. Vision is also one of the most common attributes to change through a person's use of corrective lenses. Vision testing in the field of rehabilitation can, however, be difficult and challenging. Uniform vision requirements for driving do not exist and each state determines its own vision standards. Most states have established a minimum best-corrected visual acuity level of 20/40 as qualification for an unrestricted license.[25] A few states use other minimum best-corrected visual acuity requirements ranging from 20/45 to 20/70.[26] European requirements also vary and illustrate the arbitrary nature of these standards.[27] The minimum standard of 20/40 visual acuity is based on a 1925 recommendation from the American Medical Association's Section on Ophthalmology.[28] A total of 42% of the states require binocular visual fields of at least 140 degrees and the remainder do not have visual field requirements.[25] Most Department of Motor Vehicle (DMV) agencies use automated vision testers such as the Titmus Vision Tester, Optic 2000, and the Keystone Vision Tester (Figure 21-1).

All of these instruments test vision using backlit transparencies or illuminated cards at simulated distances of 20 feet. Many individuals have appropriate vision to meet the state standards, but the test instrument is unable to accurately measure their actual abilities. Individuals with cerebral palsy often experience difficulty in binocular acuity because of ocular muscle imbalances (strabismus). Individuals who have sustained a head injury also may experience the same problems and involuntary oscillation of the eyeballs (nystagmus). An ophthalmologist tests visual fields with either a perimeter ball or a series of pinlight stimuli between 30 and 70 degrees. Individuals who have a hemianopic visual field loss because of stroke[29] or others who are experiencing the progressive stages of retinitis pigmentosa may have difficulty passing the field test with these instruments.[30] Without informed advice and introduction of appropriate visual testing instru-

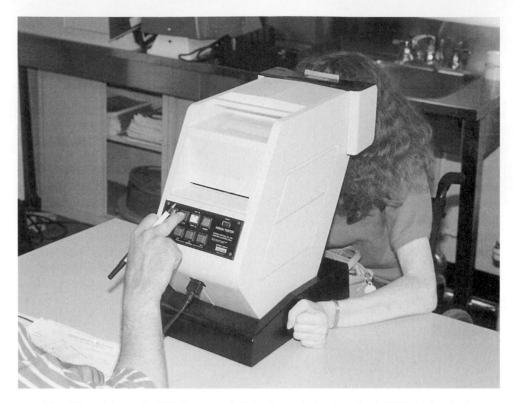

**Fig. 21-1** Driver rehabilitation specialist administering the Optic 2000 vision test.

ments, many of these individuals do not eventually drive because of poor DMV screening. Some researchers have discussed the appropriateness of these instruments to measure dynamic vision.[31] They also have studied and challenged their general reliability as a single source for license denial.[32]

### Bioptic Telescopic Spectacles

In the past 20 years, a growing number of individuals with low vision have obtained bioptic telescopic spectacles to improve their static distance acuity in the hopes of qualifying for licenses to drive motor vehicles (Figure 21-2). Estimates vary but current figures show that approximately 10 million Americans have significant visual impairments.[33] Many of these individuals have distance visual acuity in the 20/50 to 20/200 range. Persons using bioptic telescopic spectacles (BTS) for motor vehicle driving is extremely complex and controversial. The BTS that persons use for driving are mounted in the superior portion of a plastic carrier lens. The carrier lens incorporates the driver's refractive correction, as the BTS. When driving with the BTS, an individual generally views through the carrier lens and lowers the head only occasionally to use the BTS to resolve finer details, such as road sign information. Therefore the person uses the telescope for spotting purposes only and not for continuous viewing.[34]

Considerable controversy exists among various professional eye care and scientific groups about the use of these lenses. The American Association of Motor Vehicle Administrators opposes the use of spectacle mounted telescopes for visually impaired drivers,[35] as does the American Academy of Ophthalmology.[36] In sharp contrast to these positions, the American Public Health Association supports qualified visually impaired individuals using BTS.[37] The Low Vision Section of the American Optometric Association also adopted a resolution recommending that licensing of visually impaired drivers with BTS be considered on a case-by-case basis and based on the individual's performance with the BTS.[38]

Further research on the efficacy of the BTS is needed, as is careful evaluation and training with the devices within the field of driver rehabilitation. Several studies have been completed that suggest a strong correlation between training and success in the use

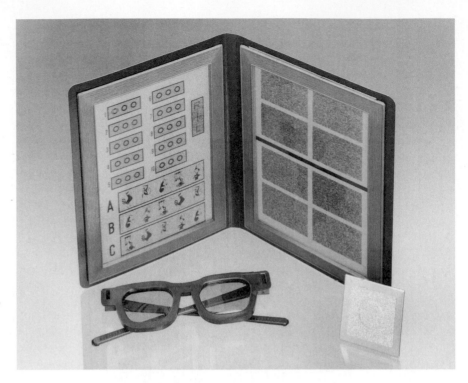

**Fig. 21-2** Bioptic lens used for driving.

of the devices.[39,40] Few programs are available that specialize in the dynamic training of these devices. A particular need exists to continue to investigate the effect of these special training programs on driving performance. Evaluation and treatment of low-vision drivers is beyond the scope of this chapter. A person can obtain further guidance and in-depth bibliographies from the American Optometric Association.[41]

### Assessment

A need exists for routine screening of vision in the clinical driver rehabilitation program. At a minimum, the trained clinician can screen out ocular imbalance problems or other elements that the automated vision testers cannot compensate for and can advise the individual to schedule a comprehensive vision examination with an eye-care professional. The clinician can administer excellent screening tools easily and recommend further testing as indicated (Figure 21-3).

### Visual Acuity

The clinician can use several tests to screen visual acuity. The least expensive and most flexible are the Sloan Letter Acuity chart and the Snellen "E" chart. A smaller hand-direction chart is helpful for aphasic or nonverbal individuals. A more expensive but excellent vision tester is the Optic 2000 automated vision tester. Keystone and Titmus also offer similar instruments. Failure of the clinician to test accurately using this instrument can alert evaluators to possible ocular motor problems, and they can use a wall chart to support or reject the initial findings.

### Visual Field Testing

A simple screening tool for visual field testing is the Vision Disk or hand disc perimeter. The device allows the clinician to test the vertical, horizontal, or oblique positions. The Optic 2000 also allows the clinician to test visual fields using a pinlight stimulus at 55, 70, and 85 degrees and at 35 degrees across the nasal septum. The advantage of the Optic 2000 is that it parallels the instrument that DMV administrations use and can alert the evaluator to possible problems related to passing the field test. Individuals also can use the test to prepare for submitting support field tests from their private eye care

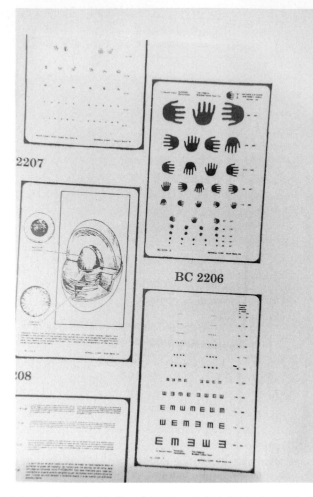

**Fig. 21-3** Vision test card with thumbing hands helpful for individuals with aphasia.

professionals. Clinicians also widely use simple confrontation techniques, which are accepted as excellent screening tools for visual fields and developing additional information on visual field scanning.[42]

### Visual Tracking and Ocular Balance

When individuals have ocular balance problems, clinicians can assess their severity. The simplest means is through direct confrontation with clinicians using two hand-held targets (pen caps or fingertips). Protocol for one standardized test is the Purdue Perceptual-Motor Survey. Another test that is helpful for clinicians to evaluate visual tracking and saccadic eye movement without the use of sophisticated instrumentation is the N.Y.S.O.A. King-Devick Test (Figure 21-4). This test is quick and easy to score, and non-eye care practitioners can administer them.

### Depth Perception and Stereopsis Tests

Related to ocular balance is depth. Several simple tests are available for this. The Far Tester is an excellent instrument that can test depth in "real space." The test assesses the individual's ability to align a pair of distant objects with millimeter calibrated accuracy and it is one of the only "real space" tests for depth. Other simulated depth-perception tests include Stereo Fly, Reindeer, and Butterfly, which test gross and fine stereopsis to help clinicians detect amblyopia, suppression, and strabismus without monocular cues. The automated vision tests also test for this feature with less specificity. Depth perception is a good visual skill but it is not essential for safe driving because the individual who has no depth perception can still judge competing distances through scanning monocular cues.

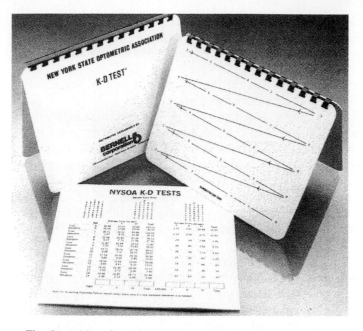

**Fig. 21-4** King-Devick test used to assess visual tracking.

The ability to identify and alert the potential driver of visual problems will assist the evaluator in recommending next step referral options and help to develop a driver profile. This will help the evaluator prepare a final recommendation for training and rehabilitation of outside testing, and administering the visual elements first also will control for other aspects of the assessment. Perhaps the most difficult aspect of evaluation and advisement is perception and cognition, which is by far the greatest element contributing to the voluntary or involuntary suspension of driving privileges.

**Perception and Cognitive Processing Screening**

Controlling for vision and vision deficits is a prerequisite for an evaluator in conducting a thorough perceptual screening. The evaluator may at first dismiss examples of the driver's perceptual deficits as inattention or clumsiness, but they may be signs of an individual's inability to process important information. Extreme perceptual deficits may result in reverse actions such as the individual stopping at green lights and going at red lights. The driver may decide to turn onto sidewalks or clearly marked one-way streets. Anecdotal reports indicate that when these situations occur, the subject may be able to describe proper conduct in each of these areas but is unable to demonstrate the ability to exercise the proper action.

Normal perception involves the apprehension, reception, and interpretation of all sensory input by the brain from within the body and from external input that senses receive (i.e., touch, vision, hearing, proprioception). When processed in an unaffected manner, this information sequences itself and a person can make decisions based on the ordering and understanding of appropriate action. Without the ability to order the information, the individual may not be able to perform various motor skills that are essential for operating a motor vehicle. Perceptual deficits may vary in type and degree based on standard human development and can be greatly affected by trauma (cerebrovascular accident [CVA], head injury), disease (multiple sclerosis, Alzheimer's), age, or developmental disability (cerebral palsy, spina bifida).

*Lack of Awareness*

Loss of awareness most often occurs with individuals who have had a CVA and in some people with brain injuries. When this occurs, the individuals may be unaware of the affected side of their bodies and may subsequently neglect them. If individuals are unaware of one side of the body, they may also neglect that side of a vehicle. Evaluators can assess this important feature through interview and confrontation and through simple letter cancellation tasks and tasks involving both sides of the body. If the evaluator suspects deficit in this area, a behind-the-wheel evaluation should focus on challenging actions at the affected side (e.g., requesting a greater number of left-hand turns and interaction at streets with moderate to high degrees of intersecting traffic).

*Depth Perception*

A depth perception problem can be an issue of ocular balance or amblyopia. The monocular driver can compensate for depth perception. If a depth perception problem exists with the brain injury associated with stroke and head injury, however, the effects can compound, and in extreme cases a physician cannot treat it. Distortion in perception in these individuals leads to balance problems in sitting and standing, but more importantly they do not know when they are sitting or standing straight.[43] This level of deficit may manifest itself by interfering with the individual's ability to maintain a constant lane attitude. The driver may drift (slow lateral movement within the lane) or weave (more rapid lateral movement within the lane) throughout an evaluation range. Lack of insight into the error is found in severe cases, and the individual will either minimize or reject the occurrence.

*Distortions in Figure Ground Discrimination*

This area of perception is a person's ability to identify and prioritize incoming visual stimuli when competing visual elements are present. The result is that a person experiencing problems in figure ground will be unable to pick out specific objects in the environment among elements found in the same field. Severe cases of this impairment are best treated when the environment is kept as uncluttered as possible. Unfortunately the driving environment cannot be artificially ordered. Drivers with this impairment may have more difficulty driving in cities than in the country or they may find that they perform well in low or no traffic environments but cannot interact in higher traffic flows.

*Apraxia*

The inability of a person to visualize internally (in the mind's eye) and then carry out complex movements that are part of driving is called *apraxia*. An example of apraxia is the earlier description of an individual stopping at a green light but being able to correctly describe the sequence verbally. Apraxia can be found in trauma to either side of the brain and is one of the most complex areas of perception. The pathophysiology of apraxia is not completely understood, but when it occurs it usually is reason for the driver to lose driving privileges.[44]

### Assessment

Assessment of visual perception and cognition is varied and diverse. Basic elements of a perceptual assessment battery include the following:

- The Motor Free Visual Perception Test (MFVPT)[45]: This is a multiple-choice test that requires the individual to point to an appropriate response. The test contains items in five categories of visual perception: spatial relationships, visual discrimination, figure-ground, visual closure, and visual memory.
- Picture completion (based on a subtest of the Wechsler Adult Intelligence Scale)[46]: This is a test of perceptual discrimination in which the individual must identify the most important missing element in each of a series of sketched figures. The abridged version is a good predictor of driving performance among individuals who have brain injuries.[47]
- Reitan's Trail Making Test[48]: This test is presented in two forms. In form A, the numbers 1 through 25 appear in randomly distributed circles on the page. The individual's task is to draw connecting lines between the circles in numeric order. In form B, the encircled numbers 1 through 13 and encircled letters A through L are randomly arranged on the page. The individual must connect the circles alternating between numbers and letters.
- Driver Performance Test II (DPT II)[49]: The DPT II is administered visually from the driver's point of view. It is a dynamic videotaped presentation with a narrator describing the circumstances of each visual scene. The individual must respond to a four-option, "priority-scaled," multiple-choice selection. Individuals receive the high-

est score if they are able to identify the most significant elements of the visual scene. Three of the five measured areas are considered perceptual, and the remaining two are considered performance or skill related.

Several other excellent instruments appear in the literature that statically test perceptual abilities.[50-52] Clinicians must isolate the perceptual skill with these clinical tools, but they must not make decisions regarding independent driving solely on the basis of these instruments. A systematic behind-the-wheel driving evaluation should always follow these static clinical tools to validate or reject their significance to driving. Many individuals may test extremely poorly on any or all of these instruments but are still able to pass the behind-the-wheel portion of the evaluation without significant error. Others will do well on these tests and drive poorly. The clinical instruments serve to validate and identify the elements of perception that may have been affected and will help guide subsequent driver rehabilitation or decisions regarding suspending driving privileges.

## Wheelchair Seating and Positioning and Driving

Clinicians often overlook seating and positioning considerations during the decision-making phases of a driver evaluation. Seating, for the purpose of this discussion, is restricted to specialized seating and the use of a wheelchair as a base for driving. Most seating clinicians will evaluate and recommend wheelchair and seating components to maximize function and guard against skin and tissue ulceration.[53,54] Adequate trunk stabilization leads to improved distal control. Many individuals with spinal cord injuries tend to hook one arm around the push rails or rely on upper extremity counterbalance for protection against tipping or falling over in the wheelchair.

Forces acting on the body in a moving van are much different than those that a person experiences while driving a powered wheelchair. Lateral and fore-and-aft acceleration can degrade performance in all human movement, but the effects are much more pronounced when limb and trunk strengths are reduced.[55] Lateral acceleration can reach 0.65 g during an evasive lane change and may reach 0.85 g in a rapid stop. The acceleration of a body in free fall is 32.24 feet per second and this is defined as 1 g. Without proper support, a driver with poor upper-body strength will not be able to remain upright and in control of the vehicle. The introduction of sensitized controls (reduced effort steering, servo gas and brake systems, and joystick control) compounds the loss of control issue. Researchers have documented vehicle control loss because of poor seating balance in case files and have roughly described it in the literature.[56]

Designers should create support modifications to ensure maximum contact with the driver control interface during typical situations and provide a support structure that is benign in the event of a collision. The modification must not interfere with the range of motion or compromise skin pressure distribution. Clinicians have achieved successful support intervention by using simple add-on hardware such as the lateral supports manufactured by Otto Bock Orthopedic Industry,[57] custom plywood and foam inserts, and molded inserts such as those manufactured by Invacare Corporation-Contour U.[58]

People should consider driving from wheelchairs as a last resort and only if they are unable to transfer into power transfer seats. Even with the resolution of the upper support issues, the much larger issue of providing safety and security in the wheelchair in the event of a collision exists. Clinicians are responsible for recommending designs that consider the wheelchair and occupant as two separate entities for every application of wheelchair driving or transportation. In other words, the clinician should ensure that the wheelchair is secured to the floor using an independently operated securement mechanism and should design and install a second securement mechanism to secure the user to the floor. This means that the driver/passenger is secured to the vehicle and not to the wheelchair, which is similar to original equipment manufacturers (OEM) vehicles in which the clinician ties the seat and shoulder belts into the floor or vehicle structure and not the seat. When a system can achieve these two goals it is termed a *Wheelchair Tiedown and Occupant Restraint System (WTORS)*.

Although simple sounding and challenging, wheelchair designers and manufacturers can create a wheelchair that they can modify to meet Federal Motor Vehicle Safety Standards (FMVSS). Several systems do exist that meet the 20 g test requirement to conform to these standards.[59] All current systems require some permanent modification to the wheelchair. The WTORS can add as much as 10 to 15 lb of hardware to the base of the wheelchair. This additional hardware is semipermanent, making the base difficult or impossible to disassemble and collapse. Therefore if an individual is in a lightweight, manual wheelchair and wants to drive from the chair, the WTORS changes the characteristics of the chair quite drastically. All WTORS require special clearance; therefore adjustments to footrests and battery mountings are often necessary. In some instances, the special mounts provide as little as ¾ inch of ground clearance, making the user's entrance through some door thresholds and negotiation of curb cuts difficult.

Finally, clinicians should consider overall head height. Most full-sized vans have roughly 53 inches of interior headroom. Drivers must maintain a functional field of view inside and outside the vehicle when considering wheelchair driving. This field of view is known as the *driver eyellipse,* and clinicians must take this into account during the vehicle selection and modification phase of planning.[60,61] Many wheelchair users sit much higher than 53 inches and some sit as high as 63 inches. Distance from the floor to the height of the eyes should be between 40 and 46 inches to provide an adequate eyellipse for most drivers (Figure 21-5).

This translates to roughly 44 to 50 inches of total head height (ground to eye + 4 inches). The seating clinician should do everything possible to minimize the ground to top-of-head clearance if the individual is planning to drive from a wheelchair. A total of 2 to 4 inches of additional headroom may be available by the clinician selecting or changing tire size or using a low-profile seating cushion. In some instances, the clinician can drop the seat into the frame using drop hooks of 2 to 3 inches. Clinicians must make these changes as early in the process as possible so that they can achieve the primary objectives of providing safe and supportive seating.

After clinicians have made every effort to minimize head height, they can make proper decisions regarding vehicle selection. If they cannot improve head height, drivers may need to restrict their options to vehicles that have independent frames (e.g., Ford and 1997 and future models of Chevrolet vans). Other options would be for drivers to consider the most costly conversion of lowered floor minivans that have been recertified to meet FMVSS. The challenge to seating and positioning professionals is to work with driver rehabilitation specialists in designing and recommending the systems and protective devices to make driving a reality.

## Considerations, Options, and Technology

At the end of World War II, many disabled veterans returned home hoping that they would be able to drive again. In the early 1940s, the War Engineering Board of the Society

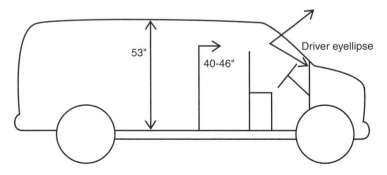

**Fig. 21-5** Proper eye-height range in full-sized van.

of Automotive Engineers developed a task group to assist in the design and development of vehicle adaptations, primarily for people with amputations. The group concluded, "that all but the worst cases of double amputations above the knee and elbow, handicapped men may safely and efficiently operate passenger cars and light trucks."[62] By August 1945, the Ford Motor Company had designed and installed over 700 free retrofit kits enabling war victims to drive using a single lever for clutch and brake.[63] For the next several years, design and development focused on the needs of the driver with lower-extremity amputations. When automatic transmissions became available, designers created and perfected mechanical hand controls. The War Engineering Board, which was later transferred to the Veterans Administration, did most of this work. Many designs were innovative and custom made, with little standardization. Public Law 91-666, enacted in 1971, required that adaptive driving aids for veterans conform to minimum safety standards.[64] This requirement was a major breakthrough for all drivers because it required manufacturers to standardize their processes and allowed for uniform safety and durability when people used the devices. Initial standards did not extend beyond simple modifications made to automobiles[65,66] but they were later extended to wheelchair lifts,[67] power-assisted steering modifications,[68] and power-assisted brake modifications.[69]

In 1983, the Society of Automotive Engineers (SAE) developed a voluntary task group, the Adaptive Device Safety Committee, which began by developing recommended practices for the manufacture and installed utility of manual adaptive driving devices. These devices included throttle, brake, and steering controls known as *Group A controls*. Essential secondary controls such as ignition/starter, gear selector, parking brake, turn signal indicator, hazard flasher, horn, wiper, dimmer, and defrost were classified as *Group B controls*. All other controls were defined and classified as *accessory controls*.[70] By 1992, the group had developed uniform terminology so that a consistency would exist in definitions within the adaptive driving industry.[71] The 1995 SAE recommended practice document-defined minimum performance and durability requirements of wheelchair lifts.[72] A subsequent report that identified a minimum compliance standard for electric lifts defined testing requirements for wheelchair lifts.[73]

Designers modifying a vehicle's structure is a radical action that can result in irreparable consequences. Structural modifications are often required to achieve the lowered floor changes needed when an individual drives from the wheelchair. The SAE developed a report that identified state-of-the-art practices in these modifications. The report provides minimum acceptable design requirements and identifies important performance criteria in planning for structural vehicle modifications.[74] In total, this document offers guidance to manufacturers, evaluators, third-party payers and other interested parties to ensure that they maintain or improve original equipment manufacturer's (OEM) structural integrity and design intent.

By the late 1990s the National Highway Traffic Safety Administration (NHTSA) began to recognize the scope and importance of applying assistive technology to motor vehicles being used on public highways. Some modifications such as the installation of mechanical hand controls are relatively simple and inexpensive. Other modifications such as the installation of servo hand controls, joysticks that control steering, acceleration and braking, or a lowering of the vehicle floor can be complex. In some cases a person altering or even removing federally required safety equipment is necessary to make those special modifications. In those cases, some individuals with a disability may be able to drive and ride in a motor vehicle and receive the benefits from the full array of federally required safety features.

On February 27, 2001 the Department of Transportation, National Highway Traffic Safety Administration published its final rule.* NHTSA identified 12 specific Federal Motor Vehicle Safety Standards (FMVSS) for which permission was granted to make

*Department of Transportation, National Highway Traffic Safety Administration: Exemption from the make inoperative prohibition, Fed Reg 66 (39), Feb 2001.*

safety features inoperative. The provision was granted if all other methods of compliance were exhausted and if the person with a disability was specifically notified that the vehicle was altered in a fashion that limited or removed certain safety features. The agency also identified 9 other FMVSS in which permission was not granted to make safety features inoperative.

Much dialogue and discussion regarding the interpretation and effect of these rules has occurred, but they are designed to ensure the public safety of individuals with disabilities and the general motoring public while not creating an undue burden on the industry. A thorough understanding of these far reaching rules will be essential for clinicians to provide sound guidance to persons with disabilities. Specific examples of the effect of these rules include the following:

- All modified vehicles will have doors that retain their OEM door latching hardware
- The fuel system and fuel delivery systems are safe and environmentally sound
- The air bags that improve safety are not haphazardly modified or disengaged

Several state Bureau of Vocational Rehabilitation agencies also have developed standards, guidelines, specifications, and criteria to guide individuals and vendors in installing appropriate adaptive driving modifications. The evaluator should consider some or all of these documents when recommending necessary equipment. A basic principle guiding this process is for evaluators to recommend the least modification to achieve a maximum amount of control. They can use an adaptive driving device hierarchy to match an individual's abilities with modification classifications.

## Class 1: OEM Sedan

A person's careful selection of features and functions in a sedan may eliminate the need for any assistive devices. Obvious choices include automatic transmission, power brakes, power steering, power seat bases, and power window motors. Two-door sedans, although rare, can help some individuals get into front seats by offering wider door openings.

## Class 2: Modified Foot Pedals

### Pedal Extensions

Individuals who are short or have right-side weakness may need modified pedals. Typical modifications include pedal extensions, which people can obtain from a variety of commercial manufacturers. They can extend the OEM pedals from 2 inches to as much as 12 inches. Preferably, clinicians should recommend the smallest car possible for individuals who are short. If mechanical extension of the foot pedals is too long or impractical, the dealer can install a pneumatic foot control onto a custom-mounting bracket to allow easy removal for access by taller drivers.

### Left-Side Accelerator Pedals

Individuals who have lost function of their right leg and foot because of amputation or paralysis can often use a left-side accelerator pedal. This modification is relatively simple and uses the right-side OEM pedal as a mechanical access link for a left-side crossover pedal mounted to the floor. Designs have changed to allow for lubrication at the floor-mounting block and, in some instances, offer a right foot stopper plate, which guards against inadvertent depression of the OEM pedal. Reported and anecdotal information suggests that although these pedals are simple, they are subject to installer and user error.[75] Clinicians should perform driver rehabilitation and careful inspection of the installation to ensure that the crossover linkage does not bind and that the user is able to operate this simple modification predictably.

## Class 3: Generic Sedan for Paraplegia

### Wheelchair Storage Device

If individuals use manual wheelchairs and are able to transfer, their choices are quite broad. Many individuals are able to transfer into the driver's seat and disassemble or fold their wheelchairs for front or rear seat (two-door sedan) storage. This type of modification was quite popular during the 1970s and early 1980s, and the Ford Motor Company and American Safety Equipment Corporation partnered in developing the improved mobility package (IMP). The IMP would allow individuals to order specially modified Ford Escorts or LTDs with custom manual wheelchairs, three-quarter front benches, built-in transfer boards, and docking stations to store the folded wheelchairs on the passenger sides of the car.[76] Unfortunately, the project was never fully developed because of poor responses from test marketing. Today, individuals who are able to transfer but unable to store their wheelchairs often use car-top wheelchair carriers. At lease two manufacturers produce these simple devices for use with X-frame, manual wheelchairs only.

### Mechanical Hand Controls

Persons use four basic types of mechanical hand controls today (Figure 21-6). Simple hand controls in this conversion area include right angle pull/push (pull down into lap for acceleration and push to firewall for brake), twist/push (twist like a motorcycle grip for acceleration and push to firewall for brake), rotate/push (rock hand control toward dash for acceleration and push to firewall for brake), and pull/push (pull toward body for acceleration and push to firewall for brake). Mechanical hand controls in this classification typically do not require grip modifications but may require installation of a hand dimmer switch (if the OEM dimmer is on a foot switch).

### Steering Spinner

Manufacturers can add steering spinner knobs, balls, or amputee rings to this classification of modification (Figure 21-7). All spinner devices should have quick disconnect hardware so that persons can remove the device easily when able-bodied drivers are using the vehicle.

### Parking Brake Extension

If the OEM sedan is equipped with a foot parking brake the manufacturer many need to add a parking brake extension to the modifications in this classification.

## Class 4: Generic Sedan for Quadriplegia

Many individuals have impairments in all four extremities. A driver with quadriplegia who retains enough residual strength to use a manual wheelchair and can successfully transfer into the driver's seat of a sedan may be able to use a generic sedan equipped for quadriplegia. This sedan typically has the same features as the Class 3 sedan, with a few additions.

### Low-Effort Steering

OEM power steering may be too difficult for a person who can push a manual wheelchair and transfer into a sedan. A person generally accomplishes low-effort steering by reducing the diameter of the OEM torsion bar so that the effort for operation is less than the OEM but more than zero effort steering (i.e., between 4.0 and 15.0 in-lb).[77] Clinicians can evaluate the individual's need for this type of modification by demonstration in the actual vehicle that the consumer intends to drive and in the clinic using specialized testing equipment such as the Baltimore Therapeutic Equipment (BTE) simulator or custom-made steering force wheel.[78]

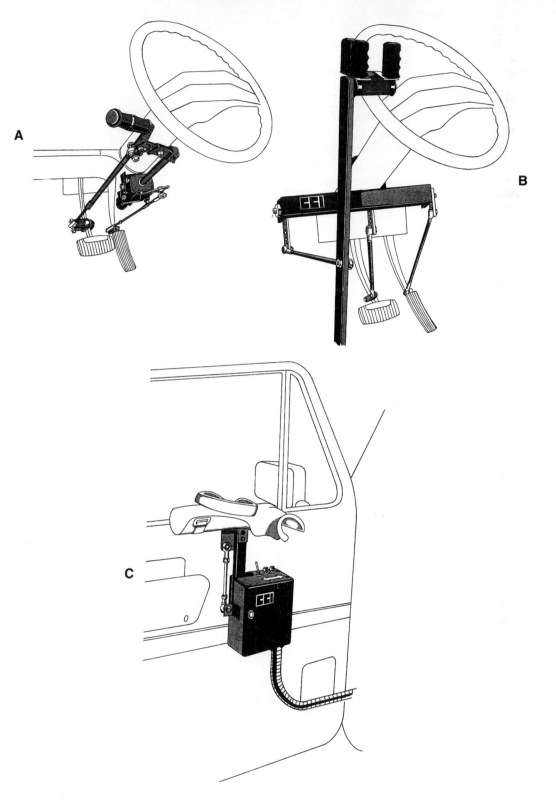

**Fig. 21-6** Hand controls for braking and acceleration. (Courtesy Creative Controls, Inc.)

## Quad Grip Mechanical Hand Controls

The clinician can modify the right angle pull/push mechanical hand control listed earlier to incorporate a u-shaped grip that allows many individuals with limited grasp to use this type of hand control. This modified grip is almost always accompanied by the use of modified headlight dimmers. A second type of push/pull hand controls is often effective

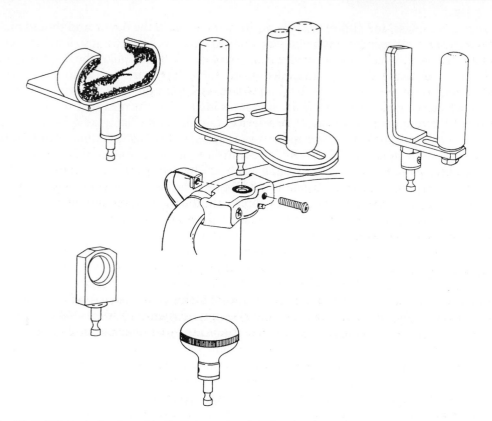

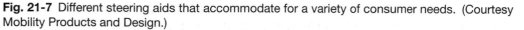

**Fig. 21-7** Different steering aids that accommodate for a variety of consumer needs. (Courtesy Mobility Products and Design.)

in allowing individuals with limited hand and arm function to use a mechanical hand control.

## Power Parking Brake

Most individuals who have upper extremity weakness do not have the strength to use a mechanical parking brake extension. Two basic types of power parking brakes are available, those that pull the park brake cable through a linear actuator and those that pull the parking brake pedal using a cable/chain on spool winch, both routinely occurring at this level of modification.

## In-Motion Secondary Controls

While in control of the vehicle, the driver must access the following five controls:

1. Turn signals
2. Headlight dimmers
3. Windshield wipe/wash
4. Horn
5. Cruise/set

Most drivers with quadriplegia have their hands roughly fitted in either a tripin steering device or a modified-grip hand control. Clinicians often modify these five in-motion controls so that the user can access them by using the right or left elbow to strike a momentary contact (toggle on/off, or timed out) switch for these functions.

## Modified Steering Devices for Persons with Quadriplegia

Three basic types of modified steering spinners are in this group, and the clinician should introduce the least restrictive spinner to the wheel. The clinician should carefully evaluate size, mass, and ability to easily position the hand in the device and should make appropriate recommendations based on demonstrated use. The least restrictive device is the flat spinner, which has a relatively low mass and size. Unlike the V-grip it has rounded ends that encircle the extended hand. The greatest problem with drivers with quadriplegia using this device is that many have entangled their fingers while completing quick steering rotations. If the flat spinner is ineffective, the next best solution is the upright V-grip spinner. The mass of this device is similar to the flat quad spinner, but the upright posts may pose a danger in even slow speed collisions. The final grip that the clinician should consider is the tripin. The clinician should introduce this type of spinner as a last resort because its mass is the greatest. The driver can have difficulty getting into the device unless properly balanced, and it poses the greatest risk of danger in an accident. It is usually restricted to use by people with the most severe disabilities in which the drivers are unable to maintain independent wrist extension. People rarely use it in this classification of modification.

## Mechanical Extensions of Secondary Dash Controls

At this level, most drivers can arrange to reach or manipulate mechanical extensions of the dash controls. This area has the most variability in method and cosmetics. If properly designed and installed, mechanical extensions are functional and provide a reasonable means of accessing controls such as headlight switches, wiper controls, heat, ventilation and air-conditioning (HVAC) levers, and radio controls.

## *Class 5: Generic Van for Drivers with Paraplegia*

Some individuals are unable to transfer into sedans but can transfer into vans using six-way, power seat bases. These individuals may need modifications found in conversion level 3, plus other assistive technology.

## Fully Automatic Lift

More than 29 types of lifts are listed for installation into full-sized vans (19 platform and 10 rotary).[2] Fully automatic lifts have existed for many years and offer an excellent means for people entering and exiting vans. The evaluator should pay considerable attention to the intended wheelchair dimensions to ensure that the user can fit onto the prescribed lift. Most of the lift manufacturers publish specification and application catalogs that can help identify appropriate items.

## Automatic Door Openers

Whenever drivers are using vans with fully automatic lifts, they must have automatic door openers to close the doors once they get in. Access switches are available through several lockable options, such as keyed outside mounted toggle switches, keyed outside lockboxes, magnetic entries, and remote control entries, which offer radio remotes to open and close the doors and operate the lift functions.

## Power Seat Base

At this level of conversion the driver is strong enough to use most of the OEM controls but is unable to transfer without the assistance of a power seat base. A power seat base eases transfer by allowing the vehicle seat to be lower than the wheelchair for transfer into the seat and higher than the wheelchair when transferring back. Installation of a power seat base has been complicated by the introduction of air bags. Chrysler, GM, and the 1997 Ford vans all have sending units for the air bag deployment system under the driver's seat. Persons cannot move or alter these units without jeopardizing the air bag system. Issues related to the air bag and a waiver provision may be granted on a case-by-case basis.[79] A person must send in each waiver separately, identifying the reason for the waiver.

## Raised Top

At this level of modification, a raised top and door openers are needed if the driver is unable to stoop into the side door opening, or if the seated head height exceeds 53 inches. Drivers should not lower the floor in this type of modification, which is considered radical and unnecessary, if they are able to transfer.

## Class 6: Generic Van for Persons with Quadriplegia

This class is one of the highest levels of technology offered to individuals with severe disabilities. This driver uses a motorized wheelchair but has some upper extremity strength. Adaptive equipment subsystem elements include several from Class 4 and 5.

## Lowered-Floor, Full-Sized Van, or Lowered Floor Minivan

Most individuals who use powered mobility sit high in their wheelchairs. This is particularly true of individuals who have sustained a spinal cord injury. At this level of conversion, the driver presumably cannot transfer. Anytime individuals sit higher than 50 inches, they will likely require vans with lowered floors. A raised top for a wheelchair driver will increase the head height but does little to increase driver visibility and interferes with the driver eyellipse. The goal of lowering the floor is for the clinician to develop optimum visibility with the least amount of floor lowering. In a full-sized, Ford van, the clinician can lower the floor roughly 4 inches, increasing head height from 53 inches to 57 inches. If the driver still requires being lower, the clinician needs to elevate the van body (usually a maximum of 2 inches) and straddle the frame (usually no more than 1.5 inches) or a combination of both. If more lowering is required, the clinician will need to raise the van body further, greatly affecting the handling because the center of gravity will change. In combination with sensitized steering and accelerator and brake controls, this can create a vehicle that is difficult to control. The recertified lowered floor minivan can offer as much as 56 inches of interior headroom but it does pose wheelchair width restrictions.[79]

## Wheelchair Tiedown and Occupant Restraint System (WTORS)

Individuals must use WTORS whenever they drive or ride as passengers from their wheelchair. The system needs to secure the wheelchair and the occupant and must meet Federal Motor Vehicle Safety Standards. WTORS is not available for all types of wheelchairs and some create a restriction in ground clearance that can tear up door thresholds and limit the terrain that the wheelchair can negotiate (Figure 21-8).

## Servo Accelerator and Brake Controls

Several servo controls are available that minimize the effort of the accelerator and brake. The introduction of these controls does not interfere with the function of the OEM pedals, and an able-bodied driver can continue to drive the van using the conventional gas and brake. Servo assist is done using electronic, pneumatic, or vacuum motors. The user must have the proper interface handle, and a designer must often create a customized handle or grip.

## Reduced-Effort Steering and Backups

Reduced effort steering can be either low effort or zero effort. Low-effort steering is defined as requiring less effort for operation than factory but more effort than a zero-effort

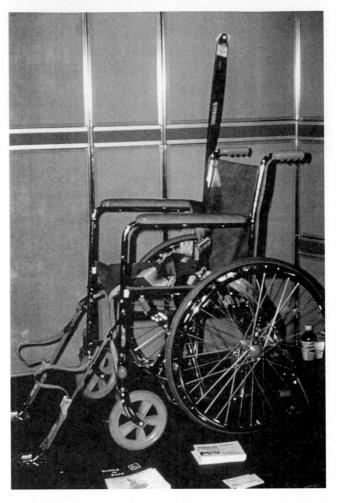

**Fig. 21-8** Manual "Q" Straint WTORS installed in a paratransit bus.

steering system (between 4.0 and 15.0 in-lb.). Zero-effort steering reduces the effort further from between 1.5 and 4.0 in-lb. The introduction of reduced-effort steering removes the vehicle's return-to-center feature and the road feel. The clinician must instruct the user in these systems because the initial user response is a tendency to continually steer the van, resulting in a drift or weave pattern.[80] The user can usually adjust for this feature, which requires several hours of training.

## Reduced Effort Brakes and Backups

In some cases, the user can still operate a mechanical hand control but lacks the strength to apply full brake. This is particularly the case if an individual is capable of using the push/pull type II hand controls fitted with a tripin interface handle. This type of mechanical control is effective when the user combines it with a reduced-effort brake modification. A hand control "lock out" is an important addition in this combination because it keeps the controls from pushing into the brake during a rapid stop by a person using the foot brake. A person should not use reduced-effort brakes in combination with servo controls.

## Relocated Dashboard Controls

In addition to the controls listed in Class 4, this class of modification often requires relocation of the dash controls with electronic relay packs. The addition of these controls can provide tailored positioning for all of the secondary dash controls plus electronic access to some of the adaptive features of the van (WTORS, emergency back-ups, lift and door operators).

## Final Classification

A final classification of modification is applied at even higher levels of impairment. This level includes joystick driving systems, multiaxis remote steering servos, and hydraulic/mechanical unilever driving systems. A person uses each of these levels in selective cases, and the clinician should evaluate it carefully. A person should receive extended evaluation or training before purchasing these systems. Many cases fail because of the problems with reliability, fit, training, and poor equipment matching.[81] The skills of OTs, PTs, physicians, engineers, and driver rehabilitation specialists (CDRS) can improve outcomes in this important aspect of assistive technology.[82]

## CASE STUDIES

### CASE 1

E.T. was a 19-year-old man whose primary disability was spina bifida. He was ambulatory using forearm crutches and periodically used a manual wheelchair. The clinical evaluation revealed that he might require considerable behind-the-wheel training. The static tests (MVPT and WAIS subtests) suggested that he had a slight deficit in figure-ground discrimination and position in space. He also demonstrated a slight perceptual delay in responding to the presented items. The clinician administered the DPT II test but aborted it after E.T. continually lost his place in the test. The clinician administered the DPT using a video format, and the speed of the visual scenes is an essential component. The clinician thought that a perceptual impairment most likely existed but thought that E.T. could compensate.

E.T. had some upper-extremity weakness. Most of the physical testing occurred in a midsized evaluation sedan equipped with factory power steering. He did not have any significant problems with this car but did require a seat cushion to elevate him in the OEM seat. He drove with a right-angle pull/push hand control and a steering spinner device. After roughly 30 hours of behind-the-wheel exposure, he passed his road test and received a restricted license. The evaluator was asked to prepare an equipment recommendation for modifying his personal car, which was a 1991 Hyundai Sonata that he planned to share with his able-bodied brother.

The clinician made the equipment recommendations based on observations in the evaluation sedan. Although E.T. learned standard power steering in a midsize sedan, the evaluator thought that the Hyundai would be more difficult to steer. This assumption was based on the general knowledge that the smaller the car, the stiffer the power steering. To lighten the steering effort, the evaluator recommended a reduced-effort, steering modification in this vehicle. The evaluator thought that the use of a seat cushion could be avoided by installing a power seat base. E.T. could have standard hand controls installed, and a removable steering spinner would allow him to keep a constant grip on the steering wheel.

When the case was reviewed, the evaluator identified several difficulties. Many cars are not able to have their steering gearbox modified to produce a reduced-effort steering system. The Hyundai did not have a conventional method of achieving this. When a car has reduced-effort steering, the "return-to-center" feature is greatly reduced or eliminated and the driver feels like the vehicle is on icy pavement. Because E.T. planned to share the car, his brother would have to learn reduced-effort steering. No power seats are available for this vehicle. One vendor planned to install a van-type power seat, but this would have interfered or eliminated the useful backseat space. Consequently, this vehicle had a hydraulic seat elevation system included as part of the OEM design and no need existed for a seat cushion or a power seat.

This simple case had a positive outcome, and the vehicle required minimal modification. The evaluator was able to produce outstanding clinical and diagnostic findings and the driver educator was able to apply guided intervention to compensate for the perceptual deficits. The case went smoothly until the evaluator had to identify modifications to the consumer's vehicle. Coordination among the evaluator, the educator, and the assis-

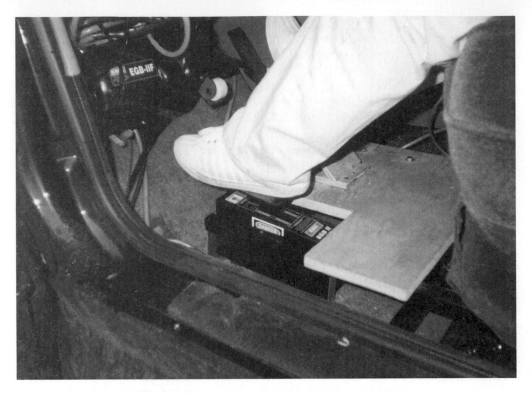

**Fig. 21-9** Left foot used to access electronic gas and brake.

tive technology specialist was necessary to address the equipment specification problems in this case.

## CASE 2

J.H. was a 26-year college senior whose primary disability was arthrogryposis. He was able to ambulate short distances but mostly used a powered wheelchair. J.H. was completing his senior year at Ohio State University and was planning to become a schoolteacher. He was extremely bright and motivated to drive. Initially, a clinician evaluated him at a large medical clinic and discovered that he was not a good candidate for driving, unless the evaluator could identify unconventional control configuration. J. H. was willing to do what was needed and traveled out of state for a clinical assessment at one of the large Driver Rehabilitation Centers in the Midwest.

A clinician conducted a brief clinical screening and found that he did not have any perceptual or cognitive impairment. His major problems were in his functional range of motion. Although J.H. had limited use of his extremities, he had limited distal use of his hands and arms. He was able to stand and ambulate for short distances. Because he was able to stand and transfer, the clinician recommended a lowered floor. The clinician could have provided a raised top, which could have achieved the same goal, but the clinician would have had to increase the overall height. Range of motion in his upper extremities was severely limited, and the clinician designed a custom, switch system for the power seat. J.H. was accustomed to using a mouth stick, so the clinician designed and installed a special switch console for use with a mouthstick. The mouthstick functions were all predriving operations. J.H. had good control of his left foot, although he had limited range of motion. The clinician decided to install and position a modified electronic gas and brake system within J.H.'s functional range that he could operate with his left foot (Figure 21-9).

J.H. steered with an electronic remote steering servo that allowed him to steer with his right elbow and shoulder. The clinician placed secondary controls for access with either the mouthstick or a single switch that emitted a tone that corresponded to one of eight intended functions (Figure 21-10). The clinician adjusted the configuration during each of several fittings, and J.H. was able to pass his road test. He has been a successful driver

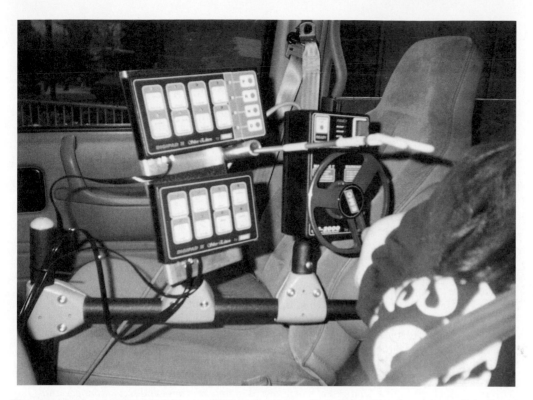

**Fig. 21-10** Mouthstick used for predriving secondary functions. Steering accomplished with wheel at right elbow location.

for more than a year, is currently a full-time teacher in a rural district, and drives his van to school every day. This case illustrates an uncharacteristic control configuration that required careful planning, positioning, and teaching. It illustrates the flexibility of existing adaptive driving controls and the need for careful evaluation.

## References

1. Butler CA, Hamada K, Kenel FC: *The AAA disabled driver's mobility guide,* Heathrow, Fla, July 1995, American Automobile Association.
2. Trace Research and Development Center: UW-Madison, Co-Net 9, Hyper-ABLEDATA, Co-Net Hyper-Able Data, ed 9, Madison, Wis, Spring/Summer 1996.
3. Help for disabled drivers, *Changing Times* 55–58, Aug 1985.
4. Simple mods enable quadriplegics to steer/brake vehicle, *Design News* 39 (8):14–16, April 25, 1983.
5. Technical News Brief: Advance concepts developed for controlling autos, *Automotive Engineering* 81 (7):21–22, July 1973.
6. Zarragh MY, Koopman R, Haraldsdottir A: *Modified steering systems for the severely disabled driver,* pp 100–102, Proceedings of the 6th Annual Conference on Rehabilitation Engineering, Washington, DC, 1983, RESNA Press.
7. Britell CA: The Unistick vehicle controller, *Paraplegia News* 41:22–24, Dec 1987.
8. Product information: As-Tech Inc, Easton, Mass; Ahnafield Corp, Indianapolis; EMC Inc, Baton Rouge, 1994–1996.
9. Chiang YP, Bassi LJ, Javitt JC: Federal budgetary costs of blindness, *Milbank Quarterly* 70 (2):319–340, 1992.
10. Butler CA, Hamada K: *AAA Digest of Motor Laws,* Heathrow, Fla, 1995, American Automobile Association.
11. Baron C: Bioptic telescopic spectacles for motor vehicle driving, *J Am Optom Assoc* 1 (62):37–41, 1991.

12. Babirad J, Mendelson L, Flis M: *Appropriate development of vehicle modification protocol for maximizing traffic safety of disabled driver*, pp 15–16, Proceedings RESNA 13th Annual Conference, Washington DC, 1990, RESNA Press.

13. Medical examination of chauffeurs, editorial, JAMA 46:1211, 1906.

14. Berens C Jr et al: Report of committee on physical standards for drivers of motor vehicles, *JAMA* 83:2094–2095, 1924.

15. NYSED Subcommittee on Driver Evaluation and Training for Individuals with Disabilities: *Final report of NYSED VESID subcommittee on driver evaluation and training for individuals with disabilities: a report to the deputy commissioner of VESID,* Sept 30, 1993.

16. NYSED VESID Subcommittee on Driver Evaluation and Training for Individuals with Disabilities: Final report to the deputy commissioner of VESID, Albany, NY, Sept 30, 1993.

17. NYSED VESID Subcommittee on Driver Evaluation and Training for Individuals with Disabilities: Final report to the deputy commissioner of VESID, Albany, NY, Sept 30, 1993.

18. NYSED VESID Subcommittee on Driver Evaluation and Training for Individuals with Disabilities: Final report to the deputy commissioner of VESID, Albany, NY, Sept 30, 1993.

19. Smith RO: *Models of service delivery in rehabilitation technology, rehabilitation technology service delivery: a practical guide,* pp 15–19, Washington, DC, RESNA Press, 1987.

20. Committee for Accreditation of Rehabilitation Facilities: 1995 standards manual and interpretive guidelines for medical rehabilitation, *CARF* 86–95A, 1995.

21. Kerr CM, Irwin E: Driver assessment and training of the disabled client, *Rehab Engineer* 323, 1990.

22. Valois T: Disabled drivers program: an OT approach, *American Occupational Therapy Association Newsletter* 5 (2):1–3, 1982.

23. Babirad J: Consent for Driver Rehabilitation/Education (form), 1996.

24. Pettis RW: Tarasoff and the dangerous driver: a look at the driving cases, *Bull Am Acad Psych Law* 20 (4): 427–437, 1990.

25. Butler CA, Hamada K: *AAA digest of motor laws: a summary of laws and regulations governing regulation and operation of passenger cars in the US, its territories, and the provinces of Canada,* Heathrow, Fla, 1995, AAA.

26. Appeal SD, Brilliant RL, Reich L: Driving with visual impairment: fact and issues, *J Vis Rehab* 4:19–31, 1989.

27. Mars S, Keightley S: Visual standard for driving and occupations, *Practitioner* 234 (1481):34–35, 1990.

28. Keeny AH: The visually impaired driver, *Am J Ophthal* 82:799–801, 1976.

29. Szylk JP, Brigell M, Seiple W: Effects of age and hemianopic visual field loss on driving, *Optom Vis Sci* 70:1031–1037, 1993.

30. Szlyk JP, Fishman, GA, Master SP: Peripheral vision screening for driving in retinitis pigmentosa patients, *Ophthalmology* 98 (5):612–618, 1991.

31. Smith, PA: *Vision and driving vision in vehicles,* pp 13–17, Proceedings of the Conference on Vision In Vehicles, Nottingham, UK, Sept 13, 1985, North-Holland.

32. Casson E: *CVNet: query on automated vision testers,* ecasson@aix1.uottaw.ca., March 10, 1996.

33. Chiang YP, Bassi LJ, Javitt JC: Federal budgetary costs of blindness, *Milbank Quarterly* 70 (2):319–340, 1992.

34. Kelleher DK: Driving with low vision, *J Vis Impair Blind* 11:345–350, Nov 1979.

35. American Association of Motor Vehicle Administrators: *Telescopic lenses,* resolution #7, Baltimore, March 1983.

36. American Academy of Ophthalmology and Otolaryngology: *Resolution on bioptic telescopic spectacles,* Alexandria, Va, 1977.

37. American Public Health Association: *Drivers license for the visually handicapped person,* policy statement #8316, Washington, DC, 1984.

38. American Optometric Association: *The use of bioptic telescopes for driving,* Position Statement of the American Optometric Association, St Louis, Aug 1982.

39. Park WL, Unatin J, Park JM: A profile of the demographics, training and driving history of telescopic drivers in the state of Michigan, *J Am Optom Assoc 66* (5):274–280, 1995.

40. Corn AL, Lippmann, Lewis MC: Licensed drivers with bioptic telescopic spectacles: user profiles and perceptions, *RE:view* XXI (4):221–230, 1990.

41. American Optometric Association Low Vision Section: *Statement on the use of bioptic telescopes for driving,* Sept 1994.

42. Trobe JD et al: Confrontation visual field techniques in the detection of anterior visual pathway lesions, *Ann Neurol 1* 10 (1):28–34, 1981.

43. Halperin EJ, Cohen BS: Perceptual-motor dysfunction: stumbling block to rehabilitation, *Maryland State Med J* 20 (7):140–142, 1971.

44. Siev E, Freshtat T: *Perceptual dysfunction in the adult stroke patient: a manual for treatment,* p 59, Thorofare, NJ, 1976, Charles B. Slack.

45. Colarusso RP, Hammil DD: *Motor free visual perception test,* Academic Therapy Publications, 1972.

46. Wechsler D: *Manual for Wechsler adult intelligence scale,* San Antonio, 1955, Psychological Corp.

47. Sivak M et al: *Perceptual cognitive skills and driving, effects of brain damage,* Ann Arbor, Mich, 1980, The University of Michigan Report No. UM-HSRI-80-3, Highway Safety Research Institute.

48. Reitan RM: *Trail making test: manual for administration, scoring and interpretation,* Bloomington, Ind, 1956, Indiana University Press.

49. Weaver JK: *Driver performance test II administrative guidelines,* Clearwater, Fla, 1990, Advanced Driver Skills.

50. Engum ES et al: Cognitive behavioral driver's inventory, *Cognitive Rehabilitation,* Sept/Oct 1988.

51. Galski T, Bruno RL, Ehle HT: Driving after cerebral damage: a model with implications for evaluation, *Am J Occup Ther* 46 (4):324–332, 1992.

52. Cossairt J: *Personal licensed vehicles, a bibliography,* Panama City, Fla, 1988, Jolan Cossairt.

53. Crenshaw RP, Vistnes LM: A decade of pressure sore research: 1977–1987, *J Rehab Res Dev* 26:63–74, 1989.

54. Jones CK: The use of molded techniques for fitting C5-6 spinal cord injured five or more years past injury (abstr). In Trefler E, editor: *Seating the disabled: third international seating symposium proceedings,* pp189–192, Memphis, Tenn, 1987, University of Tennessee Press.

55. Abnernathy CN et al: Effects of deceleration and rate of deceleration on live seated human subjects, *Trans Res Rec* N6 (46):12–17, 1977.

56. Babirad J: Considerations in seating and positioning severely disabled drivers, *Assistive Technol* 1:31–37, 1989.

57. Otto Bock Orthopedic Industry, 3000 Xenium Lane N., Minneapolis, MN 55441.

58. Invacare Corporation, 899 Cleveland Street, P.O. Box 4028, Elyria, Ohio 44036-2125.

59. Schneider LW, Melvin JW: *Sled test evaluation of a wheelchair restraint system for use by handicapped drivers* (abstr), Ann Arbor, Mich, 1978, The University of Michigan Transportation Research Institute Report No. UM-HSRI-78-57.

60. Society of Automotive Engineers: *Describing and measuring the driver's field of view,* pp 1–24, Warrensburg, Pa, rev Aug 1994, SAE Surface Vehicle Recommended Practice, J1050.

61. Society of Automotive Engineers: *Motor vehicle drivers' eye locations,* pp 1–20, Warrensburg, Pa, rev June 1992, SAE Surface Vehicle Recommended Practice, J941.

62. Driving for the disabled, *Newsweek* 87–88, July 9, 1945.

63. Amputee autoists, *Business Week* 19–20, July 27, 1946.

64. Lehneis HR: Safety achievements of disabled drivers, *Biomed Engineer* 8:438–439, 1973.

65. Reichenberger A: Automotive aids for the handicapped, *Bull Prosthet Res* 10 (22):53–54, 1974.

66. Dept of Veterans Affairs: *VA standard design and test criteria for safety and quality of special automotive driving aids (adaptive equipment) for standard passenger automobiles,* VAPC-A-7505-8, Baltimore, 1977.

67. Dept of Veterans Affairs: *VA standard design and test criteria for safety and quality of automatic wheelchair lift systems for passenger motor vehicles,* VAPC-A-7708-3, Baltimore, June 28, 1977.

68. Dept of Veterans Affairs: *VA standard design and test criteria for safety and quality of power assisted steering modification for passenger motor vehicles,* VAREC-A-8110-1, Baltimore, 1977.

69. Dept of Veterans Affairs: *VA standard design and test criteria for safety and quality of power assisted brake modifications for passenger motor vehicles,* VAREC-A-8209-1, Baltimore, 1978.

70. Society of Automobile Engineers: *Automotive adaptive driver controls, manual,* Warrensburg, Pa, rev Aug 1990, SAE Surface Vehicle Recommended Practice, J1903.

71. Society of Automobile Engineers: *Vehicle and control modifications for drivers with physical disabilities terminology,* pp 1–8, Warrensburg, Pa, rev June 1992, SAE Surface Vehicle Information Report, J2094.

72. Society of Automobile Engineers: *Design considerations for wheelchair lifts for entry to or exit from a personally licensed vehicle,* Warrensburg, Pa, issued 1995–2005, SAE Surface Vehicle Recommended Practice, J2093.

73. Society of Automobile Engineers: *Testing of wheelchair lifts for entry to or exit from a personally licensed vehicle,* Warrensburg, Pa, issued 1995–2005, SAE Surface Vehicle Recommended Practice, J2092.

74. Society of Automobile Engineers: *Structural modification for personally licensed vehicles to meet the transportation needs of persons with disabilities,* Warrensburg, Pa, issued 1995–2006, SAE Surface Vehicle Information Report, J1725.

75. Boselovic L: Runaway car had altered gas pedal, *Pittsburgh Post-Gazette* A-1, August 24, 1995.

76. In the works: auto wheelchair "Mobility Package," *J Am Ins* 50 (2):30, 1974.

77. Society of Automobile Engineers: *Terminology report J2094 for vehicle and control modifications for drivers with physical disabilities,* Warrensburg, Pa, Sept 20, 1995, SAE Adaptive Devices Committee Report.

78. Koppa RJ et al: Handicapped driver controls operability: a device for clinical evaluation of patients, *Arch Phys Med Rehab* 59:227–230, 1979.

79. *Braun Product Application Catalog,* pp A–40 – 43, 1996, The Braun Corp.

80. Risk HF: Pros and cons of the "less effort" steering and braking systems for the severely handicapped driver, *Am Correct Ther J* 34 (5):154–155, 1980.

81. Babirad J, Frost F, Flis M: *Pitfalls in van modifications for persons with quadriplegia: six case examples of failed client/technology interface,* Toronto, 1992, Proceedings of the 1992 American Spinal Injury Association.

82. Frost F, Babirad J, Bouman G: *Vehicles for disabled drivers: maximizing outcome while minimizing technology,* San Francisco, 1992, Proceedings of the 69th Annual Session of the American Congress of Rehabilitation Medicine.

# CHAPTER 22

## Lower Limb Orthotics

*Thomas V. DiBello*

## Application and Goal

In this chapter, I discuss the role that lower extremity orthoses play in the rehabilitation process. It determines who may be candidates for this technology and the way specialists might best apply that technology. An ideal outcome is one in which the orthoses provide comfort, improve function within the limits of the patient's potential, and apply the appropriate biomechanical alignment necessary to achieve a specific goal within a specific diagnosis. To demonstrate these principles, case studies will appear at the end of the chapter.

The primary objectives involved in the orthotic management of the lower limb are for specialists to provide stability, prevent deformity, and facilitate function.[1] Specialists' effective implementation of the first two goals often is in direct opposition to the third goal. The provision of stability requires that a person control or limit joint motion. The prevention of deformity requires that the person control aberrant movement that affects joint motion. In both cases, an affect on function occurs.

If normal individuals' ability to plantarflex is limited, they will have a difficult time moving through the first part of each step. Persons must compensate for this by bending the knee and hip to get the foot flat on the ground, which creates an energy-inefficient gait. If, however, a physician examines individuals with a right-side peroneal nerve palsy, they walk with gaits that require compensation for a variety of aberrations. Their feet drop when they attempt to swing them through, they are in a poor position to begin the next steps, and they begin each step on their toes instead of their heels. This creates an awkward energy-inefficient gait. A specialist's prescription of an ankle-foot orthosis (AFO) that blocks plantarflexion prevents individuals from dropping the foot during swing phase and the position of the heel for the beginning of stance thus permitting the heel, not the toe, to strike first. Additionally, this limits the chance of persons catching the dropped toe on an object and tripping. This change creates safer, more energy-efficient gaits for these individuals. Even though this device blocks several important movements at the ankle, it does not limit functionality. But by creating a safer more energy-efficient gait, the device enhances it. The progressive nature of a disease or the severity of a trauma may limit the reasonable level of function attainable. Specialists must temper the goal for the orthosis by consideration of a variety of factors. A specific functional measurement, say velocity in the previous example, may decrease so that the orthosis can serve the greater protection or stability needs of individuals.

### Function and Ability

Approximately 3% of the United States population may benefit from using some type of orthotic device.[2] A smaller percentage of that total requires a lower-extremity orthosis. Unlike prosthetic patients, function levels do not categorize users of orthoses. A broad range of individuals with many different and varied diagnoses might benefit from the use of a lower-extremity orthotic device. Some general categories include individuals with lower limb muscle weakness, spasticity, the inability to coordinate muscle movement, and skeletal deformity or weakness, any of which may be secondary to disease, trauma, or congenital defect.

Some specific diagnoses include individuals with muscular dystrophy, cerebral palsy, polio, traumatic brain injury, spinal cord injury, stroke and spina bifida. In addition, many less-common disorders exist that affect individuals' neuromuscular or skeletal systems, which may benefit from orthotic intervention.

In each case, the appropriateness of orthotic intervention depends on a particular patient's needs. These may range from lower limb positioning while they are laying, sitting, or during transfers, to stability while they are standing and performing a task, to the more demanding needs that occur during ambulation. With any form of assistive technology, its ultimate benefit depends on a variety of factors that relate to the person's needs, lifestyle, and willingness to apply the technology. Although function and comfort are of primary importance, specialists must not overlook cosmesis and usability. If a wonderfully functional orthosis is so complex or ungainly that the user rejects it, then a poor outcome results. Specialists should carefully consider the user's needs regarding the effect the device will have clinically and psychologically.

## Considerations, Options, and Technology

The most effective approach to the orthotic management of the lower limb uses a team concept. The team should include the patient, the physician, the orthotist and the physical therapist.[3] Together, they assess the patient's needs and define the immediate and long-term goals for treatment. This assessment includes their consideration of the important clinical findings involved in defining the diagnoses and prognoses and other issues including the person's cognitive abilities, coordination, motivation, living environment, vocation, and avocations. Once they complete the assessment, they may define immediate and long-term orthotic goals.

After the team formulates a general description of the orthosis, the ABC-certified orthotist determines the specific details of the orthosis design. The certified orthotist (CO) or certified prosthetist-orthotist (CPO) has a unique education that includes exposure to basic engineering principles, anatomy, physiology, pathology, biomechanics, pathomechanics, and basic materials sciences. This blend of subjects permits the CO to choose the most appropriate combinations of materials and design criterion to suit a particular person's needs.

Orthotic design and application relies on accurate specialist assessment of the lower limb. Along with an understanding of the way the disease state or trauma will affect the patient's musculoskeletal system, specialists should assess static and dynamic alignment and they must consider concomitant segment deviations. They must assess each segment from the forefoot to the hip and compare each with the norms for that segment. For instance, in the coronal plane, if the knee is in 30 degrees of valgus, the normal valgus angulation for an adult would exceed by 10 degrees and represents a segment deviation of 20 degrees. Dynamically, if the tibia fails by 10 degrees to come to vertical at midstance, this would represent a segment deviation of 10 degrees at the ankle at midstance in the sagital plane (Figure 22-1).

Once specialists observe deviation, they must assess the amount of correction possible and decide if they can reduce the joint or segment in question into the normal range. Another decision is whether specialists' attempting to hold it with an orthotic device is practical. These decisions most often involve them using observational gait analysis. In more difficult cases, they may employ video or computerized gait analysis. They observe deviations from the norm secondary to disease or trauma, and the CO's or CPO's design of the orthotic device attempts to resolve them. The valgus angulations at the knee may reach its greatest magnitude at midstance. Patients' reducing and holding the knee in a corrected position requires a device that is strong yet covers a large enough surface area to ensure that they can achieve control without excessive pressure. Therefore specialists might choose in this case a plastic knee-ankle-foot orthosis (KAFO) with metal knee joints.

Specialists much individualize the choice of materials, components, and design criterion to the specific needs of each person. They cannot generalize in terms of specific de-

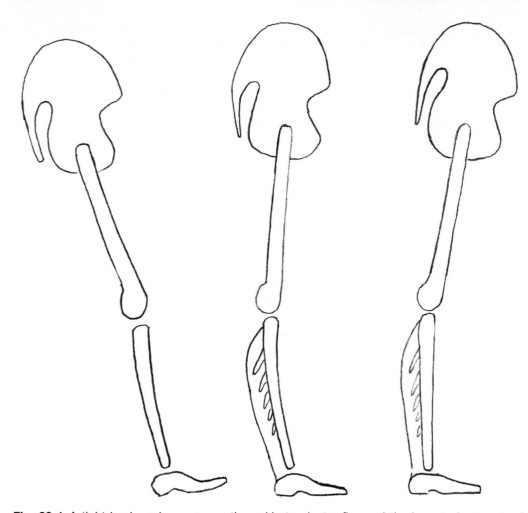

**Fig. 22-1** A tight heel cord may cause the ankle to planter flex and the knee to hyperextend through midstance.

vices for specific diagnoses or a particular component for a particular type of gait deviation. Rather, to achieve an optional result, they must design each device and choose each component based on a complete and thorough assessment.

Possibly the most important aspect involved in the successful design of an orthotic device depends on specialists' appropriate application of three-point force systems (Figure 22-2).[4] By specialists changing and adjusting the materials, device trimlines, and joint range of motion, their design applies force to correct the segment deviations that they define in the clinical analysis. Accurate application of these force systems enables the orthosis to control the limb comfortably under surprisingly high loads.

Specialists categorize lower-extremity orthoses with a nomenclature that describes the joint crossed.[5] They name the most proximal joint crossed first and then progress down the leg. A KAFO for instance crosses the three joints described (Figure 22-3). Additionally, they may add description by describing material type (i.e., metal or plastic KAFO) or function (i.e., ground reaction or solid-ankle AFO) (Figure 22-4).

Designers of orthoses for the lower limb commonly construct them of plastic, metal, or some combination. Orthotists determine the choice of one or the other or a hybrid after careful consideration and assessment of the patient's clinical status, cognitive abilities, and vocation. Once they determine this, they choose specific materials and joint componentry.

Orthotists often indicate AFOs when the problem requires control of ankle movement or alignment of the foot. Crossing the knee or hip KAFOs and hip, knee, ankle, foot orthosis (HKAFOs) enable them to effectively impart control over the movement and angular alignment of these joints.

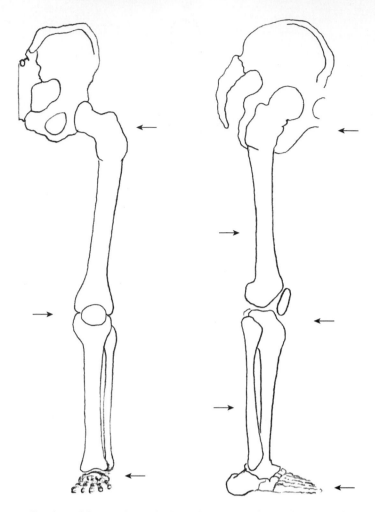

**Fig. 22-2** The application of forces through the orthosis are directed to provide optimal effect by coupling each directional force with opposing forces in the opposite direction.

Componentry for the hip, knee, and ankle permit individuals to move these joints in the orthosis. The design of the component permits the orthosis to assist, resist, move through a specific range, or completely stop motion at that joint. Orthotists may construct these joints of plastic, aluminum, steel, or titanium, which offer them many options. The orthotists' choice of a particular joint component plays an important part in the overall design and must blend well with the orthotic goal that they establish for a particular person. In addition to the joint componentry, the thigh, calf, and foot sections are also a critical part of any lower extremity orthosis (Figure 22-5). They may construct these of leather, thermoplastic, or composite materials and they typically form these over a mold of the person's extremity. They obtain the mold from a plaster impression of the limb.

The maintenance of this technology is basic. Users of orthoses should keep them clean. They should wipe it daily with a washcloth to prevent a buildup of dirt or grime. They can wipe it occasionally with rubbing alcohol to remove any stubborn buildups. Approximately once a month, they should lightly lubricate metal mechanical joints with a household oil. Individuals should remain alert to any sudden change in the feel or sounds of the orthosis, which can indicate a broken or weakened component. They should have an orthotist check the device promptly when this occurs. Furthermore, users should visually inspect the device for any loose or broken parts. They should examine the skin under the brace for any bruises or abrasions and report them promptly along with pain or discomfort. Finally, people with orthoses should return to the orthotist every 6 to 12 months, depending on level of activity, for a thorough check of the device.

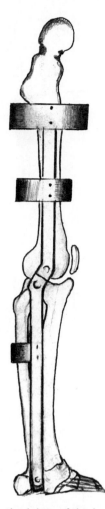

**Fig. 22-3** This metal orthosis crosses the joints of the knee, ankle, and foot and is designated a K (knee), A (ankle), F (foot), and O (orthosis).

## Outcomes and Social Validation

The rehabilitation team plays an important part in ascertaining whether they have met the goals for a particular patient. The ability of the orthosis to meet the requirements of protection, stability, and function within the parameters that the team defines determines its efficacy.

In examining successful outcomes, specialists should often remember that what other members of the team consider a successful outcome may differ from the outcome of the users. Users will judge the device in very practical terms. Specialists can ask the following questions:

- Are users able to apply the device easily?
- Are they able to do more with it than without it?
- Has the device eliminated pain or discomfort?
- Do users feel safer in it?
- How do users perceive their appearance in it?
- Does the device fit under clothing?
- In a general way, has the device improved the quality of life?

Often the answers for some or all of these questions define the value the orthotic device holds for the person. Specialists should remember that no matter how well the device meets the functional goals of the team, if they have failed to consider the practical implications that wearing the device will impose on the users, they will likely fail in providing

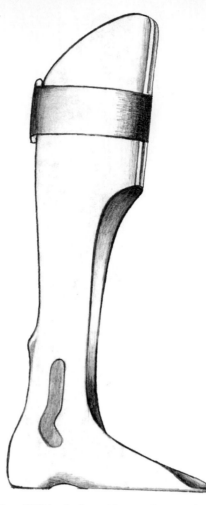

**Fig. 22-4** This ground reaction AFO is designed to create an extension moment at the knee by controlling the forward movement of the tibia at midstance. It depends on its rigid ankle and high anterior section to do this effectively.

a device that provides a strong, positive outcome. This will always be challenging for practitioners. Simply, specialists strapping a mechanical device to their patients' lower limb will always have strong social implications.

At the time of fitting, orthotists assess the fit and function of the orthosis. They check overall construction, they review the design criterion to ascertain whether they constructed the device to specification and whether it matches the guidelines of the prescription. Throughout the fitting procedure, they adjust the orthosis to improve its fit and function. This may involve them heating and reshaping the plastic, recontouring metal components, trimming and padding the device, or adjusting the shape of the sole of the shoe to smooth out the gait of users. Finally, they assess the overall result and make a judgment as to whether the orthosis is optimal for patients in this application and meets the goals and objectives of the team. Orthotists meeting these goals defines a successful outcome.

U.S. society has made important gains in terms of accepting and recognizing that people must not judge physically challenged citizens on their appearance or by the equipment they use to move through their environment, but rather on the merits of their abilities. Orthotists must consider the amalgam of all these issues in managing patients' orthotic needs. Their appreciation of these factors may result in an adjustment in the design or component selection process that improves acceptance without compromising fit or function.

These issues have become more important in the changing health care environment. Demographic studies show that the overall growth of the population and the ag-

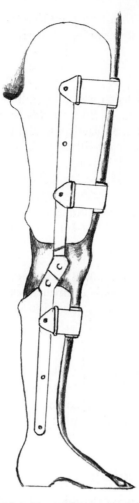

**Fig. 22-5** The plastic thigh, calf, and ankle sections permit the orthosis to transmit forces and therefore control the extremity effectively.

ing of the baby-boom generation results in an increased demand for lower-extremity orthotic services in the future.[6] The demands of the managed-care industry for improved outcomes challenges orthotists to achieve optimal fit, function, and user acceptance of the device. The relative value the device has in terms of its cost directly relates to its ability to successfully meet the clinical and practical needs of patients using it. If they perceive that the orthosis has had a positive affect on their life, they will assign a high value to it.

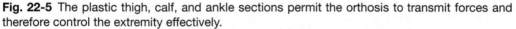

## CASE STUDIES

### CASE 1

#### *Application and Goal*

B.J. is a 14-year-old boy whose football coach noticed he was walking strangely. His right ankle was turning inward abnormally. The coach sent him to his family physician who referred him to a neurologist who made the diagnosis of Charcot-Marie Tooth disease. At the orthotic department, B.J. had a 20-degree valgus angulation of his right ankle on weight bearing. Additionally, his forefoot angulated into adduction and during ambulation, his foot dropped through swing phase. He therefore hiked his right hip and flexed his knee to clear but he was prepositioned poorly for stance, initiating it with his toe, not his heel. He had passive range of motion only to 90 degrees at the right ankle. He reported difficulty running and that he was recently tripping and falling.

### Function and Ability

The team's goals were to reduce B.J.'s tripping and falling and to position his foot to retard contracture and deformity. Because of B.J.'s already limited range, the team determined that a solid-ankle AFO constructed of plastic with the ankle set at 90 degrees would serve his needs most effectively. This AFO would hold his rear foot and forefoot in a corrected position. In addition, it would block his drop foot during swing phase thus reducing his tendency to hike his hips and flex his knee. Doing so would reduce his chances of tripping and falling and create a safer gait. This device would also preposition his foot for stance phase and permit him to approach the ground with heel first, not his toe.

### Considerations and Options

After careful static and dynamic gait analysis, orthotists assessed the specific segmental deviations that existed in B.J. They took an impression in plaster of the foot, ankle, and leg below the knee, manipulating each segment into a corrected position.

### Technology

They used plastic to fabricate this orthosis. They chose it for its ability to comfortably wrap around the foot and hold it and the ankle in a corrected position. Also, it is lightweight and more cosmetic, an important consideration for this 14-year-old. The ankle will be rigid for maximal control during midstance and they will make the toe of the orthosis more flexible to permit a smooth transition through heel off and toe off.

### Outcomes and Social Validation

B.J. ambulated comfortably in his new orthosis. He cleared through stance nicely with good prepositioning for stance. He had nice stability during midstance and transitioned well through the second half of stance phase. This device created a safer, more stable gait for B.J. and should reduce tripping and falling substantially. Additionally, it will hold his foot in a nicely corrected position and should retard the progression of contracture and deformity.

### CASE 2

### Application and Goal

D.M. is a 52-year-old successful lawyer who is active in the community and who contracted polio at age 3. The virus left him with muscle weakness in his right lower extremity. At a young age, a CO fitted him with an AFO; at 12 years of age, he self-eliminated his orthosis. He has walked without an orthosis or any type of external support since that time. D.M. came to the clinic with a chief complaint of right knee pain and an increase in tripping and falling. The specialists graded his dorsiflexors as fair, his quadriceps as poor, and his hip flexors as fair. He had a steppage-type gait, hiking his right hip to clear that foot; his right knee hyperextended 20 degrees at midstance.

### Function and Ability

The specialists' goals for D.M. were ambulation without pain and diminished tripping and falling. They determined that he should be able to function at a level equal to the one he enjoyed before the onset of knee pain. Additionally, this orthosis should reduce the abnormal hip movement and may reduce the likelihood of hip and low back pain in the future. The clinic team determined that a plastic KAFO with posteriorly offset free knee joint and articulated ankle with free dorsiflexion and a plantarflexion stop would best serve D.M.'s needs. They used plastic to reduce weight and to spread the forces more evenly across his lower limbs. The posteriorly offset knee joint would harness the ground reaction forces and create a knee that was less likely to buckle. This device would block foot drop during swing phase and reduce hyperextension during stance. Additionally, after fitting the orthosis, they determined that D.M. would have several sessions of physical therapy with a physical therapist familiar with gait training postpolio syndrome patients.

## Considerations and Options

After static and dynamic gait analysis, orthotists assessed the specific segmental deviations that existed and began to formulate the initial design characteristics of the KAFO. They took an impression of the involved extremity with special care to achieve optimal alignment. From this impression, they made a mold and modified it to best achieve the desired control.

## Technology

D.M. will ambulate most effectively if they maintain optimal alignment. The foot section should control the abduction of the forefoot and eversion of the heel present in this person. The ankle joint should provide an adjustable plantar flexion stop but permit free movement into dorsiflexion. The knee joint should be free moving but block hyperextension at 5 degrees. A posteriorly offset axis of rotation at the knee will permit D.M. to stand safely without firing his weakened quadriceps muscle (Figure 22-6). The proximal end of the KAFO will be an ischeal containment design that permits a moderate amount of weight transfer during stance phase or during standing. This orthosis will use a thermoplastic shell with metal components at the knee joint and plastic components at the ankle (Figure 22-7).

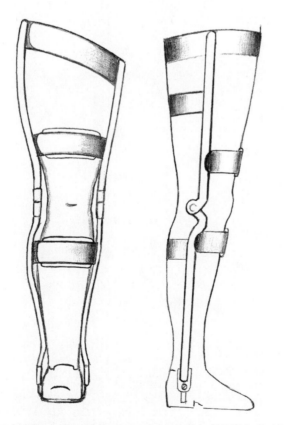

**Fig. 22-6** The center axis of rotation of the knee joint in this KAFO is behind the midline of the leg. This joint design and its placement on the leg create a tendency for the joint to remain extended through the middle of stance phase.

## Outcomes and Social Validation

D.M. ambulated comfortably without pain in the orthosis. After gait-training therapy sessions, specialists diminished his abnormal hip movement by nearly 50%. They reduced hyperextension to 5 degrees thus preventing any further deterioration of the knee joint. D.M. reported that specialists nearly eliminated his tripping and falling. The cost of this device would be more than offset by the cost of a fracture resulting from a fall because of his foot drop. The value to this person of a return to his normal level of activity without pain was incalculable.

## CASE 3

## Application and Goal

R.A. is a 62-year-old man who suffered a right CVA causing left hemiparesis approximately 6 weeks ago. He was progressing in therapy. However, he was having difficulty standing and taking steps. He was unable to effectively preposition his foot and ankle to stand. As he attempted to approach the floor, his foot forcefully inverted and supinated and his knee flexed.

To walk, people must first be able to stand thus the team's orthotic goal for R.A. was to provide stability in standing. Secondly, the orthosis should permit weight transfer over the left foot to permit initiation of gait and then swing phase clearance as he takes a step.

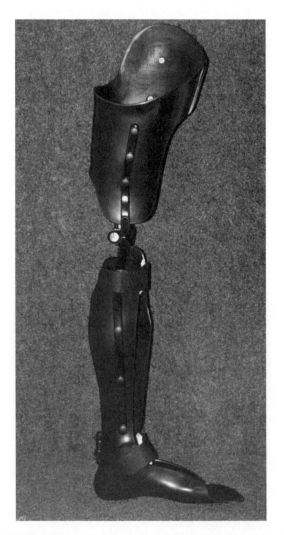

**Fig. 22-7** This plastic KAFO has metal posteriorly offset knee joints and plastic ankle joints with an adjustable plantar flexion stop.

## Function and Ability

How far R.A. would progress in his recovery was unknown to the team. However, without the stability that an AFO provides, he will have difficulty effectively developing a safe gait pattern.

## Considerations and Options

Although at some point in R.A.'s recovery he may be able to use an orthosis with an articulated ankle joint, the primary function of this orthosis were to provide stability. Absence of contracture and fluctuating edema were important considerations for specialists in the choice of AFO design.

## Technology

R.A.'s forceful posturing into inversion and supination required a device that can effectively control his foot and ankle comfortably. The most appropriate design able to affect this level of control, while stabilizing the ankle in the sagital and coronal planes, was a plastic solid ankle design (Figure 22-8). Specialists had to take the impression for this device with R.A.'s foot and ankle fully corrected. They applied correcting forces along the medial aspects of the forefoot and rearfoot and just above the lateral malleolus (Figure 22-9). R.A.'s height and weight helped specialists determine the type and thickness of plastic to use. In this case, they chose a $\frac{3}{16}$-inch polypropylene.

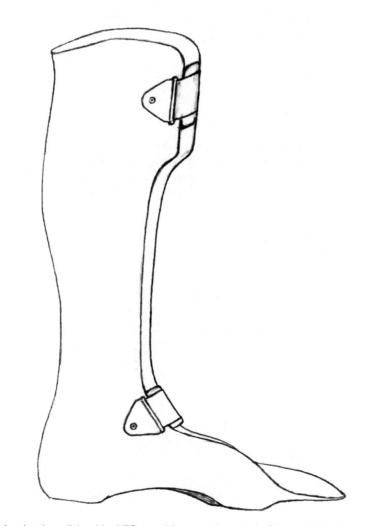

**Fig. 22-8** This plastic solid ankle AFO provides good control of the ankle in the sagittal, coronal, and transverse planes.

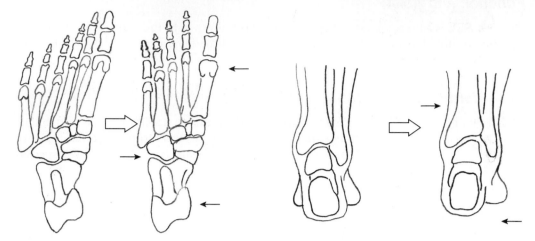

**Fig. 22-9** The trimlines of the orthosis will permit application of forces to realign and the foot and ankle.

## *Outcomes and Social Validation*

Without this orthosis, R.A. will have difficulty progressing to a functional gait. His current condition places his ankle and foot at risk of injury. His inability to stand and take a step over a stable base of support makes tripping and falling likely. This orthosis will mediate these problems, permitting him to progress through gait training and increase the likelihood that he will be able to reach his full recovery potential.

## References

1. Gage JR: *Gait analysis in cerebral palsy,* p 177, London, 1991, MacKeiht Press.
2. Shurr DG, Cook TM: *Prosthetics and orthotics,* Norwalk, Conn, 1990, Appleton and Lange.
3. Cary JM, Lusskin R, Thompson RG: Prescription principles. In Thompson R, editor: *Atlas of orthotics: biomechanical principles and applications,* St Louis, 1975, Mosby.
4. Smith LK, Weiss EL, Lehmkuhl DL: *Brunnstom's clinical kinesiology,* ed 5, Philadelphia, 1996, FA Davis.
5. Harris EE: A new orthotic terminology: a guide to its use for prescription and fee schedules, *Orthot Prosthet* 27: 6–9, 1973.
6. Neilsen CC: *Issues affecting the future demand for orthotists and prosthetists,* 1996, study prepared for the NCOPE.

# PART 5

$\bullet\bullet\bullet\bullet\bullet\bullet\bullet\bullet\bullet\bullet\bullet\bullet\bullet\bullet\bullet\bullet\bullet\bullet\bullet\bullet\bullet\bullet\bullet\bullet\bullet\bullet\bullet\bullet\bullet\bullet\bullet\bullet\bullet\bullet\bullet\bullet\bullet\bullet\bullet\bullet\bullet\bullet\bullet\bullet\bullet\bullet\bullet\bullet\bullet\bullet\bullet\bullet$

## Technologies for Environmental Access

$\bullet\bullet\bullet\bullet\bullet\bullet\bullet\bullet\bullet\bullet\bullet\bullet\bullet\bullet\bullet\bullet\bullet\bullet\bullet\bullet\bullet\bullet\bullet\bullet\bullet\bullet\bullet\bullet\bullet\bullet\bullet\bullet\bullet\bullet\bullet\bullet\bullet\bullet\bullet\bullet\bullet\bullet\bullet\bullet\bullet\bullet\bullet\bullet\bullet\bullet\bullet\bullet\bullet$

*Michael L. Jones*

People do not live in a vacuum. Much of their daily life involves responding to and interacting with the environment. The meaning of environment in this context includes the multitude of external stimuli, including other people, places, and things, which affect functioning of individuals. The relationship between the environment and users is well established. Most theories of human development, for example, are founded on the belief that progressive development is the result of interactions with the environment and peoples' efforts to accommodate to and control surroundings.

Environments may be facilitating or handicapping to people with respect to functioning. A well-lit room, for example, facilitates activities that involve sight. A dark room handicaps sight. Although humans have a great capacity for adapting to many handicapping features in the environment, most people with disabilities are at a distinct disadvantage in adapting to their environment. By definition, disability refers to limitations in peoples' performance of everyday activities—interactions with the environment—resulting from functional impairments. In current use, the term *handicap* refers to the following[1]:

> ... circumstances that place individuals at a disadvantage relative to their peers when viewed from the norms of society. The classification of handicap deals with the relationship that evolves between society, culture and people who have disabilities.

This distinction between disability and handicap makes clear the role of external, societal factors, including architectural and attitudinal barriers in creating and also eliminating handicaps for people with disabilities. In a truly supportive, accessible environment, disabilities do not have to present handicaps.

This part deals with environmental access—the extent to which an environment can support or impede independent functioning. Environmental access is concerned with the *context* of functioning. Unlike much of rehabilitation and assistive technology, which focuses on returning, supplementing, or replacing lost functioning, efforts of people to promote environmental access involve the design of products and the arrangement of space to accommodate diminished functioning. Rather than fix the person with a disability, the focus of environmental access is fixing the handicaps by removing the barriers that unusable products and environments present.

In fact, the extent to which the environmental context for use of the technology either supports its use or poses significant and persistent handicaps determines the success of many assistive technology interventions. A motorized wheelchair can afford great mobility to the person whose physical impairment prevents walking, but a flight of stairs presents an insurmountable handicap to the person using it. An augmentative communication device may allow a user to simulate speech, but a computer-controlled phone answering system may not accommodate the slower reaction time associated with a person's use of the communication device. Conversely, products and environments designed to accommodate diminished functioning may reduce or altogether eliminate a person's need for assistive technology interventions. For example, most televisions sold in the United States today include the circuitry necessary to display closed captioning. A user may turn captioning on or off through the television's installation menu thus avoiding the need to install a special decoder box.

The chapters in this part provide people practical concepts and technologies for enhancing their environmental access. Drawing from the fields of human-factors engineering, industrial design, architecture, and landscape architecture, the authors explain the way specialists can make the environmental context for disabled peoples' home lives, work, and play more usable. A common theme that emerges from the concepts and examples is the bonus benefits resulting from peoples' improved environmental access. Designs that are well thought out and more usable for people with disabilities are also safer and easier for *all* people to use.

Rehabilitation professionals can readily appreciate the advantages of more *universally* usable products and environments. Most people are sensitized to the barriers that inaccessible environments present and wonder why so much of the built environment is designed and constructed with so little thought of accessibility. Fortunately, several market factors are emerging that are likely to increase future demand for more usable products and environments.[2] First, improvements in medical and rehabilitation practice over the past 20 years have had a pronounced effect on mortality rates among people who experience catastrophic injuries or illnesses resulting in severe disabilities. As a consequence, a growing prevalence of disability in our society exists. Second, demographic trends such as the American population getting older because of the large population of baby boomers reaching late middle age and older and healthier life expectancies among older people suggest that the prevalence of disability (or at least diminished functioning) will continue to grow. And third, federal legislation such as the Americans with Disabilities Act and Fair Housing Amendments Act provide a legal mandate to make environments more accessible and usable by people with disabilities.

As diminished functioning becomes more prevalent in society, the accessibility of everyday products and environments will take on even greater importance. As rehabilitation professionals responsible for mitigating the consequences of diminished functioning, practical knowledge about environmental access is an important part of assistive technology tool kits. With an emphasis on *universal* design, people with disabilities, their children, and their parents and all people who receive greater environmental access can have an easier life.

## References

1. World Health Organization: *World Health Organization international classification of impairments, disabilities, and handicaps: a manual of classification relating to the consequences of disease,* Geneva, Switzerland 1980, World Health Organization.
2. Jones ML, Sanford JA: People with mobility impairments in the United States today and in 2010, *Assistive Technol* 8:43–53, 1996.

# CHAPTER 23

# Environmental Access in the Workplace

*James Mueller*

## Occupation Identity

In work-oriented cultures such as the United States, personal identity depends heavily on occupation. Nearly 2 million American workers every year sustain disabling injuries or illnesses that temporarily affect their ability to work and thus fundamentally change their identities. Hundreds of thousands of them leave the workplace permanently, which is expensive and wasteful. About two thirds of Americans with disabilities are unemployed, placing an enormous burden on them and their families. Concurrently, their former employers have the burden of replacing them and paying disability benefits, and taxpayers must help fund public benefit programs for them such as Social Security Disability Income (SSDI).

For example, repetitive motion injuries account for 52% of occupational illness, 93 million lost workdays annually, and $25 billion in costs. Back injuries affect 2% of the workforce each year and account for 25% of workers compensation costs.

## Disability

The workplace is the site of 1.8 million injuries per year. Each year, 780,000 employees become physically disabled and remain out of work for at least 5 months. Average permanently disabled employees cost their employer $154,400 in benefits, insurance costs, and lost productivity through age 65. However, not all disabilities occur in the workplace:

- Approximately 70% of all people with disabilities are not born with them but develop them during their lives. As more people live longer, the likelihood of experiencing disability during their lifetimes increases.
- More than 3 million Americans each year survive severe auto accidents, sports injuries, strokes, and heart attacks. From 1960 to 1990, the mortality rate from strokes declined by 65% and from heart disease by 47%.
- Medical progress has had a positive and profound effect on treatment of illness and accidents that a short time ago were fatal. Between 1900 and 1980, the survival rate for spinal cord injured individuals improved from 10% to 80%.

## Paying for Disabilities

People in government and business have been much more willing to pay cash benefits than provide assistance to help disabled workers return to productive employment. According to a 1995 study by the U.S. General Accounting Office, for every $100 that they pay in cash benefits to disabled persons, the Social Security Administration spends only a dime for rehabilitation services. Among private businesses, the total of insurance costs, replacement expenses, and workers' compensation and other disability benefit payments resulting from work disability reached $160 billion in 1992. This total is expected to reach

$200 billion per year by the turn of the century. Although the Americans with Disabilities Act and its predecessor, the Rehabilitation Act of 1973, have boosted the employment *rights* of people with disabilities, they have had little effect on the employment *level* among people with disabilities. However, increasingly common occupational injuries such as repetitive stress and back pain and the steadily aging workforce ensure that disability will continue to be a common concern among American workers and their employers.

## Reasonable Accommodation Is a Bargain

Compared with the enormous cost of paying disabled employees not to work, programs making accommodations to bring them back to their jobs is a bargain. According to the Job Accommodation Network, 78% of accommodations cost $500 or less. For every $1 spent on job accommodation, the employer gets back at least $30 in savings. Furthermore, job accommodations usually benefit co-workers without disabilities. On-site job analysis often reveals risks of reinjury to the returning disabled worker that are also hazards to other employees.

Accommodations planned with this in mind bring employers the double benefit of accommodating and preventing disability. For example, one task that workers performed in a metal fabrication shop was to cut a roll of metal tape into 9-inch lengths. They typically did this task by kneeling on the floor, judging the proper tape length by eye, and holding the tape with one hand while cutting it with tin snips in the other hand. To accommodate a disabled worker's functional limitations in doing these tasks, the employer fabricated a king-sized tape dispenser from plywood. This dispenser held the tape roll securely in a position, which allowed the worker to perform the task in a standing position. The metal tape slid under a roller and onto a cutting guide with a stop exactly at 9 inches from a slot for the tin snips. Because the guide stabilized the tape, the worker was able to use both hands if needed to cut accurately and safely. With this modification, the disabled worker was immediately faster, safer, and more accurate in doing this task than previous workers had been. Needless to say, the employer wasted no time in duplicating this design for other employees, saying, "Why didn't we do it this way in the first place?"

Low-cost, common-sense accommodations such as these are the rule rather than the exception. The reason so many workers with disabilities fail to return to work is not known. Approximately 27% of the 8,506 Title I complaints filed with the Equal Employment Opportunity Commission during the first year of the ADA alleged failure to provide reasonable accommodation. One answer lies in the loss of control felt by employee and employer during the course of peoples' disabilities.

## The Medical Approach to Work Disability

With each successive day off of work because of injuries or illnesses, employees with disabilities become less connected to their workplaces, physically and psychologically. Their identities begin to have less to do with their jobs than their medical conditions. Their physicians shape their daily routines now more than their supervisors. Within months, their identities evolve from active employee to employee/patient to patient/employee and, ultimately, to full-time patient. For example, employees out of work for 6 months with a back injury have only a 50% chance of ever returning to work. After 12 months, they only have a 20% chance of ever returning to work and after 24 months, their probability of ever returning to work is about 2%.

When the subject of people returning to work arises, a medical professional, who often knows little more about the patient's job than what that person has volunteered during the initial office visit, becomes responsible for making all judgment. Unless full recovery is anticipated, the physician can only guess the way the employee will manage on the job. If any doubt exists about reinjury, the physician extends time off for the individual.

A physician's goal for medical treatment of a patient is maximum recovery. Usually the employer simply waits until the physician determines that the patient has reached the goal before considering a plan for return to work. This extends the rehabilitation process and may even preclude it if enough time passes in which the employee's skills atrophy or the job changes sufficiently to negate the value of the employee's experience.

## Matching Worker Abilities to Job Requirements

Many employees recovering from disabling injuries or illness can and should return to work during recovery if the medical staff emphasizes what the employee *can* do rather than what the patient *cannot* do. This requires a rehabilitation approach that is functionally based rather than medically based to begin the progression from patient back to employee.

Several models exist for the medical staff identifying when and the way to begin the return-to-work process. One model that J.L. Mueller, Inc. uses involves two nearly identical forms. One form defines the working conditions and functional characteristics of the job, as seen by a variety of individuals. These usually include the immediate supervisor and coworkers and the disabled person. The other form defines the tasks and conditions under which the individual may work safely. The medical professionals involved and the disabled person complete this form. For example, the metal fabrication worker mentioned in the previous example had to perform several tasks in the fabrication of components for window frames. The essential functions of the job involved the tasks, skills, and working conditions indicated on the Employer's Description of Job Requirements (Figure 23-1). The Physician's Statement of Ability to Work describes worker's abilities (Figure 23-2).

By comparing these two completed forms, everyone involved realizes that Toni can obviously meet or exceed the job requirements except in items 1, 3, 6, 34, 35, 48, 49, and 52. These reflect her difficulty in processing information and manipulating and her limitation of balance. These mismatched items also define job requirements in conflict with the abilities of the individual and clearly denote the need for job accommodation. With this information, Toni's supervisor began to assess the way to assess each of these accommodation issues.

Job and worker matching formats such as these are useful in the return-to-work process because they use clinical knowledge of the person's functional capabilities but do not compromise the confidentiality of the doctor/patient relationship. Concurrently, they offer the medical professional a snapshot of the working conditions and requirements of the job from more than just the patient's perspective.

Used together, these forms clearly reveal any need for job accommodations for the employee. The employer is able to accommodate specific conflicts between what the job requires and what duties the employee can safely perform. Using this information, the employer is able to explore more options for temporary or transitional placement, rather than the traditional and often controversial light duty assignments.

## Job Accommodations for Everyone

The most successful job accommodations are those that successfully accommodate the disabled worker and also help to reduce the risk of disability among co-workers. At the minimum, job accommodations for workers with disabilities should be transparent or have no effect at all on co-workers or customers.

Examples of the dual benefits of successful job accommodation are numerous. Employers experiencing these benefits commonly ask, "Why didn't we do this in the first place?" Employers who formerly viewed employees as "different" because of their disabilities suddenly see them as effective templates for improvements in job and workplace design.

The Enabler system was developed to aid designers of products and environments in integrating the needs of elderly and disabled people. This approach emphasizes many

Job title __Fabricator Assistant__     Company __Carter Windows__

The essential functions of this job involve the following tasks, skills, and working conditions:

| Psychologic factors | Continuously | Frequently | Occasionally | Rarely | Never |
|---|---|---|---|---|---|
| 1. Working alone | X | | | | |
| 2. Working with others | | | X | | |
| 3. Following instructions | | X | | | |
| 4. Supervising others | | | | | X |
| 5. Performing repetitive tasks | X | | | | |
| 6. Keeping work pace/deadlines | X | | | | |
| 7. Making decisions | | | | X | |
| 8. | | | | | |

| Environmental factors | Continuously | Frequently | Occasionally | Rarely | Never |
|---|---|---|---|---|---|
| 9. Noise | X | | | | |
| 10. Vibration | | | X | | |
| 11. Abrupt temperature change | | | X | | |
| 12. Heat (up to 80°F) | | X | | | |
| 13. Cold (down to 60°F) | | X | | | |
| 14. Wetness | | | | X | |
| 15. Dampness | | | X | | |
| 16. Dryness | | | X | | |
| 17. Fumes, odors | | | X | | |
| 18. Solvents | | | | X | |
| 19. Acids, bases | | | | | X |
| 20. Oils | | | X | | |
| 21. Toxins | | | | | X |

| Sensory tasks | Continuously | Frequently | Occasionally | Rarely | Never |
|---|---|---|---|---|---|
| 22. Seeing close (inspecting) | | X | | | |
| 23. Seeing far (observing) | | | X | | |
| 24. Seeing to sides | | | X | | |
| 25. Seeing colors | | | X | | |
| 26. Speaking | | | X | | |
| 27. Hearing speech | | | X | | |
| 28. Hearing mechanical sounds | X | | | | |
| 29. Sensing odors | | | X | | |
| 30. Sensing by touch | | X | | | |

| Body Movements | Continuously | Frequently | Occasionally | Rarely | Never |
|---|---|---|---|---|---|
| 31. Sitting | | | | X | |
| 32. Standing | X | | | | |
| 33. Walking | | X | | | |
| 34. Bending/stooping | | X | | | |
| 35. Squatting/kneeling | | X | | | |
| 36. Crouching/crawling | | | | X | |
| 37. Twisting at waist | | | X | | |
| 38. Reaching above shoulders | | | X | | |
| 39. Reaching below knees | | X | | | |
| 40. Lifting/carrying up to 20 lb | | | X | | |
| 41. Pushing/pulling up to 40 lb | | | X | | |
| 42. Climbing ladders | | | | X | |
| 43. Climbing stairs | | | X | | |
| 44. Sweeping/mopping | | | X | | |
| 45. Operating foot controls | | | | | X |

| Manual tasks | Continuously | Frequently | Occasionally | Rarely | Never |
|---|---|---|---|---|---|
| 46. Grasping with one hand | | X | | | |
| 47. Grasping with both hands | | X | | | |
| 48. Manipulating with one hand | | | X | | |
| 49. Manipulating w/both hands | | X | | | |
| 50. Writing | | | | X | |
| 51. Using keyboard | | | | | X |
| 52. Using hand tools | X | | | | |
| 53. Operating power tools | | | | X | |
| 54. Operating shop machinery | | | | | X |
| 55. Twisting/wringing | | | | X | |
| 56. Scrubbing/washing/polishing | | | | X | |
| 57. Scraping | | | X | | |

| Driving | Continuously | Frequently | Occasionally | Rarely | Never |
|---|---|---|---|---|---|
| 58. Driving car | | | | | X |
| 59. Driving truck | | | | | X |
| 60. Driving inplant vehicles | | | | | X |

For further information, contact __Gayle Trevor__ GT

Address _____

Phone __516-555-7897__     Date __11/09__

**Fig. 23-1** Employer's description of job requirements. (Courtesy J.L. Mueller, Inc.)

This patient, _Toni Davila_ may begin work on this date: __11/10__

He/she may perform the tasks and work under the conditions indicated below:

| Psychologic factors | Continuously | Frequently | Occasionally | Rarely | Never |
|---|---|---|---|---|---|
| 1. Working alone | | | | X | |
| 2. Working with others | X | | | | |
| 3. Following instructions | | | X | | |
| 4. Supervising others | | | | X | |
| 5. Performing repetitive tasks | X | | | | |
| 6. Keeping work pace/deadlines | | | X | | |
| 7. Making decisions | | | | X | |
| 8. | | | | | |

| Environmental factors | Continuously | Frequently | Occasionally | Rarely | Never |
|---|---|---|---|---|---|
| 9. Noise | X | | | | |
| 10. Vibration | X | | | | |
| 11. Abrupt temperature change | X | | | | |
| 12. Heat (up to 90°F) | X | | | | |
| 13. Cold (down to 60°F) | X | | | | |
| 14. Wetness | X | | | | |
| 15. Dampness | X | | | | |
| 16. Dryness | X | | | | |
| 17. Fumes, odors | X | | | | |
| 18. Solvents | X | | | | |
| 19. Acids, bases | X | | | | |
| 20. Oils | X | | | | |
| 21. Toxins | X | | | | |

| Sensory tasks | Continuously | Frequently | Occasionally | Rarely | Never |
|---|---|---|---|---|---|
| 22. Seeing close (inspecting) | X | | | | |
| 23. Seeing far (observing) | X | | | | |
| 24. Seeing to sides | X | | | | |
| 25. Seeing colors | X | | | | |
| 26. Speaking | X | | | | |
| 27. Hearing speech | X | | | | |
| 28. Hearing mechanical sounds | X | | | | |
| 29. Sensing odors | X | | | | |
| 30. Sensing by touch | X | | | | |

| Body Movements | Continuously | Frequently | Occasionally | Rarely | Never |
|---|---|---|---|---|---|
| 31. Sitting | X | | | | |
| 32. Standing | X | | | | |
| 33. Walking | X | | | | |
| 34. Bending/stooping | | | | X | |
| 35. Squatting/kneeling | | | | X | |
| 36. Crouching/crawling | X | | | | |
| 37. Twisting at waist | X | | | | |
| 38. Reaching above shoulders | X | | | | |
| 39. Reaching below knees | | | X | | |
| 40. Lifting/carrying up to 40 lb | | X | | | |
| 41. Pushing/pulling up to 40 lb | | X | | | |
| 42. Climbing ladders | | | | X | |
| 43. Climbing stairs | | | X | | |
| 44. Sweeping/mopping | X | | | | |
| 45. Operating foot controls | X | | | | |

| Manual tasks | Continuously | Frequently | Occasionally | Rarely | Never |
|---|---|---|---|---|---|
| 46. Grasping with one hand | | X | | | |
| 47. Grasping with both hands | | X | | | |
| 48. Manipulating with one hand | | | | X | |
| 49. Manipulating w/both hands | | | | X | |
| 50. Writing | | X | | | |
| 51. Using keyboard | | X | | | |
| 52. Using hand tools | | X | | | |
| 53. Operating power tools | | | | X | |
| 54. Operating shop machinery | | | | X | |
| 55. Twisting/wringing | | X | | | |
| 56. Scrubbing/washing/polishing | | X | | | |
| 57. Scraping | | X | | | |

| Driving | Continuously | Frequently | Occasionally | Rarely | Never |
|---|---|---|---|---|---|
| 58. Driving car | | | | | X |
| 59. Driving truck | | | | | X |
| 60. Driving inplant vehicles | | | | | X |

This patient's condition is likely to change ____ Yes _X_ No

Physician ___Dr. E. Luhler___

Address __7609 E Calaloo Blvd.__

Phone __516-555-1224__           Date __11/09__

**Fig. 23-2** Physician's statement of ability to work. (Courtesy J.L. Mueller, Inc.)

human functional characteristics that specialists should consider in designing products and environments for human use. The Enabler offers a way for specialists to deal with the functional effects of disabilities without getting tangled in medical jargon or compromising, confidential medical information.

The demands of the environment determine the effect of each of these functional characteristics as much as a person's level of functional ability. For example, the effect of a limitation of balance is far more significant for a high-rise building construction worker than for a data-entry operator, even though the level of limitation may be similar.

Since its development in the 1970s, many specialists have adapted the Enabler system widely. Mueller[1] adapted this concept for use in the *Workplace Workbook 2.0*, an illustrated

## BOX 23-1

### The Functional Characteristics of Disabilities

*Difficulty in Processing Information:* An impaired ability to receive, interpret, remember, or act on information

*Limitation of Sight:* A difficulty in reading newsprint-size copy with or without corrective lenses and extends to "legal blindness" (but not total blindness)

*Total Blindness:* The complete inability to receive visual signals

*Limitation of Hearing:* A difficulty in understanding normal speech (but not total deafness)

*Total Deafness:* The complete inability to receive auditory signals

*Limitation of Speech:* A capability of only slow or indistinct speech or nonverbal communication

*Susceptibility to Fainting, Dizziness, and Seizures:* May be spontaneous or inducible by environmental factors such as sudden sounds or flashing lights, resulting in loss of consciousness, balance, or voluntary muscle control

*Incoordination:* Limited control in placing or directing extremities, including spasticity

*Limitation of Head Movement:* A difficulty in looking up, down, and/or to the side

*Limitation of Sensation:* An impaired ability to detect heat, pain, and/or pressure

*Limitation of Stamina:* Fatigue, shortness of breath, and/or abnormal elevation of blood pressure resulting from mild exercise or sensitivity to chemicals

*Difficulty Lifting, Reaching, and Carrying:* Impaired mobility, range of motion, and/or strength of upper extremities

*Difficulty in Manipulating:* Impaired hand or finger mobility, range of motion, and/or strength

*Inability to Use Upper Extremities:* Complete paralysis, severe incoordination, or bilateral absence of upper extremities

*Difficulty in Sitting:* Excessive pain, limited strength, range of motion, and/or control in turning, bending, or balance while seated

*Difficulty in Using Lower Extremities:* Slowness of gait and difficulty in kneeling, sitting, rising, standing, walking, and/or climbing stairs or ladders

*Limitation of Balance:* A difficulty in maintaining balance while standing or moving

*Modified from Mueller J: The workplace workbook 2.0, Amherst, MA, 1992, HRD Press.*

## TABLE 23-1

*Functional Disability Characteristics*

| The Enabler | The Workplace Workbook 2.0 |
|---|---|
| Difficulty interpreting information | Difficulty in processing information |
| Severe loss of sight | Limitation of sight |
| Complete loss of sight | Total blindness |
| Severe loss of hearing | Limitation of hearing |
| | Total deafness |
| | Limitation of speech |
| Prevalance of poor balance | Susceptibility to fainting, dizziness, and seizures |
| Incoordination | Incoordination |
| Limitations of stamina | Limitation of head movement |
| Difficulty moving head | Limitation of sensation |
| | Limitation of stamina |
| Difficulty reaching with arms | Difficulty in lifting, reaching, and carrying |
| Difficulty in handling and fingering | Difficulty in manipulating |
| Loss of upper extremity skills | Inability to use upper extremities |
| Difficulty bending and kneeling | Difficulty in sitting |
| Reliance on walking aids | Difficulty in using lower extremities |
| Inability to use lower extremities | Limitation of balance |
| Extremes of size and weight | |

*Modified from Mueller J: The workplace workbook 2.0, Amherst, MA, 1992, HRD Press.*

guide to reasonable accommodation and assistive technology for employers. For this resource, the Enabler's 15 functional characteristics were amended so that employers could use them in making job accommodations for employers with disabilities (Box 23-1 and Table 23-1).

Many job accommodations for disabled workers who are experiencing one or more of these functional characteristics are also useful for co-workers without disabilities. Wherever possible, such as in buildings or modified facilities, builders should integrate these features into the design of the environment. This way, accommodations for employees who develop disabilities later can be minimized.

## *Universal Design Concepts Used in the Workplace[1]*

### Flooring

Selection of flooring materials by employers affects the ability of all workers to navigate the workplace safely and with minimum effort. Color codes in pathways and work areas and contrasts in color and texture can aid blind and visually impaired employees and visitors unfamiliar with the workplace. Conversely, extreme or sudden changes in texture or grain of materials such as from carpeting to glazed tile can cause falls for people with balance limitations or workers carrying packages or simply not paying attention.

Pathway design can also help people with cognitive or mobility limitations and new visitors. Loops that return to a central starting point are preferable to dead-end hallways, which require people retracing unfamiliar routes.

### Storage

Planning for access to stored materials by employers can minimize the risks involved in lifting, carrying, and maneuvering them by the workers. Employers should locate the bulkiest and most-used materials as close as possible to the area in which their employees need them or they should store them in mobile containers, preferably at the height at which employees will use them. By providing transfer surfaces, employees can slide materials rather than lift their full weight.

The design of containers is also important. Size and weight should not restrict the vision or balance of workers. Employers should balance and stabilize loads within the container. Instruction labels on containers help workers plan the way to lift them safely. Workers may have an especially difficult time lifting and carrying heavy objects at one end of a carton. They can suddenly lose their balance when they tilt the contents of a carton.

## Tool Design

Designers can design manual tools and tasks to minimize the risks of repetitive and cumulative trauma. Wherever possible, tools should be configured to allow users to remain in as neutral a position as possible. For example, users should "bend the tool, not the wrist" and avoid reaching while using tools. Tools should be as usable for left-handed workers as for right-handed workers, which also allows them to change hands occasionally.

Tool grip range should be 2 to 4 inches. Activation force should be no greater than 7ft-lb and distributed over the largest possible hand surface. Users should have a few seconds of relaxation for every few minutes of sustained effort, and vibration that they transmit through the grip should be minimized. Tools should be as light as practical, and employers should suspend or counterbalance any tools heavier than 2 lb. Shoulder straps or hand loops can also reduce users' efforts of gripping the tool.

## Characteristics of Effective Job Accommodations

Most job accommodations are simple and involve minimal cost, especially when employers apply principles of universal design to workplace design. However, this does not mean that inexpensive accommodations are reasonable and expensive accommodations are not. The most successful accommodations include the following:

- Effective: The solution enables individuals with disabilities to do their job productively and safely. An effective accommodation does not substitute for individuals but enables them to use their own abilities.
- Transparent: The solution either has no effect on co-workers, customers, and other aspects of the business or has a positive effect in improving productivity and/or safety.
- Timely: Individuals can implement the solution in a reasonable time frame.
- Durable: The solution is useful and flexible enough to remain effective throughout the employees' service. Individuals can readily accomplish maintenance and modifications necessary because of business or technology changes.

Reasonable workplace accommodations are likely to be a compromise among these criteria. For example, a business may spend less money to relocate an employee who uses a wheelchair to a ground-floor office than to invest in an elevator to transport the person to the usual work site. Or, the workplace environment may be less disruptive if the business invests in a document scanner rather than restructuring jobs so that a co-worker can read documents to a blind employee. Each employer must select the best solution from a number of accommodation alternatives.

## Examples of Effective Job Accommodations

Real businesses have applied assistive technology to workplace access and job accommodation. The following examples are organized from the simplest ("no-tech") solutions to the most complex ("hi-tech") applications. Many times, the simplest possible technologies tend to be the most successful accommodations. The simpler the technology, the greater the emphasis on the abilities of the employee. After all, the capabilities of the employee should be the focus of accommodation, not the capabilities of technology. No-tech, low-tech, and high-tech applications each have their appropriate use.

## When No Technology Is the Best Technology

Many employers have successfully accommodated employees with disabilities without the use of any technology. They can use training programs, task restructuring, job sharing, flexible scheduling, and task modification to improve the fit between the job requirements and the worker's abilities.

### Training

A credit card billing center hired an individual through a job placement agency for people with disabilities. This individual had difficulty processing information and therefore needed frequent supervision when learning the new tasks of the job. After analysis of the job duties, the agency received approval from the employer to allow one of the agency's job coaches to work alongside the individual during the probationary period.

At first, the job coach performed most of the work, with the new employee observing. In time, the new employee took over more of the tasks, with the job coach offering guidance when needed. At the end of the probationary period, the employer assessed performance without the job coach present to confirm the new employee's readiness to perform the job unassisted. By this time, the employee, the co-workers, and the supervisor were confident of success.

### Job Sharing

Local businesses successfully contracted a sheltered employment agency, who developed teams of workers with a variety of abilities and limitations, for grounds maintenance. Working independently on location, the workers required reliable supervision, performed manual labor, and operated equipment. These disabled workers shared the cognitive and physical tasks according to their abilities. They were successful as a team, although no single worker was capable of all cognitive and physical tasks.

### Alternative Methods

Because of a back injury, an employee of a small manufacturing facility that fabricated steel doors and frames was restricted from some of the essential duties of the job. His physician had restricted him from lifting greater than 25 lb, but the extrusions he used to make the frames were up to 12 feet long and 70 lb each. This employee, like his co-workers, had become accustomed to lifting and carrying the extrusions to the circular-saw platform, where co-workers measured and cut them to size.

Upon examination of the fabrication procedure, the employer decided that no reason existed for the employer to lift the metal. A co-worker leaned the extrusions against the factory walls and carried one end. This enabled him to drag them along the floor without carrying their full weight. The force needed to move a 12-foot extrusion by a worker dragging it along the floor was less than 25 lb.

Although this dragging was initially considered lazy, supervisors acknowledged that it would be a reasonable accommodation for a worker with lifting restrictions.

## Applying Readily Available, Conventional Technology

### Commercial Products

A chemical plant worker with limitations of stamina resulting from a pulmonary condition was unable to return to his former job. His physician restricted him from walking long distances and performing other strenuous physical tasks. In addition, the worker did not have adequate pulmonary strength to use the conventional respirators that all plant employees in his area needed. One of the plant's subcontractors explored similar jobs. The subcontractor provided pickup trucks for its teams to use in traveling the plant grounds. The plant management persuaded the subcontractor to make the employee a member of one of the teams. The plant's physician also worked with the plant's safety equipment specialist to locate a powered respirator for the employee to use within the limits of his pulmonary capacity.

## Using Commercial Products in a New Way

A cardiologist with a back injury was unable to maintain his practice because of pain from bending over patients while performing 45- to 90-minute angioplasty and arteriogram procedures. The cardiologist, who stood with the positioned patient to accommodate accurate positioning of the diagnostic equipment, usually performed these procedures. Throughout the procedures, the cardiologist wore an 18-lb lead apron to protect himself from radiation that the equipment emitted. Electronic manufacturing technicians who inspect circuits throughout the workday provided a height-adjustable stool with a chest support. Because of this application, it was available in clean-room materials suitable to a surgical environment. This stool offered the cardiologist support for leaning forward, similar to that of a chair turned backward. After experimenting with several different configurations of seat, back, and base designs, the physician then selected one that minimized his pain.

## Modifying Commercial Products

A government employee with quadriplegia resulting from spinal cord injury needed a stable yet easily movable computer keyboard. During the workday, she became fatigued from using the keyboard in only one position. Occasionally, she needed to push it out of the way entirely and use the desk space for working with source documents and input data using voice recognition software. A technician modified a pivoting computer monitor arm by adding a platform to hold the keyboard (Figure 23-3). The technician applied a removable sticky mat to hold it stable. The sturdy construction and secure attachment of the monitor arm to the desk made the basic product an ideal starting point

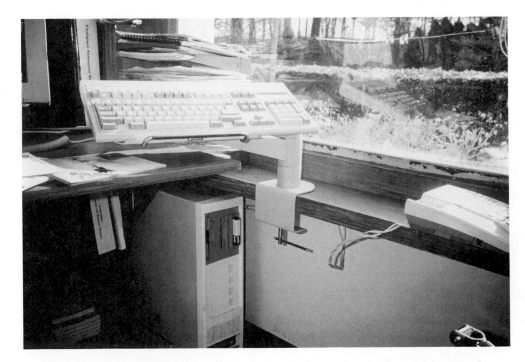

**Fig. 23-3** Swing-away keyboard support fabricated from modified monitor stand.

for developing this accommodation. With the use of this tool, she was able to use her keyboard at her ideal height and angle yet pivot it easily out of the way whenever needed.

A restaurant kitchen worker was having difficulty weighing serving sizes accurately for packaging and cooking later. Because of her height and cognitive and visual limitations, she had difficulty reading the dial scale. The employer placed the scale on a stand fabricated from plastic and added bright tape to the dial to indicate the most common weights that she measured. This modification also was helpful for her co-workers.

## Using Simple Assistive Technology

An office worker with limited coordination had difficulty using the telephone, writing messages, and performing other desktop tasks without either bumping equipment or holding the item stable with one hand. The employer provided a sticky mat material for the desk surface, placing all materials on top. With this removable mat, the worker could take messages on a note pad with one hand because all materials were stable.

## Fabricating Simple Technology

Because of congenital absence of extremities, a computer data entry trainee who used a mouthstick found it impossible to independently perform simultaneous keystrokes such as for "shift," "alt," and "control" functions. At the time, "sticky-key" software was expensive, and locking levers that a technician permanently attached to the keyboard would have slowed other trainees. A technician designed and fabricated temporary levers for the trainee's machine to lock the function keys (Figure 23-4). The technician attached these levers to the machine with Velcro fastening tape so that the other trainees could easily remove and replace them as needed.

An office worker's limited coordination required that he perform all tasks with his right hand. He used an electric wheelchair for mobility. Even with the addition of levers to all doors in his workplace, he had complications opening the latch and pushing the doors open sufficiently to drive his wheelchair through before the hydraulic closers slammed the door on him. A co-worker who found a bicycle handgrip that slid easily over the door levers suggested a simple solution to this problem (Figure 23-5). He added

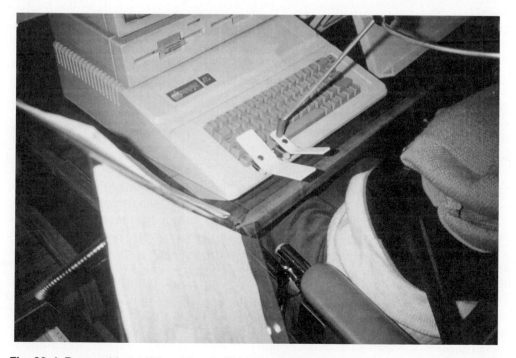

**Fig. 23-4** Removable "shift" and "control" locking levers for keyboard use with head pointer.

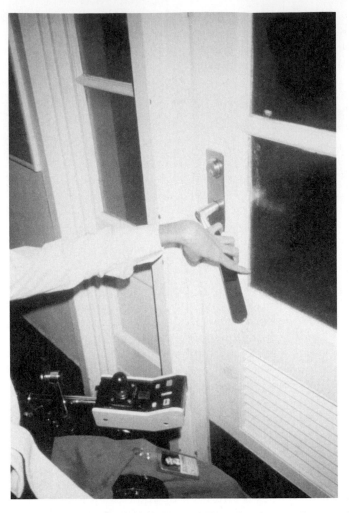

**Fig. 23-5** Bicycle grip with weighted end to hold door level open for one-handed wheelchair user.

lead weight to one end until it was heavy enough to hold the door latch open. Carrying this simple tool with him, he was able to fix the door latch in the open position so that he could simply push the door open with this wheelchair.[2]

## High-Tech Accommodations

### Commercial Products

An executive vice-president of a national consulting firm experienced limited central vision and light adaptation resulting from a degenerative eye condition. Although he required high lighting levels for close work, he resisted installing a number of task lamps. Because his office was regularly the site of high-level meetings and negotiations, he determined that any accommodations should be as unobtrusive as possible. He also expressed concern that high lighting levels would make eye adjustment to lower levels of light difficult when he left his desk. After carefully laying out his office furniture according to his work needs and usable peripheral vision, a technician designed a system of low-voltage, halogen track lights. These lamps are extremely small and unobtrusive, and a designer added baffles to prevent glare from the high-intensity light. The system included dimmers, which gave him flexibility in locating the ceiling fixtures along the tracks and aiming them wherever needed. The result was a professional atmosphere and fully adjustable lighting to accommodate his changing visual needs.

A physician restricted the full-time work of a dental hygienist, who experienced cumulative trauma. The hand motions required for dental cleaning were strenuous and repetitive and the small grip size of dental tools required tight grasping. At the request of her disability insurer, the employer explored job accommodations. The employer determined that a powered scaler could minimize the strenuous and repetitive tasks of dental cleaning. This handheld tool uses ultrasound (high-frequency sound waves) to remove most of the deposits from the teeth, leaving little manual work for the hygienist. The handpiece also has a larger grip size than conventional steel instruments. Although investment in this equipment was high, the insurer and the dental office recognized the benefits.

## High-Tech Assistive Technology

The hospital where a nurse worked as a quality assurance specialist required that she visit all patient floors each day to monitor treatment. These specialists usually made written notes on preprinted forms that they delivered to the data-processing department for input into the hospital's central data system. Her physician restricted her from writing or typing more than 1 hour per day, which made performance of her essential and usual duties impossible. The hospital explored and rejected several simpler accommodation approaches before evaluating the voice-recognition technology for hands-free data input. At the time, many fixed workplaces had used available voice-recognition software but not in a mobile application. The staff located and tested a notebook computer compatible with the software requirements on a variety of patient floors, with widely varying ambient noise levels. After they solved a series of hardware and software problems, the mobile system enabled the nurse to return to her job. She began on a limited schedule and increased it to full time, as she, her co-workers, and her patients became comfortable with the technology.[3]

## High-Tech Fabrication

In a contact lens manufacturing plant, workers handled lenses for the many required inspections, which meant thousands of manual repetitions per workday. As a result, workers were beginning to experience cumulative and repetitive trauma injuries preventing them from continuing to perform these jobs. To minimize manipulation, they used vacuum tools in place of tweezers. The employer provided a low-power, laboratory vacuum pump at each station. With these vacuum tools, however, workers sealed and released the vacuum with the index finger. Consequently, thousands of index finger movements simply replaced thousands of other manual operations, and the injuries continued. The employer took molds of many hands and fingers. From these measurements, designers fabricated finger-ring tools of surgical silicone, with stainless steel vacuum tubes and a choice of silicone suction tips (Figure 23-6). This design allowed workers to slide the tool over the index finger, eliminating all gripping. With the use of this tool, they simply pointed to the lenses and the tool did the rest. They controlled the vacuum with a knee or foot switch so that they could also eliminate this finger movement. After a series of trials and redesigns, the employer made this vacuum tool available to workers to minimize the effects of repetitive motion on the job.

## Future Tech

Because of the ever-increasing rate of technological advances, many things are becoming technologically possible. Major manufacturers of hardware and developers of software are aware that people with disabilities are a major portion of the workforce and are likely to remain so. Society must constantly reinforce and expand this awareness to other fields of workplace access and technology, including landscape and building architects, facility

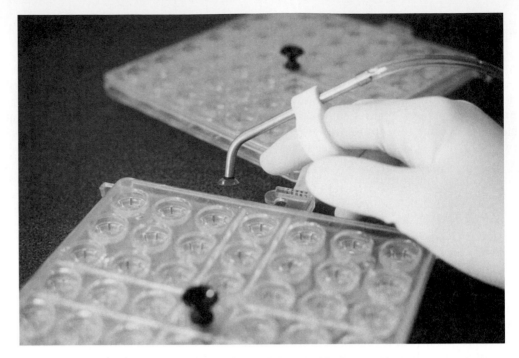

**Fig. 23-6** Finger-ring vacuum pickup tool for contact lenses.

managers, interior designers, product designers, and graphic designers. By instilling a universal design approach among those responsible for the development of work environments and products, employers will have less of a need for accommodating workers with disabilities later. In addition, those accommodations that employers are required to implement will be much more likely to be "reasonable accommodations."

## Successful Workplace Access

In each of the job accommodation examples, the solution that the employer implemented was only one of the possible alternatives. In most of these cases, the accommodation made the workplace safer or more productive for co-workers and prompted managers to ask, "Why didn't we do this a long time ago?" That question is logical because all employees usually face the difficulties that disabled employees face to some degree.

In each case, the employer and the employee with the disability had to weigh the effectiveness of the accommodation, its cost, its effect on co-workers and other aspects of the business, the timeliness of putting it in place, and the likelihood that it would be a long-term solution. This cooperation between employer and employee is even more important to success than the impressive capabilities of modern technology or the cleverness of the technologist.

## References

1. Mueller J: *The workplace workbook 2.0,* 1992, Washington, DC, HRD Press.
2. Enders A, Hall M: *Assistive technology sourcebook,* Washington, DC, 1990, RESNA Press.
3. Miller H: *Designing for accessibility: beyond the ADA,* video and applications guide, Zeeland, MI, 1995, Herman Miller.

# CHAPTER 24

# Home Environments, Automation, and Environmental Control

*Michael L. Jones*
*Jon Sanford*

Home is more than just a place to live. It is a place where people spend most of their days, where they grow up, and where they grow old. Many people take for granted the simple, everyday activities that they do at home such as turning on a light, walking down the stairs, or taking a bath. For people with disabilities, such routine household activities that structure daily life can be far from routine. If people have limitations in physical or sensory functioning, the home and many of its features can pose serious barriers in daily life.[1-2] The same, simple tasks that young, healthy adults expect to perform can often cause physical and emotional pain and discomfort, require extraordinary amounts of time to complete, and pose real hazards for many older or disabled people. Individuals are frequently forced to abandon activities unnecessarily or perform them in a dangerous manner.

Lawton's environmental press model[3] offers an important perspective to specialists for conceptualizing the problems that many disabled people experience with routine household activities. In the model, Lawton[3] describes these problems as the result of the interaction between an individual's functional capabilities (competence) and the demands that the environment (environmental press) places on the individual. When functional capabilities and environmental demands do not match, such as when an individual's level of functioning declines but the home environment does not change, the model predicts negative effects. The greater the severity of functional loss, the greater the effect of the environment on an individual's behavior. Thus when environmental demand exceeds a person's competency to attempt a task, the individual is not able to complete the task, no matter how routine.

Home modifications can reduce environmental demands in several ways. Modifications can reduce a person's amount of assistance to perform routine household activities. For example, a modified bathroom with a roll-in or "wet area" shower can allow a wheelchair user to shower without the need for assistance in transferring in and out of the tub. Modifications also can often reduce a person's need for or enhance the use of assistive technology. For example, a person using a walker needs ample floor space for maneuvering. However, handrails in key locations may completely eliminate the person's need for a walker. Lastly, modifications can enhance a person's safety (e.g., handrails to reduce the risk of falls), fire safety (e.g., visual and audible smoke alarms), and security (e.g., a voice-activated phone system and motion sensor-activated flood lights).

## Application and Goals

Home modifications for people with disabilities are adaptations to the living environment intended to enhance the quality of life by minimizing physical and emotional stress, enhancing autonomy and control, reducing home-care needs and costs, and increasing safety in completing activities of daily living (ADL). People can make the following modifications:

1. Replacing or adding fixtures, appliances, or features in the home such as installing a track lift system or raised toilet seat or replacing doorknobs with lever handles
2. Changing or adding to the structure such as widening doorways or adding a ramp
3. Automating environmental controls such as adding a movement sensor-activated light that operates automatically when someone enters the room.

For people with disabilities, modifying their homes to make them livable is an attractive goal for several reasons. Unlike strategies that target individuals and attempt to directly or indirectly modify their abilities (e.g., restorative therapy), home modifications are intended to reduce environmental demands and thus enable people with disabilities to function more effectively. The principles of people achieving livability also are applicable to all types of housing, including apartments and single-family residences and manufactured or site-built dwellings. Lastly, adapting living environments is a routine part of peoples' lives, whether they add a bathroom to accommodate the needs of growing children or aging parents. Finally, people can modify their homes in most cases without specialized equipment or unique designs. Most modifications to improve individuals' functioning enhance the convenience and safety of the home for other household members as well as guests.

## Function and Ability

People with disabilities are not a homogeneous group nor are their living environments. People differ in the nature and extent of their limitations, in the number and types of activities that are problematic, and in the types and severity of difficulties they experience with a given activity. For example, ambulatory individuals with lower body limitations and those with upper body impairments often experience difficulty bathing. People with lower body limitations may have difficulty getting in and out of the tub because of problems lifting their legs over the side of the tub, whereas people with upper body impairments may have difficulty reaching the controls to turn the water on or adjusting the flow and temperature of the bath water.

Specialists should not expect that all people with disabilities need generic design solutions such as a 5-foot turning radius and 32-inch wide doorways, which people need for wheelchair access to the bathroom. Most of these generic accessibility solutions derive from building codes and are intended to provide as many people as possible with basic accessibility to public buildings. As a result, generic accessibility solutions only usually meet some needs of some people at home. A preferred alternative to generic solutions is for people to customize their home environment to address their specific abilities and difficulties.

A number of reasons exist for the importance of individualized modifications. The environmental press model suggests that individuals achieve optimum outcomes when the environment presents them with manageable demands. Modifications that do not match the needs of individuals may result in the following two undesirable consequences:

1. They may fail to eliminate unmanageable demands, resulting in the need for assistance to complete these activities.
2. They may eliminate manageable demands, resulting in a reduced sense of personal competency.

Furthermore, home modifications require a financial investment. Few assistance or reimbursement programs cover the total cost of home modifications therefore people who need modifications must pay for at least some portion of the cost. Generally, the cost-effectiveness of home modifications is greater when people identify modifications on the basis of need.

Relating functional difficulties with household activities to specific features of housing design can be a formidable task for specialists. However, when they break the activities into task components, they can more readily understand them. Task performance spans individuals' abilities to access and use particular rooms, appliances, or fixtures that they need to complete activities.[4] For example, bathing involves a person approaching the tub, turning on the water, adjusting the temperature, getting into the tub, and reaching for the soap. An ambulatory person who experiences difficulty with bathing may only have problems with the task of getting in and out of the tub. This person may not have any problems with other bathing tasks such as turning the water on and off.

## Considerations and Options

One difficulty in specialists identifying appropriate home modifications that correspond to different functional limitations is the lack of a framework that provides practical, detailed links between problems with the performance of routine activities to specific aspects of housing design. In assistive technology, specialists have developed a conceptual framework that connects routine tasks with specific home modifications to individualize home modification efforts.[2]

The conceptual framework links peoples' activity performance to housing design features and permits specialists to assess routine household activities and evaluate the environmental features people use in each activity (Table 24-1). The framework distinguishes specific activities (e.g., bathe, shower) in 13 activity domains (e.g., personal hygiene). Each activity is subdivided into its component and requisite tasks (e.g., turning on the water, regulating water temperature, getting in the tub, grabbing the soap, etc.). These tasks are linked to particular design features. A number of different design features are related to the performance of any given activity. For example, whether people can independently bathe depends on such task-related design features as the location of the tub relative to other fixtures in the bathroom (space design) and the type and location of faucet handles (product design).

### Domains and Activities

The activity domains include not only "basic" and "instrumental" ADL that rehabilitation professionals typically assess but also the routine activities that are necessary for people to function in and maintain their homes (see Table 24-1). Activities are constituted by tasks that specialists readily understand in terms of the functional capabilities they require and related design features in the home. They use a task analysis to identify a design-relevant task sequence for each activity. The tasks capture required functional capabilities such as body movements, position changes, and sensory responses inherent in task performance. Focusing on tasks permits specialists to identify precise functional problems that individuals encounter in performing routine activities.

### Performance Features and Required Dimensions

Most often, task-related problems are the result of demands that several different characteristics of the environment create. Characteristics of spaces, products, and controls (e.g., size, shape, color, weight, etc.) create functional demands. For example, the floor space available in front of a tub, called the *area of approach,* determines how accessible the tub is to a wheelchair user. The height of a tub determines how high an ambulatory person must lift the feet to get into the tub. The type, location, and complexity of the water controls determine how usable the controls are to a person with limitations in reach, grasp, or cognition.

Fortunately, accessible products and environments share many common characteristics. For example, usable products tend to be those that require little precise hand movements to operate. An able-bodied person can easily use a lavatory faucet that a young child or an older person with arthritis can easily use. These accessible characteristics can be described as *performance features* and *required dimensions.*

TABLE 24-1
*Conceptual Framework: Examples of Task-Design Relationships*

| Design-Relevant Tasks | | | Task-Relevant Design Features | | |
|---|---|---|---|---|---|
| Activity Domain | Activity | Tasks | Space | Product | Controls/Hardware |
| *Personal Care* | | | | | |
| Hygiene | Bathe/shower | Dress/undress | Bathroom | Tub/shower | Seat, drain, faucet, shower head, soap dish, shelves |
| | | Turn water on/off | | | |
| | | Regulate water temperature | | | |
| | | Transfer | | | |
| | | Reach/grab soap, shampoo, etc. | | Grab bars | |
| | | Wash self | | | |
| | | Reach/grab towel | | Towel rack | |
| | | Transfer | | | |
| | Use toilet | Transfer | | Toilet | Seat, handle |
| | | Dress/undress | | Grab bars | |
| | | Reach toilet paper | | Toilet paper holder | Toilet paper roller |
| | | Wipe self | | | |
| | | Flush | | Storage cab or drawer | Handle, door/drawer pulls |
| | | Use personal hygiene products | | | |
| | | Transfer | | | |
| *Motor Activities* | | | | | |
| Ambulation | Get in/out of home | Place key in lock | Exterior | Driveway | |
| | | Grasp/turn key or latch | | Path | |
| | | Grasp handle | | Stairs/ramp | Handrails |
| | | Turn handle or depress latch | Entry | Door | Handle, locks |
| | | Push/pull door open | | Threshold | |
| | | Enter/exit home | | | |

*Control of Ambient Conditions*

| Thermal comfort | | | | | |
|---|---|---|---|---|---|
| Regulate temperature | Central system | Read temperature | All | Thermostat | Display controls (buttons, slide, dial, etc.) |
| | | Reach thermostat | | | |
| | | Program or set thermostat | | | |
| | Room unit | Adjust dampers, diffusers | Floor or wall registers | | Lever controls |
| | | Turn equipment on/off | Radiator, A/C unit, ceiling/attic/room fan | | Button, switch, knob, etc. |
| | | Adjust temp/fan settings | | | |
| Maintenance | Change filter | Open filter housing | Furnace | | Filter housing |
| | | Remove old filter | | | |
| | | Place new filter in housing | | | |
| | | Replace housing | | | |
| | Relight pilot | Open/remove furnace cover | | | Furnace cover |
| | | Turn furnace off | | | Furnace/pilot control |
| | | Turn to pilot | | | |
| | | Depress button and hold down | | | |
| | | Light match/lighter | | | |
| | | Light pilot | | | |
| | | Release button | | | |
| | | Turn knob to on position | | | |

A performance feature specifies how a product should operate. A common performance feature associated with environmental access is closed-fist operation. Closed-fist operation means that a person with a closed fist, using no grip and applying no more than 5 lb of force, can operate the product or feature. For example, a person can easily operate a lever door handle or a lever faucet using a closed fist, whereas another person cannot easily operate a doorknob and a round faucet control.

A required dimension specifies minimum or maximum dimensions of a product or space (e.g., the 5-foot diameter minimum turning area for wheelchairs or the 48-inch maximum height for light switches). Most required dimensions are based on accessibility for wheelchair users, because most critical accessible dimensions for wheelchairs also accommodate the needs of persons with other disabilities and those who are not disabled. Specialists should think of space in three dimensions when considering the required dimensions for access. The height of light switches and other controls (and therefore the required reach from people in a seated position) and the height of changes in level of floor surfaces (e.g., the "curb" that the threshold of a doorway creates) are just as important as the availability of sufficient floor space for approach and use.

Rehabilitation professionals should consider performance features and required dimensions when assessing the functional limitations of a particular user. They should understand limitations in manual dexterity, reach, and mobility to help them determine the importance of performance features and required dimensions associated with particular activities in the home.

## Technology

People engage in three basic tasks when modifying the home: (1) replacing or adding fixtures, appliances, or features in the home, (2) restructuring or adding space, and (3) automating environmental controls. To accommodate particular users, they may need any or all of these approaches. The first approach might include individuals replacing door hardware or faucets, adding grab bars or tub seats, or purchasing new telephones with volume control. Individuals restructuring space can be the most and the least expensive approach. They can build additions or move walls to reconfigure interior space, which can be expensive but necessary in some instances. Conversely, they can rearrange furniture in rooms or convert a downstairs study into a bedroom at little or no cost.

Home automation, electronic controls to automate many household functions, has great potential for making homes more usable. People can use timers, photocells, or motion sensors to activate lights or appliances automatically, rather than having to manually operate controls. They can use power line carrier (PLC) electronic control systems, which consist of inexpensive wireless remote controls and plug-in modules, to control lamps and switches anywhere in the house from single or multiple locations.

People have a much easier time manipulating programmable thermostats, another simple technology modification, than its manually operated predecessor. Not only does it reduce the need to adjust the temperature in the home as frequently but also the buttons that people use to change the temperature on these thermostats are more user-friendly and require much less fine motor coordination than the slide controls on manual thermostats. Finally, electronic keys, remote controls, and keypads offer alternatives to traditional lock and key mechanisms, which require a great deal of precision and fine motor control to operate.

Specialists recommend accessibility features in housing, based on knowledge of what makes products and environments more usable and more appealing to all users (Table 24-2). Although every person's needs and preferences are different, this list offers an important starting point and typifies universal design in the home environment. The listed features are biased toward individuals with mobility impairments because the required dimensions that work for them also typically work for other users. The features are designated as "structural" or "nonstructural" to indicate when peoples' addition of features to an existing home requires significant structural modifications such as tearing down walls.

## TABLE 24-2

### *Universal Design Features in Home Modifications*

|  | Structural | Nonstructural |
|---|:---:|:---:|
| **Entrances** | | |
| • Accessible route from vehicle drop off or parking | x | |
| • Maximum slope of 1:20 to entry door | x | |
| • Covered entryway | x | |
| • 5-×5-foot minimum maneuvering space | x | |
| • Package shelf or bench to hold parcels, groceries, etc. | | x |
| • Full-length sidelight at entry door | x | |
| • Movement sensor light controls | | x |
| • 5 lb maximum force to open doors | | x |
| • Ambient and focused lighting (at keyhole) | | x |
| • High visibility address numbers | | x |
| **General Interior Features** | | |
| • 32-inch minimum clear door opening width | x | |
| • 18-inch minimum space at latchside of door | x | |
| • Flush threshold (maximum of ½-inch rise) | x | |
| • Lever door handles | | x |
| • Adjustable height closet rods and shelves | | x |
| • Accessible route (42-inch minimum) throughout | x | |
| • 5-×5-foot maneuvering space in all rooms | x | |
| • Light switches at 44/48-inch maximum height | x | |
| • Electric receptacles at 18-inch maximum height | x | |
| • View windows at 36-inch maximum sill height | x | |
| • Crank operated (casement) windows | x | |
| • Loop handle pulls on drawers and cabinets | | x |
| • High contrast, glare-free floor surfaces and trim | | x |
| **Bathroom** | | |
| • 30-×48-inch area of approach in front of all fixtures | x | |
| • 18-inch maneuvering space at both ends of tub or shower | x | |
| • Integral transfer seat in tub or shower | x | |
| • Grab bars in tub/shower and around toilet | | x |
| • Offset controls in tub or shower | x | |
| • Adjustable height shower head | | x |
| • Lever-type faucets | | x |
| • Mixer valve with pressure balancing and hot water limiter | | x |
| • Toilet centered 18 inches from sidewall | x | |
| • 33-inch lavatory counter height | x | |
| • Knee space under lavatory | x | |
| • Mirror to backsplash at lavatory | | x |
| **Kitchen** | | |
| • 30-×48-inch area of approach in front of all appliances | x | |
| • Knee space under sink and near cooktop | x | |
| • Variable height work surfaces | x | |
| • Stretches of continuous counter for sliding heavy objects | x | |
| • Contrasting border treatment on countertops | | x |
| • Full-extension, pull-out drawers | | x |
| • Pull-out shelves in base cabinets | | x |
| • Adjustable height shelves in wall cabinets | | x |
| • Full-height pantry cabinets for up and down storage | x | |
| • Front-mounted controls on appliances | | x |
| • Cooktops with staggered burners | | x |
| • Lever-type faucets | | x |
| • Glare-free task lighting | | x |

## Entrances

A person should have accessible parking available on a handy route from parking to the entrance. The parking space should be at least 10 feet wide to permit a person to transfer to and from a wheelchair. The accessible route should be level (no more than 1:20 grade) and have a smooth, hard (preferably paved) surface.

If steps or other impediments exist making reaching the front door difficult to the person, specialists should know the amount of rise from parking or grade to the entry door. If the rise is not too great, a builder can add a gently sloping (1:20 grade) walk by berming up to the front door. A slope steeper than 1:20 can be dangerous for a person who has gait problems or who uses mobility aids such as a walker. Therefore the owner could consider a ramp if the rise requires greater than a 1:20 slope. At a minimum, 1 foot of ramp is required for every 1 inch of rise (a 1:12 grade). A level area (ideally 5 × 5 feet) should exist at each end of the ramp and at 30-foot intervals along the course of the ramp to provide safe "rest areas" for a person with limited stamina. Based on these requirements, room should exist on the property for a person to ramp up to the entrance door if needed. Even when a ramp is a practical solution, it is not aesthetically pleasing and often becomes the most predominant feature in the front yard. Instead of a ramp, a person could have electrically powered mechanical lifts installed.

At each entry, a covered, level landing with minimum dimensions of 5 × 5 feet provides a person protection from the weather and sufficient space for maneuvering. The builder should place railings, curbs, planters, or benches at all drop offs. A package shelf is also a good addition for a person to place items while opening the door. The entry doorway should be at least 36 inches wide with a low (maximum of ¼-inch) or flush threshold. Any vertical edge (anything greater than 45 degrees) of the threshold cannot exceed ¼ inch, and a sloped edge cannot exceed ½ inch. The door should require no more than 5 lb-force to open and a lever-type handleset is preferred. Alternatively, a power-door operator that the person can activate by a switch, keypad, or motion detectors facilitates opening the door. Regular height and low peepholes improve security. A more attractive alternative is to install full-length fixed windows on one or both sides of the front door. Lighting should appear at the entry and along the path to the entry along with a lighted doorbell and sufficient illumination on the lockset. The person should consider installing a motion sensor to activate lights at the entry when someone approaches.

## General Interior Features

Doorways should be wide enough for a person to pass through, should provide adequate floor space to open the door, and should have easy-to-use handles and flush thresholds for ease in passing through. Typically, doors should have a minimum of 32-inch clear distance between stop molding for hands and elbows of a person who uses a wheelchair to pass through (all doors should be 36 inches wide when possible). Pocket doors, swing-away hinges, or removable doors provide 32-inch clear openings on doors that are 32 inches wide. At least 18 inches of clearance on the latch side of the door is needed to permit a person to open the door from a wheelchair or while using a walker. If insufficient space is available on the latch side such as is typical in a bathroom the person should consider a reversing door swing when sufficient space exists on the opposite side of the door. Doors that require latches should have lever handles.

Sufficient turning space in circulation areas is critical for a person to move around the home. Ideally, a person should have a 5 × 5-foot turning area in each room. In addition to having a circular clear space a person can accomplish this in several ways. Two overlapping 3- × 5-foot areas form a T-shape, which provide enough space for a person to make a full 180-degree turn in a wheelchair (Figure 24-1). A 5- × 5-foot space only exists for the "footprint" of a wheelchair. People need less space once they clear the footrests and require even less space once they clear the armrests (Figure 24-2). Thus cabinets, shelves, and wall-hanging fixtures such as a sink can protrude over the 5- × 5-foot space if the builder provides adequate clearance for the foot rests.

Hallways that are at least 42 inches wide enable a person in a wheelchair to easily make a 90-degree turn into or out of a 32-inch door opening. Hallways that are 48 inches

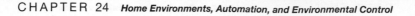

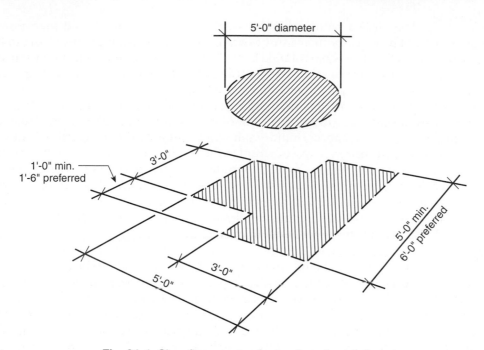

**Fig. 24-1** Clear floor spaces for turning wheelchairs.

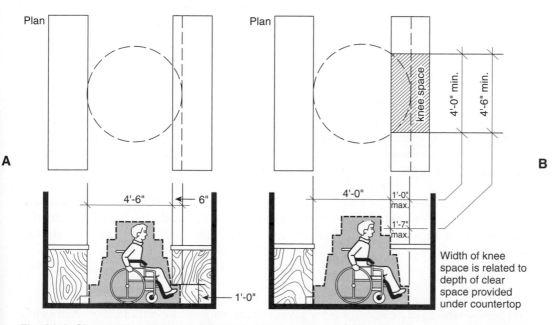

**Fig. 24-2** Clear turning space at different heights. **A,** Clear turning space between cabinets with enlarged toe space. **B,** Clear turning space between cabinets with wider-than-minimum knee space.

wide permit a wheelchair user and someone walking to easily pass each other. A person also is less likely to bang and gouge the walls with the wheelchair. Rub rails and a 12-inch high baseboard of carpet or cork also prevent gouging. Handrails along the walls help to provide assistance for an ambulatory individual with mobility or visual difficulties. Stairs should have handrails on both sides for a person's support and should be well lit to minimize the potential for falls.

In closets, the person should consider using adjustable-height closet rods and shelves. These are not only more practical for a wheelchair user and a young child but also increase storage space. A variety of closet storage systems are available at most home-improvement centers. A builder should mount all light switches, electrical outlets, and thermostats should be between 18 inches and 48 inches on the wall (44 inches if the user must reach across a counter top). The person should consider installing motion-sensor controls for switches that are difficult to reach. These controls fit into the same receptacle as a standard switch. They activate the lights when someone enters the room and are especially convenient in kitchens, bathrooms, hallways, and stairways to light the way at night.

Similar to wall-mounted controls, a person's ability to operate a window depends on sufficient clear floor space for approach and usable hardware located within reach. A 2-foot, 6-inch deep × 5-foot, 0-inch wide space in front of the window permits either a person's side or parallel approach. The person should also contemplate window height. A sill no higher than 36 inches permits a wheelchair user to easily see out the window. Hardware should not be located higher than 48 inches and the person should carefully select it to match the user's ability. Casement windows with crank handles are easier to operate than double-hung windows. Locks that protrude are easier to operate than locks that are small or recessed into the frame. Similar to doors, a person can adapt windows with power operators.

To facilitate opening drawers or cabinet doors, persons should use loop handles that do not require gripping, which they can operate with one or several fingers. For people with partial loss of vision, they way they see contrast between objects and backgrounds is also important in selecting colors for countertops, appliances, and floors. When visual contrast is low such as a white plate on a white counter, individuals who are partially sighted can have difficulty locating objects on counters, appliances, or floors. This can result in persons spilling food, breaking dishes, or knocking things onto floors. They should therefore choose kitchen colors to provide sharp, visual contrast from dishes, pots, and other utensils that they use to prepare or serve food.

Floor surfaces should be glare free and provide reasonable contrast with adjacent trim finishes. People with low vision and older people will be able to detect surfaces more easily. If used, carpet should provide a firm, not spongy, floor surface. This is accomplished using low-pile carpet and commercial padding.

In-home communications are often a problem for people with sensory and mobility problems. In most cases, PLC modules provide people with the simplest and most effective solution. For people with hearing impairments, they can configure systems so that lights flash or loud beepers sound when the doorbell rings. For people with mobility impairments, builders can install wireless call buttons, which can activate chime modules, anywhere in the home. When the modules detect the signal, chimes sound to indicate that an individual may need assistance. A more sophisticated solution to in-home communications is the telephone Key System Unit (KSU), which can add intercom capability to a home phone system. As a result, people can use phones as whole-house paging systems, room-to-room intercom systems, door intercoms, and doorphones. With this latter device, when people activate the doorbell, the phones ring.

## Bathroom

For people who have problems ambulating, transferring in and out of wheelchairs or to and from toilets or tubs are often the most difficult tasks that they must perform. However, when they must complete these tasks in bathrooms with insufficient space, they can become so time consuming and difficult that independent use of bathrooms is impractical, if not impossible. Although space is an important issue, people can use bathrooms more efficiently if fixtures are in appropriate places (even in small areas). Ideally, builders should provide a 30-inch × 48-inch area of approach in front of all bathroom fixtures, and these spaces may overlap. Also, people need 18 inches of maneuvering space at both ends of tubs or showers to provide easy access to the water controls and to transfer seats at the rear of tubs or showers.

A variety of specialty tubs and showers are available. However, people with ambulatory impairments most commonly use the following three types of bathing fixtures:

1. Standard bathtubs with built-in or removable transfer seats
2. Shower stalls with transfer seats

3.  Roll-in showers, also referred to as *wet areas*, that are large enough to accommodate wheelchairs

A builder can provide a 15-inch deep transfer surface at the rear of the tub, which makes a person's transition to or from the tub easier. The surface enables an individual to sit, rest, and assume a more comfortable and advantageous position for lowering into or rising out of the tub. When independent transfer is not possible, a person frequently uses a number of assistive devices such as a hydraulic seat powered by water pressure, a portable boom lift, or an overhead track lift. These devices are designed to lower the individual into the tub, to remain in the tub while the individual is bathing, and to raise the person out of the tub afterward.

For individuals who do not want or cannot lower themselves into the tub, they often use removable tub seats. Users can attach these seats with suction cups or clamp them to the side of the tub and they can easily remove them to enable other household members to use the bathtub. Depending on the needs of an individual user, some seats are available that extend out over the side of the tub and provide a transfer surface, whereas others merely provide a seat in the tub itself.

Although originally designed for people who use wheelchairs, transfer showers provide greater safety for many individuals who cannot or do not want to stand for the entire time that they are showering. A typical transfer shower is 3 feet × 3 feet and includes an L-shaped folding seat at the same height as the wheelchair seat on the wall opposing the controls. Ideally, these showers have no curbs and include an L-shaped grab bar on the wet wall (wall with controls). The omission of the curb enables the user to angle the wheelchairs into the shower close to the seat and also prevents a step over for a person who may be ambulatory but unsteady. The grab bar is positioned to provide support as the user transfers out of the wheelchair and slides across the seat to the corner where the walls provide lateral support. The grab bar also provides a place for individuals with poor motor control to support the arms while operating the controls located just above the bar.

A self-contained 5-feet × 5-feet wet area shower provides sufficient space for people in wheelchairs to maneuver and enough space for personal assistance, if necessary. Where space is limited, designers can make wet area showers to permit people to perform several functions in the same space. For example, the wet area can contain a tub or toilet, or when circumstances dictate, the entire bathroom can serve as the wet area shower. In such cases, the builder should waterproof the entire floor area, which should slope gently to a drain. As is the case with bathtubs, the designer's positioning of grab bars depends on the abilities and preferences of the user and the layout of the wet area (e.g., the inclusion of other fixtures that require grab bars in the wet area). Controls should be conveniently located for the user, and hand-held showers should be adjustable with a hose that is long enough to reach all areas in the shower.

Regardless of users' ability, taking a bath or shower is much safer when grab bars are available. The location of the grab bars should vary according to functional need and individual preference. For example, individuals who are ambulatory or semiambulatory and can stand to get in and out of tubs may need vertical grab bars to lower themselves into tubs or to pull themselves up to standing positions to get out. In contrast, individuals who need to transfer from wheelchairs may use horizontal grab bars for support while sliding out of the chair and to the tub. The locations of horizontal bars depend on where individuals position the wheelchairs relative to the tub, which in turn depends on available space and user preference.

Builders should fit tubs or showers with "off-set" water controls, located nearer the outside edge so that people can operate them while they are seated in wheelchairs outside of the fixture. A young child or older adult who can turn on and adjust the water before getting into the tub can more easily reach the controls. Builders can mount a hand-held showerhead, in which the user can adjust the height of the head, on a slide bar. Lever handles typically work best because they do not require fine motor control, and an individual can operate them with a closed fist. As an added safety feature, the person should consider having the builder install a mixer valve for the tub and shower that has a hot-water limiter (a device that mechanically or electronically limits the water temperature) and a pressure balancer (controls for hot or cold water surges when someone flushes the toilet).

The most critical issues when a person uses the bathroom are the location of the toilet relative to the type of transfer an individual prefers, the positioning of grab bars, and the provision of sufficient clear floor space to enable the preferred transfer. For example, a person who is semiambulatory or has some lower-body functioning often performs a front transfer that requires pulling up to a standing position, pivoting, and lowering to a seated position. To facilitate this type of transfer, builders should place the toilet where grab bars are available on both sides (e.g., side-mounted bars on walls on both sides of the toilet, rear-mounted bars that flank the toilet, or seat-mounted grab bars). Sufficient clear floor space also must be available in front of the toilet. In contrast, an individual who is nonambulatory typically prefers a side approach and transfer; therefore the toilet should sit where a grab bar can appear opposite the approach side so that an individual can grasp the bar with the preferred hand and pull across the toilet. Regardless of the type of transfer technique the individual uses, the toilet should appear 8 inches from one or both side walls to permit adequate room for the installation of grab bars. The toilet typically appears 15 inches from the side wall, which makes the space between the toilet and grab bar cramped.

In addition to maneuvering space and grab bars, seat height can also affect a person's toilet use. Seats that are too low are difficult not only for an ambulatory individual to raise or lower the body but also for a wheelchair user who may be able to lower the body onto the toilet but cannot raise back up to the height of the wheelchair seat. In contrast, seats that are so high and prevent the feet from touching the floor can be uncomfortable or create safety risk for a person with balance disorders. Therefore for an ambulatory and semiambulatory person the seat height should permit the feet to contact the floor. For a person who is nonambulatory the seat height should be at the same height as the wheelchair seat.

Regardless of whether builders mount a lavatory on the wall set into a cabinet or on a pedestal, sufficient knee space must appear below the fixture (29 inches minimum from the floor to the bottom surface of the front apron) and a maximum height of 33 inches for the top surface. These allowances enable individuals who use wheelchairs to pull underneath the lavatory and to reach the faucet handles. The open space below the lavatory where the drain and water supply lines appear should not be left exposed to avoid individuals from accidentally scalding themselves. Builders insulating these lines or adding skirts below the lavatory that angles to the wall solve this problem.

Although tubs, toilets, and lavatories are the major sources of problems for people with disabilities, builders often do not notice the locations of supporting elements such as mirrors, soap holders, towel bars, and storage areas, which can be the source of discomfort and frustration for disabled people. For people who use wheelchairs, mirrors must be low on the wall so that the bottom is no higher than 40 inches from the floor (ideally down to the backsplash of the counter). In addition, for people with vision loss, the mirrors should hang so that users do not have to lean across a lavatory but can get as close as necessary. Soap holders, towel bars, and storage for the sink and tub should appear within the reach limits of the particular user. Finally, the toilet paper roll should not hang where users must twist or turn and reach behind themselves and should be within easy reach to their sides or fronts.

## Kitchen

The kitchen is the most complex space in the home. Moreover, because the tasks that people perform in the kitchen are as diverse as their functional abilities, modifications are not the same for all people with disabilities. Of all the rooms in the home, the kitchen should have sufficient space to enable someone in a wheelchair to turn around. In addition, a minimum of 2 feet, 6 inches × 4 feet, 0 inches clear floor area should appear in front of each appliance. This accommodates forward and side approaches that are necessary for persons to complete the variety of tasks associated with each appliance. For instance, a person taking food from a refrigerator is easier from a side reach, whereas using the water dispenser in the door might be easier using a forward reach. Knee spaces that are at least 27 inches high, 30 inches wide, and 19 inches deep should appear under cook tops, sinks, workspaces, and beside ranges, wall ovens, and dishwashers to enable a person to reach a necessary item and to work comfortably. The various requirements for clear floor space are not necessarily additive. Where possible, floor space at appliances, under counters, and for turning can overlap.

The height of work surfaces is also an issue for people who cannot stand on their feet to complete kitchen-related tasks. The standard counter height of 36 inches is too high for either wheelchairs or standard kitchen chairs, although an ambulatory individual could use a barstool. However, no single height is appropriate for all tasks or for all users. One individual might prefer a 30-inch high sink to be able to see down to the bottom, whereas another individual might prefer 34 inches for food preparation. Moreover, individuals who stand to complete kitchen tasks share the kitchen, low counters can be uncomfortable for them. The most common solution is for segments of the counters to be at different heights to accommodate differing needs. A second solution is for manually or motor-driven adjustable height counters to be in the kitchen, including sinks and cook tops that individuals can raise or lower quickly. The owner also should consider the availability of stretches of continuous countertop surfaces, particularly on either side of the sink and cook top, enabling them to slide heavy objects from one location to another rather than pick them up. A contrasting border treatment on the countertops is useful for people with low vision, which makes distinguishing the countertop edge easier, particularly if low visual contrast exists between the countertop and adjacent cabinets or floor.

Accessible storage is another important consideration in kitchen design. Reach is the key limiting factor in people using upper and lower kitchen cabinets. Upper cabinets are too high and lower cabinets and drawers are either too low or too deep. The owners can have the builders make several modifications that can reduce storage problems such as lowering upper cabinets, using full-extension drawers, and providing pull-out shelves and lazy-Susan turntables in base cabinets. A full-height pantry cabinet provides plenty of accessible storage otherwise lost when individuals cannot reach wall cabinets.

For people who cannot stand or have upper-body limitations, their reach, strength, and fine motor control may limit the ability to use appliance controls. People can minimize reach limitations by using appliances with controls located on or near the front. They also should consider range or cook tops with staggered placement of burners, which eliminates their need to reach over hot burners to grasp pots or pans on back burners. Builders can wire other appliances such as a range hood or a disposal to a switch on the front face of the base cabinet. People often have difficulty operating controls that require fine motor control such as stove knobs, which they can only operate by pushing and turning at the same time. Appliances with electronic controls are typically easier to use. Similar to programmable thermostats, people operate these appliances by push buttons that require only one simple manipulation, which does not require a great deal of strength or degree of precision. Similarly, lever handles on sink faucets eliminate the need for people to grip or be precise.

For people with low vision, controls that provide tactile or auditory feedback are most effective. A knob that is shaped like a pointer and has click stops provides such feedback. In addition, high-contrast labeling and raised markers provide information for individuals regardless of the amount of vision they have. Alternatively, electronic controls such as those mentioned previously can also be effective for people with vision impairments. Individuals with vision loss should avoid touch-sensitive controls because they have difficulty distinguishing between settings unless a tactile overlay is available. Buttons provide tactile feedback and are easier to operate. Glare-free task lighting (e.g., which track lights or recessed lights provide over the counter top) instead of or in addition to ambient lighting makes visual tasks much easier for people working in the kitchen.

## Bedroom

Similar to other rooms in the home, the bedroom should have sufficient space for a wheelchair or for an individual with difficulty ambulating to maneuver safely. In most cases, the bed is the most dominant feature in the room. As a result, the size and location of the bed quite often dictates how accessible the room is. Builders should provide at least 36 inches between pieces of furniture for wheelchair passage. Space on both sides of the bed permit a wheelchair user to travel around the bed to change linens or make the bed.

All local building codes require bedrooms to have a window for emergency exit. Because this precaution typically will not help a person with a disability, the bedroom should have its own exit door to the exterior. When this is not possible, two interior routes from the bedroom should be present or at least one accessible route that does not pass by or through the kitchen, utility area, or other likely places of a fire. For safety and convenience, the owner should place telephones, emergency call buttons, alarm controls, and other environmental control systems within reach of the bed. In addition, a sufficient number of accessible electrical outlets should appear adjacent to the bed to accommodate a variety of power-operated assistive devices that an individual might use. Such devices might include an adjustable bed, a power lift, or an oxygen concentrator. The owner may also need the outlets for recharging a battery for a powered mobility device.

## Laundry Room

Unlike kitchens, which designers plan well, laundry facilities are often an afterthought, located in whatever leftover space is large enough to hold a washer and a dryer. As a result, insufficient room often exists for people with mobility impairments to move. Also, lighting is generally poor, which makes seeing appliance controls or the laundry difficult for people with vision loss. However, even when the space is well configured, people who use wheelchairs typically have difficulty seeing or reaching into top-loading appliances and reaching across the appliances to the controls located on the rear panel.

Builders can make several modifications to address these problems, even in small spaces. Front-loading appliances may help people who use wheelchairs, although people with ambulatory impairments, gait and balance disorders, and difficulty bending will have a harder time using them. For wheelchair users the direction of door swings on front-loading appliances may also cause problems in small spaces in which maneuvering a wheelchair is difficult. In addition, front-loading dryers are common, whereas front-loading washers are not, and the machines that are available are typically expensive. Moreover, front-loading machines do not facilitate use of rear-mounted controls. Alternatively, a ramped platform in front of the appliances has the effect of lowering the appliance by raising the user. Where possible, the floor below a top-loading washer can have a recess to achieve the same result. In either case, a wheelchair user can look and reach into the appliance or across to the controls. The owner can therefore add a shelf to place laundry while transferring it from the washer to the dryer, especially in spaces where maneuvering is difficult and where moving clothes directly without repositioning the wheelchair may not be possible.

For people with vision impairments, lighting in the utility area may be critical. Fluorescent lighting that will be spread evenly in the space should replace bare bulb fixtures thus eliminating glare and dark areas, especially on the control panels. Text on control panels should contrast highly with the background, with dark text on a lighter background preferred. Owners can apply raised markings to settings that they use most frequently.

CASE STUDY

### *Background*

T.R. is a 72-year-old housewife who had degenerative lumbar disease for the past 9 years. The degeneration of the discs resulted in bone rubbing against the nerve, leaving T.R. in intense, chronic pain 24 hours a day. Movement and vibration exacerbated the pain, which made moving around, climbing stairs, or riding in a car for long periods difficult. Although she could still walk, arthritis in her spinal column, knees, and ankles made ambulating without severe pain difficult. She had three surgeries and expected to eventually lose the use of one and perhaps both legs. Because of her condition, T.R. spends most of the day lying on her bed and only getting up during meals. This sedentary lifestyle resulted in her loss of muscle tone and stamina, making most physical activities extremely tiring and painful.

T.R. lived with her husband in a typical ranch-style house. Although having all the living spaces on one level facilitated her movement through the house, she had a number of problems that resulted from the home's design (Figure 24-3). In the bathroom, T.R. needed to sit in a chair while showering. Even though she could still stand, she had difficulty maintaining her balance and turning because she had nothing to hold onto in the shower. She had trouble standing at the lavatory and getting on and off the toilet. Because of the steeply sloped lot, the front of the house was more than a half story above grade and the rear entrance was one full story above grade, making it difficult for T.R. to get to the street and the garage. As a result, even though she could get out of bed and walk for short periods, she was virtually housebound. Because of the difficulty in getting out of the house and the pain associated with riding in a car, she was often unable to travel to undergo hydrotherapy, which her physician recommended. Finally, although T.R. spent most of her time in bed, her bedroom was so small that it could only accommodate a full-size bed, with little room for people to visit.

Because of the difficulty of working with the site, many friends and the architect advised T.R. that moving rather than modifying her existing home would be easier and perhaps less expensive. However, similar to many older individuals, the couple lived in their home for many years and did not want to move. In addition, they were willing to bear the cost and inconvenience of modifying the house. Fortunately, the major changes to the master bedroom and bath and the exterior of the house provided T.R. with greater mobility, safety, and freedom, while increasing the value of the house.

## Goals

Based on the difficulties that T.R. had, the goals for specialists' modifications were to facilitate T.R.'s independence with bathing, going to the bathroom, and engaging in other personal hygiene activities, getting in and out of the house, using the bedroom for living

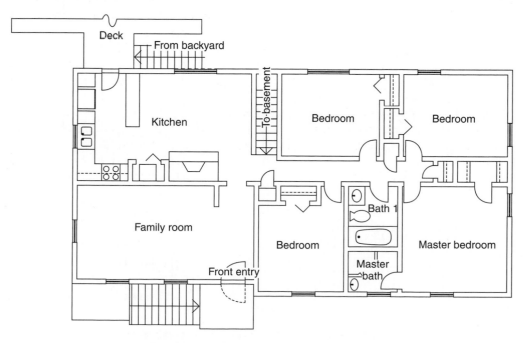

**Fig. 24-3** Before plan of T.R.'s residence.

and entertaining, and adding a hot tub for hydrotherapy. Despite problems that she had with other activities in her home, including meal preparation, cleaning, and laundry, they did not consider modifications for these activities. T.R. and her husband knew that no matter how supportive the environment was or how much assistance people provided, T.R. would have to have too much energy to engage in these activities. Because these were activities that someone else could do, the specialists thought that investing in modifications that would address those activities that T. R. did herself were more important.

### Modifications

Builders modified the master bedroom and bath and the front entry by constructing an addition that enlarged the bedroom and bath and added a deck adjacent to the bathroom (Figure 24-4). Because the house was so high above grade, the most difficult problem for the builders to address was access to the street. Fortunately, the street and main floor of the house were essentially on the same level, with the grade of the front yard well below the street and the main floor. The builders ramped the new deck down to a wooden bridge, which spanned the front yard and connected to the existing sidewalk (Figure 24-5).

They converted the old master bath into a 5-feet × 7-feet curbless, wet-area shower so that T.R. would not have to step over a curb and, eventually, would be able to roll in with a wheelchair. The shower included a seat and grab bars so that T.R. could sit or stand. (Figure 24-6). The additional space added to the bathroom also made the presence of a lavatory possible where she could sit (with the assistance of a rolling office chair) and grab bars at the toilet to enable her to get up and down by herself (Figure 24-7). The new addition provided enough space in the master bedroom to accommodate a larger bed and a home entertainment center. They also incorporated a large bay window into the front of the house, providing T.R. with a view of the street and trees in the front yard (Figure 24-8).

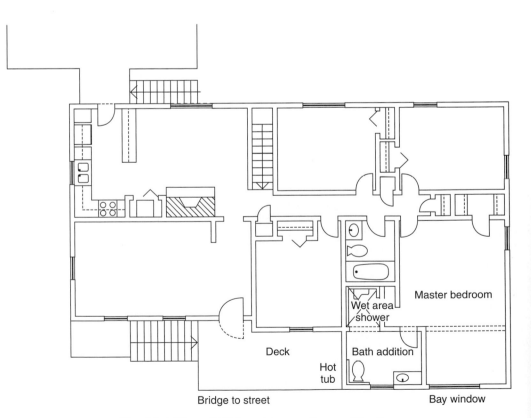

**Fig. 24-4** Plan of T.R.'s residence after modification.

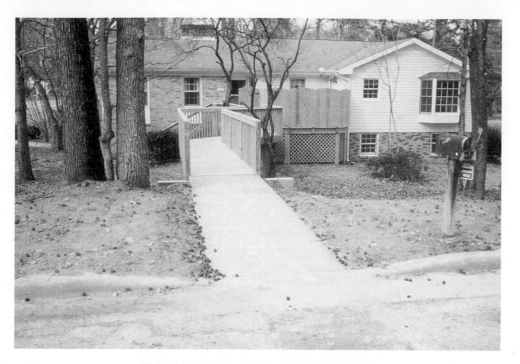

**Fig. 24-5** Wooden bridge leads to sidewalk.

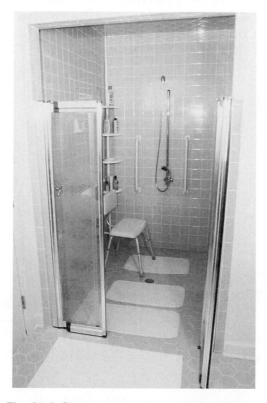

**Fig. 24-6** Shower area with seat and grab bars.

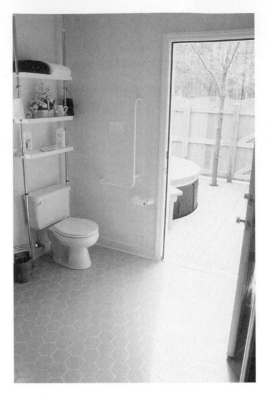

**Fig. 24-7** Toilet area with grab bars.

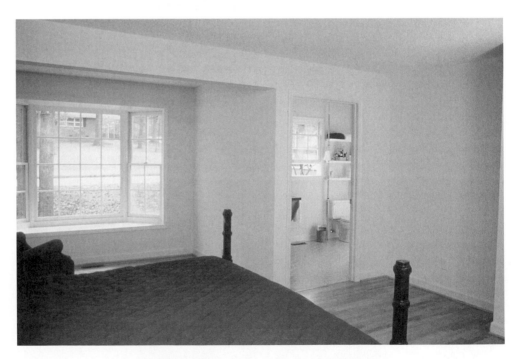

**Fig. 24-8** Bay window at front of T.R.'s house.

## *Lessons Learned*

More than 2 years has passed since the builders completed the project, and T.R. is able to do considerably more with less pain. In this regard, the project has been a great success. Often, home modifications are too clinical or specialized and may actually detract from the home's value. Fortunately, the modifications enhanced the value of the house by making it larger, adding amenities such as a larger master bedroom, a larger master bath, a more elegant shower area, and a hot tub. Even though this was an expensive project (approximately $45,000), it was not as expensive as it would have been had builders modified other areas of the house. For T.R., like many other older individuals, total independence in all routine household activities was not a realistic goal. Instead, choosing goals that were important, realistic, and within her budget and physical limitations was crucial.

Finally, little things can make big differences in quality of life, even if they do not improve functioning. Few, if any, specialists would have recommended making T.R.'s bedroom larger after functional evaluations. However, quality of life means more than just functional independence. In this case, T.R. wanted to be able to see her seven grandchildren regularly and maintain some contact with the outside world through the bay window. Therefore although the additional size of the master bedroom did not enhance her ability to perform any routine activity, the size, perhaps more than any other change, enhanced quality of life and made the home more enjoyable.

## References

1. Christenson MA: *Aging in the designed environment,* New York, 1990, Haworth Press.
2. Connell BR, Sanford JA: Individualizing home modification recommendations to facilitate performance of routine activities. In Lansprey S, Hyde J, editors: *Staying put: adapting the places instead of the people,* Amityville, NY, 1997, Baywood Publishing.
3. Lawton MP: *Environment and aging,* ed 2, Albany, NY, 1986, Center for the Study of Aging.
4. Feuerstein M et al: Hands on architecture: a typology for designers and researchers. In Harvey J, Henning D, editors: *Proceedings of eighteenth annual environmental design research association conference,* Ottowa, 1987.

# CHAPTER 25

# Adaptive Aids for Self-Care and Child Care at Home

*Christine R. Jasch*

## Application and Goal

*Equipment* is a tool that people use to complete tasks safely and efficiently. A hammer, for example, is a piece of equipment that helps the user complete the task of putting a nail through a board. Although a person can complete this task without a hammer by using a rock or a slab of wood, the hammer enables the user to complete the task more safely and efficiently.

Adapted equipment that meets the needs of persons with disabilities also are tools that they use to complete tasks safely and efficiently. A sock donner, for example, is a piece of equipment that helps the user put on a sock. Although other methods to address this task exist, such as a person using the assistance of another person, struggling to use the conventional method, or deciding to go without socks, the sock donner enables the user to address the task more safely, efficiently, and independently. For a person with a disability, adaptive equipment can often be the difference between independence and dependence. With the right tool, a person may be able to perform a task that is otherwise impossible, difficult, or tiring.

The goal of issuing or fabricating adaptive equipment is for the therapist to find the right tool to complete the task safely and use energy efficiently. Sometimes multiple pieces of equipment are useful for various tasks. Too much equipment, however, can be overwhelming and confusing for the user. Researchers have identified specific criteria to assist with evaluating and selecting equipment.[1] Assistive devices should be effective, affordable, operable, and dependable. To eliminate having a closet full of unused and unwanted equipment, the potential user and therapist should be certain of the equipment's potential success (Box 25-1).

## Function and Ability

Many equipment options are available to meet specific needs. Generalizations help pinpoint the specific equipment needs. Kohlmeyer[2] provides a starting point for clinicians in determining appropriate equipment based on deficits as follows:

Patients with range of motion limitations must compensate for lack of reach and joint excursion. Extended handles, reachers, and elastic or Velcro closures are several options. Compensation principles for decreased strength are to use gravity-assisted, lightweight, or electrical devices and to change body mechanics by using leverage. Incoordination in the form of tremors, ataxia, athetoid, or choreiform movements can cause difficulty in completing activities of daily living. Stabilizing proximal limb segments, weighting distal segments, and providing a safe environment help compensate for lack of balance and fine-motor skill. Patients with decreased hand function may use orthoses, universal cuffs, or straps to perform activities of daily living. The major compensatory technique for patients with hemiplegia is stabilization to substitute for the role normally assumed by the affected

## BOX 25-1

*Evaluating the Suitability of Assistive Equipment for a Particular Person*

Is the user open to using an adapted method?

Does the user have the appropriate motor and cognitive function to optimally use this equipment?

Can the user don/doff the equipment in a timely manner?

Can the user use the equipment for optimal task performance?

Can the user obtain the equipment in a reasonable time for a reasonable cost?

Can the user provide proper cleaning and needed maintenance to the equipment to maximize its functional life?

Is the equipment durable?

Can the equipment be replaced or repaired and if so, by whom?

Will this equipment be adaptable to meet the changing needs of normal development or improvements or declines in physical function?

Is the equipment functional in a variety of settings?

Is the equipment cosmetically appealing?

Does the equipment meet the user's goals?

side. Secured objects, Dycem, and adaptive techniques are common options. Patients with low endurance should use energy conservation and work simplification techniques, such as prioritization, organization, pacing, and utilization of equipment that improves efficiency.

## Considerations, Options, and Technology

Consumers, users, and clients have several equipment options, many of them low tech, for various self-care areas. Occupational therapy uses ". . . interventions designed to . . . promote health, prevent injury or disability and. . . . improve, sustain, or restore the highest possible level of independence . . ."[3] An occupational therapist understands the physical deficits and necessary compensations and is familiar with available equipment and resources. Occupational therapists are skilled at the selection and fabrication of adaptive equipment and can teach users about it.

This section addresses personal self-care by dividing it into several areas. Each begins with task definitions and breakdowns and possible equipment suitable for each task. Although each section lists many equipment options, the lists are not all inclusive. A variety of equipment options exist for each task depending on the deficit that requires compensation and the intact abilities still available. Most equipment is readily available and easy to use. However, some equipment requires fabrication.

Unless otherwise noted, therapists can obtain all the equipment listed from one of three major equipment resources available to occupational therapists: Sammons Preston, North Coast Medical, and Smith & Nephew Rolyan. All sources are listed in the reference list at the end of the chapter. Also, many other companies manufacture adaptive equipment. Some of this equipment is exclusive to companies that specialize in one or two types of equipment. At the end of each section is a list of unique equipment that is unusual in design, hard to find, or one of a kind.

### Feeding

Feeding and eating involves a person's ability to set up food, to use appropriate utensils and tableware, to bring food or drink to the mouth, and to suck, masticate, cough, and swallow.[4] Feeding equipment can vary from the simple (built-up foam padding added to a fork) to the complex (an electromechanical self-feeder). Ideally, any feeding aid will be portable so that a person may use it in a variety of settings such as at home, at a

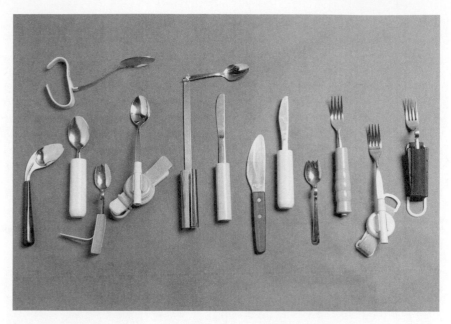

**Fig. 25-1** Utensils are available with various adaptations to meet different needs.

friend's house, or at a restaurant. The aid also will be flexible or interchangeable with other utensils to allow independence when the person eats a variety of foods.

## Utensils

Utensils are adaptable to meet the needs of individuals with decreased elbow, wrist, or finger range of motion (ROM), and/or decreased strength and coordination. Adaptive utensils can be categorized in the following ways (Figure 25-1):

- Modified handle accommodates for various grasping difficulties, ranging from a built-up utensil to accommodate decreased grasp to a strap to hold a utensil in place for an absent grasp
- Modified length accommodates decreased ROM in the elbow or shoulder
- Modified angle or curve to the handle accommodates decreased wrist function
- Weighted handles compensate for coordination difficulties
- Swiveled utensil accommodates decreased ROM of the wrist or forearm

## Drinking Aids

Cups with a variety of shaped handles, two handles, lids, weighted cups, and nose cutouts are available to accommodate for a person's decreased grasp, coordination, and limited ROM. Long straws, straw holders, and one-way straws can assist a person with decreased neck or trunk range. Wheelchair cup holders make transporting liquids easier for a person.

## Plate Guards

Plate guards are plastic or metal rings that wrap around a plate to provide an edge to assist the user in scooping food onto the utensil.

## Modified Plates or Bowls

Several types of modified plates or bowls are available. They are shaped with one side contoured to provide the user assistance with scooping. Some styles have skid-proof bottoms to eliminate the possibility of the dish sliding (Figure 25-2).

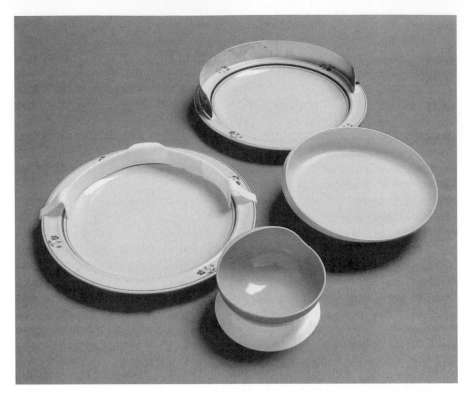

**Fig. 25-2** Plate guards and scoop bowls provide an edge to help place food on the utensil.

## Surface

To prevent a dish from slipping across the table or lap tray, the user can apply nonslip materials such as Dycem to the bottom surface. These materials are available in round, square, or placemat-shaped pads or in rolls that allow the user to cut the material to size.

## Unique Feeding Equipment

### Sandwich Holder

A sandwich holder assists the user with no hand function to eat a sandwich. The user places a long, thin handle into a utensil holder, and plastic jaws that a rubber band secures grip the sandwich. A person also may use this device to eat thin pizza.

### Mobile Arm Supports (MAS)

Also known as a *balance forearm orthosis* (*BFO*) or *ball bearing feeder*, the MAS provides help to a person with decreased upper extremity (UE) strength. By supporting the forearm and providing a smooth gilding motion, the MAS eases the hand-to-mouth motion. The basic unit attaches to a wheelchair via a bracket. However, tabletop models are available for an ambulatory individual with weak upper extremities. A therapist can add various adjustments and optional pieces to assist the user who has weak deltoids and biceps. The MAS requires installation and setup by a professional who will most likely be an occupational therapist.[5]

### Self-Feeder

For individuals without arm function, self-feeders provide a method of feeding with the setup done by another individual. The Winsford Feeder is a battery-operated and switch-activated device that can move food from a plate or a bowl up to the mouth level of a seated person. When activated by a switch, the arm of the self-feeder moves to the plate surface and a food pusher pushes the food onto the utensil. The arm is then

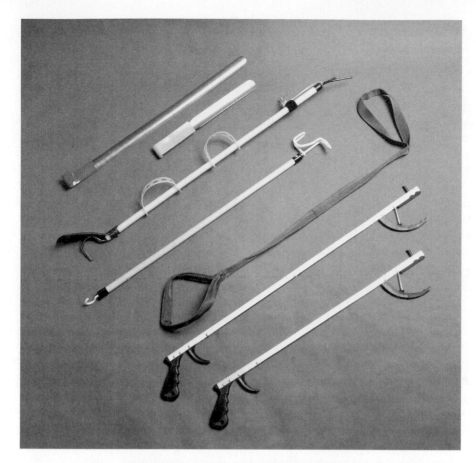

**Fig. 25-3** Examples of dressing equipment.

lifted to be within mouth range. The user then takes the food from the utensil and the process repeats. A single switch located near the chin or head activates this equipment. A therapist can place an alternative plate switch wherever movement is available, for example, a finger or foot.

## Dressing

*Dressing* refers to a person's ability to select appropriate clothing, obtain clothing from a storage area, dress and undress sequentially, and fasten and adjust clothing and shoes.[4] The act of dressing can be a task that requires a person to have physical agility and a considerable amount of endurance.

## Clothing Aids

### Dressing Sticks

Dressing sticks assist a person with limited ROM, muscle strength, and endurance. They are available in a variety of types and lengths to accommodate specific deficits. The standard stick has a plastic s-shaped hook on one end designed to hook and pull a piece of clothing. A c-shaped hook is on the opposite end. This allows a person to don pants without bending. For example, an individual with limited hip flexion can don a pair of pants by hooking the pants on the end of the dressing stick, lowering it to the floor while grasping the opposite end of the stick, and working the foot into the pants leg. Built-up foam handles and plastic hand guards assist people who have limited grasp. Options include a dressing stick and shoehorn combination, dressing stick and sock-aid combination, and a collapsible version for travel (Figure 25-3).

### Reachers

A person can use reachers to assist with donning pants. The trigger-handle type often provides control a dressing stick cannot. An individual can grasp, release, and regrasp the clothing as required. Various sizes and styles are available.

### Leg Straps and Leg Lifters

Available prefabricated or easily made of webbing, leg straps and leg lifters can ease bed mobility tasks such as a person moving the legs on and off the bed. A bed ladder provides loops of webbing, which ease a person rolling in bed. Webbing can be sewn into pants to provide a person without hand function a method to pull them up. Hooks can be added to webbing, which can be attached to the belt loops of a pair of pants. Wearing gloves made for pushing wheelchairs provides additional friction for the person with weak or limited hand function. To ease donning of pants, the wearer can try larger sizes to eliminate tight fit. Clothing specifically designed for wheelchair users allows extra room in the hips and waist and has dressing loops sewn into pants and conveniently located pockets (Figure 25-4).[6]

### Fasteners

*Buttonhooks and Button Extenders*

Buttonhooks help a person manipulate buttons and are helpful for individuals with limited coordination, only one-hand use, or limited fine motor strength. A buttonhook consists of a metal loop extending from a base or handle, which varies in size and shape to meet individual needs. The user feeds the metal loop through the buttonhole, hooks the button, and then pulls it through the buttonhole. Button extenders are useful at the cuffs of sleeves. Once secured, they allow a person to don or doff a shirt without buttoning or unbuttoning the cuff.

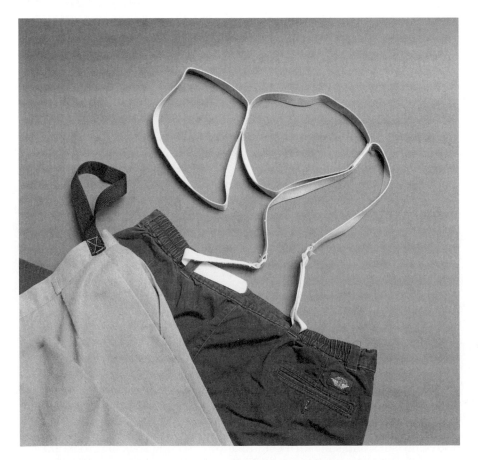

**Fig. 25-4** Pant loops can hook onto the belt loops or can be sewn in.

*Zipper Pulls*
Zipper pulls are designed to provide assistance with zippers for people with limited or no hand function.

## Socks and Shoes
*Sock Aids*
To ease the task of donning a pair of socks, a person can choose from a variety of sock aids. Designed to reduce the need for bending, they are also helpful for persons with weak hand function. They are usually made of lightweight plastic, and the user slides the sock onto the sock aid. Grasping the attached cord, the user lowers the sock aid to the foot and slides the sock around the toes. By pulling on the cord, the user can pull the sock onto the foot. They are available in many styles to meet individual needs. Styles include hard or flexible plastic, nylon covered to reduce friction, a wide base to accommodate larger feet, one or two cords for pulling, foam or hook handles, and a pantyhose aid (Figure 25-5).

*Shoehorns and Shoelaces*
Several shoehorn types are available. They differ in length and type of handle and may be made of either plastic or steel. Shoe fasteners vary from elastic shoelaces to clips that hold the laces tight. Elastic shoelaces allow a person to don or doff the shoe without tying and untying the laces. Some versions lace and tie and look like regular laces and others require no tying.

## Unique Dressing Equipment
*Jobst Stocking Donner*
The Jobst Stocking Donner assists a person don tight-fitting vascular stockings. The individual must be able to manipulate the stocking around the device. However, the person can perform this task at waist or chest level. The metal frame holds the stockings open while the individual pulls on the handles.

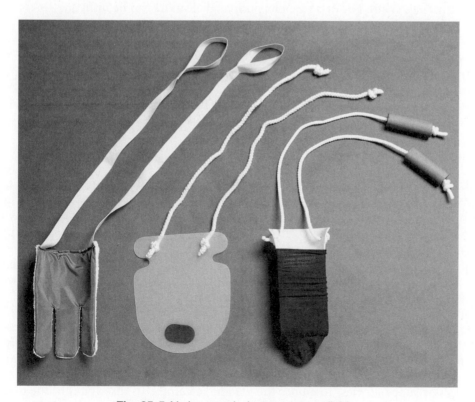

**Fig. 25-5** Various sock donners are available.

## *Toileting*

*Toileting* refers to a person's ability to obtain and use supplies, clean oneself, transfer to and from the toilet, and maintain toileting position on a bedpan, toilet, or commode.[4] Toileting is a highly private and personal act and a person usually desires optimal independence.

## Toileting Equipment for Those with Mobility Impairments

### Commode Seats and Chairs

For people with limitations in mobility, raised toilet seats, grab bars, and bedside commodes are good options for functionality and safety. If sitting and standing from a standard commode seat is difficult, a person has a wide range of raised toilet seats to choose from. Most people raise the sitting surface 4 inches. However, a person can find seats that add 2 inches and adjustable seats that add up to 6 additional inches. If a person needs handrails, they are available attached to certain models of raised toilet seats. A person also can purchase them individually. Stand-alone commode chairs are useful for persons with limited mobility. A person can place them near the bed for nighttime use or in the shower as a shower chair. To meet specific needs, commode seats are available with removable or adjustable handrails to facilitate easy transfer and height adjustments.

### Urinals

Hand-held urinals are available for men and women and are helpful for persons with limited mobility to empty their bladders from beds or chairs. Some urinals have been designed with extended necks to decrease spillage when persons use them from sitting positions.

## Hygiene Management

Persons with limited or no upper extremity function usually only need equipment for hygiene management. For these people, perirectal cleaning can be difficult.

### Toilet aids

A variety of toilet-aid devices are available. They are designed to assist a person with limited hand function or upper extremity ROM to manipulate and secure toilet paper to perform hygiene. Styles include tongs, spring clip, an S-shaped hook, and a small cup-shaped head with recessed serrations. Various lengths are available to meet individual needs (Figure 25-6).

### Water Systems

A bidet also can be a helpful cleaning method. Bidets provide a stream of water to properly clean the perirectal area. Systems are available that attach to a standard toilet and require little-to-no fine motor control. They receive water supply either from a nearby sink or the toilet tank, and persons can adjust them and place the controls where they want. The water can provide effective cleansing for any person with limited upper-extremity function, especially a bilateral upper-extremity amputee. If using equipment is not preferred or equipment is not available, an individual can use one simple method such as laying toilet paper on the rim of the toilet seat and rubbing against the paper.

### Equipment for Individuals with Dysfunctional Bowel or Bladder

If individuals are unable to voluntarily empty the bladder or bowel, they must use alternative methods. In conjunction with physicians and/or nurses, individuals usually determine these methods. Adaptive equipment can assist those individuals who cannot manipulate the standard medical equipment they need for the procedure, such as catheters or suppositories. To empty the bladder, a catheter is inserted into the bladder via the urethra. For an individual with limited fine motor skills or limited mobility, equipment may be able to ease the task.

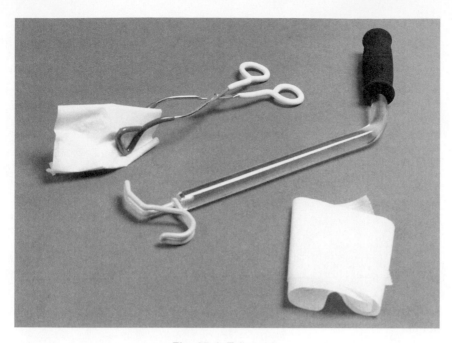

**Fig. 25-6** Toilet aids.

To assist self-catheterization, a standard hair clip can be mounted in splinting material and attached to a universal cuff positioned in the palm of the hand (Figure 25-7, *A*). Using wrist pronation and supination, the hair clip can be closed around the catheter, providing a secure grip of the catheter. A catheter inserter can assist an individual with decreased hand function (Figure 25-7, *B*) (see Unique Toileting Equipment below. While seated in a wheelchair, the individual can use a bungee cord, which can ease clothing management when preparing for catheterization. One end of the bungee cord can be hooked onto a part of the wheelchair or any other fixed surface, and the other end can secure the pants, pulling them away and freeing up both hands for catheterization.

An individual with dysfunctional bowels, such as a person with a spinal cord injury (SCI), may use a method called *digital stimulation* to stimulate a bowel movement. An individual without sufficient arm placement or hand control may use a digital bowel stimulator. With proper instruction, the client inserts the tool into the rectum to provide the required stimulation. If a suppository is necessary, a suppository inserter can help. Both of these tools are available with a long handle or a short handle (Figure 25-8).

### Unique Toileting Equipment
*Spil-Pruf Urinal*
The Spil-Pruf Urinal is designed with an extended neck and a special spill-proof spout that prevents leaks and helps reduce odor. An o-ring gasket and a special one-way flow spout prevent leakage.

*Catheter Inserter*
The catheter inserter is designed for individuals with limited hand function, such as a C6, C7 SCI. It consists of a c-handle that the user supports in one palm and a straight handle connected by a spring clip, which holds the catheter stable. By applying pressure to the handle, users can open the clips thus releasing the catheter and allowing them to regrasp the catheters in another location.

*Lubidet*
The Lubidet provides personal hygiene with a warm water wash and warm air dry for effective, hands-free cleansing of the perirectal area. It is mounted onto a standard toilet with the nozzle fitting between the existing toilet seat and bowl.

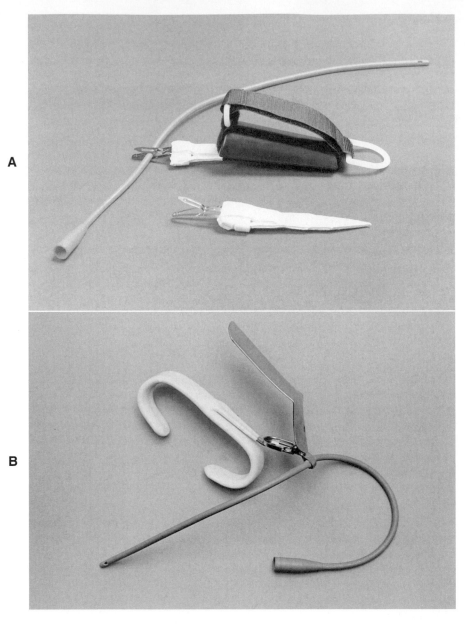

**Fig. 25-7 A,** A hair clip mounted in splinting material and held in a utensil cuff can stabilize a catheter for insertion. **B,** Catheter inserter.

*Pneumatic and Electric Leg Bag Openers*

Pneumatic and electric leg bag openers offer independence with leg bag management. Once set up, the user can open the valve of the leg bag by activating a switch that is either pneumatic or electric. The valves remain open as long as the user activates the switch. This equipment requires the user to position the end tubing over a toilet or other receptacle.[7,8]

## Bathing

*Bathing* refers to the skills a person needs to obtain and use supplies, soap, rinse, and dry all body parts, maintain bathing position, and transfer to and from bathing position.[4] The shower or bathtub are inherently unsafe and present bathers with many obstacles and risks. The task of bathing is physically taxing and requires physical agility and endurance. Optimally, bathing equipment helps provide a safe environment that maximizes independence and provides energy conservation opportunities.

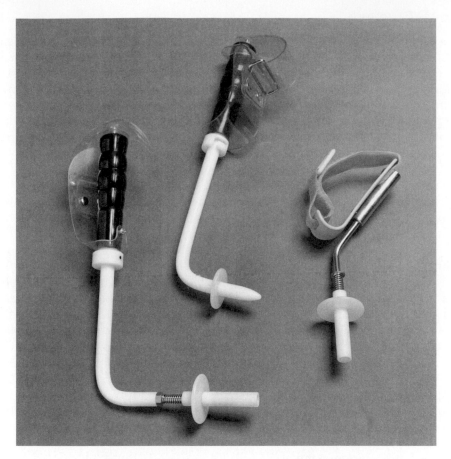

**Fig. 25-8** Digital stimulator and suppository inserter.

## Seating Aids and Lifts

A variety of bath benches and chairs are designed to allow an individual to sit during a shower. They range from the simple bath bench to the powered seat.

### Simple Options

The user can place a bath bench (no backrest) and a bath chair (with backrests) in the tub or shower stall. Bath boards fit across the top edges of the tub, and transfer benches extend over the side of the tub to assist with transfers.

### More Elaborate Options

The user can roll rolling shower chair into an accessible shower stall or use powered seats that lower and raise a person in the tub.

Most bath chairs and benches are height adjustable, have rubber or suction tips, and are waterproof. Some have optional commode cutouts and grab-bar attachments available. To meet individual needs, a person can mount some shower seats to the wall of a tub or shower and fold them out of the way when they are not in use. The user should consider the total weight of the person using the bench when deciding on a bath chair. Although most benches accommodate up to 250 lb, some benches can accommodate 300 lb.

For the more dependent individual, mechanical transfer lifts are available that mount to the side of the tub. The seat then swings over the tub and lowers the person into the bath water.[9] More elaborate lifts are the ceiling mounted lifts that allow individuals to lift themselves out of a wheelchair and into the tub.[10]

## Personal Care Aids

Once a person is in the shower or tub, the bathing task is easier with a hand-held shower nozzle. Basic models have a rubber suction-cup end that fits over most tub faucets. Other models require installation onto the shower arm. A person can mount most models within reach of a sitting person. Some models have on/off valves to allow control of this function at the handle.

For people with sensory loss, hand-held shower nozzles can direct the spray onto an area with intact sensation for temperature testing. The user can install scald guards and can regulate the temperature to decrease the chance of accidental burns.

### Grab Bars

A person can clamp tub grab bars onto the side of the tub to assist with tub entry and exit. Wall grab bars or a handgrip can provide a secure, nonslip handhold. The user must install these wall grab bars into the wall tile of the tub.

### Sponges and Brushes

Long-handled sponges and brushes are available with various handles, lengths, bends, shapes of sponges, and functions. Two examples are a foot brush with a specially designed sponge tip for cleaning the feet and a soaper sponge with a built-in soap holder. Wash mitts eliminate the need for the person's hand-grasp function to hold onto a wash cloth or bar of soap. A suction cup soap holder can help an individual with decreased hand function to hold soap.

### Liquid Soap

Liquid soap dispensers can be helpful to a person with decreased upper-extremity function to dispense soap and shampoo.

### Bedside Bathing Equipment

For people who want to wash their hair out of the tub or shower, shampoo trays made of lightweight plastic are available that bridge the space between the individual and the sink to ease hair washing at the sink. Shampoo basins and trays allow a person to wash the hair while in bed. Special cleansers are available that require no water for body and hair cleansing.[11]

## Unique Bathing Equipment

### EZ-Bathe

The EZ-Bathe is an inflatable vinyl tub that allows a person to receive a thorough bed bath or bed shower. The user lies on the deflated tub that an assistant inflates with a wet-and-dry vacuum. The inflated tub surrounds the person allowing an assistant to collect water around the person. A long, hand-held hose allows an assistant or the individual to direct the flow of the water. Afterward, a drain hose empties the tub.

### Bath-O-Matic Hydrocushion

The Bath-O-Matic Hydrocushion lowers the user to the bottom of the tub for a bath. Once filled with water, the cushion provides a firm surface for the user to transfer to. The user then drains the cushion. This lowers the person to the floor of the tub and fills the tub with water. To exit the tub, the user refills the cushion with water and returns to the sitting position. Similarly, the Aqua-tech Bath Lift (Clarke Health Care Products Inc.) uses waterpower, and the Bathmaster bath lifting aid uses battery power to lift and lower an individual into and out of the tub.[12]

### Rubbermaid Bath Bench

The Rubbermaid Bath Bench is a sturdy, lightweight, adjustable bath seat. It features a large sitting surface with built-in storage for a hand-held shower spray and soap dish accessory. The seat height is adjustable from 17 inches to 22 inches. The user can add a backrest for additional support. Although most bath seats accommodate up to 250 lb, the Rubbermaid Bath Bench can accommodate 300 lb.[13]

### Quantum Bath Chair

The Quantum Bath Chair is a compact, collapsible, bath chair that a person can use for regular bathing and travel. The chair is made with durable yet lightweight polyvinyl chloride (PVC) plastic with stainless steel hardware. The user does not need tools for folding, transporting, or adjusting. It features a commode cutout, a reversible for left or right transfer, and a carrying case.[14]

## *Grooming*

*Grooming* refers to the skills a person needs to obtain and use supplies to shave, apply and remove cosmetics, wash, comb, style, and brush hair, care for nails and skin, and apply deodorant. *Oral hygiene* refers to a person obtaining and using supplies, cleaning the mouth and teeth, and removing, cleaning, and reinserting dentures.[4] Grooming tasks include the most personal self-care tasks. Each individual has preferences about the way to perform these tasks. Society views proper grooming as a requirement, but a person with decreased arm or hand function may have difficulty grooming. Although brushing teeth and combing hair appear to be simple tasks, they require a person to have adequate upper-extremity ROM, strength, coordination, and endurance. Equipment is available to assist individuals to maintain their grooming habits.

## Teeth Care

The ability for a person to independently brush teeth without equipment requires several of the following skills and abilities:

1. Adequate shoulder and elbow active/passive range of motion (A/PROM) to reach the mouth
2. Supination, pronation, and wrist movement sufficient to turn the brush to reach all teeth
3. Enough upper-extremity strength to apply pressure to the teeth
4. Adequate grasp to hold the brush and squeeze the toothpaste tube
5. Coordination to apply the toothpaste and brush the teeth

For people who lack one or many of these skills and abilities, equipment is available to compensate. A universal cuff can hold a toothbrush. To rotate the brush, the user can pull the toothbrush out of the cuff, turn the brush with the teeth and tongue, and reinsert the brush. A rotation universal holder can stabilize a toothbrush in the palm of the hand and provide the rotation needed to reach all teeth. A battery-powered toothbrush can compensate for decreased strength and/or endurance and may provide a more thorough cleaning. For people with dentures, they can use suction denture brushes. Once stabilized on the countertop with the suction cups, the user who has one hand or decreased coordination can rub the dentures against the bristles.

To apply the toothpaste, a person can use a toothpaste dispenser. Two types are available: one for squeezing tubes and one for pump-style dispensers. Both are designed to make putting toothpaste on a brush easier for individuals with limited finger/hand function. Other methods that a person can use are pushing on the tube with one hand while it rests on a countertop or bringing the tube of toothpaste up to the mouth, applying bilateral palmar pressure, and dispensing the toothpaste directly into the mouth. To complete the task of flossing, a Y-shaped dental floss holder allows the floss to be strung between its projections.[15] A universal cuff can support the straight end if needed.

## Hand and Face Care

A person needs functional hand strength, shoulder and elbow ROM, and coordination for equipment-free face and hand washing. Liquid soap dispensers can ease the task of a person manipulating a bar of soap and are available in the grocery store. A wash mitt may be easier for a person with limited hand strength or coordination to wash with than a wash cloth. The user can stabilize a suction brush to assist cleaning under nails, especially for someone who can only use one hand or with decreased hand strength. The user can mount a nail-clipper/file onto a board to provide stabilization or use a battery-operated nail trimmer. Nail file holders provide a built-up handle that can assist an individual with limited grasp.

## Hair

Long-handled combs and brushes are available for individuals with limited ROM. Brushes with a Velcro strap and D-ring can stabilize the brush in the palm of the hand of someone with limited grasp (Figure 25-9). The user can mount a hair dryer onto a wall for hands-free operation.

## Shaving

A universal, electric razor holder assists the individual with limited grasp to stabilize an electric razor. The user can secure disposable razors in a universal cuff. A rotating razor holder can help reach difficult areas. To dispense shaving cream, a shaving-cream dispenser handle clamps onto a can of shaving cream to allow a person to dispense the cream with a lever handle (Figure 25-10). A variety of mirrors are available to assist with all grooming tasks.

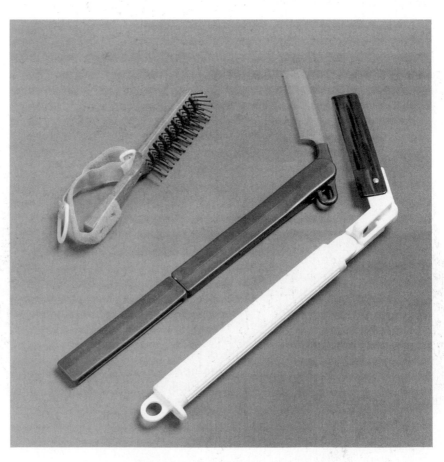

**Fig. 25-9** Hair-care equipment.

## Unique Grooming Equipment

### The Turn-Round Universal Holder

The Turn-Round Universal Holder can accommodate a variety of grooming items such as a razor, toothbrush, brush, and comb. It features a rotating holder that allows the accessories to change position easily while performing the task. Accessories snap in and out of the holder, which is helpful for individuals with limited grasp and ROM.[16]

### The Pistol-Grip Remote Toenail Clipper

For use by individuals with limited ROM or flexibility, the Pistol-Grip Remote Toenail Clipper is a toenail clipper mounted onto a standard reacher. The user operates the clippers by the grip at the handle of the reacher.[17]

## *Functional Communication*

*Functional communication* refers to equipment or systems that enhance or provide communication, such as writing equipment, telephones, typewriters, communication boards, call lights, emergency systems, Braille writers, augmentative communication systems, and computers.[4] Because of the high-tech nature of augmentative communication systems, Braille writers and computers, these subjects appear in other chapters.

## Writing

Traditionally, a person needs to hold a writing device to write and needs to hold the reading material and turn the pages to read. Writing is a personal and individual task. People have their unique writing styles (penmanship) and comfortable methods of holding a writing tool. A person's individual method of holding a writing tool is based on the size and function of the fingers and hand. This influences the style and legibility of the writing and writing endurance. For persons with full hand movement, a variety of built-up writing aids are available to reduce the pressure they need to hold a writing tool thus easing the fatigue.

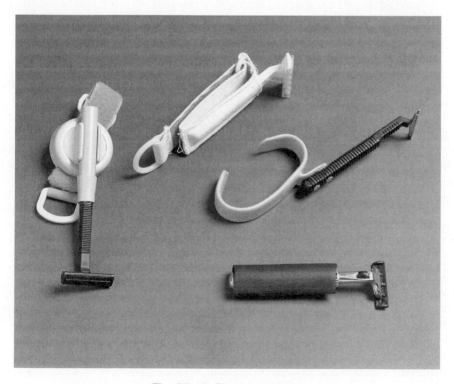

**Fig. 25-10** Shaving options.

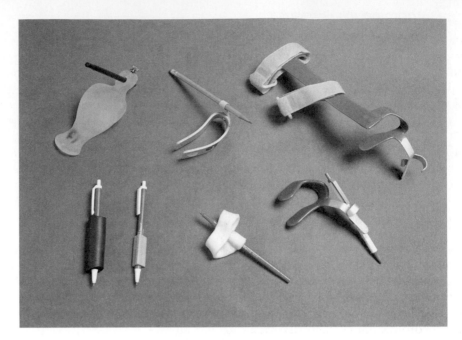

**Fig. 25-11** Writing equipment.

For people with decreased hand strength and/or joint deformities, specially designed writing tools and built-up pens are available to accommodate many needs. These pens are curved or shaped to better fit the contours of a hand with joint deformities. For people with limited control, the weighted pen and the magnetic wrist hold-down are designed to stabilize the hand thus reducing excessive movement (Figure 25-11). For people without hand function, they can use cuffs and splints to hold writing tools in their proper position. These are commercially available or can be fabricated to fit individual need. Clipboards and writing boards can help stabilize a piece of paper for a one-handed writer. Dycem sheets or pads also can help stabilize paper.

## Reading

### Book Holders

A variety of book holders are available to assist a person with limited motor function or endurance. They stabilize a book for hands-free reading and are available for table top, bed, or lap positioning. Persons can use Dycem to stabilize a magazine or a book on a surface. Persons with limited UE arm movement can use a BFO in conjunction with a writing splint. Persons without functional UE movement or endurance can use a mouthstick to complete a writing task (see Mouthsticks on p. 442). Powered page turners are another option for people with limited UE function. These devices usually hold a book or magazine in an upright position. When a person activates a switch either by sip/puff or touch, the turner turns the page in the direction chosen.[18] Unfortunately, these devices do not generally work well on newsprint.

## Telephone Use

A person who independently uses a telephone is connected to the world. This common tool increases the spectrum of contact with potential people, places, and things that could become part of that person's life. It markedly reduces a person's feelings of isolation and provides a means of regular communication with family and friends and access to services and information. Most importantly, a telephone is a means for a person to receive response in an emergency. For this reason alone, a person with a disability should have independent telephone access.

### Low Tech/Low Cost

Today's telephones offer a variety of disability-friendly features and are readily available at discount and electronic stores. Stored memory buttons and redial eliminate the need for a person to use the keypad. Answering machines, Caller ID and auto call back can assist the person who has difficulty reaching the phone before the caller hangs up. The user can add a hook-like support to provide a way for an individual with weak or no hand function to hold a phone. Typically made for a standard handset, the support wraps around the receiver. For "princess-type" phones, with the keypad in the handset, a cuff can be fabricated out of low-temperature plastic and secured onto the back of the receiver with Velcro. A gooseneck can hold a telephone receiver in position for those with weakness. Used with a phone flipper that can be purchased or fabricated at home, the gooseneck can provide independent phone access to a person with independent mobility to the phone "station."

#### *Speakerphones*

A person can use a speakerphone to provide phone access without requiring the individual to pick up the receiver. Speakerphones are readily available at most retail stores and, if needed, specialty phones designed for the disabled also are available (see Unique Communication Equipment on p. 443).

#### *Cordless Phones*

Using a cordless phone can offer the portability needed for a person with mobility impairments. A person can transport the cordless phone around the home in a walker bag, crutch pouch, wheelchair bag, or simply on the lap in the wheelchair.

#### *Headset Phones*

A person can achieve private conversation and hands-free stabilization of the receiver by using a headset phone. A large variety of headset types are available to accommodate many preferences and physical needs. Cordless headset phones are available that allow the user mobility throughout the home and convenient phone access.

For those with hearing impairments, a number of services and pieces of equipment are available. For instance, flashing lights can be attached to notify the person of an incoming call. Volume amplifiers increase the volume through the receiver. Telecommunication devices for deaf users (TDD) and teletype (TTY) phones offer communication options to persons with hearing or verbal communication difficulties. By using a small keyboard, the user can type and read a conversation. Many features on different models are available to best meet an individual's needs (see Chapter 12).[19]

## Typing and Computer Access (Low Tech)

Many high-tech hardware and software programs are available to ease computer access (see Chapter 7). Low-tech options for keyboard typing access also exist.

### Low Cost and Low Tech

#### *Typing Sticks*

A typing stick may assist an individual with limited hand function and can meet each individual's preferences, such as for pronated or neutral forearm positioning. All typing sticks have a rubber tip to prevent it from slipping off the key. A person also can use mouthsticks for keyboard access (see Mouthsticks on p. 442).

#### *Keyguards*

A keyguard, which provides a guide to the correct key, can enhance standard keyboard access.[20] Made of plastic, keyguards provide a person with support and guidance for accurate keyboarding while leaving the keyboard in complete view. The tapered holes of the keyguard assist the single-finger typist, mouthstick or headstick typist, or typist with limited control to target any desired key and decrease and eliminate accidental entries.

#### *Alternative Keyboards*

Ergonomic keyboards are designed to eliminate strain and pain that can develop from a person using straight standard keyboards. To properly use a standard keyboard, the person's wrist may overextend and encourage ulnar deviation. Multiple versions are available and are all designed to fit the typist.[21-23] With proper alignment and comfortable positioning, an individual should experience less pain and has the potential for increased productivity. A number of wrist pads and arm supports are available to provide support to the wrist and forearm therefore putting less strain on these joints.

*Mouthsticks*

Mouthsticks are devices designed to perform a variety of functions. A mouthstick consists of a mouthpiece, mouthstick shaft, and tip. Most mouthsticks provide a standard adult or pediatric bite plate. If needed, a dentist can fabricate a custom bite plate. The shaft varies in length and angle depending on the functional needs and abilities of the individual. The mouthstick tip is the functional component of the mouthstick. Some mouthsticks allow for the user to change tips depending on the current task. Others have fixed tips, requiring multiple mouthsticks to meet the needs of specific tasks. A variety of mouthsticks are available to fit each individual's motor ability and functional needs (Figure 25-12).

A person can use mouthsticks to perform a variety of communication, leisure, and community tasks. These tools are most likely to be considered for individuals with limited UE function such as those with high-level SCI, amyotrophic lateral sclerosis (ALS), muscular dystrophy (MD), or severe arthritis. Good head and neck ROM and strength, good mouth opening and closure function, functional endurance and motivation enhances functional use of a mouthstick. Independence with mouthstick use is directly proportional to available functional range, strength, and endurance. The stronger the movements and farther the range, the more independent the user will be. For people with limited head and neck function, they can use mouthsticks in limited environments and with precise setup. Functional mouthstick use requires training and appropriate selection of mouthstick and docking station.

Independence of mouthstick use requires a functional, reachable docking station (a location for the user to place the mouthstick when not in use) and accessibility of the environment. Neck ROM, strength, and the specific activity determine placement of the docking station. Docking stations can include commercially available stations, those fabricated by a therapist to meet specific needs, or a homemade station such as an empty soup can or cup (Figure 25-13 and Table 25-1).

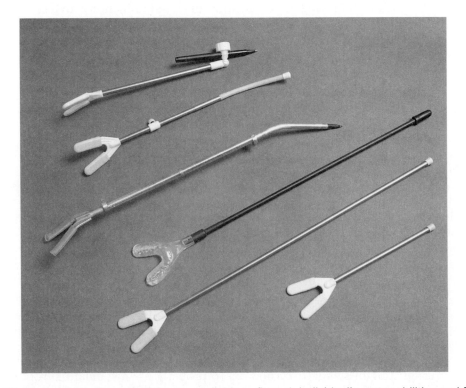

**Fig. 25-12** A variety of mouthsticks are available to fit each individual's motor abilities and functional needs.

## Unique Communication Equipment

### Handi-Tracker

A Handi-Tracker is a writing aid for those with use of one hand or decreased strength.[24] This aids a person's writing by stabilizing the paper and the person can accomplish this with a clipboard or tape. The Handi-Tracker writing aid can make any paper temporarily self-sticking. Supplied in a dispenser, the continuous roll of adhesive attaches to the back of a paper before the user secures it on a table or other writing surface. Afterward, the user can remove it.

### Dialogue RC

Dialogue RC is a remote-controlled telephone that allows the user to answer and make outgoing calls by simply pressing a remote switch. Once activated by the remote switch, the phone scans through up to 20 memory buttons at variable speeds. When the user activates the switch a second time, the corresponding preprogrammed number is dialed. If the switch is not activated after three rounds of scanning, the first number is automatically dialed, making this phone ideal for emergency situations. The phone also has voice-activated answering, a person can use it as a standard speakerphone, and it can accommodate a headset.[25]

## *Home Management*

Home management is considered a work activity and consists of clothing care, cleaning, meal preparation and cleanup, shopping, money management, household maintenance, and safety procedures.[4] Some management tasks are complex and involve multiple physical components.

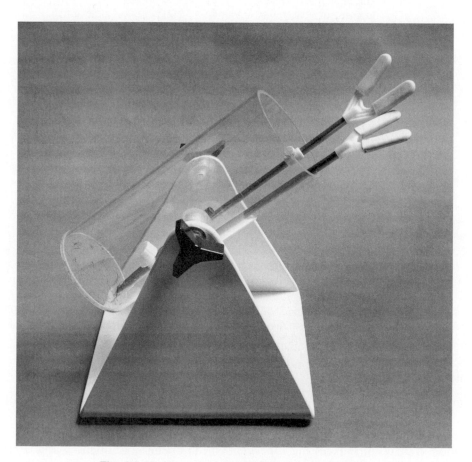

**Fig. 25-13** The swivel mouthstick docking station.

TABLE 25-1

*Various Uses of Mouthsticks and Possible Setups*

| Task | Mouthsticks | Possible Setup |
|------|-------------|----------------|
| Phone use | Wand<br>Protracting tip<br>Bendable mouthstick<br>Implement holder with eraser tip<br>Extensions for independence with rubber tip | Gooseneck phone holder<br>Phone flipper<br>Speaker phone |
| Page turning | Wand<br>Bendable page turner<br>Extensions for independence with rubber tip<br>Vacuum wand<br>Implement holder with eraser tip | Reading material placed on flat surface (table/laptray) or book holder |
| Moving papers on a desktop | Extensions for independence with rubber tip<br>Implement holder with eraser tip<br>Bendable page turner<br>Wand<br>Vacuum wand | Level, uncluttered work surface |
| Writing | Extensions for independence with pen tip<br>Implement holder with pen, marker, or pencil | Pen/pencil or marker tipped mouthstick<br>Book holder<br>Paper secured by tape or clipboard |
| Typing | Protracting tip<br>Wand<br>Bendable page turner<br>Implement holder with eraser tip<br>Extensions for independence with rubber tip | Keyboard positioned at an angle<br>Mind keyboard or sensitive touch keyboard<br>"Sticky keys" activated |
| Playing cards | Vertical pincher<br>Straight or bent mouthstick with straight pin secured at the tip | Cards held by card holder<br>Holes punched in each card<br>Cards held by card holder |
| Painting | Implement holder with paintbrush<br>Extensions for independence with paintbrush tip | Easel<br>Properly positioned paints |
| Remote buttons on ECU or TV/VCR | Protracting tip<br>Bendable wand<br>Implement holder with eraser tip<br>Extensions for independence with rubber tip | Laptray or overbed table<br>Book holder used for proper angle if needed |
| Elevator buttons/ automatic doors | Protracting tip<br>Bendable or wand<br>Implement holder with eraser tip<br>Extensions for independence with rubber tip | Properly positioned docking station secured onto wheelchair |

*Courtesy Extensions for Independence, 555 Saturn Blvd, Suite B-368, San Diego, CA, 92154, 619-423-7709; Adlib Inc, 5142 Balsa Ave, Suite 106, Huntington Beach, CA, 92649, 714-895-9529.*

## Cooking Aids

To complete cooking tasks, a number of products are available that will assist an individual who has use of one hand or decreased hand function. Cutting boards designed with corner guards enable users to push food against them for support. Food spikes can hold food in place for safe cutting. One-handed can openers, jar openers, and vegetable peelers are available. A pan holder stabilizes a pan on the stove to ease stirring for a person, and a suction bottle-brush can assist a person with washing dishes. A variety of adapted knives are available to assist persons with a weak grip, arthritic deformities, or use of one-hand. Jar openers range from nonslip Dycem pads to wall-mounted electric jar openers. These devices are designed to assist with a variety of disabilities ranging from limited use of two hands to arthritis. Other miscellaneous devices designed to help individuals with limited upper extremity functions in the kitchen include items to help open a soda can or bottle, milk cartons, boxes, close zipper bags, or seal food packages. A person can often use convenience devices such as blenders, food processors, grinders, mixers, table-top toasters, oven/broilers, and microwave ovens to perform otherwise difficult tasks and to save time and energy in the kitchen.

### Reachers

Reachers can extend a person's functional reach. Used to pick up items from the floor or cabinets, a person can use reachers for dressing tasks as well. A variety of reachers have been designed to meet individual needs. The basic reacher consists of a trigger end that a person grasps, a shaft of various lengths, and a pincher end, which grasps the desired item. After grasping the item, the user holds the trigger and pulls the item into reach.

### Wall Switches

Wall switch extenders consist of a plastic rod or plate that extend 6 to 12 inches below an existing wall switch. They allow a wheelchair user or an individual with limited upper extremity ROM to operate a wall switch without raising an arm. Rocker-type light switches are commercially available at most hardware stores. These can provide a large switch activation surface area. An outlet extender raises an existing outlet within reach of a wheelchair user or an individual with limited bending capabilities.

### Miscellaneous Household Helpers

Key holders, doorknob turners, plug pullers, and tap turners are also available to ease specialized tasks.[26]

## Unique Homemaking Equipment

### JarPop

JarPop is a device that the Fred Sammons catalog offers, which assists in releasing the vacuum inside of an unopened jar. This release makes opening the jar easier for the user.

### Open Up

Open Up electric jar and bottle opener mounts under the cabinet and allows for easy jar or bottle opening for an individual who has use of only one hand or limited hand function. When the user presses a jar or bottle lid into the cone-shaped mechanism, the motor turns the cone, thereby opening the container.

### The Electric Iron Safety Guard

The Electric Iron Safety Guard can help reduce the risk of burns while a person is ironing. A person with sensory or visual deficits can use the safety guard to guide the movement of the iron without the risk of getting burned. This device is made of two plastic rods that surround the edges of the iron.[27]

### The Etwall Compact Trolley

The Etwall Compact Trolley is a small-wheeled cart that helps a person transport hot or heavy items from one surface to another. It features a compact size and a conveniently located push handle for the ambulatory user.

## *Child Care*

Parenthood is an exciting experience filled with joy and frustrations. For parents with disabilities, frustrations are often compounded by physical limitations. *Child care* refers to the tasks involved with persons providing for children, such as giving physical care, nurturing, communication, and doing age-appropriate activities.[4] All parents receive support from many people to help them raise their children, including grandparents and other relatives, babysitters, and teachers. Parents with disabilities may need the additional assistance of others for personal care tasks such as bathing, dressing, and feeding. Childcare adaptations should be considered for the parents with disabilities and relatives and friends with disabilities.

Most of the equipment in this section will benefit those with young children. As the child grows, a person's need for self-care equipment decreases and the need for disciplinary measures and cooperative behavior increases. This section includes equipment and adaptation ideas that are readily available or easily fabricated. Often times, household adaptations or readily available infant/toddler products can assist a disabled individual perform a component of child care more easily. Standard infant/toddler products are available through mail order catalogs or general retail outlets.[28-29] The user and, if possible, an occupational therapist should assess functional application of the equipment before purchase to meet specific needs. Two excellent resources for fabricated equipment to meet specific needs is *Adaptive Parenting Equipment: Idea Book*[30] and *Adaptive Baby Care Equipment: Guidelines, Prototypes & Resources.*[30a] These resources illustrate items that have been specially fabricated to provide solutions to common problems that parents with disabilities face.

## Furniture

### Cribs
Several options are illustrated in the idea book for parents who are wheelchair users. A crib is also commercially available which features swing out gates.[31] For an ambulatory parent with limited use on one side, a standard crib's side locks can be replaced with magnetic childproofing locks. A foot-released crib may also be helpful.

### Changing Tables
A desk or table can be set up as the changing and dressing area with a changing pad and organizational dividers to hold diapering and dressing supplies. The user should secure the changing pad to the table or desk surface, which should include a safety strap.

### Feeding Equipment
A user can place a bouncy chair or infant carrier on a secure table or the floor to help position a child for feedings. High chairs with a swing-away tray or one-handed release latch are also available.

### Bathing
The user can place infant bath seats in a sink for easy access or position them on a stable table near a water source. A person uses bath seats in the bathtub, which can provide some positioning and stabilization assistance. Either way, a person should never leave a child in the tub without supervision.

## Childproofing

Childproofing is a difficult task for some parents with disabilities. They must consider that by blocking the child's access to a drawer, cabinet, or room they may be blocking access for themselves. Several types of latches are available to keep children from opening cabinets and drawers. The Tot-Lok system uses a magnetic "key" to open the latch. A person can easily manipulate or mount this key into a splint.

## Transport

A person can use a bassinet with wheels, a stroller, or wagon to transport an infant from each room within the home. The wheelchair user can wrap half moon-shaped cushions around the waist, which may provide the needed support for an infant or toddler to lay or sit on the lap. The wheelchair user can wear a "fanny pack" filled with towels to provide a cushion or seat for a child with adequate trunk control. Slings and baby carriers allow a person to carry a child in a variety of positions, which assist the ambulatory parent who has adequate balance but use of only one arm or who must use a cane or crutch. A wheelchair user also can use these devices to support children on the lap. Once the child can sit up independently, a wheelchair user also can use a common easy-locking luggage strap as an additional "seat belt" for the child sitting on the lap. If a child is wearing overall-type clothing, the parent can feed the seat belt through the straps. The parent must take care to ensure the buttons or snaps are secure and that the front portion is not near the child's neck.

## Feeding

### Bottles

The user should stabilize a bottle before pouring liquid in it by placing it in a coffee mug. By using liquid formula, the person can eliminate the need to manipulate powders. Newer models of bottles are available that keep the formula and water separated until use. With the twist of the cap, the user releases the formula can serve it without further manipulation, which is helpful when traveling or for nighttime feedings. If powdered formula is used, a person can use a plastic food container to store the formula in premeasured portions. The person can make these portions ahead of time to ease the task of manipulating formula. For nighttime feedings, the person can mix premeasured water and formula at the bedside, or the person can keep a minirefrigerator or bottle cooler at bedside. The person can then use an electric bottle warmer to warm the bottle, which eliminates the need to get out of bed to prepare a bottle. The bottle warming system keeps two bottles cool and can warm a bottle.

### Breastfeeding

Breastfeeding is ideal because it eliminates the need for a person to prepare, manage, and clean bottles. Proper positioning can create a relaxing environment and help eliminate a person's problems with fatigue. A number of commercially available cradle-style carriers can help hold the child in position if the mother prefers to sit in a chair while feeding. The mother can prop pillows up to hold the infant while breastfeeding when sitting or laying down. Special pillows designed to make breastfeeding more comfortable also are available. Pillows for mothers with twins have a larger lap surface area and may be particularly helpful for persons with disabilities. Assistance from a lactation consultant can assist if positioning or latching problems and questions exist.

### Solid Foods

Once the mother introduces solid foods, Velcro bibs may be easier to manipulate than a draw string bib. An oversized t-shirt can also serve as a bib. A person can purchase multiple types of jar openers to assist with opening baby food jars.

## Diapers

Diaper wraps designed for use with cloth diapers can cover cloth and disposable diapers. They are available with Velcro closures, and a person can make loops out of webbing material. A person can add plastic D-rings for the individual who has limited hand function. A person can use a diaper service to deliver and pick up a week's supply of cloth diapers, which results in fewer grocery and garbage items but requires more frequent diaper changes. Disposable diapers are available with Velcro closures that allow less frequent diaper changes but add groceries and more garbage.

## Outcomes and Social Validation

Multiple studies have shown that people are using adaptive equipment in the home at percentages ranging from 29% to 86% of the time.[32-35] Reasons for discarding equipment include "improved physical function" and "alternative solutions found."[33] Careful consideration of when and where to issue equipment could effect the use of equipment at home. Gitlin and Burgh[36] identified six considerations therapists used when issuing an assistive device during the rehabilitative stage. They found therapists first identified the correct equipment based on patient-focused considerations such as physical abilities and interests and functional importance and external factors such as device characteristics, availability, and payment concerns. The next steps involved matching the equipment with an appropriate activity, timing the introduction, instructing about the device, and reinforcing its use.

In the end, equipment use is a personal choice influenced by convenience, functionality, and improvement of quality of life. One issue therapists often face is helping people find a balance between achieving a high level of functional independence and the quality of their time and effort. Functionality and time influence on quality of life in individual ways. An example is a man with a C6 spinal cord injury who can dress himself using a variety of activities of daily living (ADL) equipment. For him, this task consumes almost an hour. With the help of another person, he could complete it in 10 to 15 minutes. To him, this independence in completing his morning routine adds quality to his life. However, to another individual with a similar injury, this hour adds up to time and energy the person would rather spend at work, with kids, or at leisure. These are personal choices individuals must make when considering the way the adaptive equipment will add to their abilities. The equipment may be as simple as a buttonhook or as complex as an automatic feeder. Successful use of equipment is a personal decision and depends on the way it effects a person's quality of life.

## CASE STUDY

### CASE 1

K.G. was a 28-year-old woman with MD that resulted in generalized weakness in all extremities and endurance limitations. She was unable to lift her arms above her head but could reach her mouth if something supported her elbow. She had full ROM in her hands, but her grasp was weak. K.G. was disabled since birth and described herself as a "gadget junkie." She lived in an accessible condominium with her parents who shared responsibilities of personal care with her personal care attendant. K.G. worked part time at an insurance company.

K.G. drove her powered wheelchair with a standard joystick. She received assistance for dressing because she said, "It would take me all day and I have more important things to do." She liked to wear clothes designed specifically for wheelchair users because they were more comfortable. She groomed herself in her accessible bathroom. She used a battery-operated toothbrush to compensate for her upper-extremity weakness. "A friend designed a strap that helps hold the toothbrush in my hand," she reported. To care for her hair, she used another practical approach, "I use a long-handled comb and keep my hair short because it's easier." K.G. used a shower chair for bathing. A long-handled sponge and liquid soap allowed her to independently bathe her arms, torso, and legs. She received assistance to wash her hair and back. A long-handled utensil and straw helped with eating. "Everything I drink is through a straw, even hot tea," she said. "I have someone else cut meat for me; I've tried rocking knifes but they take too much time and effort."

Most of her gadgets help her around the house. A reacher helped pick items off the floor. A plastic light extender allowed her to operate the wall switch. A short dowel rod with a rubber pencil grip at the end helped her turn on her computer and feed paper into the printer. She used a portable desktop with a beanbag bottom designed for reading books (available at most large bookstores) to support items such as the telephone, a laptop computer, or a drink while she sat in bed. She used a speakerphone for some of her phone calls tend attached a phone in her room to a gooseneck phone holder for private phone conversations. K.G. said the following[37]:

It's the little things that can sometimes make a big difference. Like a tab grabber for a can of soda. I've always hated that these were marketed as a luxury for women to prevent nail breakage. For me, it gives me the leverage I need to open a soda by myself. Whether it's finishing school, getting my first job, or problem solving something as simple as opening a can of soda myself, nothing replaces the feeling of accomplishment.

# References

1.  Batavia AI, Hammer GS: Toward the development of consumer-based criteria for the evaluation of assistive devices, *J Rehab Res Dev* 27 (4): 425-436, 1990.
2.  Kohlmeyer KM: Assistive and adaptive equipment. In Hopkins H, Smith H, editors: *Willard and Spackman's occupational therapy*, ed 8, pp 316-320, Philadelphia, 1993, JB Lippincott.
3.  American Occupational Therapy Association: Uniform terminology for occupational therapy, ed 3, *Am J Occup Ther* 48 (11): 1047-1054, 1994.
4.  American Occupational Therapy Association: Uniform terminology for occupational therapy, ed 3, *Am J Occup Ther* 48 (11): 1047-1054, 1994.
5.  Jaeco Orthopedic Specialties, P.O. Box 75, Hot Springs, AR 71902, 501-623-5944; also Fred Sammons.
6.  JC Penney Home Health Care and Easy Dressing Catalog, P.O. Box 2021, Milwaukee, WI, 53201-2021, 800-222-6161.
7.  RD Equipment, Inc, 230 Percizal Dr, Barnstable, MA, 02668, 508-362-7498.
8.  Warren Technologies, 2008 Spring Rd, Stoughton, WI, 53589, 608-249-1234.
9.  Hoyer Chrome Bath lift, Guardian Products Inc, 4175 Guardian St, Simi Valley, CA, 93013, 800-255-5022.
10. CM Assist Lift & Transfer System, Columbus McKinnon Corporation, Mobility Products Division, 140 John Hames Audubon Parkway, Amherst, NY 14228-1197, 800-888-0985; SureHands, Handi-Move International, Pine Island, NY 10969, 800-724-5305; Barrier Free Lifts, 9230 Prince William St, Manassas, VA 22110, 800-582-8732.
11. Peri Wash Body Cleanser, Bedside Care.
12. Clarke Healthcare Products Inc, PIIP-ICM building, 1003 International Drive, Oakdale, PA 15071-9223, 412-695-2122.
13. AliMed obese equipment section, AliMed, Inc, 297 High Street, Dedham, MA 02026, 800-225-2610.
14. Innovative Medical Incorporated, P.O. Box 4780, Overland Park, KA 66204, 913-642-5106.
15. Floss Aid, Maddok, Inc, Pequannock, NJ, 07440-4926, 800-443-4926.
16. Turn around Universal Holder, Maddok, Inc.
17. Pistol Grip Remote Tocnail Clipper, Maddok, Inc.
18. Touch Turner, 443 View Ridge Dr, Everett, WA 98203, 206-252-1541.
19. HiTech Group International, 8160 Madison, Burr Ridge, IL 60521, 800-288-8303.
20. Tech-Able, Inc, 1112A Brett Dr, Conyers, GA 30094, 770-922-6768.
21. LS&S Group, P.O. Box 673, Northbrook, IL 60065, 800-468-4789, and most computer hardware stores.
22. AliMed Inc, 297 High Street, Dedham, MA 02026, 800-225-2610.
23. LS&S Group, P.O. Box 673, Northbrook, IL 60065, 800-468-4789.
24. Maddok, Inc, Pequannock, NJ 07440-4926, 800-443-4926.
25. Ameriphone, Inc, 12082 Western Ave, Garden Grove, GA 92841, 800-874-3005.
26. Plug Puller, Maddak, Inc.
27. Electric Iron Safety Guard, Maddak, Inc.
28. The Right Start, Right Start Plaza, 5334 Sterling Center Drive, Westlake Village, CA 91361-4627, 800-548-8531.
29. One Step Ahead, P.O. Box 517, Lake Bluff, IL 60044, 800-274-8440.
30. DeMoss A et al: *Adaptive parenting equipment: idea book I*, Berkeley, Calif, 1995, Through the Looking Glass.
30a. Vensand K et al: *Adaptive baby care equipment: guidelines, prototypes & resources*, Berkeley, Calif, 2000, Through the Looking Glass.
31. 5-1 Safety Converting Crib, Babee Tenda, 123 S. Belmont Blvd., Kansas City, Mo 64123, 816-231-2300.
32. Bynum H, Rogers JC: The use and effectiveness of assistive devices possessed by patients seen in home care, *Occup Ther J Res* 3:181-191, 1987.

33. Garber SL, Gregorio TL: Upper extremity devices: assessment of use by spinal cord-injured patient with quadriplegia, *Am J Occup Ther* 44:126-131, 1990.
34. Geiger CM: The utilization of assistive devices by patients discharged from an acute rehabilitation setting, *Phys Occup Ther Geriatr* 9 (1):3-25, 1990.
35. Rogers JC, Figone JJ: Traumatic quadriplegia: follow-up study of self-care skills, *Arch Phys Med Rehab* 61:316-321, 1980.
36. Gitlin LN, Burgh D: Issuing assistive devices to older patients in rehabilitation: an exploratory study, *Am J Occup Ther* 49:994-1000, 1995.
37. KG interview, Chicago, 1996.

## Resources

Adlib, Inc, 5142 Balsa Ave, Suite 106, Huntington Beach, CA 92649, 714-895-9529.

AliMed, Inc, 297 High Street, Dedham, MA 02026, 800-225-2610.

Ameriphone, Inc, 12082 Western Ave, Garden Grove, GA 92841, 800-874-3005.

Clarke Healthcare Products, Inc, PIIP-ICM building, 1003 International Drive, Oakdale, PA 15071-9223, 412-695-2122.

CM Assist Lift & Transfer System, Columbus McKinnon Corporation, Mobility Products Division, 140 John Hames Audubon Parkway, Amherst, NY 14228-1197, 800-888-0985.

Extensions for Independence, 555 Saturn Blvd, Suite B-368, San Diego, CA 92154, 619-423-7709.

Guardian Products, Inc, 4175 Guardian St, Simi Valley, CA 93013, 800-255-5022.

HiTec Group International, 8160 Madison Burr Ridge, IL 60521, 800-288-8303.

Innovative Medical Inc, P.O. Box 4780 Overland Park, KS 66204, 913-642-5106.

JC Penney Home Health Care and Easy Dressing Catalog, P.O. Box 2021, Milwaukee, WI 53201-2021, 800-222-6161.

LS&S Group, P.O. Box 673, Northbrook, IL 60065, 800-468-4789.

Maddok, Inc, Pequannock, NJ 07440-4926, 800-4926.

North Coast Medical, Inc, 187 Stauffer Boulevard, San Jose, CA 95125-1042, 800-821-9319.

One Step Ahead, P.O. Box 517, Lake Bluff, IL 60044, 800-274-8440.

R.D. Equipment, Inc, 230 Percizal Dr, Barnstable, MA 02668, 508-362-7498.

Sammons Preston, Inc, P.O. Box 5071, Bolingbrook, IL 60440-5071, 800-547-4333.

Smith & Nephew Rolyan, One Quality Drive, P.O. Box 1005, Germantown, WI 53022-8205, 800-558-8633.

SureHands, Handi-Move International, Pine Island, NY, 800-724-5305; Barrier Free Lifts, 9230 Prince William St, Manassas, VA 22110, 800-582-8732.

Tech-Able, Inc, 1112A Brett Dr, Conyers, GA 30094, 770-922-6768.

The Right Start, Right Start Plaza, 5334 Sterling Center Drive, Westlake Village, CA 91361-4627, 800-548-8531.

Touch Turner, 443 View Ridge Dr, Everett, WA 98203, 206-252-1541.

Warren Technologies, 2008 Spring Rd, Stoughton, WI 53589, 608-249-1234.

# CHAPTER 26

## Recreation and Play Environments

*Susan M. Goltsman*

## Application and Goal

A quality play and learning environment is more than just a collection of play equipment. The entire site with all its elements—from vegetation to storage—can become a play and learning resource for all children whether they have disabilities or not.

Play is more than having fun. It is a process through which children develop their physical, mental, and social skills. It is value laden and culturally based. In the past, most of these play experiences occurred in unstructured places that children chose. Depending on the types and severities of disabilities and the attitudes of parents, children with disabilities had less access to these free-range play settings in the neighborhood and had limited choices for usable play settings. Today, however, because of working parents and safety concerns for children after school, informal play happens in created, designated areas. These play areas are usually attached to public settings and private institutions, such as schools, parks, housing, and shopping centers. Although this setting is more controlled and less natural, more opportunities for children with disabilities should exist because it is intentionally created.

A good play area that is designed to integrate children with and without disabilities consists of a range of settings carefully layered onto a site. The settings contain one or more of the following elements: entrances, pathways, fences and enclosures, signs, play equipment, game areas, land forms and topography, trees and vegetation, gardens, animal habitats, water and sand play areas, loose parts, gathering places, stage areas, storage places, and ground covering and safety surfacing (Figure 26-1). In any play area design, each play setting varies in importance, depending on community values, site constraints, and location. The way people use these elements also determines the degree of accessibility and integration possible in that environment. However, in designing a play space of any size, designers must consider the full range of settings.

Diversity and opportunities within the setting are the keys to integration and access in a play area. To be developmental, play must present a challenge as part of its value and every part of the environment should not be expected to be physically accessible to every user. Therefore a play area must support a range of challenges that are mental and physical. Physical challenge within the play area must be part of a progression of challenges that foster an individual's skill.

Conversely, the available social experience must be accessible to all people (Figure 26-2). Unlike a physical challenge, which a child must earn through effort to be developmental, the opportunity for social interaction should be easy. Social integration is the basic reason a play area must be accessible to children of all abilities. If the play area truly services a range of users, then it is considered universally designed.

## Function and Ability

The use of assistive technology (AT) in a play area is primarily considered part of the whole design. AT in terms of a play area would be considered design elements, such as a transfer deck or handholds or a raised area to provide access to a sand or water play area.

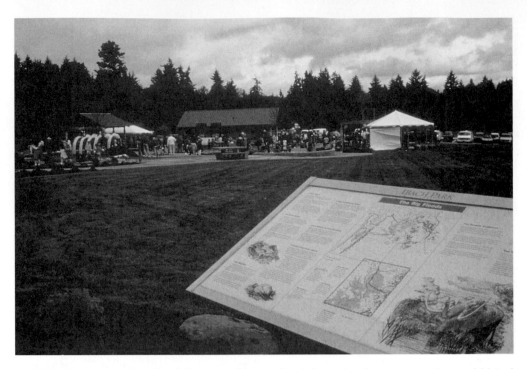

**Fig. 26-1** An interpretive sign informs residents about the natural resource value and historic context of the site.

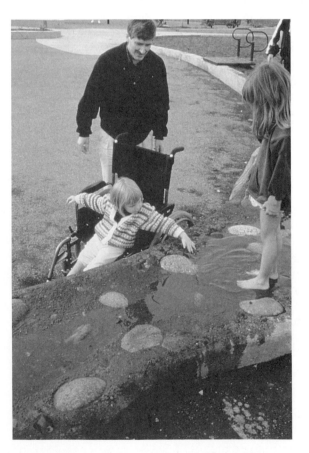

**Fig. 26-2** One side of the waterway is at ground level; the other side is at side reach height for a child who uses a wheelchair.

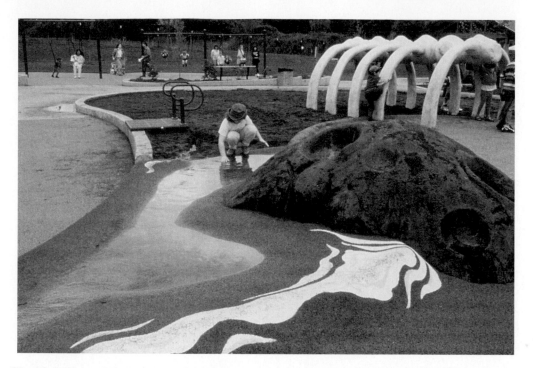

**Fig. 26-3** The water goes around the meteor and drops into the sand. Behind the child, off to the left, is a transfer platform that facilitates a transfer from a wheelchair into the sand.

Provision of a multilayered play area provides opportunities for children who have varying abilities to interact and learn from each other. These types of elements help the play setting to be usable by a wider variety of children, promoting universal design.

Many different designers such as landscape architects, therapeutic recreation specialists, and landscape contractors create a universally designed play area integrating the needs of all children into play area design. Diverse physical and social environments are key to achieving this (Figure 26-3). Obtaining physical diversity means placing a broad range of challenges within the play setting. Doing this allows more children to participate, make choices, take on challenges, develop skills, and, most importantly, have fun together.

Social diversity is closely linked to physical diversity. Contact among children of different abilities naturally increases in play areas that are open to a wider spectrum of users. This interaction is particularly critical for children with functional limitations who are often denied these social experiences. Although every part of a play area may not be physically accessible to all, the social experience must be.

## Considerations and Options

To create an integrated play area, designers must keep the following ideas in mind:

- Consider the many ways in which children of different abilities can interact.
- When arranging the play area, integrate accessible play equipment with the rest of the play setting. Placing less challenging activities directly next to those requiring greater physical ability will encourage interaction among all users.

Provide an accessible route that connects every activity area and every accessible play component in the play setting. (A play component is an item that provides an opportunity for play. It can be a single piece of equipment or part of a larger composite structure.) Although not every play component will be physically accessible to everyone, enabling all children to be near the action provides the opportunity, choice, and possibility to communicate with others. This is a major step toward integration.

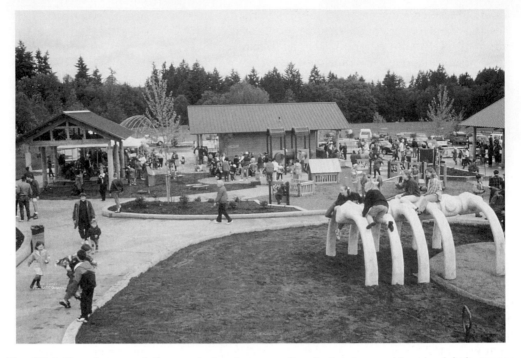

**Fig. 26-4** The ribcage of the mastodon has one rib missing to provide wheelchair access through and under the structure. A rubber surface connects with the sand to allow the wheelchair user access to the structure.

Ensure that at least one of each kind of play component on the ground is accessible and usable by children with mobility disabilities. Likewise, at least half of the play components elevated above ground should be accessible. Access on and off of equipment can be eased with ramps, transfer platforms, or other appropriate methods of access. Remember that ramps and transfer systems can also serve as physical challenges and should be designed so that they add to the play environment's diversity.

Make sand play accessible by providing raised sand areas or installing a transfer system into the sand (Figure 26-4). Note that raised sand areas, which provide space underneath for wheelchairs, provide severely limited play experiences because the necessary clearance keeps the sand depth at a minimum. Providing a transfer system into the sand area will allow users to enjoy full-body sand play.

Make portions of gathering places accessible to promote social interaction. These areas are important areas of interaction and allow groups of people to play, eat, watch, socialize, and congregate. Include accessible seating, such as benches with backrests and arm supports, so that people of varying abilities can sit together.

Follow safety guidelines that outline important parameters such as head entrapments, safety surfacing, and use zones. At times, however, provisions for safety and accessibility can conflict. For example, a raised sand shelf could be considered hazardous because the shelf is 30 inches off the ground. To strictly follow the safety requirements, a non-climbable enclosure along the edge of the shelf would have to be constructed, which would defeat the whole purpose of the design. In such cases, seek solutions that provide other means of access or that mitigate the safety hazard, such as installing rubber safety surfacing on the ground below the shelf.

## Technology

A universally designed play setting is not high tech; it is design tech. The AT is more in the realm of good anthropometric data, user-based design guidelines and performance criteria, accessible components, such as transfer systems for manufactured equipment, and firm, resilient surfacing. The options for a designer creating a universally designed play area are all based on low technology, innovative thinking, and problem solving. Certain design solutions, especially new ones, may require a designer and manufacturer to fabricate and manufacture in a state-of-the-art factory. They should share ideas in the manufacture of play components. Users, designers, and manufacturers can work together to advance this relatively new area of environmental design.

## Accessible Routes of Travel within a Play Setting

Because play is primarily a social experience, accessible routes through a play setting must connect all types of activities. A path that connects the accessible play elements within a play-area setting is essential. Without this connection, children with disabilities can be too easily isolated from their friends who do not have disabilities. The accessible route within a play setting avoids problems caused by circulation design flaws and promotes social interaction. The surface of the route must be firm, stable, slip resistant, safe to crawl on, within the use zone of equipment, and resilient as described by the American Society for Testing and Materials (ASTM F1292) performance standard.

Many routes through the space contribute to a good play setting. A route may be the play experience. Pathways can support wheeled toys, running games, and exploration and can be play elements. To be accessible, pathways require good surfaces and correct grades (1 up to 20) and cross slopes (2% or less.) The quality of the pathway system sets the tone for the environment. Pathways can be wide with small branches, long and straight, or circuitous and meandering. Each type creates different play behaviors and experiences. Minimum routes or auxiliary pathways through a play experience are exempt from the strict requirements of the primary accessible route of travel. Therefore they can promote the range of challenges necessary for a variety of developmentally appropriate play experiences.

If an auxiliary pathway is less than 100 feet, it does not have to conform to accessible route requirements. Where items of equipment are used to provide more than one similar play activity and they are located next to each other, a minimum of one piece of the play equipment is required to be accessible for the primary, intended use of the activity. For example, if four swings are in a group, one must be on accessible surfacing so that persons who require a firm and stable safety surface can approach it. Where more than one of the same piece of play equipment exists but are not in close proximity and persons are to use them for the same purpose, each should be accessible. If a firm, stable, slip-resistant surface is not provided over the entire surface of the play setting, then criteria for accessible route design applies (Box 26-1).

## Play Equipment

Most equipment settings stimulate large muscle activity and kinesthetic experience, but they can also support non-physical aspects of child development. Equipment can provide opportunities to experience height and can serve as landmarks to assist orientation and wayfinding. They may also become rendezvous spots, stimulate social interaction and provide hideaways in hiding and chasing games. Small, semi-enclosed spaces support dramatic play, and seating, shelves, and tables encourage social play. Designers should consider many factors when choosing manufactured play equipment for a recreation area (Box 26-2).

Play equipment is designed to provide physical challenge and social interaction. For equipment to be appropriate for different skill levels, it must offer graduated challenge opportunities. Access up to, onto, through, and off equipment should also provide a variety of challenges appropriate to the ages of intended users.

### Access onto Elevated Play Equipment

Ramps onto play equipment are play components, and designers must design them to fit into the play structure. If the play equipment or play area as a whole has more than 20 elevated play activities, then a ramp is required to access a minimum of one half of the play

## BOX 26-1

*Accessible Route Design*

1. An accessible route must be provided to and for the intended use of the different activities within the play area.
2. The accessible route should be a minimum of 60 inches wide but can be narrowed to 36 inches if it is in conjunction with a play activity.
3. The cross slope of the accessible route of travel should not exceed 1:50.
4. The slope of the accessible route of travel should not exceed 1:20.
5. If the slope exceeds 1:20, it is a ramp. A ramp on the accessible route of travel on the ground plane should not exceed a slope of 1:16. All other ramp conditions found in ADAAG apply except for the handrail requirements. Ramps onto play equipment are exempt from this requirement.
6. If the accessible route of travel is adjacent to loose fill material or if a drop exists, then the edge of the pathway should be treated to protect a wheelchair from falling off the route and into the loose fill material. This can be accomplished by beveling the edge with a slope that does not exceed 30%. A raised edge will create a trip hazard for walking children. If this route is within the use zone of the play equipment, the path and the edge treatment should be made of safety surfacing that meets ASTM F1292.
7. Changes in level along the path should not exceed ½ inch.
8. Where egress from an accessible play activity occurs in loose fill surface that is not firm, stable, and slip resistant, a means of returning to the point of access for that play activity should be provided. Also, the surfacing material should not splinter, scrape, puncture, or abrade the skin when being crawled on.
9. Auxiliary pathways should have a minimum width of 36 inches. If this 36-inch wide route is longer than 100 feet, a 60-inch turn-around area must be present in which two wheelchair users can pass every 100 feet. For play purposes, an auxiliary path may be textured or bumpy for a maximum length of 20 feet. Any texture may be used. Grades can be extreme, and bumps will be determined by safety, not accessibility. Vegetation may overhang the pathway below 80 inches, but the vegetation must not be woody or thorny as that may puncture or abrade the skin.

component on the structure or structures. One half of those components that are accessible by ramp should be similar to those elevated components that are not accessible by ramp. A ramp longer than 12 feet is a spatial and visual imposition on the landscape and cannot be effectively integrated into the play opportunities. Ramps also may become barriers to play because they can constrict circulation and flow. At this time, a ramp is the only known safe way that a child who cannot leave the wheelchair can access elevated equipment.

If the width of the ramp is 60 inches or greater, then all ADAAG requirements apply except for the handrail requirements. Criteria apply if ramp width is less than 60 inches (Box 26-3).

### Transferring onto Equipment

People in wheelchairs may transfer themselves onto play equipment at a transfer platform. A transfer platform is one way to access equipment by leaving a wheelchair. The transfer platform must be on an accessible path of travel. A designer must provide a clear, level area or turning space on one side of the transfer platform to allow for a front or side transfer (Box 26-4).

### Equipment and Play Components on the Ground

In the place equipment is provided on the ground, children with disabilities must be able to access and use at least one of each similar play activity. The accessible play activities on the ground should be adjacent to an accessible route of travel. A surface that is firm, and stable, and slip resistant, and in which within the use zone of the equipment is resilient as described by the ASTM F1292 performance standard, should surround an accessible

## BOX 26-2

*Play Equipment Considerations*

1. Properly selected equipment can support the development of creativity and coopera- tion, especially structures that incorporate sand and water play. Play structures can be converted to other temporary uses such as stage settings. Loose parts can be strung from and attached to the equipment for backdrops or banners for special events and dramatic play activities. Equipment settings must be designed as part of a comprehen- sive multipurpose play environment because isolated pieces of equipment are ineffec- tive.
2. Equipment should be properly sited, selected, and installed over appropriate shock- absorbing surfaces. Procedures and standards for equipment purchase, installation, and maintenance must be developed. A systematic safety inspection program must be implemented. Site and program supervision standards must also be developed, and accident and incident records must be kept. Parents and caregivers must be warned about the dangers of strangulation when loose clothing gets caught on equipment and about the effect of extreme weather on equipment and surfacing safety.
3. A number of well-documented safety issues exist related to manufactured play equip- ment. Falls, entrapments, protrusions, collisions, and splinters have all occurred. These issues must be addressed in the design, maintenance, and supervision of the play equipment. ASTM has a set of standards that are the standard of care of the United States. These are ASTM 14 for play equipment and ASTM 1292 for protective surfacing under play equipment.
4. Equipment should be accessible but must be designed primarily for children, not wheel- chairs. Transfer points should always be marked visually and tactually. Take care not to create hazards when providing access, for instance, adding ramps that can be used for skate boarding. Using synthetic surfacing can provide access to, under, and through the equipment for children in wheelchairs. Getting to be in the center of the action may be as important as climbing to the highest point for some children.
5. Play equipment provides opportunities for integration, especially when programmed with other activities. Play settings should be exciting and attractive for parents and chil- dren. Adults accompany children to the park or playground more often now than in the past; therefore designing for parents using wheelchairs is equally important.

## BOX 26-3

*Criteria for Ramp Width Less Than 60 Inches*

1. Minimum width must be 36 inches.
2. Cross slope must not exceed 1:50.
3. Running slope must not exceed 1:12.
4. Ramp run or length must not exceed 12 feet.
5. Landings at bottom and top of ramp run should be a minimum of 60 inches in diameter.
6. Landings that contain play activities should include a minimum of 30 inches by 48 inches of clear space where a wheelchair user may park and play at the component. A parked wheelchair must not reduce the circulation path to less than 36 inches.
7. The edges of ramps and landings should have a means of preventing wheelchairs from falling off the landing.
8. Handrails should be provided on each side of the ramp at 26 to 28 inches above the ramp surface.
9. Where ramp access is provided to an elevated play component, wheelchair parking spaces may overlap with turning space.

ground level play activity. When children crawl on surface material, it should not cut, scrape, or abrade the skin.

The place play activities provide the same experience and are near each other, people must be able to access a minimum of one. In recognition of the diversity of equipment that a designer can place on the ground in a play area and the need to promote social in-

BOX 26-4

*Specifications for Transferring onto Equipment*

1. The deck used as a transfer platform should be 11 to 14 inches above the ground when designed for use by children who are 2 to 5 years old and 14 to 17 inches above the ground when designed for use by children who are 5 to 12 years old.
2. The minimum clear width of the deck used in the transfer system should be 24 inches, and the minimum depth of the platform should be 14 inches.
3. A means to assist the child in transferring, such as a grab bar or handhold, should be provided.
4. Adjacent steps or decks from the transfer platform that are used to move through the equipment should have a maximum rise of 6 inches for children under 5 years old and a maximum rise of 8 inches for children over 5 years old.
5. Decked platforms may be used in the transfer system as transfer platforms or with transfer platforms (steps) to provide access.
6. The transfer system must be made of a material that will not cut, scrape, or burn the skin when children slide over it.
7. A minimum of one 30-inch by 48-inch wheelchair parking space should be provided adjacent to the transfer platform off of the route of travel. Wheelchair parking spaces may overlap with turning spaces. The parking space at the transfer platform should accommodate a minimum of one wheelchair and should not reduce the circulation path to less than 36 inches. If additional parking spaces are added, each one should be 30 inches wide by 48 inches long and should be adjacent to the accessible route of travel.
8. A space that allows a wheelchair to turn around should be provided at the base of the transfer platform. The turning space should be off the accessible route of travel and have a clear space of 60 inches in diameter or a T-shaped area.
9. Berms or natural hills may be used to provide an accessible route of travel up to and onto the equipment. These features must conform to applicable safety standards.

teraction while not unnecessarily duplicating play components, only one of each type of component on the ground needs to be accessible.

## Equipment and Play Activities Elevated above the Surface

A larger play structure is defined as having 20 or more elevated play components. The place 20 or more elevated play components on a composite structure appear or the place 20 or more elevated play components at one site serving the same age group appear, people will need a ramp and transfer system.

Many play areas, such as those in home daycare centers and restaurants, are small, have limited space, and cannot accommodate a ramp. Therefore the number of play activities on a structure is a means of determining the size of the structure. A total of 20 elevated play components seems to be in the range for a midsized composite play structure that will have enough space around it to accommodate a ramp and enough space on it to accommodate larger numbers of children.

A designer does not need to duplicate every elevated play activity that people cannot directly access by ramp at a level with vertical access. All play components may not be accessible to all users. This is consistent with the need for diversity of challenges among the developmental needs of different ages and ability levels. However, some of the same type of play experiences should be accessible to provide as much equality as possible. Similar play experiences do not necessarily mean people will duplicated the experiences. Simply, through the use of design creativity, designers should try to establish challenging play experiences. For example, a guardrail is not considered a play component but a barrier. A pipe wall is a barrier but can also be an activity because of the amount of enclosure. Decks, steps/ladders, posts, and other structural components should be excluded. All activity panels with the same level of challenge are considered similar. For example, two or more tic-tac-toe panels are unnecessary and undesirable.

### Slides

In the place a slide experience is provided, users should be able to have at least one slide that is accessible by ramp. The designer may use a transfer system with a ramp to enable the use of the slide. The sliding experience is one activity on the play area that requires height to participate. Swinging, climbing, and rocking can occur in a play area on the ground. A designer cannot duplicate some types of slides at lower heights. Therefore some latitude must occur when the designer is considering alike and similar sliding experiences. An important goal for the designer is to provide the experience or sensation of sliding.

### Swings

The designer should surface one swing in each group of swings with accessible, protective surfacing (Figure 26-5). Two functions are necessary for swing access: (1) swinging, which provides a person access up to the swing to transfer onto it and (2) pushing, which provides a place for a person to push from a firm, stable, slip-resistant, and resilient surface. A designer also should consider seats that provide body support (Box 26-5).

## Water Play Areas

Water in all its forms is a universal play material because people can manipulate it in many ways. People can splash it, pour it, float objects in it, and mix it with dirt to form "magic potions." Permanent or temporary, the multisensory effect of water makes a substantial contribution to child development. Water settings include hoses in sandpits, puddles, ponds, drinking fountains, bubblers, sprinklers, sprays, cascades, pools, and dew-covered leaves.

If water play or rubber waves are provided, a part of the area must be wheelchair accessible (Figure 26-6). If children manipulate the water source, all children should be able to use it (Figure 26-7). If a designer provides loose parts such as buckets and children have access to the equipment storage, then the storage should also be accessible to all children. When water is provided for play, many dimensions apply (Box 26-6).

## Sand Play Areas

Children will play in dirt wherever they find it. Using props, such as a few twigs, a small plastic toy, or a few stones, children can create an imaginary world in the dirt, around the roots of a tree, or in a raised planter. The sandbox is a refined and sanitized version of dirt play and functions best if it retains dirt play's qualities. The designer should provide intimate, small group spaces, adequate play surfaces, and access to water and other small play props.

If a sand play area is provided, part of it must be accessible. Important elements are clear floor space, maneuvering room, reach and clearance ranges, and operating mechanisms for control of sand flow. When children use products such as buckets and shovels in the sand play area, storage places should be at accessible reach range. Raised sand play is a limiting play experience because of the way a designer must construct a raised play area. To provide a place for the wheelchair under the sand shelf, little depth of sand is available for play. Therefore a raised sand area by itself is not a substitution for full-body sand play. A designer should make all sand play opportunities on the site so that all children can use it as much as possible.

## Sand at Ground Level

If the sand area is designed to allow children to play inside the area, the designer should provide a place within the sand play area in which a participant can rest or lean against a firm, stationary back support in close proximity to the main activity area. Any vertical surface that is a minimum height of 12 inches and a minimum width of 6 inches can provide back support, depending on the size of the child. Back support can be a boulder,

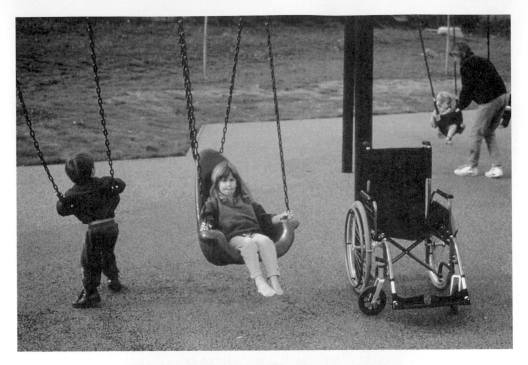

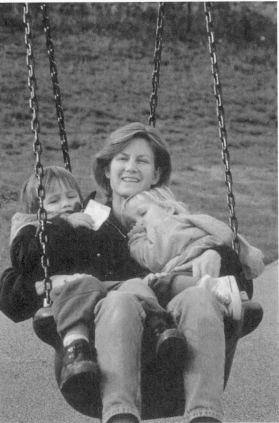

**Fig. 26-5** A variety of swing types allows for choices so that everyone can find a place to swing.

a log, or a post that is holding up a shade structure. A transfer system into a sand area may also be necessary if the area is large and contains a variety of sand activities. A transfer system would be appropriate if no areas of raised sand play exist in the primary activity area or if the sand area is more than 100 square feet and the raised sand area tends to isolate accessible sand play activities.

## BOX 26-5

### *Swing Requirements*

1. One swing in each group of swings should be surfaced with accessible, protective surfacing.
2. A 30-inch by 48-inch parking space for a wheelchair is required outside of the swing seat use zone.
3. A continuous, firm, stable, slip-resistant, and resilient surfacing under the full arch of the swing should be provided. If the accessible surfacing is going to extend beyond the 30 inches to the front of the swing, it should then extend to the entire use zone. A child falling on the edge where the unitary and loose fill materials come together could be injured.
4. Two turn-around spaces along the route of the swing are required. One is necessary for accessing the swing seat and one for pushing the swing 4 feet beyond the maximum extension of the swing arch.
5. Other designs that meet the intent of the concept are acceptable. Presently, no swing seats exist that conform to current safety standards and allow a wheelchair user to remain in the chair while swinging. Therefore assistance is needed for transferring onto swing seats.

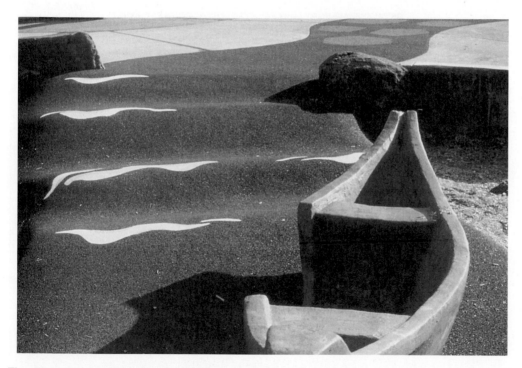

**Fig. 26-6** The Native American "redwood" canoe accommodates a wheelchair user, and the rubber waves provide an exciting ride down the river.

## Raised Sand Play

When raised sand is provided, the following clearance ranges apply:

- Top height to sand: 30 to 34 inches maximum
- Under clearance: 27-inch minimum
- Side reach: 36 to 20 inches
- Forward reach: 36 to 20 inches
- Clear space for wheelchair: 36 by 55 inches

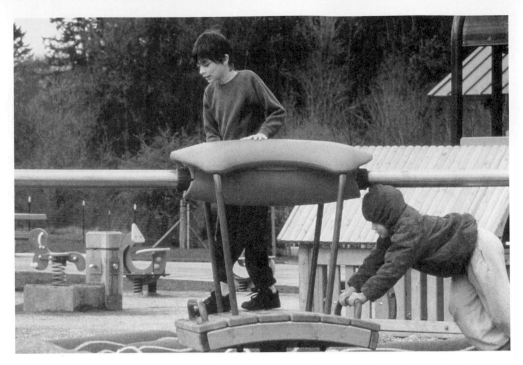

**Fig. 26-7** The ferry is child powered with places for standing or sitting on the movable platform.

BOX **26-6**

*Dimensions for Water-Play Areas*

1. Forward reach: 36 inches by 20 inches
2. Side reach: 36 inches by 20 inches
3. Clear space: 36 inches by 55 inches. The clear space should be located at the part of the water play area where the most water play will occur. If the water source is part of the active play area and children turn the water on and off, then it must be accessible. If the water source is part of a spray pool, the area under the spray should be accessible. Accessibility should involve the dimensions for clear space and reach.
4. Clearance ranges: top height to access water 30 inches maximum, under clearance 27 inches minimum

## Shade Sand Areas

Depending on the site conditions and the amount of sand play, shade may be necessary. If shade is required by site conditions, a variety of means, such as trees, tents, umbrellas, structures, etc may provide it. This advisory requirement for shade is based on site context, program, and users. Some shade in or around sand is usually desirable.

### Gathering Places

To support social development and cooperation, children need comfortable gathering places. Parents and play leaders need comfortable places for sitting, socializing, and supervising.

If gathering places are provided, a portion of each of them should be accessible. A gathering place contains fixed elements to support playing, eating, watching, talking, or assembling for a programmed activity and should serve people of all ages.

## Seating

*Formal seating* refers to manufactured site furniture. Informal seating can be rocks, logs, and other parts of the natural environment. Only formal seating must adhere to the following criteria, and they apply only if a designer provides it:

- Along accessible routes: Where benches are provided in a play area setting for rest and recreation by adults and children, these should be adjacent to the accessible route to activities. A total of 50% all benches must be accessible and 25% of them should have a backrest and arm supports. Arm supports need to meet ASTM requirements for entrapment. The bench layout should offer a place for a wheelchair user to converse with the bench user that is out of the path of travel.
- Along auxiliary routes: Where benches are provided along an auxiliary route, a minimum of 1% or 50%, whichever is greater, should include a backrest and arm supports. Issues include height of seat, parking space for a vacated wheelchair, and clear ground space. Where seating is used as part of a program area in combination with work or eating tables, benches used by children should have the following heights:
  Prekindergarten: 8 to 12 inches (203 to 305 mm)
  Kindergarten and older: 12 to 17 inches (305 to 432 mm)
- Fixed benches: A variety of seat choices should be available in fixed benches.
- Seat space: A minimum of 2% or 10%, whichever is greater, should have one accessible seat space.

## Tables

In the place tables are provided, the designer should provide a variety of sizes and seating arrangements as follows:

- Tables, counters, and work surfaces for children who use wheelchairs should have clear knee space 24 inches (610 mm) high, 24 inches (610 mm) deep, and 30 inches (760 mm) wide.
- The tops of tables and work surfaces used by children should be a maximum of 2 inches (51 mm) higher than the upper end of the knee clearance range from the floor or ground. Every fixed picnic table installed should be an accessible design, even if it is not on an accessible path of travel. Dimensions for children are 27 inches minimum clear underneath, 12 inches of depth, 30 inches maximum to top of table, and 36-inches wide space for the chair.
- Temporary or portable tables should comply with this requirement to the maximum extent feasible.

### Game Tables

Game tables provide a place for two to four people to play board games. In the place fewer than five game tables are provided, a minimum of one four-sided game table should include an accessible space on one side. Height and clearance would be similar to the previous table requirements for children. In the place five or more game tables are provided, a minimum of one or 10%, whichever is greater, of the tables should have two accessible seat spaces.

## Storage

If storage is supplied as part of a gathering area and children use the storage, accessible shelves and hooks should be a maximum of 36 inches above the ground. The amount of storage is depends on program requirements.

## Shade

Shade may be desirable for gathering areas in the place people participate in activities over a long period. Depending on the site context, trees, canopies, or trellises can provide shade.

### Garden Settings

A powerful play and learning activity, gardening allows children to interact with nature and each other. A designer can adapt garden beds and tools so that children with disabilities can use them. Scent gardens are attractive to all children and have a special appeal to children with low vision.

A designer primarily uses gardens in play areas to provide a program with the activities of planting, tending, studying, and harvesting vegetation. Depending on the type and height of plantings, planter boxes may require a raised area for access or a transfer point. A garden must provide a minimum of one accessible gardening area.

### Raised Gardens

If a raised area is provided, the following guidelines apply:

- The raised area should be located as part of the main garden area. The program determines the amount of raised area, but a minimum of 10% of the garden should be raised.
- The edge should be raised above the ground surface to a minimum of 20 inches and a maximum of 30 inches.
- The garden growing area should require access either by side or by forward reach 12 to 36 inches above the ground.

### Ground-Level Gardens

If children are required to sit in the dirt to garden, a designer should provide a transfer point that enables a participant to transfer into the garden.

### Potting and Maintenance Areas

Potting and preparation areas should require access either by forward or side reach. The amount of area that the designer makes accessible depends on the program. At least one workstation for potting should be accessible.

### Garden Storage

Storage areas for the garden should provide access for children who use wheelchairs. Hooks and shelves should be a maximum of 36 inches off the ground.

### Circulation

Aisles around the garden should provide access for movement and work. A designer should provide a minimum of 44 inches on a main aisle so that a child using a wheelchair or walker can get to the garden. This larger aisle should also provide access to the accessible gardening spaces.

### Vegetation, Trees, and Land Forms

Vegetation, trees, and topography are important features in a play setting. The designer should integrate them into the flow of play activities and spaces, or they can be play features.

Land forms help children explore movement through space and provide for varied circulation. Topographic variety stimulates fantasy play, orientation skills, hide-and-go-seek games, viewing, rolling, climbing, sliding, and jumping. Summit points must accommodate wheelchairs and provide support for other disabling conditions.

Trees and vegetation comprise one of the most ignored topics in the design of play environments, yet they are two of the most important elements of integration because everyone can enjoy and share them. Vegetation stimulates exploratory behavior, fantasy, and imagination. It is a major source of play props, including leaves, flowers, fruit, nuts, seeds, and sticks. It allows children to learn about the environment through direct experience.

Designers and program providers should emphasize integrating plants into play settings rather than creating separate nature areas. For children with disabilities, the experience of being in trees can be replicated by the designer incorporating trees that a wheelchair can roll into or under. The designer can create an accessible miniforest by planting small trees or large branching bushes.

If vegetation trees and/or landforms are used as a feature, the designer should provide a means for access up to and around the feature. The designer also must select tree grates and other site furniture that support or protect the feature so that wheels, canes, and crutch tips are not entrapped.

## Animal Habitats

A person's contact with wildlife and domestic animals stimulates a caring and responsible attitude toward other living things, provides a therapeutic effect, and offers many learning opportunities. Play areas can provide the chance for children to care for or observe domestic animals. Existing or created habitats for insects, aquatic life, birds, and small animals should be protected. Planting appropriate vegetation will attract insects and birds.

## Entrances and Signage

Entrances are transition zones that help orient, inform, and introduce users to the site. They are places for congregating and for displaying information. However, not all play areas have defined entrances. Sometimes a designer can provide entry to a play area from all directions.

Signs can be permanent or temporary, informative, and playful. Expressive and informative displays use walls, floors, ground surfaces, structures, ceilings, sky wires, and roof lines on or near a play area to hang, suspend, and fly materials for art and education. Signage is a visual, tactile, or auditory means of conveying information and it must communicate the message "All users are welcome." A designer can use appropriate heights, depths, colors, pictures, and tactile qualities to make signs accessible. Signs should be graphic, tactile, and written. In an environment used by children, signs should primarily communicate graphically. Talking signs are also good. A designer must apply all other ADAAG provisions.

## Fences, Enclosures, and Barriers

An enclosure is a primary means of differentiating and articulating the child's environment. For example, fences can double back on themselves to provide small social settings. Fences, enclosures, and barriers protect fragile environments, define pathways, enclose activity areas, and designate social settings. Low fences should be play elements, and the designer must consider them as such. The entrance to an enclosure should be clearly visible and also should be wide enough for wheelchair passage. This width is 36 inches minimum, although 48 inches is preferable.

## Safety and Access

In the place equipment or any play element is provided, access to equipment must conform to existing safety requirements, such as ASTM F1487, when those requirements are based on actual risk and anthropometric data. If the conflict between safety and access can be demonstrated and documented, the designer can use safety criteria to modify access considerations. The designer can use access criteria to modify safety criteria if an unsafe condition exists.

## BOX 26-7

*Design Requirements Discussed with Community Members*

1. Documentation of the accessible route of travel should be provided.
2. Documentation of the accessible point of access for elevated equipment and an accessible egress for elevated equipment should be provided when egress occurs on a surface that is not firm, stable, and slip-resistant. Documentation of the provision of a means of return to the point of ingress from the point of egress should be provided.
3. Where 20 or more elevated play components are provided, documentation of the provision of play components which are accessible by ramp and are similar to play components that are not accessible by ramp should be provided.
4. Where 20 or more elevated play components are provided, documentation of the provision of play components, which are accessible by transfer systems and are similar to play components, which are not accessible by transfer systems should be provided.

### Consultation and Documentation

Every new play area that the designer develops requires consultation between the organization that operates the play area, the selected manufacturer and/or designer, and all potential users of the environment, including people with disabilities who reside in the community. Participation is important in new projects, especially if the play area is a community asset. As part of the design process, the designer should discuss requirements with community members and the decisions they reach need to become part of the records for the play area (Box 26-7).

## Outcome and Social Validation

Play is the raw material of education that helps children to express, apply, and assimilate knowledge and experience. A rich play environment can encourage all children to take those first experimental steps toward growth and development. Laws recently enacted to protect and promote the rights of persons with disabilities have now created the market demand and social acceptance of an all-inclusive, universally designed play environment.

To fully support child development and integrate children with and without disabilities, the designer should augment a well-designed play environment with a risk management program and professional play leadership. Part of the play leader's job is to set up, manipulate, and modify the physical environment to facilitate creative activity. Because the environment can either support or hamper play, designers must learn the way they can best empower children through design.

When evaluating the effectiveness of AT, the designer should look key elements, such as a diversified play environment that provides more opportunities for children of various abilities. The end products are improved physical and mental health and an enhanced learning environment available to all children. Although scientific research in the area of AT for play and recreation is limited, anecdotal references serve as sources of information that validate the relevance and need for such technology.

## CASE STUDY

### CASE 1

### Specific Application: Ibach Park

Ibach Park is a 19.86-acre neighborhood park that is owned and operated by the city of Tualatin Parks and Recreation Department. The design and development of the park reflects the benefits desired by community residents who were active participants in the design process. Park features include a three-fourths acre play area that reflects the rich heritage of Tualatin from prehistory to early settlement days, preteen play area, soccer field, softball field, tennis courts, basketball court, picnic areas, open-turf area, Hedges Creek greenway trail development and restoration, interpretive signage, restrooms, and parking. Although unique in its specific elements, the play area is a typical Moore Iacofano Goltsman (MIG) project in three major respects: (1) the local community helped with the design, (2) the play area integrates children of varying abilities, and (3) the goal was not only to provide a space for physical stimulation but also to create an environment that encourages social and intellectual development.

## DESIGN PROCESS

To ensure that as many community members as possible would have an opportunity to contribute their ideas, visions, and goals to the site design, a series of five workshops took place. Participants included residents, members of the Tualatin Parks and Recreation Advisory Board, and members of the Tualatin Disabilities Advisory Board. As part of the public participation process, a design charrette was held to involve residents in identifying the future benefits that would be provided at the park. From these public meetings, the design concept for the site was identified based on the site's archeologic context. This concept was then overlaid with the functional requirements for a neighborhood park, including active and passive recreational opportunities. Other overall goals for the park included safety, security, accessibility, environmental preservation and education, and ease of maintenance.

The design team worked closely with the city's maintenance staff during the design process to reduce operational costs. Some features designed to reduce costs included special court surfacing on tennis and basketball courts, timed release of water for water play features, the use of synthetic safety surfacing in the play area, plant selection, and the design of mow strips to facilitate equipment use. Restroom doors have timers that can be set to automatically lock and unlock, reducing personnel costs. Sand-based softball and soccer fields are designed for year-round use with complete underground drainage and irrigation to increase playing time and user safety.

## CHILDREN'S PLAY AREA

Based on the desired benefits identified by community members and the results of the community design charrette, the design team developed an interpretive design concept for the Ibach play area. The accessible play area reflects the city's rich heritage. Children learn about the history of Tualatin from prehistory to early European settlement days through interactive play. They reenact historic events in play settings. The play area was designed to meet the developmental needs of preschool and school-age children and to allow children with and without disabilities to have equal access to play opportunities. The final design provides play area users with an interactive tour through the history of Tualatin that allows people to experience the city's past. The play area includes three distinct areas reflecting significant historic periods: prehistory, Native American, and early European settlement. A watercourse of real and simulated water runs through the entire play area, symbolizing the historic effect the Tualatin River has had on the life of the city and its people. In areas in which real water was not feasible, the river flow is continued symbolically by blue, synthetic safety surfacing. A segment of the river is a water play element that allows children to turn on the river flow by pressing against a bollard. The water flows into a riverbed, which is at the ground level on one side and at a raised height on the other side to allow water play while a person is in a wheelchair or is standing.

The prehistory area begins at a high, rocky area, simulating a mountain such as Mount Hood, which a person can view from this site. It contains a child-sized version of the meteor that landed on earth millions of years ago and was carried west to Tualatin by the surging waters of the Bretz Floods more than 15,000 years ago. In addition, an archeologic dig allows children to unearth fossil rocks and fern prints and explore a giant mastodon ribcage, giving them a wonderful sense of discovery. Not only do children get to see what happens when they scrape away a layer of earth to discover fossils but also

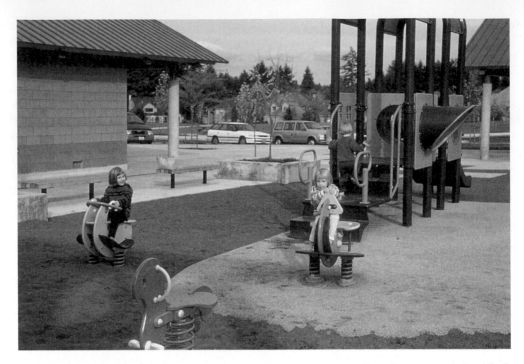

**Fig. 26-8** The farm is for younger children with spring horses pulling the wagon train. All play equipment components are wheelchair accessible.

they can develop a better concept of the natural world and the history of life. The mastodon ribcage also is an excellent climbing structure. One missing rib permits wheelchair access.

Replicas of Native American petroglyphs signal the change from prehistory to Tualatin's Native American history. This area contains a circle of drums that allow children to create music. Each drum is a different height so that children can play standing or sitting. A dugout canoe that has been cut out to accommodate wheelchairs allows children to experience the way the Native Americans might have traveled the river to catch fish or look for a better hunting ground.

At the Pioneer Settlement, young children can play in log cabin-style play houses, prepare breakfast at the sand tables, harness a team of horses to pull a covered wagon, ride a ferry across the Tualatin River, or care for the family milk cow (Figure 26-8).

Children can view the play environment from the swing area, which is entirely covered with accessible safety surfacing and includes a bucket swing for young children or children with disabilities. Located at a distance from the play area for younger children is a separate area that allows active play and "hanging out" space for youth ages 10 to 14. Both play areas meet state-of-the-art safety standards.

The final design for the Ibach Park play area symbolizes the collective memory of generations of Tualatin inhabitants. What makes this play area unique is its translation of history into an interactive, educational resource that provides play and learning opportunities through a person's direct interaction with the natural and built environments. This results in a diversity of play opportunities and environments that allow children of all abilities to discover, learn, and have fun.

Since its grand opening in May 1996, Ibach Park has attracted users from throughout the region and has won many prestigious awards. Among them was its selection by the National Endowment for the Arts and the National Building Museum as one of 50 projects nationwide that exhibit excellence in universal design.

## Suggested Readings

American Society for Testing and Materials: *Standard consumer safety performance specification for playground equipment for public use,* West Conshohocken, Pa, 1993, 1995, ASTM.

Center for Accessible Housing: *Recommendations for accessibility standards for children's environments,* Raleigh, 1992, North Carolina State University.

Moore RC, Goltsman SM, Iacofano DS: *Play for all guidelines: planning, design and management of outdoor play settings for all children,* Berkeley, Calif, 1993, MIG Communications.

PLAE, Inc: *Universal access to outdoor recreation areas: a design guide,* Berkeley, Calif, 1993, MIG Communications.

US Architectural and Transportation Barriers Compliance Board: *Americans with Disabilities Act Accessibility Guidelines (ADAAG): accessibility requirements for new construction and alteration of buildings and facilities covered by the ADA,* Washington, DC, 1991, Access Board.

US Architectural and Transportation Barriers Compliance Board: *Recommendations for accessibility guidelines: recreational facilities and outdoor developed areas,* Washington, DC, 1994, Access Board.

# Index

*References with t denote tables; f denote figures; b denote boxes.*